Download Your Included Ebook Today!

Your print purchase of *Essentials of Clinical Infectious Diseases, Second Edition*, **includes an ebook download** to the device of your choice—increasing accessibility, portability, and searchability!

Download your ebook today at:
http://spubonline.com/infdis2E
and enter the access code below:

1316TS5W6

demosMEDICAL
An Imprint of Springer Publishing

springerpub.com

Essentials of Clinical Infectious Diseases

Second Edition

William F. Wright, DO, MPH
University of Pittsburgh Medical Center
Harrisburg, Pennsylvania
Former Assistant Professor
Division of Infectious Diseases
Department of Medicine
University of Maryland School of Medicine
Baltimore, Maryland

demosMEDICAL
An Imprint of Springer Publishing

Visit our website at www.springerpub.com

ISBN: 978-0-8261-2727-3
ebook ISBN: 978-0-8261-2782-2

Acquisitions Editor: Beth Barry
Compositor: Exeter Premedia Services Private Ltd.

Library of Congress Cataloging-in-Publication Data

Names: Wright, William F. (William Floyd), editor. | Preceded by (work):
  Wright, William F. (William Floyd). Essentials of clinical infectious
  diseases.
Title: Essentials of clinical infectious diseases / editor, William F. Wright.
Description: Second edition. | New York: Demos Medical Publishing, an
  imprint of Springer Publishing Company, LLC, [2018] | Preceded by
  Essentials of clinical infectious diseases / William F. Wright. 2013. |
  Includes bibliographical references and index.
Identifiers: LCCN 2017053246| ISBN 9780826127273 | ISBN 9780826127822 (eBook)
Subjects: | MESH: Bacterial Infections--diagnosis | Bacterial
  Infections--drug therapy | Infection | Anti-Infective Agents--therapeutic
  use | Communicable Diseases--diagnosis | Communicable Diseases—drug
  therapy | Outlines
Classification: LCC RC111 | NLM WC 18.2 | DDC 614.5/7—dc23
LC record available at https://lccn.loc.gov/2017053246

Contact us to receive discount rates on bulk purchases.
We can also customize our books to meet your needs.
For more information please contact: sales@springerpub.com

To Susan—my beautiful wife, best friend, and the wind beneath my wings. I am the luckiest man in the world to be married to a magnificent and brilliant woman like you. Sharing our life and love along this journey together is a blessing beyond words. I am grateful for your unwavering love, faith, and support. This book is affectionately dedicated to you, without whom this second edition would not have been completed.

CONTENTS

CONTRIBUTORS

Anthony Amoroso, MD, Associate Professor, Division of Infectious Diseases, Department of Medicine, University of Maryland School of Medicine, Baltimore, Maryland

Ryan S. Arnold, MD, Former Fellow, Division of Infectious Diseases, Department of Medicine, University of Maryland School of Medicine, Baltimore, Maryland

Ulrike K. Buchwald, MD, Clinical Assistant Professor, Division of Infectious Diseases, Department of Medicine, University of Maryland School of Medicine, Baltimore, Maryland

Jason Bailey, DO, Clinical Assistant Professor, Division of Infectious Diseases, Department of Medicine, University of Maryland School of Medicine, Baltimore, Maryland

Eric Cox, MD, Former Fellow, Division of Infectious Diseases, Department of Medicine, University of Maryland School of Medicine, Baltimore, Maryland

Charles E. Davis, MD, Associate Professor, Division of Infectious Diseases, Department of Medicine, University of Maryland School of Medicine, Baltimore, Maryland

Susan L. DeBiase, BS, RN, Department of Nursing, University of Pittsburgh Medical Center, Harrisburg, Pennsylvania

Guesly Delva, MD, Clinical Assistant Professor, Division of Infectious Diseases, Department of Medicine, University of Maryland School of Medicine, Baltimore, Maryland

Bruce L. Gilliam, MD, Associate Professor, Division of Infectious Diseases, Department of Medicine, University of Maryland School of Medicine, Baltimore, Maryland

Emily L. Heil, PharmD, BCPS, Clinical Assistant Professor, Department of Pharmacy, University of Maryland Medical Center, Baltimore, Maryland

Jennifer Husson, MD, MPH, Assistant Professor, Division of Infectious Diseases, Department of Medicine, University of Maryland School of Medicine, Baltimore, Maryland

Luciano Kapelusznik, MD, Clinical Assistant Professor, Division of Infectious Diseases, Department of Medicine, University of Maryland School of Medicine, Baltimore, Maryland

David W. Keckich, MD, Former Fellow, Division of Infectious Diseases, Department of Medicine, University of Maryland School of Medicine, Baltimore, Maryland

Janaki C. Kuruppu, MD, Assistant Professor, Division of Infectious Diseases, Department of Medicine, University of Maryland School of Medicine, Baltimore, Maryland

Surbhi Leekha, MBBS, MPH, Associate Professor, Division of Infectious Diseases, Department of Epidemiology and Public Health and Medicine, University of Maryland School of Medicine, Baltimore, Maryland

Gonzalo Luizaga, MD, Former Fellow, Division of Infectious Diseases, Department of Medicine, University of Maryland School of Medicine, Baltimore, Maryland

Adrian Majid, MD, Assistant Professor, Department of Medicine, Weill Cornell Medical College, New York, New York

Shivakumar Narayanan, MBBS, Adjunct Assistant Professor, Department of Medicine, University of Maryland School of Medicine, Baltimore, Maryland

Nicole M. Parrish, PhD, MHS, D (ABMM), Assistant Professor, Division of Microbiology, Department of Pathology, Johns Hopkins University School of Medicine, Baltimore, Maryland

Devang M. Patel, MD, Assistant Professor, Division of Infectious Diseases, Department of Medicine, University of Maryland School of Medicine, Baltimore, Maryland

Robert R. Redfield, MD, Chair, Division of Infectious Diseases, Professor of Medicine, Professor of Microbiology and Immunology, University of Maryland School of Medicine, Baltimore, Maryland

David J. Riedel, MD, Assistant Professor, Division of Infectious Diseases, Department of Medicine, University of Maryland School of Medicine, Baltimore, Maryland

Stefan Riedel, MD, PhD, D (ABMM), Director, Clinical Laboratories, Johns Hopkins Bayview Medical Center; Assistant Professor, Division of Microbiology, Department of Pathology, Johns Hopkins University School of Medicine, Baltimore, Maryland

Clare Rock, MD (MB BCh), Assistant Professor, Division of Infectious Disease, Department of Medicine, Johns Hopkins University School of Medicine, Baltimore, Maryland

Neha U. Sheth, PharmD, BCPS, AAHIVE, Associate Professor, Department of Pharmacy Practice and Science, University of Maryland School of Pharmacy, Baltimore, Maryland

Leonard A. Sowah, MB BCh, MPH, Clinical Assistant Professor, Division of Infectious Diseases, Department of Medicine, University of Maryland School of Medicine, Baltimore, Maryland

Michael Tablang, MD, Former Fellow, Division of Infectious Diseases, Department of Medicine, University of Maryland School of Medicine, Baltimore, Maryland

Rohit Talwani, MD, Clinical Associate Professor, Division of Infectious Diseases, Department of Medicine, University of Maryland School of Medicine, Baltimore, Maryland

Kerri A. Thom, MD, MS, Associate Professor, Division of Infectious Diseases, Department of Epidemiology and Public Health and Medicine, University of Maryland School of Medicine, Baltimore, Maryland

John Vaz, MD, Former Fellow, Division of Infectious Diseases, Department of Medicine, University of Maryland School of Medicine, Baltimore, Maryland

William F. Wright, DO, MPH, University of Pittsburgh Medical Center, Harrisburg, Pennsylvania; Former Assistant Professor, Division of Infectious Diseases, Department of Medicine, University of Maryland School of Medicine, Baltimore, Maryland

PREFACE

We have been gratified by the popularity of the first edition of *The Essentials of Clinical Infectious Diseases*. It has been more than five years since the first edition of this book presented readers with the essential aspects of the subspecialty infectious diseases. The popular reception of the book and the rapid expansion of medical knowledge call for a new edition to assist readers through this medical transformation—*from a demystified wonder to a commonplace tool in medical education.*

This edition (a) provides technical corrections, updates, and clarifications in all 45 chapters of the original book; (b) adds six new chapter topics; (c) includes new developments that are consistent with the published peer-reviewed medical literature, published relevant clinical practice guidelines, and updated bibliographical references at the end of each chapter; and (d) elucidates subtle issues that readers and reviewers have found perplexing, objectionable, or in need of elaboration.

Our main audience remains the students and medical providers in training. However, information within this book evolved from prior formal didactic lectures or bedside clinical teaching on clinical infectious diseases, microbiology, and antimicrobial pharmacology that was delivered to help students, residents, fellows, and primary care physicians. Current basic science and clinical concepts regarding each relevant infectious disease topic are still written as a synoptic account to make these topics clear and practical for the readers of this text. Teachers who have taught from this book before should find the revised edition more lucid and palatable. We continue to adhere wherever possible to a standard pattern of description that aims to define the topic; provide an introduction that would include classification, pathophysiology, and epidemiologic information; list relevant causative microorganisms; describe the clinical aspects and approach to the topic with the physical examination and relevant laboratory methods, diagnostic imaging, and appropriate antimicrobial therapy. This updated essentials text also includes new chapters that readers will hopefully find useful beyond the basic clinical syndromes: introduction to clinical reasoning and statistics, introduction to antimicrobial stewardship, and basic approach to travel medicine.

While medicine continues to evolve and the amount of knowledge a learner must retain may seem daunting, knowing basic concepts can make the approach to a patient with a possible infection an easy and exciting task. Although this text is arranged by certain infectious disease topics, patients typically present with a constellation of symptoms and signs. Knowing basic concepts, therefore, can help clinicians arrive at the diagnosis of the disease causing the patient's symptoms and signs. This process (clinical problem solving) begins by a discussion with the patient of the chronology of events associated with the symptoms or signs experienced as well as asking appropriate relevant questions. Additionally, a complete physical examination is then performed for diagnostic clues that then lead to the formulation of the most appropriate differential diagnosis that is based on an understanding of these basic concepts. Based on the initial discussion and examination, appropriate laboratory or imaging tests are ordered to support or refute the diagnostic considerations. The goal of this text is to help guide the reader through the diagnostic evaluation as well as the process of caring for the patient with an infection.

The editor and contributing authors have collaborated to prepare chapters consistent with the peer-reviewed published medical literature, published clinical practice guidelines and their teaching, clinical, and research activities. Each chapter concludes with important medical references that may also include reference to a "classic" article regarding the infectious disease topic that can be utilized by the reader as additional reading. Through this text the authors strive enthusiastically to impart to readers a solid fundamental knowledge and approach to clinical infectious diseases that will sustain them adequately in their chosen medical professional career.

William F. Wright, DO, MPH

ACKNOWLEDGMENTS

I am very grateful to all the contributing authors for their hard work and dedication to this book and our profession. I would also like to personally thank several additional colleagues who reviewed many sections of the manuscript and/or provided many helpful suggestions. The book would not have been possible without the support and assistance of these additional individuals:

Neil Abramson, MD
Majdi N. Al-Hasan, MBBS
Andrea Chao Bafford, MD
Richard Colgan, MD
W. Christopher Ehmann, MD
Silvia M. Ferretti, DO
Samuel M. Galvagno Jr., DO, PhD
John D. Goldman, MD, FACP
John N. Goldman, MD
Richard N. Greenberg, MD
Luciano Kapelusznik, MD
Christine Kell, PhD
Matthew E. Lissauer, MD, FACS
Philip Mackowiak, MD
Michelle S. Rarick, RPh
Julie A. Ribes, MD, PhD
Ryan M. Scilla, MD
Christine N. Shiner, PharmD
Wendy Stock, MD
Jennifer W. Toth, MD
Michael Young, MD
John J. Zurlo, MD

INTRODUCTION AND BASICS OF CLINICAL REASONING

William F. Wright

I. **INTRODUCTION.** Akkadian cuneiform inscriptions from the 6th century BCE suggest that medicine of early Mesopotamian societies involved supernatural interpretations of disease with blaming of gods and ghosts frequently. Medical epistemology in Hellenistic Palestine and Greco-Roman societies from the 5th century BCE embodied the philosophical notion of both a macrocosm and microcosm. The writings of Aristotle, as well as early Greek philosophers such as Plato and Pythagoras, proposed the world, or macrocosm, was composed of the four elements of air, earth, fire, and water. This corresponded to a microcosm with the harmonious balance of four bodily elements (blood, phlegm, yellow bile, and black bile), which were known as humors. In his treatise, *On the Nature of Man*, Hippocrates introduced the classic theory of humors and their imbalances as a means of explaining disease. The Roman physician Galen endorsed this pathophysiology and further defined medicine for Medieval Western Europe. The classic theory of humors predominated medical thinking until the 19th century when both Louis Pasteur and Robert Koch provided proof of the microbial basis of disease. This ushered in the era of what would now be considered a rational scientific basis of medicine.

Modern clinical medicine and infectious diseases have dramatically changed over the past century. The practice has evolved from a healing art in which standards were based mainly on the personal experience of physicians to a discipline focused on the scientific method and evidence-based practice standards. While scientific advances serve as the evolutionary basis for the diagnostic and therapeutic approaches to common medical and infectious-disease conditions, reconciling the traditional physical diagnostic approach with contemporary diagnostic methods has been a continuous process throughout the history of medicine and clinical infectious diseases. The approach to the patient with an infectious disease is still best accomplished by a systematic method that combines the critically important comprehensive history and physical examination with the added benefits of contemporary technology. This process, the basis of the fundamental skills of medical diagnosis and treatment, strives to improve the physician's clinical reasoning and includes:

1. Understanding disease definitions, mechanisms, and patterns

2. Identifying the patient's chief complaint and performing a chronologically accurate medical history

3. Formulating a differential diagnosis based on the chief complaint and medical history (also known as the pretest probability)

4. Performing physical-examination maneuvers that will support or refute the conditions being considered in the differential diagnosis

5. Ordering appropriate diagnostic and laboratory tests and interpreting the results in relation to the differential diagnosis (also known as the posttest probability)

6. Implementing an appropriate evidence-based treatment plan

The purpose of this clinical reasoning is to establish a systematic and rational approach to medical decision making that allows the physician to explain the patient's symptoms based on one unified diagnosis (i.e., Occam's razor).

Critically important when applying this process to clinical infectious diseases are the chief complaint and an extended medical history that ideally includes antibiotic uses and allergies, past medical conditions and/or infections, sexual practices, drug use, travel destinations, occupational history, screening tests (e.g., purified protein derivative [PPD]), and vaccinations, which when taken together, provide important clues to the risk of acquiring an infection. However, one of the more difficult processes in clinical infectious diseases is the synthesis of all data including organisms identified in the microbiology laboratory to distinguish between an infectious process and colonization. Colonization is generally considered to be the presence of a particular microorganism or group of microorganisms (i.e., normal flora) in which their presence does not create a specific host immune response (i.e., infection). In contrast, infection is most commonly due to the invasion of body tissues with a particular microorganism or group of microorganisms, which elicits an immune response that results in a disease state.

II. EVIDENCE-BASED MEDICINE BASICS. A group of further categories highlighting important concepts regarding clinical reasoning and evidence-based medicine principles is listed in the following. These concepts should be kept in mind when evaluating all encountered patients, including infectious diseases, so as to provide a systematic and rational approach to the clinician's medical decision making.

A. Basics of Clinical Reasoning

1. **Differential diagnosis.** The differential diagnosis is a systematic process for considering the most likely possible causes of a patient's symptom or physical finding. This process begins with evaluating a hypothesis by matching the patient's findings with the clinician's internal understanding of disease. Most often an associative model of disease, also known as pattern recognition, is used that consists of clinical findings, illness progression, predisposing characteristics, and complications that are associated with a disease.

   Clinical hypothesis generation begins with the patient's chief complaint and a chronologic account of illness from its beginning. This approach provides valuable information and perspective on the patient's illness. It also respects the patient in allowing time to recount the story as well as provide the clinician time to think, write down some diagnoses to consider, and observe the patient for diagnostic clues. Once the patient has provided a chronologic account of the illness the clinician should ask specific questions to test each of the initial diagnostic hypotheses (e.g., cross-examination history taking). The combined patient recounted and cross-examined history (e.g., chief complaint, history of present illness, and past medical–surgical history) should generate the most hypotheses. The physical examination is then usually the time to gather objective physical clues to rank, confirm, or discard a hypothesis. Remember that a pathognomonic finding usually improves diagnostic efficiency and establishes a diagnosis for one disease, but very few of these findings exist.

When the considered hypotheses have been ranked in order of plausibility, the clinician then has to decide whether to withhold any further testing or treatment, begin treatment without further testing, or gather more information with diagnostic testing prior to beginning treatment. The choice among these three alternatives is guided by probability and utility (e.g., benefit vs. harm).

2. **Probability.** Probability in medicine is referred to as either the present state of the patient or the possibility of a future patient event. Predictors of the present state of the patient would involve information from a ***cross-sectional design study***. Predictors of a possible future event of the patient would involve information from a ***cohort design study***.

   a. **Pretesting probability.** Defined as the probability of a patient having the target disorder before a diagnostic test result is known. Mathematically, it can be calculated as the proportion of patients with the disorder divided by both those with and without the disorder expressed as a percentage.

      Pretesting probability = Disease/Disease + No disease

   b. **Posttesting probability**. Defined as the probability of a patient having the target disorder after a diagnostic test result is known. The clinician can calculate the posttesting probability of a disease using the **Bayes theorem**.

3. **The Bayes theorem.** Reverend Thomas Bayes (1702–1761), an English clergyman, developed a method of predicting probability that an event is true given that another event is true. This is referred to as the "notion of conditional probability."

   In medical terms, the Bayes theorem is the probability (P) of a medical hypothesis (H) conditional upon new information or evidence (E). It is expressed mathematically as:

$$P(H/E) = P(E/H) \times P(H)/P(E)$$

Another way of expressing this is as follows:

$$P\ (H/E) = \frac{\text{Probability of the evidence given the hypothesis} \times \text{the probability of the hypothesis}}{\text{The probability of the evidence}}$$

Therefore, using this theorem the clinician can calculate or estimate the probability of disease based upon the following: (a) pretesting probability of disease, (b) probability of a history of present illness finding and physical examination or laboratory test result conditional upon the patient ***having*** the disease (e.g., sensitivity), and (c) probability of a history of present illness finding and physical examination or laboratory test result conditional upon the patient ***not having*** the disease (e.g., specificity).

B. **Incidence and Prevalence**

Clinically relevant measures of the frequency of events are usually expressed as fractions in which the ***numerator*** is the number of patients experiencing the outcome (e.g., cases) and the ***denominator*** is the number of people in whom the outcome could have occurred (e.g., population). The measure of disease is usually expressed as the following:

1. **Incidence.** This refers to the number of new cases of disease (numerator) occurring in a population at risk for disease (denominator) in a given time frame (e.g., weeks, months, or years). Incidence is a measure of rate of disease and estimates the risk of disease.

2. **Prevalence.** This refers to the number of people possessing the clinical condition, or disease (numerator), occurring in a given population of people (denominator). Prevalence is a measure of proportion and estimates the burden of disease. *Prevalence is also called pretesting probability, the probability of disease before the test result is known.*

C. **Sensitivity, Specificity, and Predictive Values**

1. **Sensitivity (Se).** Defined as the proportion of people with the disease who also have a positive test (e.g., history of present illness in question and/or physical examination or laboratory test) for the disease in question. A sensitive test is helpful to identify or rule in disease.

2. **Specificity (Sp).** Defined as the proportion of people without the disease who also have a negative test (e.g., history of present illness in question and/or physical examination or laboratory test) for the disease in question. A specific test is helpful to exclude or rule out disease.

3. **Positive predictive value (PPV).** The probability of disease in a patient with a positive test result for the disease in question. The more specific a test is, the better will be its PPV. As the prevalence of disease in a population approaches zero, the PPV of a test also approaches zero.

4. **Negative predictive value (NPV).** The probability of *not* having the disease in a patient with a negative test result for the disease in question. The more sensitive a test is, the better will be its NPV. As the prevalence of disease in a population approaches 100%, the NPV of a test approaches zero.

SENSITIVITY AND SPECIFICITY 2×2 CONTINGENCY TABLE

Test Result	Disease		
	Present	Absent	
Positive	A	B	PPV = A/A + B
Negative	C	D	NPV = D/C + D
	Se = A/A + C	Sp = D/B + D	

C is also known as false negative.
B is also known as false positive.
Cutoff point for a test is the point on a continuum between a positive test and a negative test.

5. **Receiver operating characteristic (ROC) curve.** ROC analysis had its beginnings in observations made in Britain during World War II when radar receiver operators were being assessed on their ability to differentiate signal (e.g., enemy aircraft) from noise (e.g., flocks of birds). Its use in medicine to assess diagnostic test performance was first described by Lee B. Lusted, MD, in 1971.

In medicine, ROC is a measure of the distinguishing properties of a test for the disease in question. The curve is constructed by graphically plotting the true-positive rate (e.g., sensitivity) against the false-positive rate (e.g., 1 − specificity) over a range of possible test cutoff values. The best test cutoff value is a graphically plotted point on the scale that maximizes the sensitivity value and minimizes the false-positive rate. The overall accuracy of the test then can be described as the area under the curve (AUC).

In general, the AUC value and the quality of the test are interpreted as follows:

AUC Value	Test Quality
0.9–1.0	Excellent
0.8–0.9	Good
0.7–0.8	Fair
0.6–0.7	Poor
0.5–0.6	Fail

D. Odds, Risk, and Likelihood Ratios

1. **Odds ratio (OR).** The OR is a measure of association between an exposure and an outcome. ORs are used to compare the relative odds of the occurrence of the outcome of interest (e.g., disease or disorder), given exposure to the variable of interest in *case–control studies*. The OR can also be used to determine whether a particular exposure is a risk factor for a particular outcome and to compare the magnitude of various risk factors for that outcome.

   In *case–control studies* researchers start with two cohorts of patients, one group with the outcome of interest (e.g., case group) and one group without the outcome of interest (e.g., control group). Then researchers look retrospectively for the given exposure.

   Mathematically the OR is expressed as:

   Odds ratio = odds of disease in exposed group/odds of disease in unexposed group.

   In general, the values of OR are interpreted as:

   1. OR = 1; exposure does *not* affect odds of outcome
   2. OR > 1; exposure associated with higher odds of outcome
   3. OR < 1; exposure associated with lower odds of outcome

2. **Risk ratio or relative risk (RR).** The RR is a measure of the risk of a certain event happening in one group compared to the risk of the same event happening in another group. In a *cohort study* researchers start with two cohorts of patients, one group with the exposure and one group without the exposure (e.g., control group). Then researchers look prospectively for the outcome of interest. An RR value of 1 means there is no difference between the two groups in terms of their risk of disease, based on whether or not they were exposed to a certain substance or factor, or how they responded to two treatments being compared. An RR value greater than 1 or less than 1 usually means that being exposed to a certain substance or factor either increases

(RR greater than 1) or decreases (RR less than 1) the risk of disease, or that the treatments being compared do not have the same effects.

Mathematically these measures are expressed as:

Relative risk = risk of event (experimental group)/risk of event (control group)

Risk ratio = risk in exposed group/risk in unexposed group

3. **Likelihood ratio (LR).** It is the likelihood that a given test result would be expected in a patient with the disease in question compared to the likelihood that the same result would be expected in a patient without the disease in question. LR values are used to assess the discriminating properties of a particular diagnostic test and to also assist in selecting an appropriate diagnostic test(s) or sequence of tests. These values have the advantage over sensitivity and specificity because they are less likely to change with the prevalence of the disorder.

Mathematically these measures are expressed as:

Positive LR [LR+] = sensitivity/(1 − specificity)

Negative LR [LR−] = (1 − sensitivity)/specificity

Likelihood Ratio Value	Interpretation
Greater than 10	Strong evidence in support of diagnosis
5–10	Moderate evidence in support of diagnosis
2–5	Weak evidence in support of diagnosis
0.5–2	No clear evidence to support diagnosis
0.2–0.5	Weak evidence to refute the diagnosis
0.1–0.2	Moderate evidence to refute the diagnosis
Less than 0.1	Strong evidence to refute the diagnosis

E. Testing and Treatment Thresholds

These thresholds describe levels of probability of disease at which one should be indifferent between ordering more testing and withholding more testing or giving treatment and withholding treatment. In other words, it is the relationship between the rational willingness of the physician to either perform more testing or treat and the probability of disease. The probability of disease at which one should be indifferent between testing, giving treatment, and withholding treatment is based primarily on maximizing the patient's welfare (e.g., benefits) and reducing the patient's potential harms of testing or treatment. While each clinical scenario is different, some general rules for applying this concept may be as follows:

1. The probability of disease at or above which the physician might be comfortable treating a patient with no further diagnostic testing is 80% (0.8).

2. The probability of disease at or below which the physician might be comfortable deferring further testing or treatment is 25% (0.25).

3. The probability of disease at or above which the physician might be comfortable deferring treatment in favor of requesting more diagnostic testing is 25% to 50% (0.25–0.5).

4. The probability of disease at or above which the physician might be comfortable starting treatment in conjunction with requesting further diagnostic testing is 50% to 80% (0.5–0.8).

F. **Evaluating Published Data on Treatment**

The accepted definition of a clinical trial is *any research study in which one or more human subjects are prospectively assigned to one or more interventions (which may include placebo or other controls) to evaluate the effects of those interventions on health-related biomedical or behavioral outcomes.*

The recorded history of clinical trials begins with biblical descriptions in 500 BCE. While the evolution of clinical research traverses a long and fascinating journey, James Lind (1716–1794) is considered the first physician to have conducted a controlled clinical trial of the modern era while working as a surgeon on the British naval ship *Salisbury*. In his 1753 paper, *A Treatise on the Scurvy*, he details how he conducted a parallel arm medical experiment among scurvy afflicted seafarers. He discovered that lemons and oranges were most effective in treating the dreaded affliction. The first randomized control trial of streptomycin for treating pulmonary tuberculosis was carried out between 1946 and 1947 (published in 1948) by the Medical Research Council (MRC) of the United Kingdom (UK).

All clinical trials share basic common features:

1. **Basic structure**

   a. **Abstract.** This section presents an overview of the published article.

   b. **Introduction**. This section introduces the clinical topic with a review of previous relevant clinical trials and also states the primary and secondary research hypotheses.

   c. **Methods.** This section defines the patient population, lists the inclusion and exclusion criteria, describes the research design, defines the primary and secondary outcomes, and details the statistical methods and analysis.

   d. **Results.** This section summarizes the characteristics of each study group and describes the results of the study outcomes.

   e. **Discussion/conclusion.** This section provides an interpretation of the results in the context of previous studies, discusses the limitations and strengths of the study, and provides suggestions for future research.

2. **Phases of clinical trials.** Clinical trials are conducted in phases with each phase serving a particular purpose.

   a. **Phase I.** Initial testing of a new drug or treatment is performed on a small group of human subjects to evaluate a drug or treatment's safety, determine a certain safe dosage range, and identify side effects.

   b. **Phase II.** The new drug or treatment is tested on a larger group to determine its efficacy (e.g., whether it works under ideal circumstances).

   c. **Phase III.** Randomized controlled multicenter trials are performed on even larger patient groups to confirm effectiveness (e.g., whether the drug or therapy does more good than harm under usual care conditions).

   d. **Phase IV.** Postmarketing studies gather data on whether the drug affects population groups differently or whether there are side effects associated with its long-term use.

3. **Questions to consider when evaluating a clinical trial**
   a. **What are the study hypotheses, and are they clearly stated and relevant?** The hypotheses of interest require a definition of dependent (outcome) and independent (treatment) variables. The primary hypothesis states the effect of an independent variable on a dependent variable. The secondary hypothesis states the effect of an independent variable on a dependent variable among specified subgroups.
   b. **Is the study population adequately described?** Every trial should clearly state the inclusion and exclusion criteria, randomization procedure, and number of subjects in each group.
   c. **Are the observed differences due to chance (e.g., random error) or attributable to a true effect?** Statistical testing involves an assessment of the probability of an observed difference in outcome when there is actually no true difference between groups (e.g., false-positive rate; p value). When the p value is less than .5 the difference is considered significant and due to a true effect. When the p value is greater than .5 the difference is not considered significant and due to chance or random error.

   The probability of obtaining a significant result when a real difference exists is called the *study power*. A sample size large enough to achieve a power of 80% to 90% is desired.
   d. **Are the observed differences due to bias (e.g., systematic error)?** The most common types of bias include subject selection, outcome measures, and confounding. Confounding is defined as the modification of the true relationship between the treatment and outcome. The greatest level of evidence in support of a true outcome difference is associated with randomized, controlled clinical trials, particularly in combination with other randomized trials in a systematic fashion (e.g., meta-analysis).
   e. **Are the observed differences modified by other factors?** In general, inclusion of a variable in a multivariate model adjusts for confounding.
   f. **Are the observed differences relevant to the treatment of my patient?**

   The aforementioned information represents a basic guide for the proper design and method of conducting a trial that readers of the medical literature should consider when evaluating the published results of a clinical trial and its potential clinical application to patient care.

   This book is designed to assist physicians of any specialty and at all levels—students, residents, and attending—with the diagnosis and management of clinical infectious diseases. Within the book, we emphasize the core topics encountered by most physicians and highlight the definitions, classifications, microorganisms, clinical manifestations, physical-examination clues, contemporary diagnostic and laboratory methods, and treatment. A physician who utilizes the process outlined previously will ask the appropriate questions, elicit the pertinent symptoms and signs, order the appropriate diagnostic tests, and follow clinical reasoning to a definitive diagnosis and evidence-based treatment plan. In the end, this will result in optimal outcomes for patients and physicians alike.

BIBLIOGRAPHY

Appel LJ. A primer on the design, conduct, and interpretation of clinical trials. *Clin J Am Soc Nephrol*. 2006;1(6):1360–1367.

Fagan TJ. Letter: nomogram for Bayes theorem. *N Engl J Med*. 1975;293(5):257.

Grimes DA, Schulz KF. Refining clinical diagnosis with likelihood ratios. *Lancet*. 2005;365(9469): 1500–1505.

Grimes DA, Schulz KF. Cohort studies: marching towards outcomes. *Lancet*. 2002;359(9303):341–345.

Herrle SR, Corbett EC Jr, Fagan MJ, et al. Bayes' theorem and the physical examination: probability assessment and diagnostic decision making. *Acad Med*. 2011;86(5):618–627.

Kocher MS, Zurakowski D. Clinical epidemiology and biostatistics: a primer for orthopaedic surgeons. *J Bone Joint Surg Am*. 2004;86-A(3):607–620.

Lasko TA, Bhagwat JG, Zou KH, et al. The use of receiver operating characteristic curves in biomedical informatics. *J Biomed Inform*. 2005;38(5):404–415.

Lusted LB. Decision-making studies in patient management. *N Engl J Med*. 1971;284(8):416–424.

Richardson WS, Wilson MC, Guyatt GH, et al. Users' guides to the medical literature: XV. How to use an article about disease probability for differential diagnosis. Evidence-Based Medicine Working Group. *JAMA*. 1999;281(13):1214–1219.

Schulz KF, Grimes DA. Sample size calculations in randomised trials: mandatory and mystical. *Lancet*. 2005;365(9467):1348–1353.

Schulz KF, Grimes DA. Case-control studies: research in reverse. *Lancet*. 2002;359(9304):431–434.

2

INTRODUCTION TO ANTIMICROBIAL STEWARDSHIP

Susan L. DeBiase
William F. Wright

I. **INTRODUCTION.** Antimicrobial agents are among the most commonly prescribed medications in hospitals and outpatient community clinics. Unfortunately, a great number of these prescriptions are unnecessary or inappropriate. Abuse and misuse of antimicrobial agents have several negative consequences, including drug-related adverse events, the emergence of multidrug-resistant bacterial pathogens, the development of *Clostridium difficile* infection, the negative impact on the normal flora microbiota, and undertreatment risks. With the emergence of antimicrobial resistance, several organizations, including the Infectious Disease Society of America (IDSA), the Society for Healthcare Epidemiology of America (SHEA), and the American Society of Health System Pharmacists (ASHP), have identified antimicrobial stewardship as having an important role in healthcare environment. Antimicrobial stewardship is defined as a rational, systematic approach to the use of antimicrobial agents in order to achieve optimal outcomes.

II. **GENERAL PRINCIPLES.** In the United States, the IDSA has published guidelines for developing an institutional program to enhance antimicrobial stewardship. To be maximally effective in rationing antibiotic prescriptions, antimicrobial stewardship strategies and protocols must account for several elements strictly related to the antibiotic prescription but should also consider the need for continuous access to expertise in clinical pharmacology and infectious diseases and for transparent monitoring of antibiotic use. Additional strategies to improve antimicrobial prescribing methods include education of providers, compliance with published treatment guidelines, formulary restriction, streamlining/de-escalation of antimicrobial therapy, early intravenous to oral conversion, dose optimization, and use of antimicrobial order forms. Educational programs are particularly important and should provide adequate information about the rules for the identification of patients for whom antibiotics are necessary, the optimal timing of drug administration, and the most appropriate antibiotic regimen with the time of de-escalation or discontinuation specified. Education should also highlight the need for identification of local physician and nurse champions as well as other potential resources (e.g., pharmacy records, infection control practitioners, pharmacists, microbiologists, microbiology results, and information technology). Hospital administration and medical staff leadership must also support and contribute, even with financial support, to the application of antimicrobial stewardship principles.

III. CORE ELEMENTS. The core elements of improving antimicrobial utilization and minimizing antimicrobial resistance are important to patient safety and the greater public health. Elements common to successful antimicrobial stewardship include the following.

  A. Organizational and Leadership Commitment. Dedicating hospital and medical clinic resources to the development and implementation of antimicrobial stewardship efforts.

  B. Accountability. Appointing a physician and pharmacist level leadership team in association with dedicated multidisciplinary committee responsible for antimicrobial stewardship outcomes.

  C. Expertise. Recruiting infectious diseases providers (e.g., physicians, pharmacists, and nurses) to directly participate in the antimicrobial stewardship efforts.

  D. Implementation. The development of facility-specific guidelines to appropriate antimicrobial utilization.

  E. Tracking and Reporting. Monitoring of implemented facility-specific antimicrobial stewardship guideline measures and regular reporting of outcomes to the local leadership, committee members, and general medical community.

  F. Education. Providing regular educational programs (lectures, newsletters, etc.) infectious diseases conditions, management consideration, microbial virulence and resistance as well as optimal antimicrobial prescribing practices.

IV. SUMMARY. The discovery of penicillin in 1928, followed by its commercialization in the 1940s, ushered in the antibiotic era of medicine. Subsequent unparalleled advances in healthcare, excessive use of antimicrobial agents to eradicate infections associated with disease states that had previously rendered their treatment unthinkable, and underinvestment in the discovery and development of new antimicrobial agents have culminated in a crisis of antibiotic resistance.

> *It is not difficult to make microbes resistant to penicillin. . . . The time may come when penicillin can be bought by anyone in the shops. Then there is the danger that the ignorant man may easily under dose himself and by exposing his microbes to non-lethal quantities of the drug make them resistant.*
> —*Alexander Fleming's Nobel Prize Acceptance Lecture, 1945*

Antimicrobial stewardship is a key component of a multifaceted approach to preventing the emergence of antimicrobial resistance. Good antimicrobial stewardship involves selecting an appropriate drug and optimizing its dose and duration to cure an infection while minimizing toxicity and conditions for selection of resistant bacterial strains.

BIBLIOGRAPHY

Dellit TH, Owen RC, McGowan JE Jr, et al. Infectious Diseases Society of America and the Society for Healthcare Epidemiology of America guidelines for developing an institutional program to enhance antimicrobial stewardship. *Clin Infect Dis.* 2007;44(2):159–177.

Nagel JL, Kaye KS, LaPlante KL, et al. Antimicrobial stewardship for the infection control practitioner. *Infect Dis Clin North Am.* 2016;30(3):771–784.

Olans RN, Olans RD, DeMaria A Jr. The critical role of the staff nurse in antimicrobial stewardship—unrecognized, but already there. *Clin Infect Dis*. 2016;62(1):84–89.

Pollack LA, Srinivasan A. Core elements of hospital antibiotic stewardship programs from the centers of disease control and prevention. *Clin Infect Dis*. 2014;59(Suppl 3):S97–S100.

INTRODUCTION TO ANTIMICROBIAL AGENTS

Emily L. Heil
Neha U. Sheth
William F. Wright

I. **INTRODUCTION.** Understanding of the general factors involved with determining appropriate antimicrobial therapy for patients with an infection is an important aspect of treating clinical infectious diseases. While the preferred antimicrobial agents for the treatment of specific infections are discussed in the respective chapters, the following principles should provide guidance to the appropriate selection and use of these agents:

A. **Appropriate microbiological cultures should be obtained prior to starting antimicrobial therapy.** An exception to this rule is that empirical antibiotic therapy should be initiated immediately in critically ill, unstable patients when an infection is suspected.

B. **Accurate microbiological identification and antimicrobial susceptibility testing should be performed for the appropriate selection of antimicrobial therapy.** In general, especially for severe infections, the agent should be bactericidal to the pathogen.

C. **Appropriate selection and dosing of the antimicrobial agent should always consider patient age, weight, medication allergy history, and comorbid conditions (e.g., immunosuppression or pregnancy) as well as both hepatic and renal function.** In general, antimicrobial agents should be well tolerated and cost-effective.

II. **ANTIBACTERIAL ANTIMICROBIALS.** See Table 3.1.

A. **Aminoglycosides** (gentamicin, tobramycin, and amikacin).

1. **Activity.** These are a group of bactericidal drugs with concentration-dependent killing, a post-antibiotic effect, and can be synergistic with certain antibiotics. Most widely used for gram-negative enteric bacteria, *Pseudomonas* spp, and certain gram-positive bacteria (e.g., *Staphylococcus aureus* and *Enterococcus* spp). Aminoglycosides inhibit protein synthesis by irreversibly binding to the 30S bacterial ribosome.

2. **Resistance.** Resistance to aminoglycosides can occur via enzymatic inactivation (plasmid mediated), decreased drug uptake, and ribosomal mutation (chromosomal).

3. **Toxicity (pregnancy class D).** Therapeutic drug monitoring of aminoglycoside levels should be done to avoid nephrotoxicity (renal tubular damage) and ototoxicity and to ensure efficacy.

4. **Dosing changes with renal or hepatic failure.** Renal; once-daily dosing is associated with less nephrotoxicity.

(Text continues on page 23)

TABLE 3.1 ■ Antibacterial Agents

Target	Class	Agents	Spectrum	Adverse Effects	Pharmacology
Bacterial cell wall	Penicillins	Natural penicillins	Penicillin G (IV) Penicillin V (PO)	Good: *Streptococcus, Treponema pallidum* Moderate: *Enterococcus, Streptococcus pneumoniae*	Hypersensitivity reactions Acute interstitial nephritis GI	Very short half-life Hepatic metabolism accounts for <30%, excreted via glomerular and tubular secretion
		Penicillinase-resistant penicillins	Oxacillin (IV) Nafcillin (IV) Dicloxacillin (PO) Methicillin (IV)	Good: *Staphylococcus aureus, Streptococcus*	Hypersensitivity reactions GI Rare hepatotoxicity Acute interstitial nephritis	Highly protein bound. Hepatic metabolism accounts for ~50% of dose. Primarily excreted by the liver and to a lesser extent the kidneys
		Aminopenicillin	Ampicillin (PO, IV) Amoxicillin (PO)	Good: *Streptococcus, Enterococcus* Moderate: enteric gram-negative rods, *Haemophilus* Poor: *Staphylococcus*, anaerobes	Hypersensitivity reactions GI Rare hematologic effects	Absorbed well from the GI tract; widely distributed in tissues (especially inflamed tissue); renal excretion
		Antipseudomonal penicillins	Piperacillin (IV)	Good: *Pseudomonas, Streptococcus, Enterococcus* Moderate: enteric gram-negative rods, *Haemophilus* Poor: *Staphylococcus*, anaerobes	Similar to other beta-lactams	
		Beta-lactam/ beta-lactamase inhibitor combinations	Ampicillin/sulbactam (IV) Amoxicillin/clavulanic acid (PO) Ticarcillin/clavulanic acid (IV) Piperacillin/tazobactam (IV)	Good: *Staphylococcus aureus, Streptococcus, Enterococcus*, enteric gram-negative rods, anaerobes, *Pseudomonas* (only piperacillin/tazobactam and ticarcillin/clavulanic acid) Poor: atypicals, extended-spectrum beta-lactamase-producing gram-negatives	Hypersensitivity reactions Acute interstitial nephritis GI (diarrhea, especially with amoxicillin/clavulanic acid) Hematologic effects (thrombocytopenia with piperacillin/tazobactam) CNS toxicity (seizures) with high doses	Renal excretion beta-lactamase inhibitor component does not cross the blood–brain barrier

(continued)

14

TABLE 3.1 ■ Antibacterial Agents (*continued*)

Target	Class	Agents	Spectrum	Adverse Effects	Pharmacology
Cephalosporins	First generation	Cefazolin (IV), cephalexin (PO)	Good: *Staphylococcus aureus* Moderate: enteric gram-negative rods Poor: *Enterococcus*, anaerobes, *Pseudomonas*	GI	Highly protein bound, poor CNS penetration Primarily excreted unchanged in the urine
	Second generation	Cefuroxime (IV and PO) Cefprozil (PO) Cefoxitin (IV) Cefotetan (IV)	Good: some enteric gram-negative rods, *Haemophilus*, *Neisseria* Moderate: *Streptococcus*, *Staphylococcus* Poor: *Enterococcus*, *Pseudomonas*, anaerobes (cefoxitin and cefotetan have added gram-negative anaerobe coverage)	GI Cefoxitin/cefotetan interfere with vitamin K dependent coagulation; may increase PT/INR	Primarily renal excretion
	Third generation	Cefotaxime (IV) Ceftriaxone (IV) Cefpodoxime (PO) Cefixime (PO) Ceftazidime (IV)	Good: *Streptococcus*, *Staphylococcus aureus*, enteric gram-negative rods, *Pseudomonas* (ceftazidime only) Poor: *Enterococcus*, anaerobes	Ceftriaxone can cause cholestasis/biliary sludging Cefpodoxime interferes with vitamin K production; may increase PT/INR	Cefotaxime and ceftriaxone have the best CSF penetration Renal excretion with the exception of ceftriaxone (biliary excretion)
	Fourth generation	Cefepime (IV)	Good: *Staphylococcus aureus*, *Streptococcus*, *Pseudomonas*, enteric gram-negative rods Poor: *Enterococcus*, anaerobes	Rare convulsions (high doses in renal failure) Positive Coombs test (without hemolytic anemia)	20% protein bound, decent CSF concentrations 85% excretion unchanged in the urine
	Anti-MRSA	Ceftaroline (IV)	Good: *Staphylococcus aureus* (including methicillin-resistant), enteric gram-negative rods Poor: *Enterococcus*, anaerobes, *Pseudomonas*	GI	Ceftaroline fosamil is dephosphorylated to ceftaroline—ceftaroline and metabolite renally excreted

(*continued*)

TABLE 3.1 ■ Antibacterial Agents   (*continued*)

Target	Class	Agents	Spectrum	Adverse Effects	Pharmacology
	Carbapenems	Imipenem/cilastatin (IV) Meropenem (IV) Doripenem (IV) Ertapenem (IV)	Good: *Staphylococcus aureus*, *Streptococcus*, anaerobes, enteric gram-negative rods, extended-spectrum beta-lactamase-producing gram-negative rods, *Pseudomonas* (except ertapenem) Moderate: *Enterococcus*	Lower seizure threshold (associated with higher doses, or normal doses in patients with renal impairment, imipenem to the greatest extent)	Well distributed into body tissues; variable CSF penetration Eliminated primarily unchanged in the urine
	Monobactams	Aztreonam (IV)	Good: *Pseudomonas*, most gram-negative rods Poor: gram-positive organisms, anaerobes	Similar to other beta-lactams Renally excreted	
	Glycopeptides	Vancomycin (IV, PO)	Good: *Staphylococcus aureus* (including methicillin-resistant), *Streptococcus*, *Clostridium difficile* (PO only) Moderate: *Enterococcus* Poor: gram-negatives	Red-man syndrome (infusion-related histamine release) Thrombophlebitis Nephrotoxicity (interstitial nephritis) and ototoxicity	Poorly absorbed in the GI tract, penetrates well into most areas of the body except CNS (without meningeal inflammation) 90% excreted by glomerular filtration
	Lipopeptides	Daptomycin (IV)	Good: *Staphylococcus aureus* (including methicillin-resistant), *Streptococcus*, *Enterococcus* (including vancomycin-resistant) Poor: gram-negatives	Rare rhabdomyolysis	Long half-life Highly protein bound—poor CSF penetration Inactivated by pulmonary surfactant Primarily renal excretion

(continued)

16

TABLE 3.1 ■ Antibacterial Agents *(continued)*

Target	Class	Agents	Spectrum	Adverse Effects	Pharmacology
	Lipoglycopeptide	Telavancin	Good: *Staphylococcus aureus* (including methicillin-resistant), *Streptococcus*, *Enterococcus* (including vancomycin-resistant) Poor: gram-negatives	Most commonly taste disturbance, nausea, vomiting, and foamy urine. Rapid infusion can result in "red-man syndrome"–like reaction and so it has to be infused over 60 min	Highly protein bound as 90% of the administered drug is bound to serum albumin and has a half-life of 8 h; eliminated primarily by the kidney
	Polymyxin	Polymyxin B Colistimethate	Good: *Acinetobacter*, *Pseudomonas, Klebsiella pneumoniae*, *Escherichia coli* Poor: *Proteus*, *Providencia*, *Burkholderia, Serratia*, gram-positives	Nephrotoxicity (acute tubular necrosis) Neurotoxicity Enhancement of neuromuscular blockade	Widely distributed into body tissues, low levels in synovial, pleural, and pericardial fluid. ~25% CNS penetration with meningeal inflammation Renal excretion
Protein synthesis	Aminoglycosides	Amikacin (IV) Gentamicin (IV) Tobramycin (IV)	Good: gram-negatives, including *Pseudomonas* and *Acinetobacter* Moderate: *Staphylococcus, Streptococcus, Enterococcus* (for these gram-positives must be combined with a beta-lactam or glycopeptide) Poor: anaerobes, atypicals	Nephrotoxicity Ototoxicity Enhanced neuromuscular blockade	Not absorbed from the GI tract Poor penetration into lungs and CSF Volume of distribution correlates with volume of extracellular fluid (dose based on adjusted or ideal body weight) Excreted unchanged via glomerular filtration

(continued)

17

TABLE 3.1 ■ Antibacterial Agents (continued)

Target	Class	Agents	Spectrum	Adverse Effects	Pharmacology
	Macrolides	Clarithromycin (PO), azithromycin (PO, IV), erythromycin (IV, PO)	Good: atypicals, *Haemophilus influenzae, Moraxella catarrhalis, Helicobacter pylori, Mycobacterium avium* Moderate: *Streptococcus pneumoniae, S. pyogenes* Poor: *Staphylococcus,* enteric gram-negative rods, (azithromycin > clarithromycin), anaerobes, *Enterococcus*	GI: nausea, vomiting, diarrhea (erythromycin is the worst) Hepatic: telithromycin most severe Cardiac: QT prolongation (most with erythromycin)	Well absorbed (food reduced absorption of erythromycin); penetrates well into tissues Excreted in bile
	Lincosamides	Clindamycin (IV, PO)	Good: gram-positive anaerobes, *Plasmodium* spp Moderate: *Staphylococcus aureus* (including some MRSA), *Streptococcus pyogenes,* gram-negative anaerobes, *Chlamydia trachomatis, Pneumocystis jirovecii, Actinomyces, Toxoplasma* Poor: *Enterococcus, Clostridium difficile,* gram-negative aerobes	GI: diarrhea, *Clostridium difficile* Dermatologic: rash, SJS	90% bioavailability; penetrates most body fluids except CSF; hepatically metabolized Eliminated by urine and feces

(continued)

TABLE 3.1 ■ Antibacterial Agents (continued)

Target	Class	Agents	Spectrum	Adverse Effects	Pharmacology
	Tetracyclines	Doxycycline (IV, PO) Minocycline (IV, PO) Tetracycline (PO), Tigecycline (IV)	Good: atypicals, *Rickettsia*, spirochetes, *Plasmodium* spp Moderate: *Staphylococcus* (MRSA), *Streptococcus pneumoniae* Poor: most gram-negative rods, anaerobes, *Enterococcus* Tigecycline: in addition to the aforementioned: MRSA, VRE and most MDR GNRs	GI irritation (nausea/diarrhea) Photosensitivity Esophageal irritation Minocycline (vertigo/dizziness) Teeth discoloration Absorption is decreased with dairy products, aluminum hydroxide, sodium bicarbonate, calcium, magnesium, and iron; penetrates well into tissue metabolized in the liver Excreted in urine Tigecycline achieves low serum concentrations and should not be used for bacteremias	
	Oxazolidinone	Linezolid (IV, PO)	Good: *Staphylococcus aureus* (including methicillin-resistant), *Streptococcus* (including multidrug-resistant *Streptococcus pneumoniae*, *Enterococcus* (including VRE), *Nocardia* Moderate: some atypicals Poor: all gram-negatives, anaerobes	Bone marrow suppression Peripheral neuropathy	100% bioavailable, good CSF penetration (but bacteriostatic), hepatic metabolism Mostly nonrenal excretion
	Chloramphenicol	Chloramphenicol (IV, PO)	*Haemophilus influenzae*, *Neisseria meningitides*, *Streptococcus pneumoniae*, most gram-positive aerobes, *Rickettsia*	Reticulocytopenia, anemia, leukopenia, thrombocytopenia Gray baby syndrome	Well absorbed from GI tract, administered IV; hepatically metabolized Inactive form excreted in urine

(continued)

TABLE 3.1 ■ Antibacterial Agents *(continued)*

Target	Class	Agents	Spectrum	Adverse Effects	Pharmacology
	Streptogramins	Quinupristin/Dalfopristin (IV)	Good: MSSA, MRSA, *Streptococcus, Enterococcus faecium* Poor: *Enterococcus faecalis*, gram-negatives	Phlebitis, myalgias, arthralgias	Hepatically metabolized Hepatic, biliary, and renal excretion
DNA synthesis	Fluoroquinolones	Ciprofloxacin (IV, PO) Levofloxacin (IV, PO) Moxifloxacin (IV, PO)	Ciprofloxacin: Good: enteric gram-negative rods (*Escherichia coli, Proteus, Klebsiella,* etc.), *Haemophilus influenzae* Moderate: *Pseudomonas,* atypicals, *(Mycoplasma, Chlamydia, Legionella)* Poor: *Staphylococcus, Streptococcus pneumoniae,* anaerobes, *Enterococcus* levofloxacin/ moxifloxacin Good: enteric gram-negatives, *S. pneumoniae,* atypicals, *H. influenzae* Moderate: *Pseudomonas* (levofloxacin), MSSA Poor: anaerobes (except moxifloxacin), enterococci	GI, headache, photosensitivity Hyper/hypoglycemia, seizures, QT prolongation (dose related) Arthralgias, Achilles tendon rupture CNS: dizziness, confusion, hallucinations	Well absorbed in upper GI tract; good penetration into tissues but not CSF; minimally metabolized Renally excreted

(continued)

TABLE 3.1 ◾ Antibacterial Agents (continued)

Target	Class	Agents	Spectrum	Adverse Effects	Pharmacology
	Nitroimidazoles	Metronidazole (IV, PO)	Good: gram-negative and gram-positive anaerobes, including *Bacteroides*, *Fusobacterium*, *Clostridium* spp, protozoa including *Trichomonas*, *Entamoeba*, *Giardia* Moderate: *Helicobacter pylori* Poor: gram-positives and gram-negatives, *Peptostreptococcus*, *Actinomyces*, *Propionibacterium*	GI: nausea, vomiting, diarrhea with metallic taste, hepatitis, pancreatitis Neurologic: peripheral neuropathy (dose dependent)	Absorbed orally and rapidly; immediately distributed to ~80% of body weight; hepatically metabolized Excreted in urine and feces
	Folate antagonists	Sulfamethoxazole–trimethoprim (IV, PO)	Good: *Staphylococcus* (including MRSA), *Haemophilus influenzae*, *Stenotrophomonas maltophilia*, *Listeria*, *Pneumocystis jirovecii* pneumonia, *Toxoplasma gondii* Moderate: enteric gram-negative rods, *Streptococcus pneumoniae*, *Salmonella*, *Shigella*, *Nocardia* Poor: *Pseudomonas*, *Enterococcus*, *Streptococcus pyogenes*, anaerobes	Nausea, vomiting, diarrhea, rash, fever, headache, depression, jaundice, hepatic necrosis, drug-induced lupus, serum sickness–like syndrome, acute pancreatitis Acute hemolytic anemia (G6PD deficiency), aplastic anemia, agranulocytosis, thrombocytopenia, leukopenia Hypersensitivity	Absorbed immediately in small intestine and stomach; well distributed to CSF, pleural, and peritoneal fluids; hepatically metabolized Renally excreted

(continued)

TABLE 3.1 ■ Antibacterial Agents (continued)

Target	Class	Agents	Spectrum	Adverse Effects	Pharmacology
			Renal: crystalluria and *acute interstitial nephritis* by sulfamethoxazole leading to renal insufficiency; trimethoprim can cause creatinine excretion blockade causing false elevation in serum creatinine		
	Rifamycins	Rifampin (IV, PO), Rifabutin (PO)	Good: most *Mycobacterium* Moderate: *Staphylococcus, Acinetobacter, Enterobacteriaceae* Poor: "typical" bacteria as monotherapy	Dizziness, drowsiness, abdominal pain, diarrhea, nausea, vomiting, headache, visual change, pruritus, rash, hepatotoxicity	Completely absorbed in GI tract with a peak at 1–4 hours; 80% protein bound with good distribution; hepatically metabolized Excreted through biliary tract
Other	Nitrofurantoin	Nitrofurantoin (PO)	Good: *Escherichia coli, Staphylococcus saprophyticus* Moderate: *Citrobacter, Klebsiella, Enterococcus* Poor: *Pseudomonas, Proteus, Acinetobacter, Serratia*	GI (nausea, vomiting) Acute pneumonitis Chronic pulmonary fibrosis Peripheral neuropathy	Increased absorption with meal in small intestine; highly protein bound and distributed through tissues; metabolized in tissues Renally excreted

CNS, central nervous system; CSF, cerebrospinal fluid; G6PD, glucose-6-phosphate dehydrogenase; GI, gastrointestinal; INR, international normalized ratio; IV, intravenous; MDR GNR, multidrug-resistant gram-negative rod; MRSA, methicillin-resistant *Staphylococcus aureus*; MSSA, methicillin-susceptible *Staphylococcus aureus*; PT, prothrombin time; SJS, Stevens–Johnson syndrome; VRE, vancomycin-resistant enterococci.

B. Beta-lactams (penicillin, cephalosporin, carbapenem, and monobactam).

1. **Activity.** These are bactericidal drugs with time-dependent killing that bind penicillin-binding proteins in the bacterial cell wall and inhibit cell-wall cross-linking with relatively good activity against a variety of gram-positive and gram-negative pathogens depending on the agent. Cephalosporin antibiotics are divided into generations based on their spectrum of antibacterial activity. All beta-lactam antibiotics do not cover atypical organisms. While cephalosporin antibiotics are relatively broad-spectrum agents, none of them cover *Enterococcus* spp or *Listeria* spp. The carbapenem antibiotics are extremely broad-spectrum agents that can resist the effect of many beta-lactamases. Monobactam agents cover gram-negative organisms including *Pseudomonas* spp but lack gram-positive coverage.

2. **Resistance.** Resistance to beta-lactams is via inactivation by beta-lactamases, reduced permeability via porin proteins in gram-negative outer membranes, efflux pumps, or altered penicillin-binding proteins.

3. **Toxicity (pregnancy class B, except imipenem/cilastatin class C).** Anaphylaxis, or hypersensitivity, is the most feared reaction. Monobactams (e.g., aztreonam) are usually reserved for patients with penicillin allergy, as they have minimal cross-reactivity with other beta-lactams; however, aztreonam has a similar side chain to ceftazidime and should be avoided in patients with an allergy to ceftazidime. In general, the beta-lactams are well tolerated with minimal other adverse effects, which may include diarrhea, vomiting, seizures, acute interstitial nephritis, *Clostridium difficile* infection, and bleeding disorders.

4. **Dosing changes with renal or hepatic failure.** Renal.

C. Chloramphenicol

1. **Activity.** This agent is principally bacteriostatic and irreversibly binds to the 50S ribosomal subunit and inhibits peptidyl transferase, which consequently inhibits protein synthesis. This medication is active against most gram-positive and gram-negative aerobic organisms. This agent should not be used for urinary tract infections or infections with *Pseudomonas* spp or methicillin-resistant *Staphylococcus aureus* (MRSA).

2. **Resistance.** This includes the production of a *plasmid-mediated* enzyme (chloramphenicol acetyltransferase) that causes inactivation of chloramphenicol, the reduction of permeability through the bacterial membrane, or a mutation of the ribosomal subunit.

3. **Toxicity (pregnancy warning use with caution).** Mainly associated bone marrow suppression, aplastic anemia, gastrointestinal disturbances, and optic neuritis.

4. **Dosing changes with renal or hepatic failure.** Hepatic.

D. Clindamycin

1. **Activity.** This is a chlorine-substituted lincomycin that is bacteriostatic with time-dependent activity. It has the same binding site as macrolides and chloramphenicol and subsequently prevents protein synthesis. It is mainly used for severe anaerobic infections and may also be used to treat certain gram-positive infections (not *Enterococcus* spp) in patients with a beta-lactam allergy. It also has the ability to penetrate biofilms.

2. **Resistance.** Mechanisms of resistance include the production of an enzyme that causes inactivation, the reduction of permeability through the bacterial membrane, or a mutation of the ribosomal subunit.

3. **Toxicity (pregnancy class B).** Most commonly associated with *Clostridium difficile* superinfection.

4. **Dosing changes with renal or hepatic failure**. None.

E. **Folate Antagonists** (trimethoprim-sulfamethoxazole).

1. **Activity.** This agent acts by inhibiting the conversion of para-aminobenzoic acid (PABA) into tetrahydrofolic acid and thereby prevents microbial folic acid synthesis (an important metabolite for DNA synthesis). This mechanism results in the mostly bacteriostatic behavior of this class.

2. **Resistance.** A common resistance mechanism includes either the overproduction of PABA or the structural changes to the tetrahydropterin structure that affects the affinity of sulfonamides. It should be noted that there are high rates of resistance seen with these medications for organisms such as *Staphylococcus* spp (other than MRSA) and *Streptococcus* spp, and resistance patterns should be evaluated prior to the empiric use of these medications.

3. **Toxicity (pregnancy class C, not recommended in third trimester).** Associated with hypersensitivity reactions, Stevens–Johnson syndrome, anemia, leukopenia, hyperkalemia, and nephrolithiasis.

4. **Dosing changes with renal or hepatic failure**. Renal.

F. **Fluoroquinolones** (ciprofloxacin, levofloxacin, and moxifloxacin).

1. **Activity.** These agents are bactericidal, with concentration-dependent activity. They inhibit DNA gyrase and topoisomerase IV, which are responsible for bacterial DNA synthesis (leading to bacterial cell death).

2. **Resistance.** Mutations in the chromosomal genes of these enzymes can cause fluoroquinolone resistance.

3. **Toxicity (pregnancy class C).** Agents are associated with tendonitis/tendon rupture (higher risk in older adults, solid organ transplants, and with concomitant corticosteroids), prolonged QTc, headache, nausea, antibiotic-related diarrhea, rash, and delirium.

4. **Dosing changes with renal or hepatic failure**. Renal. Additionally, it is important to note that aluminum- and magnesium-containing products can cause a reduction in fluoroquinolone bioavailability and should be separated by 2 to 3 hours.

G. **Glycopeptide** (vancomycin).

1. **Activity.** Vancomycin is a slow bactericidal drug compared to beta-lactams and is bacteriostatic against *Enterococcus* spp. Vancomycin inhibits cell-wall synthesis by binding to the D-alanyl-D-alanine portion of cell-wall precursors.

2. **Resistance.** Resistance can occur via plasma-mediated modification of D-ala D-ala to D-ala D-lactate (resistance develops slowly).

3. **Toxicity (pregnancy class C [intravenous]; class B [oral]).** Vancomycin is associated with red-man syndrome, nephrotoxicity, prolonged QTc, and thrombocytopenia.

    4. Dosing changes with renal or hepatic failure. Renal. Therapeutic drug monitoring of vancomycin troughs is recommended.

H. Lipopeptide (daptomycin).

    1. Activity. Daptomycin is a concentration-dependent, rapidly bactericidal drug that forms transmembrane channels and causes membrane depolarization.

    2. Resistance. Resistance can be the result of altered membrane potential.

    3. Toxicity (pregnancy class B). Daptomycin is associated with myositis, constipation, and nausea.

    4. Dosing changes with renal or hepatic failure. Renal.

I. Lipoglycopeptide (telavancin).

    1. Activity. Telavancin mechanism of inhibition of cell-wall synthesis is similar to that of vancomycin. The glycopeptide core binds to the terminal acyl-D-alanyl-D-alanine chains of the cell wall with high affinity by means of hydrogen bonds and hydrophobic packing interaction.

    2. Resistance. Resistance can occur via plasma-mediated modification of D-ala D-ala to D-ala D-lactate (resistance develops slowly).

    3. Toxicity (pregnancy class C). Animal studies have shown reduced fetal weights and increased rates of digit and limb malformations. Rapid infusion can result in "red-man syndrome"-like reaction and so it has to be infused over 60 min. It also has a propensity to cause QTc prolongation similar to vancomycin.

    4. Dosing changes with renal or hepatic failure. Renal.

J. Polymyxins (polymyxin B and colistimethate [colistin or polymyxin E]).

    1. Activity. The polymyxins interfere with cell-membrane function by acting as a cationic detergent resulting in leakage of essential intracellular metabolites and nucleosides.

    2. Resistance. Resistance is not fully understood but may involve inherent genetic bacterial regulatory systems.

    3. Toxicity. Colistin **(pregnancy class C)** and polymyxin B **(pregnancy class B)** are associated with nephrotoxicity, neurotoxicity, respiratory failure, paresthesia, and vertigo.

    4. Dosing changes with renal or hepatic failure. Renal.

K. Linezolid

    1. Activity. A bacteriostatic, time-dependent antibiotic that binds to the 23S component of the 50S ribosome, which then prevents formation of the 70S complex involved with protein synthesis. This agent is most commonly used for infection with gram-positive organisms such as MRSA and vancomycin-resistant enterococci (VRE).

    2. Resistance. The most common mechanism of resistance is a mutation at the binding site; however, inhibition of linezolid to its binding site can also occur by medications with similar mechanisms of action such as chloramphenicol and lincosamides.

    3. Toxicity (pregnancy class C). This agent was first studied as an antidepressant medication that nonselectively inhibited monoamine oxidase reversibly;

therefore, there is a minimal chance that when given with a serotonin agonist the patient could be at risk for serotonin syndrome. This should be monitored if coadministered with serotonin reuptake inhibitors (e.g., selective serotonin reuptake inhibitor [SSRI] antidepressant).

4. **Dosing changes with renal or hepatic failure.** None.

L. **Macrolides** (azithromycin, clarithromycin, and erythromycin).

1. **Activity.** These agents are bacteriostatic medications that reversibly bind to the 23S rRNA located on the 50S ribosomal subunit thereby inhibiting protein synthesis.

2. **Resistance.** The mechanism of resistance is similar to that of chloramphenicol and lincosamides and includes the plasmid-mediated production of an enzyme that causes inactivation, the reduction of permeability through the bacterial membrane, or a mutation of the ribosomal subunit (methylation).

3. **Toxicity (pregnancy class B, except for clarithromycin C).** Mainly associated with gastrointestinal disturbances and antibiotic-related diarrhea (not due to *C. difficile*) but may also cause prolonged QTc (lowest associated with azithromycin).

4. **Dosing changes with renal or hepatic failure.** None.

M. **Nitroimidazoles** (metronidazole).

1. **Activity.** A concentration-dependent antibiotic that is reduced by nitroreductase to an active component that directly disrupts bacterial DNA leading to bactericidal activity (nitroreductase is produced by organisms during an anaerobic state).

2. **Resistance.** A common mechanism of resistance is when the organism produces less nitroreductase leading to less disruption in the bacterial DNA.

3. **Toxicity (pregnancy class B; avoid during first trimester).** It should be noted that patients should be counseled on the potential for disulfiram-like reactions (e.g., flushing, nausea, vomiting, headache, vertigo, dyspnea, and/or weakness) if using alcohol with this medication. Patients should be advised to refrain from alcohol during metronidazole use and up to 48 hours after the discontinuation of metronidazole. Additionally, may be associated with delirium, metallic taste, nausea, and peripheral neuropathy.

4. **Dosing changes with renal or hepatic failure.** Adjust only for severe renal failure (creatinine clearance less than 10 mL/min) and hepatic failure.

N. **Nitrofurantoin.** Currently solely utilized for urinary tract infections due to the high concentration of medication into the urinary system.

1. **Activity.** Though the mechanism is not well understood, it is proposed to directly damage bacterial DNA resulting in the medication having bactericidal activity.

2. **Resistance.** Mechanism is not well understood.

3. **Toxicity (pregnancy class B; contraindicated at time of delivery due to risk of hemolytic anemia in neonates).** Associated with acute pneumonitis reactions, prolonged use may be associated with hepatitis, interstitial fibrosis, and/or peripheral neuropathy.

4. **Dosing changes with renal or hepatic failure**. Renal. It should not be used in patients with a creatinine clearance of less than 60 mL/min due to subtherapeutic urinary concentrations and increased risk of adverse effects.

O. **Streptogramins** (quinupristin/dalfopristin).

1. **Activity.** They irreversibly bind to the 50S ribosomal subunit but have separate mechanisms by which to prevent peptide chain elongation and interfere with peptidyl transferase (e.g., protein synthesis).

2. **Resistance.** Mechanism of resistance includes modification of the drug target (i.e., ribosome) that can also cause cross-resistance with other agents (e.g., macrolides and clindamycin), efflux of streptogramins, which are also associated with cross-resistance with macrolides, and the production of enzymes that inactivate streptogramins.

3. **Toxicity (pregnancy class B).** This agent is associated with myalgia, hepatitis, and hyperbilirubinemia. This agent must be infused through a central venous catheter.

4. **Dosing changes with renal or hepatic failure.** None. However, these agents inhibit the hepatic cytochrome P450 (CYP) enzyme 3A4 (CYP3A4), which can lead to many clinically relevant drug–drug interactions that should be reviewed prior to use.

P. **Rifamycin** (rifampin, rifabutin, and rifapentine).

1. **Activity.** A group of antibiotics that inhibit DNA-dependent RNA polymerase at the B-subunit that ultimately prevents RNA elongation and thereby resulting in these agents to be bactericidal.

2. **Resistance.** A common mechanism of resistance is when the organism experiences missense mutation in the genes encoding the RNA polymerase leading to less disruption in the bacterial RNA elongation.

3. **Toxicity (pregnancy class C, except rifabutin pregnancy class B).** Associated with hepatitis, rash, leukopenia, thrombocytopenia, headache, nausea, and antibiotic-related diarrhea. Potent inducers of CYP3A4 that can lead to many significant drug–drug interactions. Patients should be counseled on the potential of urine and other bodily fluids to have a red-orange discoloration.

4. **Dosing changes with renal or hepatic failure.** Rifampin (hepatic); rifabutin (renal); and rifapentine (no data).

Q. **Tetracyclines** (tetracycline, minocycline, and doxycycline).

1. **Activity.** A group of agents that bind to the 30S ribosomal subunit resulting in the prevention of peptide chain elongation; therefore, they are bacteriostatic and have time-dependent activity.

2. **Resistance.** Common mechanisms occur with either protein pumps that remove the drug from the bacteria or mutations that occur at the binding site of the 30S subunit.

3. **Toxicity (pregnancy class D; avoid in children less than age 8 years).** These agents are associated with photosensitivity, hepatitis, nausea, vomiting, and diarrhea.

4. **Dosing changes with renal or hepatic failure**. Tetracycline (renal and hepatic); minocycline (renal); and doxycycline (absorption of these agents can be decreased when coadministered with dairy products, aluminum, calcium, magnesium, and iron).

III. ANTIFUNGAL ANTIMICROBIALS. See Table 3.2.

A. **Azole Antifungal Agents** (fluconazole, voriconazole, posaconazole, ketoconazole, and itraconazole).

1. **Activity**. These agents are fungicidal drugs that inhibit the synthesis of ergosterol, an essential component of fungal cell membranes.

2. **Resistance**. Resistance can occur via increased drug efflux or altered C-14 alpha-demethylase (enzyme essential for normal fungal membranes).

3. **Toxicity (pregnancy class C, except voriconazole class D; fluconazole for longer than one dose, class D).** These agents are mainly associated with hepatitis and gastrointestinal symptoms.

4. **Dosing changes with renal or hepatic failure.** Renal.

B. **Echinocandin Antifungal Agents** (anidulafungin, caspofungin, and micafungin).

1. **Activity**. While these agents are fungicidal against most *Candida* spp, they are fungistatic against *Aspergillus flavus* and act by inhibiting beta-glucan synthesis in the fungal cell walls.

2. **Resistance**. The mechanism of resistance includes the mutation of the enzyme that produces beta-glucan (glucan synthase) and/or the reduction of permeability through the fungal membrane.

3. **Toxicity (pregnancy class C).** They are associated with hepatitis, nausea, vomiting, fever, and drug rash.

4. **Dosing changes with renal or hepatic failure.** Hepatic. These agents do not result in adequate urinary concentrations and therefore should not be used to treat fungal-related urinary tract infections.

C. **Amphotericin Antifungal Agents**

1. **Activity**. These agents are broad-spectrum antifungal products that bind to ergosterol in fungal cell membranes causing increased membrane permeability.

2. **Resistance**. Mechanisms include alterations of ergosterol, alteration of cell-membrane composition, and altered defense mechanisms against oxidative damage.

3. **Toxicity (pregnancy class B).** These agents are commonly associated with nephrotoxicity, fevers, chills, nausea, vomiting, anemia, hypokalemia, and hypomagnesemia. The lipid formulations of amphotericin were created to reduce binding of amphotericin to human cell membranes to reduce nephrotoxicity.

4. **Dosing changes with renal or hepatic failure.** None.

D. **Flucytosine**

1. **Activity**. This agent is converted to 5-fluorouracil (5-FU) within the cell to interfere with protein synthesis by incorporating into fungal RNA. This agent

TABLE 3.2 ■ Antifungal Agents

Class	Agents	Spectrum	Adverse Effects	Pharmacology
Azoles	Fluconazole (IV, PO) Itraconazole (PO) Voriconazole (IV, PO) Posaconazole (PO)	*Candida* spp (*C. krusei* is intrinsically resistant to fluconazole, increasing fluconazole resistance with *C. glabrata*) *Aspergillus* spp, *Cryptococcus neoformans*, *Fusarium* spp, *Scedosporium apiospermum* (voriconazole) Zygomycetes (posaconazole)	Hepatotoxicity GI Visual disturbances/rare visual hallucinations (voriconazole)	Hepatic metabolism (significant drug–drug interaction potential) Fluconazole has excellent bioavailability and is the only azole with good urine penetration Good CSF penetration Oral bioavailability of posaconazole affected by food—must be administered with high-fat meals
Echinocandins	Caspofungin (IV) Micafungin (IV) Anidulafungin (IV)	*Candida* spp (higher MICs with *C. parapsilosis*), *Aspergillus* (in combination)	Relatively nontoxic Rare hepatotoxicity	Hepatic metabolism (except anidulafungin) Limited CNS, bone, and urine penetration
Polyene	Amphotericin B (IV) Liposomal amphotericin B (IV) Amphotericin B lipid complex (IV) Amphotericin B cholesteryl sulfate complex (IV)	*Aspergillus* spp, *Candida* spp (except *C. lusitaniae*), *Cryptococcus neoformans* *Blastomyces dermatitidis*	Nephrotoxicity (including magnesium and potassium wasting) Infusion-related reactions (fevers, chills) Phlebitis Anemia	Renal excretion, wide volume of distribution, highly protein bound, poor CNS penetration (still effective for cryptococcal meningitis). Lipid formulations have lower serum concentrations than conventional amphotericin B, but greater volumes of distribution.
Pyrimidine	Flucytosine (PO)	*Cryptococcus neoformans*, *Candida* spp	Bone marrow toxicity (leukopenia, thrombocytopenia) Pruritus GI	Wide volume of distribution, good CNS penetration Renal excretion

CNS, central nervous system; CSF, cerebrospinal fluid; GI, gastrointestinal; IV, intravenous; MIC, minimum inhibitory concentration.

is also converted to 5-fluorodeoxyuridylic acid monophosphate, which inhibits DNA synthesis.

2. **Resistance.** Simultaneous use with other antifungal agents has been proposed due to the high frequency of resistance. The mechanism of resistance includes production of an enzyme (cytosine deaminase) that causes drug inactivation and/or the reduction of drug permeability through the fungal membrane.

3. **Toxicity (pregnancy class C).** This agent is associated with fever, rash, nausea, vomiting, hepatitis, anemia, leukopenia, and thrombocytopenia. Levels of flucytosine should be checked for treatment greater than 2 weeks.

4. **Dosing changes with renal or hepatic failure.** Renal.

IV. ANTIPARASITIC ANTIMICROBIALS

A. **Antimalarial Heme Metabolism Inhibitors** (chloroquine, quinine and quinidine, and mefloquine).

1. **Activity.** While the mechanism of action for mefloquine is not well understood, the other agents act by binding to ferriprotoporphyrin IX to inhibit the polymerization of this heme metabolite, which then leads to accumulation of this product that is toxic to the parasite (oxidative membrane damage).

2. **Resistance.** The most accepted mechanisms include drug efflux and/or mutations in the genes that code for membrane proteins responsible for pH regulation.

3. **Toxicity (pregnancy class C; except mefloquine, class B; and chloroquine, no data).** Mefloquine is associated with vivid dreams, hallucinations, depression, psychosis, and prolongation of QTc. Quinine is associated with tinnitus, deafness, headaches, nausea, vomiting, and drug-induced lupus. Quinidine can also be associated with hemolytic anemia in patients with glucose-6-phosphate dehydrogenase (G6PD) deficiency, cardiac arrhythmias, and/or hypotension (based on the infusion rate). Chloroquine is well tolerated at normal doses but may be associated with pruritus.

4. **Dosing changes with renal or hepatic failure.** Renal (except mefloquine).

B. **Antimalarial Electron-Transport-Chain Inhibitors** (primaquine and atovaquone).

1. **Activity.** The mechanism of action for these agents involves inhibition of ubiquinone (a normal shuttling protein of the electron transport chain) resulting in a reduced interaction with the cytochrome bc_1 complex.

2. **Resistance.** The mechanism most commonly involves point mutations in the cytochrome bc_1 complex; therefore, atovaquone is usually administered with a second agent such as proguanil (a dihydrofolate reductase inhibitor) or doxycycline.

3. **Toxicity (pregnancy class C for atovaquone; no data for primaquine—avoid).** These agents are associated with headache, rash, leukopenia, hepatitis, nausea, vomiting, and diarrhea. Primaquine is particularly associated with hemolytic anemia in patients with G6PD deficiency.

4. **Dosing changes with renal or hepatic failure.** None (except Malarone).

C. Ivermectin

1. **Activity.** The mechanism of action as an anthelmintic agent includes the direct activation of glutamate-gated chlorine channels as well as to potentiate the binding of gamma-aminobutyric acid (GABA) that results in interruption of neuromuscular activity with tonic paralysis.

2. **Resistance.** No clinically relevant resistance.

3. **Toxicity (pregnancy class C).** This agent is associated with rash, dizziness, diarrhea, nausea, vomiting, and abdominal cramps.

4. **Dosing changes with renal or hepatic failure.** None.

D. Anthelmintic DNA Inhibitors (albendazole and mebendazole).

1. **Activity.** These agents inhibit beta-tubulin polymerization that disrupts DNA replication as well as nematodal motility.

2. **Resistance.** No clinically relevant resistance.

3. **Toxicity (pregnancy class C).** These agents are associated with hepatitis, anemia, leukopenia, nausea, vomiting, and diarrhea.

4. **Dosing changes with renal or hepatic failure.** None.

E. Praziquantel. Usually the drug of choice with cestode or trematode infections.

1. **Activity.** This agent is thought to cause parasite paralysis by increasing membrane permeability to calcium.

2. **Resistance.** No clinically relevant resistance.

3. **Toxicity (pregnancy class B).** This agent is associated with nausea, abdominal cramps, and headaches.

4. **Dosing changes with renal or hepatic failure.** Hepatic.

V. ANTIVIRAL ANTIMICROBIALS. See Table 3.3.

A. Viral DNA Polymerase Inhibitors (acyclovir, valacyclovir, famciclovir, ganciclovir, and valganciclovir).

1. **Activity.** These agents are activated by viral thymidine *kinase* to inhibit viral DNA polymerase and viral DNA synthesis. Ganciclovir and valganciclovir are also phosphorylated by thymidine kinase and inhibit viral DNA synthesis. Both also have more potent inhibition of cytomegalovirus (CMV) compared to acyclovir, valacyclovir, and famciclovir.

2. **Resistance.** Resistance to acyclovir is related to the presence or production of thymidine kinase, altered thymidine kinase substrate specificity, or alterations to viral DNA polymerase; however, famciclovir may be active against herpes simplex virus (HSV) that is resistant to acyclovir due to alterations in thymidine kinase. Resistance in CMV to ganciclovir can be from reduced phosphorylation of ganciclovir from a mutation encoded by the *UL97* gene or point mutations in the viral DNA polymerase encoded by the *UL54* gene.

3. **Toxicity (pregnancy class C for ganciclovir/valganciclovir; class B for acyclovir/valacyclovir/famciclovir).** These agents may be associated with seizures, tremors, renal tubular necrosis, nausea, vomiting, anemia, leukopenia, and thrombocytopenia.

4. **Dosing changes with renal or hepatic failure.** Renal.

TABLE 3.3 ■ Antiviral Agents

Class	Agents	Spectrum	Adverse Effects	Pharmacology
Neuraminidase inhibitors	Oseltamivir (PO) Zanamivir (inhalation) Peramivir (IV)	Influenza A and B, H5N1 (in vitro)	Bronchospasm (zanamivir) GI (oseltamivir)	Renal excretion
Adamantanes	Amantadine (PO) Rimantadine (PO)	Influenza A	CNS: insomnia, dizziness, lethargy, seizure (rare; amantadine > rimantadine) GI	Good PO absorption Renal excretion Amantadine crosses blood–brain barrier (rimantadine does not)
Guanosine analog	Ribavirin (PO, IV, inhalation)	Broad spectrum of RNA and DNA viruses (RSV, HCV most notably)	Anemia Fatigue Bronchospasm (inhalation) Contraindicated in pregnancy	Absorption increased with a fatty meal
Viral DNA polymerase inhibitors	Acyclovir (PO, IV) Valacyclovir (PO) Famciclovir (PO) Ganciclovir (IV) Valganciclovir (PO)	HSV-1, HSV-2, VZV, EBV (excluding famciclovir), CMV, HHV-6 (ganciclovir/ valganciclovir)	Nephrotoxicity (IV acyclovir) CNS toxicity (IV acyclovir, high doses in renal failure) Neutropenia, thrombocytopenia (ganciclovir, valganciclovir)	Valacyclovir and valganciclovir have good bioavailability CNS penetration ~50% serum (acyclovir)
Phosphonoformate	Foscarnet (IV)	CMV, VZV, HSV, influenza A	Nephrotoxicity Electrolyte imbalances	Renal excretion
Cytosine analog	Cidofovir (IV, intravitreal, topical)	CMV, HSV, VZV, EBV, HHV-6	Nephrotoxicity (significant, must coadminister probenecid) Neutropenia Metabolic acidosis GI intolerance	Renal excretion

CMV, cytomegalovirus; CNS, central nervous system; CSF, cerebrospinal fluid; EBV, Epstein–Barr virus; GI, gastrointestinal; HCV, hepatitis C virus; HHV, human herpesvirus; HSV, herpes simplex virus; IV, intravenous; RSV, respiratory syncytial virus; VZV, varicella-zoster virus.

B. Neuraminidase Inhibitors (oseltamivir and zanamivir).

    1. Activity. These agents inhibit the enzyme neuraminidase, which is essential to the influenza virus life cycle and prevents the release of new virions.

    2. Resistance. Resistance occurs from point mutations in the viral neuraminidase genes.

    3. Toxicity (pregnancy class C). These agents may be associated with bronchospasm, seizures, confusion, and hallucinations.

    4. Dosing changes with renal or hepatic failure. Renal, especially with a creatinine clearance of less than 30 mL/min for oseltamivir.

C. Adamantanes (amantadine and rimantadine).

    1. Activity. Amantadine and rimantadine act primarily by inhibiting viral uncoating as well as inhibiting the function of the M2 protein of influenza A viruses that have an effect on two different stages of viral replication.

    2. Resistance. Resistance to both amantadine and rimantadine can also occur with a single amino acid substitution at critical sites of the M2 protein.

    3. Toxicity (pregnancy class C). Rimantadine is relatively well tolerated but amantadine is associated with confusion, ataxia, blurred vision, dry mouth, hypotension, urinary retention, constipation, and livedo reticularis.

    4. Dosing changes with renal or hepatic failure. Renal.

D. Foscarnet. This agent can be used for HSV, varicella-zoster virus (VZV), and CMV infections.

    1. Activity. This agent directly inhibits viral DNA polymerase by noncompetitively blocking the pyrophosphate binding site.

    2. Resistance. The mechanism of resistance to foscarnet is via point mutations in the DNA polymerase. Mutations that lead to foscarnet-resistant CMV do not cause cross-resistance to ganciclovir or cidofovir.

    3. Toxicity (pregnancy class C). This agent is associated with nephrotoxicity, hypocalcemia (and tetany), headache, seizures, peripheral neuropathy, anemia, nausea, and vomiting.

    4. Dosing changes with renal or hepatic failure. Renal. Patients should receive preinfusion and postinfusion hydration to decrease the risk of nephrotoxicity.

E. Cidofovir. This agent is mainly used for CMV-related infections.

    1. Activity. This agent inhibits viral DNA synthesis by incorporation into the viral DNA and slowing chain elongation. Cidofovir does not rely on enzymes from the virus for phosphorylation, so it is active against acyclovir-resistant HSV strains with altered or deficient thymidine kinase. It is also active against ganciclovir-resistant CMV with the UL97 mutation.

    2. Resistance. The mechanism of resistance to cidofovir is related to mutations in viral DNA polymerase. CMV that is highly ganciclovir-resistant and has the UL54 mutation can be cross-resistant to cidofovir.

    3. Toxicity (pregnancy class C). This agent is associated with nephrotoxicity, neutropenia, visual disturbances, hepatitis, pancreatitis, and nausea.

4. **Dosing changes with renal or hepatic failure.** Renal. This agent is contraindicated with creatinine clearance less than 55 mL/min (or serum creatinine greater than 1.5 mg/dL). Cidofovir is also administered with high-dose probenecid (2 g 3 hours before and 1 g 2 hours and 8 hours after each infusion) to block the tubular secretion of cidofovir. Patients should also receive saline prehydration.

F. Ribavirin

1. **Activity.** This agent is a guanosine analog whose mechanism of action varies for different viruses. Ribavirin inhibits viral RNA polymerase but also interferes with the synthesis of guanosine triphosphate, which thereby interferes with nucleic acid synthesis.

2. **Resistance.** Rare; currently has only been documented with both the Sindbis virus (SINV) and hepatitis C virus (HCV).

3. **Toxicity (pregnancy class X).** This agent is associated with hemolytic anemia, fever, rash, nausea, diarrhea, hyperbilirubinemia, elevated serum uric acid, and leukopenia.

4. **Dosing changes with renal or hepatic failure.** Avoid with creatinine clearance less than 50 mL/min.

G. Antiretroviral Agents. See Table 3.4. A comprehensive review of the antiretroviral agents is beyond the scope of this chapter; however, a brief overview of the common classes and certain agents follows (also see Chapter 43: HIV and AIDS).

1. **Nucleoside/**nucleotide reverse transcriptase inhibitors (NRTIs)

    a. **Abacavir** is the only NRTI medication whose concentrations are not affected with renal insufficiency because of its unique pharmacokinetics. This medication should be used with caution as it can cause a hypersensitivity reaction that can present as fever, nausea, vomiting, diarrhea, abdominal pain, fatigue, myalgia, arthralgia, general ill feeling, shortness of breath, cough, and/or sore throat. Patients who are diagnosed with abacavir hypersensitivity should not be rechallenged with the medication owing to the increased risk of death.

    b. **Didanosine and stavudine** have the highest likelihood of causing symptoms that are part of the black box warning for this class of medications (Table 3.4). Owing to the significance of these toxicities, these medications should not be used together to avoid the synergistic toxic effects.

    c. **Tenofovir** is also active against hepatitis B and is the only NRTI that can cause renal toxicity (such as acute renal failure and Fanconi syndrome) and can be associated with a decrease in bone-mineral density.

    d. **Zidovudine** is the only one in its class that is likely to cause severe macrocytic anemia or neutropenia (seen as an elevated mean corpuscular volume [MCV], anemia, and darkening nail pigmentation [at higher doses]).

    e. **Lamivudine and emtricitabine** are very similar medications regarding mechanisms of action and toxicities. They are both active against hepatitis B and are associated with few toxicities. These agents should not be used in combination, and resistance to one agent confers resistance to the other agent.

TABLE 3.4 ▪ Antiretroviral Agents

Class	Agents	Adverse Effects	Pharmacology
Nucleoside(-tide) reverse transcriptase inhibitors	Abacavir (ABC) Didanosine (ddI) Tenofovir (TDF) Zidovudine (AZT) Lamivudine (3TC) Emtricitabine (FTC) Stavudine (d4T)	General side effects: fatigue, headache Black box warning: pancreatitis, lactic acidosis, peripheral neuropathy (do not use ddI and d4t together) AZT (anemia), ABC (hypersensitivity), TDF (acute renal failure)	Most are rapidly absorbed. Most are metabolized intracellularly except for abacavir, which is metabolized by alcohol dehydrogenase and glucuronosyltransferase. All are excreted renally.
NNRTIs	Efavirenz (EFV) Nevirapine (NVP) Etravirine (ETR) Rilpivirine (RPV) Delavirdine (DLV)	General side effects: rash and hepatotoxicity (higher with NVP), increase in LFTs Potential for many drug interactions May be taken without regard to food	Absorption of efavirenz, rilpivirine, and etravirine is increased with fatty foods. NNRTIs are highly protein bound. Efavirenz and nevirapine are metabolized by CYP 3A4 and 2B6. Etravirine is metabolized by CYP 3A4, 2C9, and 2C19. Rilpivirine is metabolized solely by CYP 3A4. Etravirine, nevirapine, and efavirenz are strong inducers of 3A4. They are excreted through feces and urine.
Protease inhibitors	Atazanavir (ATV) Darunavir (DRV) Fosamprenavir (FPV) Indinavir (IDV) Lopinavir/ritonavir (LPV/r) Nelfinavir (NFV) Ritonavir (RTV) Saquinavir (SQV) Tipranavir (TPV)	General side effects: GI (nausea, vomiting, diarrhea) Long-term side effects: Metabolic (dyslipidemia, insulin resistance) Physiologic (buffalo hump, protease paunch, sunken cheeks) RTV is only used now as a "booster" dose with other PIs (100–200 mg) Potential for many drug interactions Administer with food	Absorption is typically increased with food intake. Typically metabolized by CYP 3A4 but can also serve as inhibitors for this enzyme. Excretion is primarily through feces and urine.

(continued)

TABLE 3.4 ■ Antiretroviral Agents *(continued)*

Class	Agents	Adverse Effects	Pharmacology
Integrase inhibitors	Dolutegravir (DTG) Raltegravir (RAL) Elvitegravir (EVG)	Rash, SJS, TEN, nausea, headache, diarrhea, pyrexia, and rhabdomyolysis	Absorption is increased with a high-fat meal. Highly protein bound at 83%. Hepatically metabolized by UGT1A1. Primarily excreted in feces but also in urine.
Entry inhibitors	Enfuvirtide (ENF) Maraviroc (MVC)	Local injection site reactions (ENF): pain, erythema, induration, nodules, pruritus Abdominal pain, cough, dizziness, musculoskeletal symptoms, pyrexia, rash, upper respiratory tract infections, hepatotoxicity, orthostatic hypotension	Enfuvirtide is given as SC injection. It is highly protein bound and not hepatically metabolized through the CYP pathway. Maraviroc absorption is not affected by food. It is about 76% protein bound and is also a substrate for CYP3A4. It is primarily excreted through feces and urine.
Pharmacokinetic enhancer	Cobicistat (COBI)	Nausea, diarrhea, fatigue, increase in serum creatinine levels without a true decline renal function	Potent CYP3A4 inhibitor given with CYP3A4 substrates to increase concentrations. Similar to ritonavir without antiviral activity.

GI, gastrointestinal; LFT, liver function test; NNRTI, nonnucleoside reverse transcriptase inhibitor; PI, protease inhibitor; SC injection, subcutaneous injection; SJS, Stevens–Johnson syndrome.

2. Nonnucleoside reverse transcriptase inhibitors (NNRTIs)

   a. Efavirenz is likely to cause central nervous system (CNS) toxicities such as dizziness, somnolence, abnormal dreams, confusion, hallucinations, and euphoria. These toxicities are increased with fatty-food intake due to the increase in medication concentration. It should also be noted that efavirenz can cause false-positive results for cannabinoid and benzodiazepine screening tests. Resistance to efavirenz can cause cross-resistance with nevirapine and delavirdine. Finally, the half-life of this medication is much higher than that of NRTI medications ranging from 40 to 55 hours; therefore, discontinuation of this medication should be done with caution as many of the medications given in conjunction with efavirenz may not have such a long half-life.

   b. Nevirapine can cause autoinduction resulting in the need for an increase in dosage from once a day to twice a day after 2 weeks of therapy. Additionally, this agent can cause hepatotoxicity; however, it should be noted that this toxicity occurs significantly more in antiretroviral naïve female patients with a baseline CD4 cell count of greater than 250 cells/ mm^3 and greater than 400 cells/mm^3 in males.

   c. Etravirine and rilpivirine are second-generation NNRTIs that may still be efficacious when resistance develops to efavirenz, nevirapine, and delavirdine. Rilpivirine is more likely to cause CNS toxicities than etravirine.

3. Protease Inhibitors (PIs)

   a. Ritonavir should only be used to boost the concentrations of other PIs. The boosting of a PI with ritonavir occurs due to the inhibitory effects of ritonavir on the active PI metabolism. This causes a prevention of metabolism and therefore an increase in active PI concentration. Owing to the toxicities of this medication and its high potential for drug–drug interactions, ritonavir is no longer used as the primary PI.

   b. Atazanavir is least likely to cause any metabolic toxicity within this class; however, the risk begins to increase when given in combination with ritonavir. This agent is also known to cause hyperbilirubinemia (increased indirect [unconjugated] bilirubin) and is not usually indicative of hepatotoxicity. This medication also requires an acidic environment for absorption. Medications such as H2 antagonists and proton-pump inhibitors may decrease atazanavir absorption and concentration and should be used with caution.

   c. Darunavir and fosamprenavir both contain a sulfonamide moiety that may have some cross-reaction with sulfa-related hypersensitivity reactions.

   d. Indinavir can cause nephrolithiasis; to prevent this toxicity it is recommended to take up to eight glasses of fluids a day to ensure hydration.

   e. Lopinavir/ritonavir is the only PI at this time that is coformulated with ritonavir.

   f. Nelfinavir is the only PI that should not be "boosted" with ritonavir. Nelfinavir has an active metabolite and therefore the prevention of metabolism would in fact prevent efficacy of this medication.

TABLE 3.5 ■ Hepatitis Treatment Medications

Class	Agents	Adverse Effects	Pharmacology
Nucleoside (-tide) reverse transcriptase inhibitors	Lamivudine* Adefovir Entecavir Telbivudine Tenofovir* Emtricitabine*	Nephrotoxicity can occur rarely in adefovir patients Entecavir is very well tolerated similar to lamivudine Telbivudine can cause peripheral neuropathy and myopathy	Adefovir is available as a prodrug and rapidly converted to active drug in the intestines Absorption of entecavir is delayed with concurrent food intake Telbivudine, entecavir, and adefovir are not highly protein bound and are primarily excreted in the urine
Protease inhibitors	Boceprevir (BOC) Telaprevir (TVR)	BOC: anemia, dysgeusia TVR: rash, anemia, pruritus, nausea and diarrhea, rectal irritation	Absorption is increased with food. TVR must be taken with a high-fat (~20 g of fat) meal These medications are highly protein bound. They are metabolized by CYP3A4 and p-glycoprotein. They also act as an inhibitor for both 3A4 and p-glycoprotein Primarily excreted in the feces and urine

*See Table 3.4 for information on these medications.

4. Integrase Inhibitors

  a. **Dolutegravir** is a once-daily medication. It should be given twice daily with certain integrase-related mutations or when coadministered with either UGT1A or CYP3A inducers such as efavirenz, fosamprenavir/ritonavir, tipranavir/ritonavir, or rifampin.

  b. **Raltegravir** is a twice-daily medication that does not use CYP450 enzymes for metabolism decreasing its risk of drug–drug interactions with other medications.

  c. **Elvitegravir** is a once-daily medication that shares similar mutations for resistance with raltegravir. It is metabolized by CYP3A4 and requires a pharmacokinetic enhancer such as cobicistat when used.

 H. **Antivirals for Hepatitis.** See Table 3.5. A comprehensive review of the antivirals for hepatitis is beyond the scope of this chapter; however, a brief overview of the common classes and certain agents follows (also see Chapter 27: Hepatitis B and Chapter 28: Hepatitis C).

BIBLIOGRAPHY

Chemotherapy of microbial diseases. In: Brunton LL, Chabner BA, Knollman BC, eds. *Goodman and Gilman's The Pharmacological Basis of Therapeutics*. 12th ed. New York, NY: McGraw-Hill; 2011:1363–1664.

Drusano GL. Pharmacokinetics and pharmacodynamics of antimicrobials. *Clin Infect Dis*. 2007;45(suppl):89–95.

US Department of Health and Human Services Panel on Antiretroviral Guidelines for Adults and Adolescents. Guidelines for the use of antiretroviral agents in HIV-1-infected adults and adolescents. 2017:1–288. http://www.aidsinfo.nih.gov/ContentFiles/AdultandAdolescentGL.pdf

INTRODUCTION TO MEDICAL MICROBIOLOGY

Nicole M. Parrish
Stefan Riedel

I. **INTRODUCTION.** The diagnosis of infectious diseases commonly requires the use of diagnostic laboratory tests to identify the causative organism or etiology of a particular disease. *Medical microbiology is the study of interactions between organisms, such as bacteria, viruses, parasites, and fungi, and the human and/or animal host that result in infectious disease manifestations.* This chapter provides a broad overview of key concepts related to medical microbiology and common diagnostic tests used for the detection of infectious agents in clinical specimens. This information is by no means comprehensive and is not intended to provide a detailed description of each organism causing a specific disease. Such information is beyond the scope of this chapter. Rather, the information contained herein is intended to provide a framework from which a further in-depth study of medical microbiology can be pursued as a complementary discipline to infectious diseases.

II. **GENERAL PRINCIPLES.** *The most important decisions related to the successful identification of a pathogenic organism causing a disease typically occur prior to submission of the specimen to the medical microbiology laboratory.* These preanalytical considerations are essential in order to define the right type of specimen, the best approach to specimen collection, and the choice of appropriate transport media. Other factors that merit careful consideration include the following:

1. Determining which test or tests to order (based on clinical history and careful physical examination)

2. Determining which specimen(s) to collect

3. Ensuring that the specimen is labeled correctly with all of the requisite patient identifiers

4. Determining the appropriate way for the specimen to be transported to the laboratory

Ordering an inappropriate test or submitting a clinical specimen using inappropriate transport media or with significant delay may result in the inability to successfully identify the causative microorganism. In addition, patient care providers must consider that submission of additional clinical information (e.g., prior antibiotic use) can be crucial when attempting to isolate and identify a microorganism. Likewise, the specimen transport time and conditions are critical parameters influencing the success of organism isolation and identification. Since clinical samples, such as tissue and blood, contain living microorganisms, it is important to remember that the viability of those organisms may be adversely affected by a number of conditions including the type of media and pH, temperature, drying, exposure to oxygen or lack of oxygen, and prolonged transit times.

III. TYPES OF TESTS COMMONLY USED IN THE CLINICAL MICROBIOLOGY LABORATORY

A. **Microscopy.** Most infectious agents are visible only when viewed through a microscope. Thus, microscopic examination is not only one of the oldest tests utilized in the medical microbiology laboratory but also remains a cornerstone in diagnostics today. Although microscopy may lack in sensitivity and specificity compared to culture and molecular methods, it is a rapid and relatively inexpensive test method, providing for differentiation of organisms based on staining and morphologic characteristics, and is typically available at all times in many clinical laboratories. *The **Gram stain** provides for differentiation of gram-positive versus gram-negative organisms, which can be further subdivided based on morphologic characteristics (cocci, bacilli, coccobacilli, or curved; cell arrangement, e.g., clusters, pairs, tetrads).* In some cases, other staining methods are required to visualize particular organisms that cannot be seen on Gram stain owing to differences in size and the nature of the microbial cell structure. Some examples of organisms requiring an alternate stain include *Mycobacterium* spp (acid-fast and fluorochrome stains), *Nocardia* spp (modified acid-fast stain), and protozoa (trichrome stain used to visualize organisms in fecal specimens). The reader is referred to the reference list at the end of this chapter for more comprehensive information regarding microbial staining.

B. **Culture.** Almost all **medically important bacteria and fungi** can be cultivated from clinical specimens using artificial growth media. These media can be prepared as liquids (broth-based) or solids (agar-based). *Although not as rapid as direct examination of specimens, culture is by far more sensitive and specific and is still considered the gold standard in many cases. The majority of human pathogens require only 1 to 2 days of incubation for recovery on media.* Some slow-growing organisms such as *Mycobacterium tuberculosis* and some fungi require several days to weeks for recovery. Organism recovery in culture also affords the microbiology laboratory the opportunity to pursue additional testing, including antimicrobial susceptibility testing, serotyping, virulence factor detection, genotypic characterization, and molecular epidemiology testing. Recovery in culture of a given organism depends upon several factors related to the phenotypic and biochemical characteristics of the organism; an additional confounding factor may be the presence of competing microflora in the sample. Growth requirements for microorganisms include specific nutrients, temperature (most pathogens grow at 37°C whereas some organisms require 4°C, 30°C, or even 42°C), and the presence or absence of oxygen and/or CO_2. Organisms that only grow in the presence of oxygen are called **aerobes** (e.g., many bacteria and fungi); those that only grow in the absence of oxygen are called **anaerobes** (e.g., microflora of the gastrointestinal and female genital tracts); organisms that can grow under either condition are called **facultative anaerobes**; and those that grow in reduced oxygen are referred to as **microaerophiles** (e.g., *Campylobacter* spp and *Helicobacter* spp). *Some bacteria are extremely difficult to cultivate or cannot be grown in vitro (Chlamydia, Chlamydophila, Rickettsia, Anaplasma, Orientia, Ehrlichia, Coxiella, the spirochetes, and Mycobacterium leprae). For these organisms, alternate diagnostic approaches must be used, such as immunologic methods, cell culture, and molecular diagnostics* (see the following).

Viruses and some other microorganisms are obligate intracellular pathogens and, as such, cannot be cultivated using the techniques described previously.

Because growth and replication of these pathogens require living cells, three techniques have been used: inoculation of tissue or cell culture, embryonated hens' eggs, and experimental animals. *Tissue culture is the most common method used to culture viruses.* Visualization of growth can be detected by recognition of the cytopathic effect (CPE) that the virus has on the cell culture. For instance, respiratory syncytial viruses cause fusion of cells to produce multinucleated giant cells, termed syncytia. Some viruses produce proteins that are expressed on the membrane of infected cells. These viral proteins bind erythrocytes, which can be detected by testing for hemadsorption or hemagglutination. Detection and visualization of viruses that produce little to no CPE, do not possess hemagglutinins, or do not completely replicate in cell culture can be achieved through immunologic or nucleic acid probes. Both indirect fluorescent antibody (IFA) methods and direct fluorescent antibody (DFA) techniques are used for detection of specific agents (see the following section).

C. **Diagnostic Immunology.** It is not always possible to isolate a microorganism in culture or visualize it microscopically. In such cases, immunoassays are often used to detect the presence of a particular agent. *In general, immunoassays involve one of two main principles: testing for the presence of specific microbial antigens or testing for specific microbial-antigen antibodies.* These assays may involve the detection of a microbial antigen directly from a clinical specimen or the detection of a specific antigen once an organism is cultured in vitro.

   Fluorescent antibody (FA) techniques such as DFA and IFA are commonly used for the detection of specific agents. For DFA, a fluorescein-labeled antibody specific for a particular antigen is incubated with a test specimen fixed on a glass microscope slide. If the antigen is present in the specimen, a bright yellow-green fluorescence will be seen under a fluorescent microscope. For IFA, a primary, unlabeled, antigen-specific antibody and a fluorescein-labeled anti-immunoglobulin specific for the primary antibody are used. Both are incubated with the test specimen, and results are interpreted the same as for DFA.

D. **Molecular Diagnostics.** While microscopy, culture, and phenotypic characterization remain the mainstay for microbial identification in most laboratories, advances in molecular techniques have resulted in improved speed, sensitivity, and specificity for identification of some infectious microorganisms.

   Despite improving the ability to make some diagnoses, most molecular techniques are used more as research tools rather than as a standard-of-care test. *Applications of molecular methods for infectious disease testing include the identification of microorganisms or the detection of factors used to monitor disease or predict outcome. Such factors include antimicrobial resistance genes, virulence factors, and quantitation of microorganisms (e.g., viral load testing).* Traditionally, molecular testing has been widely used for the detection of viruses; however, in recent years many newer polymerase chain reaction (PCR) based methods have been developed to identify bacteria and antimicrobial resistance. Nucleic acid probe technology and the PCR have revolutionized diagnostic microbiology. Nucleic acid probe technology is based on the selection of unique genomic sequences for a particular group of etiologic agents or specific genes with subsequent cloning, synthesis, and utilization. Probes are designed to hybridize with either DNA or RNA with high specificity to complementary sequences of the target nucleic acid. Hybridization is detected by labeling the probe with radioisotopes, enzymes, antigens, or chemiluminescent compounds that can be measured through instrumentation specific for the label. PCR is based on the ability of DNA polymerase to copy a strand of DNA when two primers (oligonucleotides) bind to complementary strands of target DNA. With each cycle, the PCR product or target sequences are doubled. This technology has a wide array of applications with adaptations including real-time (RT) PCR, nested PCR, and multiplex PCR.

While molecular tests may be very sensitive tests for detecting microorganisms even at very low levels, one must consider that **false positives** from contamination (specimen or environmental) or **false negatives** from a failure of the detection process are possible. Furthermore, molecular tests only detect known, previously identified gene sequences. Recent and novel mutations in microorganisms may not be readily detected by common commercial molecular assays, as those have to be first modified to have the ability to detect the novel genetic-altered microorganism. Recent examples include the problems related to detection of methicillin-resistant *Staphylococcus aureus* (MRSA) strain with *mecA* gene dropout and novel antimicrobial resistances such as the NDM-1 beta-lactamase. Finally, from a financial perspective, molecular diagnostics are often more costly than traditional culture-based identification methods. Microbiology laboratories have to take cost analyses into consideration when deciding whether to implement molecular test methods. However, such methodologies are useful in situations in which culture-based techniques are unable to recover the organism in vitro, or for instances when current laboratory methods may have low sensitivities and specificities or are simply too time-consuming with long turnaround times for test results.

IV. SUMMARY. The microbiology laboratory plays an essential role in the diagnosis, prognosis, and ultimately the treatment of patients with infectious diseases. At this time, however, the "perfect" single diagnostic test for identification of a microorganism does not exist. Therefore, the detection and identification along with determination of antibiotic susceptibility require multiple tests or combinations of tests for confirmation of the infectious etiology of a disease. Newer, molecular technologies provide a great addition to the laboratory's testing repertoire and may improve the efficiency and speed of infectious disease testing in the future.

BIBLIOGRAPHY

Anaissie EJ, McGinnis MR, Pfaller MA. *Clinical Mycology*. 2nd ed. Philadelphia, PA: Churchill Livingstone Elsevier; 2009.

Barrett JT. *Microbiology and Immunology Concepts*. Philadelphia, PA: Lippincott-Raven Publishers; 1998.

de la Maza LM, Pezzlo MT, Shigei JT, Peterson EM. *Color Atlas of Medical Bacteriology*. Washington, DC: ASM Press; 2004.

Flint SJ, Enquist LW, Krug RM, et al. *Virology, Molecular Biology, Pathogenesis, and Control*. Washington, DC: ASM Press; 2000.

Garcia LS. *Diagnostic Medical Parasitology*. 4th ed. Washington, DC: ASM Press; 2001.

Knipe DM, Howley PM. *Fields Virology*. 5th ed. Philadelphia, PA: Lippincott Williams & Wilkins; 2007.

Larone DH. *Medically Important Fungi*. 4th ed. Washington, DC: ASM Press; 2002.

Mandell GL, Bennett JE, Dolin R. *Principles and Practice of Infectious Diseases*. 7th ed. Philadelphia, PA: Churchill Livingstone; 2010.

Persing DH, Tenover FC, Versalovic J, et al. *Molecular Microbiology: Diagnostic Principles and Practice*. Washington, DC: ASM Press; 2004.

Versalovic J, Carroll KC, Funke G, et al. *Manual of Clinical Microbiology*. 10th ed. Washington, DC: ASM Press; 2011.

5

FEVER OF UNKNOWN ORIGIN

William F. Wright

I. INTRODUCTION

A. **Classic Fever of Unknown Origin (FUO) Definition.** A temperature record on multiple occasions that is greater than 38.3°C (101°F) for more than 3 weeks' duration despite 1 week of logical diagnostic evaluation in the hospital.

B. **Revised Classic FUO Definitions and Further Classifications.** A fever lasting more than 3 weeks with recordings greater than 38.3°C (101°F) despite logical diagnostic evaluation during 3 days in the hospital or three outpatient clinic evaluations.

1. **Classic FUO.** Defined previously with the most common etiologies within three main categories: infection, malignancy, or collagen vascular disease.

2. **Nosocomial FUO.** Usually a fever occurring in a patient who has been hospitalized for at least 24 hours without a defined source prior to admission or 3 days of evaluation. The more common etiologies of a nosocomial fever include urinary tract infections, catheter-related infections, pneumonia, *Clostridium difficile* colitis, pulmonary embolism, deep vein thrombosis (DVT), septic thrombophlebitis, gastrointestinal bleed, or medication-induced fever.

3. **Neutropenia FUO.** A recurrent or persistent fever in a patient with neutropenia (absolute neutrophil count less than 500 cells/mm^3 or 0.5×10^9/L) despite 3 days of logical diagnostic evaluation. The more common etiologies include nosocomial etiologies (as mentioned previously) as well as opportunistic bacterial infections (see the following), aspergillosis, candidiasis (e.g., hepatosplenic candidiasis), or herpes simplex virus/varicella–zoster virus (HSV/VZV).

4. **HIV-related FUO.** A recurrent or persistent fever for greater than 4 weeks in a patient seropositive for HIV despite 3 days of logical diagnostic evaluation in the hospital. The more common etiologies include *Mycobacterium avium–intracellulare* complex (MAC), cytomegalovirus (CMV), *Pneumocystis jirovecii*, lymphoma, Kaposi sarcoma, toxoplasmosis, *Cryptococcus*, or medications.

II. CAUSES OF FUO. While greater than 200 possible causes for FUO have been reported, the following lists are the more common causes to be considered initially. A cause may not be found in as many as 20% to 30% of cases. **The causes are listed by the three main etiologic categories:**

A. Infection. This group of causes has been estimated to occur in 28% of FUO cases. The etiologies to initially consider include:

1. **Tuberculosis** (*Mycobacterium tuberculosis*; pulmonary and extrapulmonary disease; see Chapter 14)

2. **Abdominal or pelvic abscess** (most common cause in the elderly age group)

3. **Sinusitis** (most commonly with chronic infections or hospitalized patients with nasogastric tubes)

4. **Dental abscess** (usually oral bacterial flora and may or may not be associated with a recent dental procedure)

5. **Endocarditis** (most commonly culture negative endocarditis)

6. **Osteomyelitis** (most commonly chronic osteomyelitis)

7. **Hepatitis or chronic biliary tract infections** (see Chapters 26–28)

8. **Prostatitis** (especially with a recent prostate procedure and is characterized by chronic pelvic pain)

9. **HIV infection or sexually transmitted disease** (see Chapters 42 and 43)

10. **CMV** (especially in immunocompromised patients)

11. **Epstein–Barr virus** (EBV; especially following posthematopoietic stem cell transplantation)

12. **HSV or VZV** (most commonly associated with reactivation infections in immunocompromised patients)

13. **Rocky Mountain spotted fever (RMSF) or Lyme disease** (*Rickettsia rickettsii* or *Borrelia burgdorferi*; usually associated with outdoor activities and a tick bite)

14. **Q fever** (*Coxiella burnetii*; associated with exposure to farm animals [cattle, sheep, or goats] and is characterized by flu-like symptoms with fevers, pneumonia, and hepatitis)

15. **Brucellosis** (*Brucella* spp; associated with exposure to animals [goats, sheep, bison, or swine] and is characterized by intermittent fevers, gastrointestinal symptoms [e.g., nausea, abdominal pain], and joint effusions)

16. **Leptospirosis** (*Leptospira interrogans*; usually associated with rodents or colonized dogs [the organism resides in the renal tubules and is shed in the urine] during recreational activities and is characterized by malaise, headaches, myalgias, abdominal pain, and conjunctival erythema)

17. **Psittacosis** (*Chlamydophila psittaci*; usually associated with birds, especially parrots, and is characterized by fevers, chills, malaise, myalgias, and nonproductive cough)

18. **Malaria** (*Plasmodium* spp; transmitted by the *Anopheles* mosquito and usually characterized by periodic fevers, chills, and rigors)

19. **Leishmaniasis** (a group of obligate intracellular parasites that are transmitted by sand flies [genera *Phlebotomus* and *Lutzomyia*]; commonly associated with cutaneous lesions [e.g., a necrotic ulcer] but can be associated with fevers, chills, diarrhea, weight loss, and hepatosplenomegaly)

20. **Babesiosis** (*Babesia* spp; an intraerythrocyte parasitic infection transmitted by the bite of an *Ixodes* tick and characterized by fevers, chills, night sweats, fatigue, weakness, and anemia)

21. **Enteric fever** (*Salmonella enterica*, serovar Typhi; associated with travel and characterized by fevers, headaches, myalgias, malaise, and gastrointestinal pain)

22. **Toxoplasmosis** (*Toxoplasma gondii*; most commonly a reactivation infection in immunocompromised patients)

23. **Rat-bite fever** (*Streptobacillus moniliformis*; patients have an exposure to rats and the disorder is characterized by fevers, headaches, chills, polyarthralgias, and a maculopapular rash on the hands and/or feet)

24. **Cat scratch disease** (*Bartonella henselae*; a disorder characterized by fevers and localized adenopathy with an exposure to cats)

25. **Whipple disease** (*Tropheryma whippelii*; a disorder characterized by fevers, arthralgia, abdominal pain, chronic diarrhea, weight loss, and generalized lymphadenopathy)

26. MAC (usually associated with fevers and cavitary pulmonary disease in immunocompromised patients)

27. ***Pneumocystis jirovecii* pneumonia** (almost exclusively associated with acute hypoxic pneumonia in immunocompromised patients, especially AIDS patients with a CD4 cell count below 200 cells/mm^3)

28. ***Cryptococcus neoformans*** (commonly associated with chronic corticosteroid use or immunocompromised patients and usually presents as fevers with meningitis or pulmonary pneumonia)

29. **Aspergillosis** (*Aspergillus* spp; opportunistic pathogens that can be associated with fevers and pulmonary cavities or endocarditis)

30. **Candidiasis** (*Candida* spp; opportunistic pathogens that can be associated with fevers and catheter infections, endocarditis, or hepatosplenic candidiasis)

B. **Malignancy.** This group typically accounts for 17% of cases. The etiologies to initially consider include:

1. **Leukemia** (more commonly chronic leukemia)

2. **Lymphoma** (most common cause in this group—Hodgkin's and non-Hodgkin's lymphoma)

3. **Renal cell carcinoma**

4. **Colorectal cancers**

5. **Myelodysplastic syndrome**

6. **Pancreatic carcinoma** (most commonly not associated with biliary or pancreatic duct obstruction)

7. **Metastatic cancer with or without known primary**

C. **Collagen Vascular Disease.** This group is estimated to account for 21% of cases. The etiologies to initially consider include:

1. **Temporal arteritis** (more common over the age of 50)

2. **Rheumatoid arthritis**

3. **Systemic lupus erythematosus (SLE)**

4. **Polymyalgia rheumatica**

5. **Vasculitis**

6. **Polychondritis**

7. **Polymyositis**

8. **Adult Still disease or adult juvenile rheumatoid arthritis**

9. **Sjögren syndrome or Behçet syndrome**

D. **Miscellaneous.** This group accounts for 5% to 10% of cases. The etiologies to initially consider include:

1. **Crohn disease or ulcerative colitis**

2. **Thyroiditis**

3. **Sarcoidosis**

4. **Amyloidosis**

5. **Gout or pseudogout**

6. **Addison disease**

7. **Hemochromatosis**

8. **Medications.** The fever usually resolves within 2 to 5 days of discontinuation of the medication. More common medications to consider include:

   a. **Antibiotics** (penicillin, cephalosporin, sulfonamide, tetracycline, and rifampin)

   b. **Anticonvulsants** (phenytoin, carbamazepine, and barbiturates)

   c. **Antihistamines**

   d. **Nonsteroidal anti-inflammatory drugs (NSAIDs)**

   e. **Iodine and iodide agents** (e.g., contrast dye)

III. **CLINICAL MANIFESTATIONS OF FUO.** While documentation of fever is required to establish the diagnosis of FUO, there is no significant relationship between the fever pattern and underlying etiology. However, some associations have been suggested:

A. **Double Quotidian Fever.** Defined as a fever with two peaks within 24 hours; conditions to consider include endocarditis, malaria, military *Mycobacterium tuberculosis,* adult Still disease, and leishmaniasis.

B. **Sustained Fever.** Defined as a continuously elevated temperature and most commonly associated with central nervous system (CNS) injury (e.g., stroke, bleed) or pneumonia (most commonly secondary to a gram-positive pathogen).

C. **Pel–Ebstein Fever.** A daily fever that resolves only to recur again with a similar pattern; consider Hodgkin's disease.

D. **Periodic or Relapsing Fever.** Consider endocarditis, malaria, lymphoma, Lyme disease, RMSF, or rat-bite fever.

E. **Early Morning Fever Spike.** Consider *Mycobacterium tuberculosis*, polyarteritis nodosa, brucellosis, or salmonellosis.

In general, there are no classic symptoms or signs pathognomonic for a particular FUO etiology, and conditions or causes may be a typical or atypical presentation for a particular disease. It should also be emphasized that no symptom or sign be regarded as irrelevant in a patient suspected of FUO.

IV. APPROACH TO THE PATIENT WITH FUO

A. **History.** The most important initial approach to the patient with FUO is documenting the fever and recording a complete, accurate, and comprehensive history. **Physicians must be meticulous and systematic when obtaining information for the following key elements:**

1. **Age.** Certain illnesses may be more likely associated with particular age groups (e.g., malignancy, temporal arteritis, and intra-abdominal abscess may be more likely in persons over the age of 50).

2. **History of present illness.** While most patients exhibit atypical manifestation, it is important to establish in chronological fashion the onset of symptoms and events that may be related to the fever.

3. **Past medical history.** This area should focus on any recent or chronic medical illness or infection; any prior diagnosis of malignancy; any prior surgery or complication related to surgery; and any implanted prosthetic device, prosthetic valve, pacemaker or implantable defibrillator, cosmetic implanted surgical device, indwelling venous catheter, or implanted vascular graft.

4. **Medications.** A complete list of prescription, over-the-counter, and herbal medications should be documented. Drug-related fevers are more common in the elderly and HIV seropositive patient groups.

5. **Allergies.** Medication allergies may suggest a drug fever while environmental allergies may suggest an atopic condition.

6. **Social history.** This should include information about the patient's country of origin, immigration status, prior country or state of residence, travel history (with relevant exposure, vaccination, and prophylaxis history), vaccination status, occupation and occupational risks, smoking status, alcohol and drug exposure, hobbies or leisure activities, pet or animal exposure, dietary (usual or unusual) habits, and sexual activity.

7. **Family history.** It is important to establish any recent or prior illness in family members and any unusual hereditary cause for fever (e.g., familial Mediterranean fever).

B. **Physical Examination.** A complete physical examination should be performed with attention to all body systems. While physicians should be meticulous and conduct the examination in a systematic approach, repeat examinations are often helpful as diagnostic clues may be either atypical or obscure for the cause of the FUO. Areas of the physical examination that require careful attention and common associations include:

1. **Dermatologic examination**

a. **Rose spot** (typhoid or psittacosis)

b. **Hyperpigmentation** (hemochromatosis, Addison disease, or Whipple disease)

c. **Petechial rash** (RMSF)

d. **Erythema multiforme** (Lyme disease)

e. **Vesicular rash on an erythematous base** (HSV or VZV)

2. **Cardiovascular examination.** A new diastolic murmur or change with existing murmur may suggest **endocarditis** or **atrial myxoma**

3. **Oral–pharyngeal examination**

a. **Gingivitis and/or poor dentition** (odontogenic infection or HSV)

b. **Mucous membrane ulcers** (inflammatory bowel disease, Behçet disease, or HSV [most commonly located on the vermilion border])

c. **Tongue tenderness** (amyloidosis or temporal arteritis)

4. **Abdominal examination**

a. **Hepatomegaly** (alcoholic liver disease, lymphoma, hepatoma, relapsing fever, Q fever, typhoid fever)

b. **Splenomegaly** (leukemia, lymphoma, rheumatoid arthritis, sarcoidosis, alcoholic liver disease, endocarditis, CMV, EBV, brucellosis, RMSF, psittacosis, or typhoid fever). *Fever and hepatosplenomegaly in a neutropenia patient should raise concern for hepatosplenic candidiasis.*

5. **Lymphatic examination.** While lymphoma, adult Still disease, Whipple disease, HIV, toxoplasmosis, CMV, EBV, or tuberculosis present with generalized lymphadenopathy, cat scratch disease is usually associated with a localized adenopathy.

6. **Musculoskeletal examination**

a. **Joint pain** (gout or pseudogout, SLE, rheumatoid arthritis, rat-bite fever, Lyme disease, Whipple disease, or brucellosis). *Joint pain or arm pain in children associated with raising the arms above the head may suggest Takayasu disease.*

b. **Calf tenderness** (DVT, polymyositis, or RMSF)

c. **Costovertebral tenderness** (perinephric abscess or pyelonephritis)

d. **Spine**

i. **Bruit** (tumor or arteriovenous [AV] fistula)

ii. **Tenderness** (vertebral osteomyelitis, endocarditis, brucellosis, or typhoid fever)

e. **Sternal tenderness** (leukemia, myeloproliferative disorder, osteomyelitis, or brucellosis)

f. **Thigh tenderness** (brucellosis or polymyositis)

g. **Cartilage tenderness (**polychondritis, Raynaud syndrome, or CMV)

h. **Trapezius tenderness** (subdiaphragmatic abscess)

7. **Ophthalmologic examination**

a. **Subconjunctival hemorrhage** (endocarditis)

     b. Uveitis (SLE, Behçet disease, sarcoidosis, adult Still disease, or tuberculosis)

     c. Conjunctivitis (histoplasmosis, tuberculosis, cat scratch disease, chlamydia infection, or SLE)

     d. Conjunctival suffusion (leptospirosis, RMSF, or relapsing fever)

     e. Dry eyes (Sjogren syndrome, polyarteritis nodosa, SLE, or rheumatoid arthritis)

8. **Vital signs**. While most vital signs are nonspecific to the cause of FUO, the pulse should increase 15 to 20 beats/min for each 1-degree increase in core body temperature greater than 39°C. A lower than normal increase (or no increase) is termed *relative bradycardia*. Causes include:

     a. Beta-blockers or drug fevers

     b. CNS-related disease (e.g., hemorrhagic stroke)

     c. Typhoid fever

     d. Malaria

     e. Leptospirosis

     f. Psittacosis

C. Laboratory Studies. There is no diagnostic gold standard workup for the etiology of FUO. While the following represents a minimum diagnostic evaluation, laboratory testing or imaging should be guided by findings from a complete history and physical examination.

1. **Complete blood count (CBC) with differential cell count.** Leukocytosis may suggest infection or leukemia. Leukopenia may be associated with leukemia, lymphoma, or tuberculosis. Thrombocytosis (greater than 600,000 mm³) may be associated with cancer, bone marrow disease, tuberculosis, or infections with yeast or molds.

2. **Peripheral blood film/thick and thin films.** Nucleated red blood cells (RBCs) in the absence of hemolysis may suggest bone marrow disease. Films may also be helpful to identify morphologic abnormalities, hemolytic changes, *Babesia* spp, and malaria.

3. **Basic metabolic panel.** Routinely ordered but nonspecific. An elevated calcium level may suggest cancer or pseudogout. An elevated uric acid level may suggest gout.

4. **Liver functions test.** Alkaline phosphatase may be most important as it may be elevated with temporal arteritis, thyroiditis, or tuberculosis. Abnormal liver enzymes may also suggest alcoholic liver disease, biliary tract and hepatic cirrhosis, liver abscess, hemochromatosis, EBV, or CMV.

5. **Thyroid-stimulating hormone (TSH).** Abnormalities may suggest thyroiditis.

6. **Urinalysis and microscopy.** Routinely ordered but nonspecific for etiologies of FUO. Blood may suggest glomerulonephritis, urinary tract cancer, and urinary tract infection (especially with pyuria). Pyelonephritis may be suggested by the presence of white blood cell casts.

7. **Blood and urine cultures.** Routinely ordered as three sets of blood cultures and a clean-catch midstream culture.

8. Prostate-specific **antigen (PSA).** Elevations may be associated with prostate cancer, bacterial prostatitis, *Cryptococcus*, or extrapulmonary tuberculosis.

9. Erythrocyte **sedimentation rate (ESR).** Nonspecific test that is elevated with infections (greater than 70 mm/hour may suggest osteomyelitis) or inflammation (e.g., temporal arteritis).

10. **Antinuclear antibodies and rheumatoid factor**

11. **HIV antibody**

12. **CMV serology or serum polymerase chain reaction (PCR)**

13. **EBV heterophile antibody test or serology**

14. **Viral hepatitis serology** (especially when considering chronic hepatitis B or C infections)

15. **Q fever, RMSF, Lyme disease, brucellosis, leptospirosis, Whipple disease, as well as rat-bite fever and cat scratch disease serology** might be useful depending on the exposure risk.

16. **A skin purified protein derivative (PPD) or interferon gamma release assay (e.g., QuantiFERON-TB Gold)** is important for tuberculosis screening.

D. **Radiography Studies**

1. **Plain-film chest imaging.** A two-view chest image is routinely ordered that may be helpful to identify tuberculosis or malignancy.

2. **CT scan.** Imaging of the abdomen and pelvis with contrast is important early in the evaluation as two of the most common causes of FUO are intra-abdominal abscesses and lymphoproliferative disorders.

3. **Echocardiography.** Transthoracic or transesophageal imaging in association with the review of Duke criteria is important for the evaluation of endocarditis (see Chapter 7).

4. **Ultrasonography.** A noninvasive imaging study that may be helpful to evaluate biliary tract or pelvic etiologies for FUO.

5. **Venous Doppler study.** A noninvasive imaging study that may be helpful to evaluate for venous thrombosis.

V. **TREATMENT.** The treatment for FUO consists of identifying the underlying cause and formulating a treatment plan for that particular condition.

BIBLIOGRAPHY

High KP, Bradley SF, Gravenstein S, et al. Clinical practice guideline for the evaluation of fever and infection in older adult residents of long-term care facilities: 2008 update from the Infectious Diseases Society of America. *Clin Infect Dis.* 2009;48(2):149–171.

Laupland KB. Fever in the critically ill medical patient. *Crit Care Med.* 2009;37(7 suppl):S273–S278.

Mourad O, Palda V, Detsky AS. A comprehensive evidence-based approach to fever of unknown origin. *Arch Intern Med.* 2003;163(5):545–551.

O'Grady NP, Barie PS, Bartlett JG, et al. Guidelines for the evaluation of new fever in critically ill adult patients: 2008 update from the American College of Critical Care Medicine and the Infectious Diseases Society of America. *Crit Care Med.* 2008;36(4):1330–1349.

Tolia J, Smith LG. Fever of unknown origin: historical and physical clues to making the diagnosis. *Infect Dis Clin North Am.* 2007;21(4):917–936.

LEUKOCYTOSIS

William F. Wright

I. INTRODUCTION

A. Definition. An increase in the circulating white blood cell (WBC) counts of greater than **11,000 cells/mm³ (11 × 10⁹/L)**; however, the upper limits of normal vary depending on the population assessed and the equipment utilized.

B. Normal Physiology of WBC Production. Pluripotent stem cells within the bone marrow develop into leukocytic stem cells of which the various lineages of WBCs develop with the assistance of specific **cytokines** and **growth factors.** The leukocyte lineages include:

1. **Granulocytes**

   a. **Neutrophils.** Typically account for 50% to 75% of the leukocyte population and are the most important defense against bacterial pathogens. They are produced in the bone marrow under the influence of granulocyte colony-stimulating factor (GCSF), granulocyte macrophage colony-stimulating factor (GM-CSF), macrophage colony-stimulating factor (M-CSF), and interleukin 3 (IL-3). There are three pools of neutrophils with the circulating pool having a normal count range of **1.8 to 7.7 × 10⁹/L** or **1,800 to 7,700 cells/mm³.**

      i. Marrow pool (largest pool of reserve neutrophils)

      ii. Tissue pool (similar to the circulating pool but residing in tissue)

      iii. Circulating pool (divided into a *freely circulating pool* that is counted and a noncounted *marginated pool* that loosely adheres to the vascular endothelium. The life span of a noncirculating neutrophil is 1–2 weeks.)

   b. **Eosinophils.** Typically make up 5% to 10% of the leukocyte population and are important for parasitic, allergic, or neoplastic illnesses. These cells are produced in the bone marrow under the influence of GM-CSF and IL-3 and IL-5 for a normal circulating count of **200 cells/mm³** or **0.2 × 10⁹/L.**

   c. **Basophils.** Typically the least common granulocyte with a normal circulation count of **less than 200 cells/mm³** or **0.2 × 10⁹/L.** These cells are related to tissue mast cells and are important for immediate or cutaneous hypersensitivity reactions.

2. **Monocytes.** Typically make up 3% to 8% of the leukocyte population. They are produced in the bone marrow under the influence of GM-CSF and M-CSF and released into the circulation for a normal count of **300 cells/mm³** or **0.3 × 10⁹/L.** Migration of monocytes into tissues produces **macrophages**.

3. **Lymphocytes.** Typically compose 30% to 35% of the circulating WBC population with a normal count of **1,000 to 4,000 cells/mm³** or **1.0 to 4.0 × 10⁹/L.** Three types of lymphocytes include:

   a. **T cells.** These cells are produced in the bone marrow under the influence of IL-2 and IL-15 and are important for **cell-mediated immune responses.**

   b. **B cells.** These cells are produced under the influence of IL-7 and are important for **antibody production**.

   c. **Natural killer (NK) cells.** These cells are called "natural killer" cells because of their role in destroying virus-infected cells or HLA-incompatible cells.

C. **Pathophysiology of Leukocytosis.** Two basic mechanisms operate to cause an increased circulating WBC count:

   1. **Leukocytosis with a normal bone marrow.** This is also known as a **secondary leukocytosis** and reflects the appropriate response of normal bone marrow to an external process such as infection, inflammation, drug, or toxin. An **elevated neutrophil count (i.e., neutrophilia)** occurs as a result of releasing both the marginated pool and marrow-pool neutrophils. Release of marrow-pool neutrophils are typically less mature forms of neutrophils known as **band cells** and **metamyelocytes**, commonly referred to as a "left-shift" leukocytosis. Finally, secondary leukocytosis is characterized by changes in the more mature neutrophils seen on a peripheral blood smear: toxic granulation, Döhle bodies, and cytoplasmic vacuoles.

   2. **Leukocytosis with an abnormal bone marrow**. This process is also known as a **primary leukocytosis** and likely reflects either a lack of maturation of stem cells (e.g., acute leukemia) or more mature WBCs (e.g., chronic leukemia) that is either a congenital or acquired disorder. Primary leukocytosis may be associated with:

      a. WBC count greater than **30,000 cells/mm³** or **30 × 10⁹/L** and differentiated from a true **leukemoid reaction** (see Section II.A.1).

      b. Associated anemia and/or thrombocytopenia; however, these findings may also occur with secondary leukocytosis.

      c. Lymphadenopathy, hepatomegaly, and/or splenomegaly.

      d. Petechia, purpura, hemorrhage, fatigue, and weight loss.

II. **NEUTROPHILIA.** A leukocytosis with an increased neutrophil count greater than **7,700 cells/mm³** or **7.7 × 10⁹/L**; however, the upper limits of normal vary depending on the population assessed and the equipment utilized. While infection is the most important consideration, the differential diagnosis also may include:

A. **Neutrophilia With an Abnormal Bone Marrow**

   1. **Leukemoid malignancy.** An elevated number of immature neutrophils greater than **50,000 cells/mm³** or **50 × 10⁹/L** but with a normal leukocyte alkaline phosphatase determination and absent Philadelphia chromosome.

2. **Leukocyte adhesion deficiency.** An increased neutrophil count due to an abnormal expression of the adhesions CD116 and CD18 that inhibits the ability of neutrophils to migrate from the bloodstream to sites of infection.

3. **Hereditary neutrophilia.** An autosomal dominant condition that results in neutrophilia and splenomegaly.

4. **Familial cold urticaria and neutrophilia.** A congenital syndrome associated with neutrophilia, fever, urticaria, and muscle and skin tenderness on cold exposure.

5. **Chronic idiopathic neutrophilia.** Chronic unexplained neutrophilia in healthy persons.

B. **Neutrophilia With a Normal Bone Marrow**

1. **Acute infection.** Most commonly seen with acute bacterial infections.

2. **Chronic inflammatory illnesses** (e.g., rheumatoid arthritis, vasculitis, inflammatory bowel, gout).

3. **Physical and emotional stress.** Most commonly a transient neutrophilia as a result of neutrophil demargination in response to strenuous exercise, seizures, surgical anesthesia, and injection of epinephrine.

4. **Medications**

   a. **Corticosteroids.** Stimulate release of neutrophils from the marrow and marginated pools without an increased proportion of immature cells (i.e., band cells). Corticosteroids also inhibit neutrophil migration from the circulation to tissue.

   b. **Beta-agonists.** Release neutrophils from the marginated pool.

   c. **Lithium.** Same mechanism as beta-agonists.

   d. **Tetracycline.** Same mechanism as beta-agonists.

   e. **Hematopoietic growth factors.** Typically used following stem cell transplantation and stimulate the bone marrow.

5. **Hemolytic anemia or immune thrombocytopenia.**

6. **Trauma.** Neutrophilia results from elevated endogenous glucocorticoids.

7. **Pregnancy.** This is associated with a slight increase in total neutrophil count due to the physiologic change and stress related to pregnancy as well as hormonal changes.

8. **Hyperthyroidism**

III. **LYMPHOCYTOSIS.** An increased circulating lymphocyte count greater than **4,000 cells/mm^3** or **4.0 × 10^9/L**; however, the upper limits of normal vary depending on the population assessed and the equipment utilized. While viral-related infections are the most important consideration, the differential diagnosis includes:

A. **Lymphocytosis With an Abnormal Bone Marrow**

1. **Acute lymphocytic leukemia**

    2. Chronic lymphocytic leukemia

    3. Non-Hodgkin's lymphoma

B. Lymphocytosis With a Normal Bone Marrow

    1. Relative lymphocytosis. An elevated lymphocyte count occurs during the first year of life and then gradually declines to adult levels.

    2. Viral infections

       a. Epstein–Barr virus (EBV) infection. Characterized by large atypical CD8 T lymphocytes and NK cells in the blood.

       b. Cytomegalovirus (CMV) infection

       c. Viral hepatitis

       d. Mumps, roseola, rubeola, and rubella

       e. Herpes simplex and herpes zoster. Also occurs with varicella infections.

       f. Influenza A

       g. HIV infection

    3. Bacterial infections. Lymphocytosis is rarely observed with bacterial infections. Bacterial infections associated with this finding include:

       a. Pertussis

       b. Tuberculosis

       c. Brucellosis

       d. Syphilis

       e. *Rickettsia* infections

    4. Parasitic infection. Lymphocytosis can be associated with toxoplasmosis.

    5. Connective tissue disorders (e.g., rheumatoid arthritis, systemic lupus).

    6. Hyperthyroidism and thyrotoxicosis

    7. Addison disease

    8. Splenomegaly. Most commonly occurs in association with EBV infections but may occur with malaria, tuberculosis, and endemic fungal infections (e.g., histoplasmosis) as a result of lymphocyte proliferation in the splenic white pulp.

IV. MONOCYTOSIS. An increased circulating monocyte count greater than **300 cells/mm³** (0.3×10^9/L) or an elevated absolute monocyte count greater than **900 cells/mm³** (0.9×10^9/L); however, the upper limits of normal vary depending on the population assessed and the equipment utilized. Monocytosis usually results from chronic infection or inflammatory conditions. The differential diagnosis includes:

A. Monocytosis With an Abnormal Bone Marrow

    1. Acute monocytic leukemia

    2. Juvenile myelomonocytic leukemia. Most commonly occurs in children less than 4 years of age.

    3. Myeloproliferative disease of monosomy 7

   4. Cyclical neutropenia or congenital agranulocytosis

B. **Monocytosis With a Normal Bone Marrow**

   1. Neutropenia recovery following chemotherapy

   2. Tuberculosis

   3. Bacterial endocarditis

   4. Brucellosis

   5. Listeriosis

   6. Trypanosomiasis

   7. Invasive fungal infections (e.g., aspergillosis, histoplasmosis)

   8. Rheumatoid arthritis and systemic lupus erythematosus

   9. Sarcoidosis

   10. Inflammatory bowel disease (e.g., ulcerative colitis)

   11. Hodgkin's lymphoma and non-Hodgkin's lymphoma

   12. Malignancy (e.g., gastric or ovarian cancer)

V. **EOSINOPHILIA.** An increased circulating eosinophil count greater than **200 cells/mm^3 (0.2 × 10^9/L)** or an absolute eosinophil count greater than **500 cells/mm^3 (0.5 × 10^9/L)**; however, the upper limits of normal vary depending on the population assessed and the equipment utilized. Most causes are related to inflammatory disorders, allergic or atopic disorders, parasitic infections, or malignant diseases. The differential diagnosis includes:

A. **Eosinophilia With an Abnormal Bone Marrow**

   1. Chronic myelogenous leukemia

   2. Polycythemia vera

   3. Myelofibrosis

B. **Eosinophilia With a Normal Bone Marrow**

   1. Parasitic infections

   2. Rheumatoid arthritis and systemic lupus erythematosus

   3. Sarcoidosis

   4. Adrenal insufficiency (e.g., Addison disease)

   5. Hodgkin's lymphoma and non-Hodgkin's lymphoma

   6. Allergic bronchopulmonary aspergillosis

   7. Coccidioidomycosis

   8. Chronic tuberculosis

   9. Asthma, atopic dermatitis, allergic rhinitis, drug-medication reaction, vasculitis, and Churg–Strauss syndrome

   10. Eosinophilia–myalgia syndrome. Most commonly associated with dietary supplements of **tryptophan.**

   11. Leprosy

12. **Scabies**

13. **Bullous pemphigoid**

14. **Hypereosinophilic syndrome.** Typically associated with eosinophilia for greater than 6 months, organ dysfunction (e.g., asthma, sinusitis, neuropathy, vasculitis, and pulmonary infiltrates), and exclusion of other etiologies.

VI. BASOPHILIA. An unusual cause of leukocytosis but associated with an elevated basophil count greater than **200 cells/mm³ (0.2 × 10⁹/L)**; however, the upper limits of normal vary depending on the population assessed and the equipment utilized. The differential diagnosis includes:

A. Basophilia With an Abnormal Bone Marrow

1. **Chronic myelogenous leukemia**

2. **Polycythemia vera**

3. **Myelofibrosis**

4. **Mast cell leukemia.** Associated with an elevated number of circulating mast cells and neutrophils.

B. Basophilia With a Normal Bone Marrow

1. **Influenza infection**

2. **Varicella infection**

3. **Tuberculosis**

4. **Rheumatoid arthritis**

5. **Ulcerative colitis**

6. **Hodgkin's lymphoma and non-Hodgkin's lymphoma**

7. **Hypothyroidism**

8. **Ovulation**

9. **Estrogen supplements**

10. **Hemolytic anemia**

11. **Splenectomy**

BIBLIOGRAPHY

Abramson N, Melton B. Leukocytosis: basics of clinical assessment. *Am Fam Physician.* 2000;62(9):2053–2060.

Stock W, Hoffman R. White blood cells 1: non-malignant disorders. *Lancet.* 2000;355(9212): 1351–1357.

INFECTIVE ENDOCARDITIS

Jennifer Husson
William F. Wright

I. INTRODUCTION

A. Definition and Classification. Endocarditis is defined as a microbial infection involving the endocardial surface of a natural (native) heart valve or an artificial (prosthetic) heart valve.

B. Pathology. It is characterized by a ***vegetation*** that is a collection of microorganisms and cellular debris (e.g., platelets, fibrin, and inflammatory cells) that commonly results from colonization of damaged valvular endothelium by circulating microorganisms with specific adherence properties. Vegetations can occur in the following locations (from most common to least common):

1. Heart valves

2. Chordae tendineae

3. Endocardium

4. Endothelium

5. Septal cardiac abnormalities

II. RISK FACTORS FOR INFECTIVE ENDOCARDITIS.
While rheumatic heart disease was once the predominate risk factor, degenerative aortic- and mitral-valve disease predominates as the most common cause of native-valve endocarditis, except in developing countries where rheumatic heart disease is still common. Additional risk factors include:

A. Intravenous drug use (IVDU)

B. Poor dental hygiene

C. Diabetes mellitus (poorly controlled)

D. Hemodialysis and chronic kidney disease

E. HIV infection (most commonly associated with IVDU)

F. Mitral-valve prolapse (usually associated with mitral regurgitation severity and thickened mitral-valve leaflets)

G. Previous endocarditis

H. Long-term indwelling catheter (e.g., peripherally inserted central catheter [PICC] line)

I. Prosthetic heart valve. Early prosthetic infections usually occur within 2 months of surgery and are higher in mechanical valves.

J. Men are infected more than women

III. CLINICAL MANIFESTATIONS OF INFECTIVE ENDOCARDITIS. The clinical manifestations are variable but depend on the duration of illness (acute vs. chronic), microorganism, age of the patient (young vs. old), location (aortic and mitral valve vs. tricuspid valve), and underlying comorbid medical history (e.g., renal failure, diabetes).

A. **Fever; defined as greater than 38°C.** Present in the majority of patients (96%) and typically associated with chills, night sweats, weight loss, malaise, and/ or anorexia. However, fever may not be prominent in immunocompromised patients, including those with heart failure, renal failure, liver failure, prior antibiotics, and older adults.

B. **Murmurs.** Found in greater than two thirds of patients (68%). Most commonly these are preexisting murmurs, but a worsening of old murmurs or a new valvular regurgitation murmur might be more suggestive of endocarditis.

C. **Splenomegaly.** Can be observed in approximately 11% of cases.

D. **New or Changing Back Pain and Joint Pain.** May indicate septic emboli from an underlying endocarditis.

E. **Peripheral Manifestations.** These include:

1. **Splinter hemorrhages** have been observed in 8% of cases and are located on fingernails and toenails. They are typically linear and red or brown. The more proximal the splinter hemorrhage is located in the nail the more suggestive of endocarditis, as digital trauma can cause distal splinter hemorrhages.

2. **Roth spots** (retinal hemorrhages) and **conjunctival petechiae** (conjunctival hemorrhages) have been observed in 2% and 5% of cases, respectively.

3. **Osler nodes** have been observed in 3% of cases and are *tender* subcutaneous nodules located on the fingertips or palms.

4. **Janeway lesions** have been observed in 5% of cases and are *nontender* erythematous, hemorrhagic lesions on the palms or soles.

F. **Cough, Dyspnea, or Pleuritic Chest Pain.** May occur as a result of septic emboli in isolated right-sided endocarditis or heart failure in left-sided endocarditis.

G. **Stroke Syndrome.** May occur as a result of septic emboli to the brain or ruptured mycotic aneurysm. (A mycotic aneurysm is a septic embolus to the arterial vasa vasorum.)

IV. MICROBIOLOGICAL CAUSES OF ENDOCARDITIS. While the majority of patients with endocarditis will have identification of a microbial pathogen, a minority of patients will not have a pathogen identified by routine microbiological methods (e.g., culture-negative endocarditis). *The most common reason for culture-negative endocarditis is prior antibiotics.*

A. **Most Common Causes of Culture-Positive, Native-Valve, and Prosthetic-Valve Endocarditis.**

1. *Streptococcus* **(viridans).** Observed in as many as 17% of cases and most commonly involve *S. sanguis, S. mitis, S. mutans,* and *S. gallolyticus (bovis)* groups with native-valve endocarditis and typically late (greater than 12 months) prosthetic-valve endocarditis.

   Isolation of an *S. gallolyticus (bovis)* group pathogen warrants colonic evaluation for associated colonic malignancy.

2. *Staphylococcus aureus.* Most common pathogen (31% of cases) with both native- and prosthetic-valve types.

3. **Coagulase-negative** *Staphylococcus* **species.** Observed in as many as 11% of cases and commonly involves *S. epidermidis* with cases of prosthetic-valve endocarditis; however, *S. lugdunensis* is also rarely associated with both native- and prosthetic-valve endocarditis.

4. *Enterococcus* **spp**. *E. faecalis and E. faecium* are the major pathogens and are considered the third leading cause of infective endocarditis (an estimated 10% of cases). Most commonly occur in older adults with native-valve endocarditis but can occur at any stage in prosthetic-valve endocarditis.

5. **Gram-negative aerobic bacillus species.** *E. coli and Pseudomonas aeruginosa* account for the majority of cases. Rare pathogens for native-valve and prosthetic-value infection but typically occur in early prosthetic-valve endocarditis.

6. **Gram-positive aerobic bacillus species.** *Corynebacterium species and Bacillus species.* Rare pathogens occurring most commonly with indwelling cardiovascular devices and intravenous drug abuse, respectively, but can also occur at any time with prosthetic-valve endocarditis.

7. *Streptococcus pneumoniae.* Infection can rarely occur as a native-valve (aortic valve most commonly) endocarditis in middle-aged men with chronic alcoholism that also may involve pneumonia and meningitis (i.e., Austrian syndrome).

8. *Streptococcus pyogenes* **and groups B, C, F, and G beta-hemolytic streptococci**. These organisms are uncommon causes of infective endocarditis.

B. **Common Causes of Culture-Negative Endocarditis.** When blood cultures remain negative in patients suspected of endocarditis, consider the following causes and consult the clinical microbiology laboratory. Culture-negative endocarditis accounts for approximately 10% of cases overall and may reflect one of two situations: patients exposed to antimicrobial agents just prior to the diagnosis of infective endocarditis and infection caused by fastidious microorganisms. Some of the more common fastidious microorganisms include the following:

1. *Abiotrophia* **spp**, *Granulicatella* spp, or nutritionally variant streptococci.

2. *Bartonella* **spp**. *B. henselae* are usually associated with cat exposure or cat scratch disease, and *B. quintana* are usually associated with homeless persons.

3. *Coxiella burnetii* **(Q fever).** Typically associated with veterinarians or livestock exposure.

4. **HACEK organisms.** *Haemophilus* spp, *Aggregatibacter* spp, *Cardiobacterium hominis, Eikenella corrodens,* and *Kingella* spp. These organisms are found in the oral flora and typically grow by 7 days in standard automated-culture systems and have been observed in as many as 2% of cases.

5. *Chlamydia psittaci*

6. *Tropheryma whipplei*

7. *Legionella* **spp**

8. *Brucella melitensis or B. abortus*

9. **Fungi.** Account for as many as 2% of cases and most commonly involve *Candida* spp or *Aspergillus* spp. Standard automated-culture systems are often able to grow *Candida* spp.

V. COMPLICATIONS OF ENDOCARDITIS

A. **Heart Failure.** This is the most common complication (32% of cases) that is commonly associated with aortic-valve endocarditis and is the result of infection-related valvular damage.

B. **Pericarditis and/or Cardiac Abscess.** Abscesses are observed in an estimated 14% of cases and typically associated with prosthetic valves manifesting as conduction abnormalities.

C. **Embolic Phenomenon.** Events have been observed in approximately 17% to 23% of cases of infective endocarditis.

1. **Stroke.** Observed in 17% of cases and usually the result of septic emboli and/or mycotic aneurysm rupture; 90% occur in the middle cerebral artery (MCA) territory.

2. **Splenic abscess** as a result of septic emboli.

3. **Septic arthritis or vertebral osteomyelitis** as a result of septic emboli.

VI. APPROACH TO THE PATIENT.
The diagnosis of endocarditis involves a complete history (to determine risk factors) and physical examination in conjunction with laboratory and radiographic data (echocardiogram).

A. **History.** Obtain history about risk factors (e.g., IVDU), cardiovascular history (e.g., valvular disease), and any recent surgery, procedure, or indwelling catheter.

B. **Physical Examination**

1. **Head, eyes, ears, nose, and throat (HEENT) examination** (to detect Roth spots or conjunctival petechial).

2. **Cardiovascular examination** (to detect murmurs or heart failure).

3. **Pulmonary examination** (to detect heart failure).

4. **Dermatologic examination** (to detect signs of peripheral manifestations).

5. **Neurologic examination** (to identify focal deficits). Intracranial mycotic aneurysms are an uncommon complication that results from septic embolization of vegetations to the arterial vasa vasorum or intraluminal space, particularly at arterial branching points. The distal MCA branches are most commonly involved, resulting in subarachnoid or intraventricular hemorrhage manifesting sometimes as severe headache, altered sensorium, or focal neurologic deficit. *Streptococcus* species and *Staphylococcus aureus* account for the majority of cases.

6. **Musculoskeletal examination** (to identify osteomyelitis or septic arthritis).

C. **Laboratory Studies**

1. **Blood cultures.** At least three sets of blood cultures (an aerobic and anaerobic blood culture bottle defines one set of blood cultures), drawn at least 1 hour apart, from different anatomical sites should be obtained prior to the initiation of antibiotics. *Improved culture results are obtained with more*

blood volume and cultures taken coincident with fever spikes. It is reasonable to obtain at least two sets of blood cultures every 24 to 48 hours until the bloodstream infection (bacteremia) has resolved.

2. **CBC.** Leukocytosis and anemia may be present.

3. **Complete metabolic profile (CMP).** Patients may have renal or liver failure.

4. **Erythrocyte sedimentation rate (ESR)/C-reactive protein (CRP).** Nonspecific tests that may be elevated with infective endocarditis in as many as 61% to 62% of cases.

5. **Serum brain natriuretic peptide (BNP).** To evaluate for heart failure.

6. **Serum antibodies.** Most helpful to identify the cause of culture-negative endocarditis for *Bartonella* spp, *Coxiella* spp, *Chlamydia* spp, *Tropheryma whipplei*, and *Brucella* spp.

7. **Serum beta-D-glucan and/or *Aspergillus galactomannan*.** May be helpful to identify fungal causes of endocarditis.

8. **Urinalysis.** Typically demonstrates glomerulonephritis, but urinary antigen tests can also be helpful to identify *Legionella* serogroup-1 or histoplasmosis. Hematuria has been observed in approximately 26% of cases.

9. **ECG.** Abscesses may manifest as conduction abnormalities seen on ECG.

10. **Serum rheumatoid factor (RF).** The origin of RF is unclear; however, it is typically an autoantibody directed at the FC portion of immunoglobulin G (IgG), particularly IgG1. RFs occur during the course of various infections such as leprosy, tuberculosis, trypanosomiasis, visceral larva migrans, infectious mononucleosis, influenza A, viral hepatitis, and cytomegalovirus infection, and have been observed to occur in 5% of cases of infective endocarditis.

D. **Radiology.** Echocardiography is the technique of choice for investigating endocarditis. Intracardiac vegetations are most commonly found on mitral values (41%) followed by aortic values (38%), tricuspid valves (12%), and pulmonary valves (1%).

1. **Transthoracic echocardiography (TTE).** Has a sensitivity of 60% to 70% in low-risk patients and should be performed in all cases of suspected infective endocarditis.

2. **Transesophageal echocardiography (TEE).** More invasive than TTE but has an increased sensitivity of 75% to 95% with specificity of 85% to 98%. Additionally, TEE is particularly helpful in patients with prosthetic valve endocarditis and perivalvular abscesses as well as mitral-valve vegetations.

Performing a TEE before a TTE has been recommended for patients with prosthetic valves, complicated infective endocarditis (suspected paravalvular abscess), and possible infective endocarditis as defined by Duke's modified criteria; but other reasons may include:

a. *High initial risk for infection:* prosthetic valves, congenital heart disease (CHD), prior infective endocarditis, new murmur, heart failure, or stigmata of endocarditis.

b. *Difficult to interpret TTE:* patients with chronic obstructive pulmonary disease (COPD), obesity, and/or thoracic surgery.

3. **CT scanning or multislice CT angiography with three-dimensional (3D) construction**. Usually indicated for the evaluation of intrathoracic or intra-abdominal mycotic aneurysms.

E. **Modified Duke Criteria for Assessing Patients With Suspected Endocarditis.** Overall, the criteria provide agreement with the diagnosis in 72% to 90% of cases and have a high negative predictive value (see Table 7.1). Cases are defined as either:

1. **Definite endocarditis**

   a. Two major criteria

   b. One major plus three minor criteria

   c. Five minor criteria

2. **Possible endocarditis**

   a. One major criterion and one minor criterion

   b. Three minor criteria

VII. TREATMENT

A. **Antimicrobial Therapy.** (See Table 7.2.) Non-HACEK gram-negative bacilli (e.g., *E. coli* and *Pseudomonas* species) are typically treated with a beta-lactam antimicrobial and either an aminoglycoside or fluoroquinolone for 6 weeks with early cardiac valvular surgery evaluation.

B. **Indications for Surgery.** Combined medical and surgical therapy may improve survival among the following patients:

1. Valve dysfunction resulting in symptoms and signs of heart failure

2. Uncontrolled infection despite maximal medical therapy; typically defined as persistent bacteremia or fever lasting greater than 5 to 7 days

3. Infection with highly resistant organisms or particular unusual pathogens such as *Pseudomonas, Brucella,* or *Coxiella*

4. Fungal infection

TABLE 7.1 ■ Summary of the Modified Duke Criteria for Endocarditis

Major Criteria	Minor Criteria
Typical organism found in two separate blood cultures; >12 hr apart	Predisposing cardiac condition or injection drug use
Persistently positive blood cultures	Fever greater than 38°C
Single blood culture with *Coxiella* or IgG titer greater than 1:800	Vascular phenomena; arterial emboli, mycotic aneurysm, intracranial hemorrhage, Janeway lesions, and conjunctival hemorrhage
New valvular regurgitation	Positive blood culture not meeting major criteria or evidence of an infection with an organism consistent with infective endocarditis
Echocardiogram with vegetation	Immunologic phenomena; glomerulonephritis, Osler nodes, Roth spots, and rheumatoid factor

TABLE 7.2 ■ Antimicrobial Therapy

Organism	Therapy	Duration
Streptococcus	**A. Native Valve:**	2–4 weeks
	1. PCN MIC less than 0.12 mcg/mL penicillin G 2–3 million U IV q4–6 (for a total of 24 million U per day) *or* ceftriaxone 2 g IV q24 *or* vancomycin 15 mg/kg IV q12 *plus* gentamicin 3 mg/kg IV q24 *(for a duration of 2 weeks)*	4 weeks 6 weeks 6 weeks
	2. PCN MIC between 0.12 and 0.5 mcg/mL, same as earlier, *plus* gentamicin 3 mg/kg IV q24 *(for a duration of 2 weeks)*	
	3. PCN MIC greater than 0.5 mcg/mL ampicillin 2 g IV q4 *or* penicillin G 3–5 million U IV q4 *or* ceftriaxone 2 g IV q24 *or* vancomycin 15 mg/kg IV q12 *plus* gentamicin 3 mg/kg IV q24 *(for a duration of 6 weeks)*	
	B. Prosthetic Valve: penicillin G 4–6 million U IV q4–6 (for a total of 24 million U per day) *or* ceftriaxone 2 g IV q24 *or* vancomycin 15 mg/kg IV q12 *plus* gentamicin 3 mg/kg IV q24 *(for a duration of 6 weeks)*	
Staphylococcus	**A. MSSA:** nafcillin 2 g IV q4 *or* oxacillin 2 g IV q4 or cefazolin 2 g IV q8 *with or without gentamicin 3 mg/kg IV q24* **(for a duration of 3–5 days)**	6 weeks 6 weeks 6 weeks
	B. MRSA: vancomycin 30 mg/kg/24 hours *or* daptomycin 6 mg/kg IV q24	
	C. Prosthetic Valve: same as above but with rifampin 300 mg PO q8 *plus* gentamicin 1 mg/kg IV q8 *(for a duration of 2 weeks)*	
Enterococcus	**A.** *Enterococcus* **sensitive to PCN, gentamicin, and vancomycin:** ampicillin 2 g IV q4 *or* penicillin G 3–5 million U IV q4 *or* vancomycin 15 mg/kg IV q12 *plus* ntamicin 1 mg/kg IV q8 *or* ampicillin 2 g IV q4 plus ceftriaxone 2 g IV q12	4–6 weeks 4–6 weeks
	B. *Enterococcus* **resistant only to gentamicin:** ampicillin 2 g IV q4 *or* penicillin G 6 million U IV q4 *or* vancomycin 15 mg/kg IV q12 *plus* streptomycin 7.5 mg/kg IV q12	
	C. *Enterococcus* **resistant to PCN, gentamicin, streptomycin, and vancomycin:** typically divided by organism	8 weeks
	1. *E. faecium*: linezolid 600 mg IV/PO q12 *or* quinupristin-dalfopristin 7.5 mg/kg IV q8	
	2. *E. faecalis*: ampicillin 2 g IV q8 *plus* either imipenem-cilastatin 500 mg IV q6 *or* ceftriaxone 2 g IV q12	

(continued)

TABLE 7.2 ■ Antimicrobial Therapy (*continued*)

Organism	Therapy	Duration
Bartonella	**A. Native Valve:** ampicillin 2 g IV q6 *plus* gentamicin 1 mg/kg IV q8 *or* vancomycin 15 mg/kg IV q12 *plus* gentamicin 1 mg/kg IV q8 *plus* ciprofloxacin 1,000 mg PO q24 **B. Prosthetic Valve:** vancomycin 15 mg/kg IV q12 *plus* cefepime 2 g IV q8 *plus* rifampin 300 mg IV q8 *with* gentamicin 1 mg/kg IV q8 *(for a duration of 2 weeks)*	4–6 weeks 6 weeks
HACEK	Ceftriaxone 2 g IV q24 *or* ciprofloxacin 1,000 mg IV q24 *or* ampicillin–sulbactam 3 g IV q6	4 weeks
Coxiella burnetii	Doxycycline 100 mg PO q12 *plus* hydroxychloroquine 600 mg PO q24	1.5–3 years
Fungi	Lipid-based amphotericin B 3–5 mg/kg IV q24 *plus* flucytosine 25–37.5 mg/kg PO q6 *plus* surgical resection	6–8 weeks after surgery

HACEK, *Haemophilus* spp, *Aggregatibacter* spp, *Cardiobacterium hominis, Eikenella corrodens,* and *Kingella* spp. MIC, minimum inhibitory concentration; MRSA, methicillin-resistant *Staphylococcus aureus;* MSSA, methicillin-susceptible *Staphylococcus aureus*; PCN, penicillin.

5. Prosthetic-valve endocarditis

6. Perivalvular abscess, valve dehiscence, severe valvular regurgitation, perforation, rupture, or fistula

7. Large vegetations (relative indication), particularly mobile vegetations greater than 10 mm

8. Recent neurologic complication (this is a relative contraindication for immediate surgery and in most cases surgery is delayed for 3 to 4 weeks)

C. **Anticoagulation.** There is *no known benefit for anticoagulation*, including routine aspirin use, in cases of infective endocarditis. Recommendations for anticoagulation include the following:

1. Discontinue all forms of anticoagulation for mechanical prosthetic-valve endocarditis for at least 2 weeks.

2. Initiation of aspirin or another antiplatelet agent as adjunctive therapy is not recommended.

3. Long-term antiplatelet therapy may be continued during infective endocarditis with NO bleeding complications.

D. Once antimicrobial therapy is completed, TTE or TEE should be repeated for a new baseline.

VIII. PROPHYLAXIS

A. **Cardiac Indications for Prophylaxis.** Current recommendations are based on cardiac conditions that have the highest predisposition to the acquisition of endocarditis and cardiac conditions associated with the highest risk of adverse outcome from endocarditis among the following patients:

1. Prosthetic cardiac valve or prosthetic material used for cardiac valve repair

2. Previous history of infective endocarditis

3. CHD that includes the following:

   a. Unrepaired cyanotic CHD, including palliative shunts and conduits

   b. Completely repaired congenital heart defect with prosthetic material or device, whether placed by surgical or catheter intervention, during the first 6 months after the procedure (*endothelialization of prosthetic material typically occurs within 6 months after the procedure*)

   c. Repaired CHD with residual defects at or adjacent to the site of a prosthetic patch or prosthetic device

4. Cardiac transplantation recipients who develop valvulopathy

B. **Dental Procedure Indications for Prophylaxis.** Prophylaxis for endocarditis is reasonable for ***ALL*** dental procedures that involve manipulation of gingival tissue or the periapical region of teeth or perforation of the oral mucosa (Table 7.3). Dental procedures and/or events that ***DO NOT*** need prophylaxis include:

1. Routine anesthetic injections through noninfected tissue

2. Obtaining dental radiographs

3. Placement of removable prosthodontic or orthodontic appliances

4. Adjustment of orthodontic appliances

5. Placement of orthodontic brackets

6. Shedding of deciduous teeth

7. Bleeding from trauma to the lips or oral mucosa

TABLE 7.3 ■ Antimicrobial Prophylaxis Regimens for Dental Procedures

Situation	Agent	Single-Dose Regimen *Provided 30–60 minutes prior to the procedure*	
		Adults	Children
Oral	Amoxicillin	2 g	50 mg/kg
Unable to take oral	Ampicillin or	2 g IM or IV	50 mg/kg IM or IV
	Cefazolin/Ceftriaxone	1 g IM or IV	50 mg/kg IM or IV
Able to take oral but allergy to ampicillin or other penicillins	Cephalexin* or	2 g	50 mg/kg
	Clindamycin or	600 mg	20 mg/kg
	Azithromycin/ Clarithromycin	500 mg	15 mg/kg
Unable to take oral and allergy to ampicillin or other penicillins	Cefazolin/Ceftriaxone or	1 g IM or IV	50 mg/kg IM or IV
	Clindamycin	600 mg IM or IV	20 mg/kg IM or IV

*Cephalosporin antimicrobial agents should NOT be used in patients with a history of anaphylaxis, angioedema, or urticaria with ampicillin and/or other penicillins.
IM, intramuscular; IV, intravenous.

BIBLIOGRAPHY

Baddour LM, Wilson WR, Bayer AS, et al. Infective endocarditis in adults: diagnosis, antimicrobial therapy, and management of complications: a statement for health care professionals from the American Heart Association. *Circulation.* 2015;132:1435–1486. doi:10.1161/CIR.0000000000000296

Beynon RP, Bahl VK, Prendergast BD. Infective endocarditis. *BMJ.* 2006;333(7563):334–339.

Hoen B, Duval X. Infective endocarditis. *N Engl J Med.* 2013;368(15):1425–1433.

Li JS, Sexton DJ, Mick N, et al. Proposed modifications to the Duke criteria for the diagnosis of infective endocarditis. *Clin Infect Dis.* 2000;30(4):633–638.

Murdoch DR, Corey R, Hoen B, et al. Clinical presentation, etiology, and outcome of infective endocarditis in the 21st century, The international collaboration on endocarditis-prospective cohort study. *Arch Intern Med.* 2009;169(5):463–473.

Mylonakis E, Calderwood SB. Infective endocarditis in adults. *N Engl J Med.* 2001;345(18):1318–1330.

Wilson W, Taubert KA, Gewitz M, et al. Prevention of infective endocarditis: guidelines from the American Heart Association, by the Committee on Rheumatic Fever, Endocarditis, and Kawasaki Disease. *Circulation.* 2007;116:1736–1754.

Wright WF. Central venous access device-related Bacillus cereus endocarditis: a case report and review of the literature. *Clin Med Res.* 2016;14(2):109–115.

INFECTIOUS MYOCARDITIS

William F. Wright

I. INTRODUCTION

    A. Definition. A nonischemic inflammatory condition of the myocardium, most commonly as the result of a viral illness.

    B. Classification. Most classification schemes for myocarditis are complex and divided by etiology, histology, immunohistology, and clinicopathology categories. The clinicopathology categories are most useful clinically and include:

        1. Acute myocarditis. Cardiac symptoms (e.g., heart failure symptoms) present for *more than 2 weeks without* hemodynamic compromise or a distinct viral illness prodrome.

        2. Fulminant myocarditis. Cardiac symptoms (e.g., heart failure symptoms) present for *less than 2 weeks associated with* hemodynamic compromise and a distinct viral illness prodrome.

        3. Chronic myocarditis. Heart failure associated with a dilated left ventricle and immunohistology evidence of myocardial inflammation.

    C. Epidemiology. The true incidence and prevalence of myocarditis are unknown, but it has been detected in as much as 9% to 16% of routine postmortem examinations. Myocarditis is associated with a slight male predominance and is estimated to be the cause of *sudden cardiac death* in 2% to 42% of cases.

    D. Risk Factors. No specific risk factors for myocarditis are reported.

II. CAUSES OF MYOCARDITIS. Myocarditis can result from infectious microorganisms, antimicrobials, cardiac toxins, immune-mediated conditions, and systemic disorders.

    A. Infectious Microorganisms

        1. Viral pathogens. Viruses and postviral-related immune responses remain the most common cause of myocarditis. Common pathogens include:

           a. Parvovirus B19 (*most common viral pathogen*)

           b. Coxsackievirus B, poliomyelitis virus, and echovirus

           c. Adenovirus, influenza A virus, and mumps virus

           d. Epstein–Barr (EBV) virus, cytomegalovirus (CMV), herpes simplex virus (HSV), and human herpesvirus (HHV) 6

           e. Hepatitis C virus

   f. HIV

   g. Dengue virus and yellow fever virus

   h. Rubella, rubeola, varicella, and variola

2. **Bacterial pathogens.** Common pathogens include:

   a. *Staphylococcus* spp and *Streptococcus* spp

   b. *Corynebacterium diphtheriae, Clostridium tetani, Actinomyces* spp, and *Nocardia brasiliensis*

   c. *Neisseria gonorrhoeae* and *Neisseria meningitidis*

   d. *Mycobacterium tuberculosis*

   e. *Treponema pallidum* (syphilis), *Borrelia burgdorferi* (Lyme disease), and *Leptospira*

   f. *Rickettsia rickettsii* (Rocky Mountain spotted fever [RMSF]) and *Coxiella burnetii* (Q fever)

3. **Parasitic pathogens.** Common pathogens include:

   a. *Trypanosoma cruzi* (Chagas disease), *Toxoplasmosis gondii, Plasmodium* spp (malaria), and *Leishmania* spp

   b. *Echinococcus granulosus, Trichinella spiralis, Schistosoma* spp, and *Strongyloides stercoralis*

4. **Fungal pathogens.** Common pathogens include:

   a. *Cryptococcus neoformans* and *Candida* spp

   b. *Aspergillus* spp

   c. *Histoplasma capsulatum, Coccidioides immitis, Blastomyces dermatitidis,* and *Sporothrix schenckii*

B. **Cardiac Toxins.** Some agents that have a direct toxic effect on the myocardium include: alcohol, arsenic, anthracyclines (cancer chemotherapy), carbon monoxide, copper, iron, lead, and cocaine.

C. **Antimicrobial Therapy, Medication, and Other Related Reactions.** Some agents include antibiotics (most commonly penicillins, cephalosporins, tetracyclines, and sulfonamides), diuretics, lithium, tetanus toxoid, benzodiazepines, tricyclic antidepressants, and insect or snake bites.

D. **Systemic Disorders**

1. **Autoimmune diseases.** Rheumatoid arthritis, systemic lupus, Kawasaki disease, Crohn disease, ulcerative colitis, scleroderma, dermatomyositis, myasthenia gravis, and sarcoidosis.

2. **Hypereosinophilic syndromes.** Loffler syndrome, Churg–Strauss syndrome, and *eosinophilic myocarditis* (e.g., hypersensitivity reaction or parasitic infection).

3. **Chronic medical conditions.** Insulin-dependent diabetes, thyrotoxicosis, and pheochromocytoma.

III. **PATHOPHYSIOLOGY OF MYOCARDITIS.** While a number of infectious and noninfectious causes are associated with myocarditis, viral myocarditis predominates as the most common cause and best explains the pathophysiology of this condition. Conceptually, viral myocarditis is characterized by three phases:

A. **Acute Phase.** This phase is initiated in the first 2 weeks after infection by introduction, or reactivation, of a viral pathogen in a host followed by hematogenous or lymphangitic spread to reach the myocardium (this phase is also initiated by direct or indirect cardiac toxins). Viral or other microbial pathogens gain entry followed by proliferation within the myocytes resulting in cytopathic effects, myocyte death, release of cytokines/chemokines, and activation of the innate immune response (i.e., macrophages and CD4/CD8-positive T lymphocytes).

B. **Subacute Phase.** This phase is characterized by an adaptive immune response (i.e., antibody production) to *both viral and cardiac proteins* that results in further myocyte injury and reduced contractile function (i.e., left ventricular dysfunction). Most patients eliminate the viral or microbial pathogen, have a decline in immune response, and recover cardiac contractile function.

C. **Chronic Phase.** This phase is characterized as a persistent immune response in some patients associated with myocardial fibrosis and remodeling leading to *dilated cardiomyopathy.*

IV. **CLINICAL MANIFESTATIONS OF MYOCARDITIS.** The clinical presentation varies among adults and children but can range from an asymptomatic course to a fulminant illness associated with cardiogenic shock or sudden death.

A. **Adults.** While the clinical manifestations are variable, frequently adults experience a viral prodrome characterized by fever, maculopapular rash, myalgias, arthralgias, fatigue, dyspnea, palpitations, decreased exercise tolerance, or gastrointestinal symptoms (e.g., nausea or diarrhea). Additional manifestations include:

1. **Syncope/palpitations.** May occur as the result of new-onset atrial or ventricular arrhythmias or atrioventricular conduction blocks.

2. **Chest pain.** May mimic typical angina (i.e., pressure pain that is constant) but may also be more typical for pericarditis (e.g., substernal or left precordial pleuritic chest pain with radiation to the scapula).

3. **Heart failure symptoms.** Patients with fulminant myocarditis usually present with more severe symptoms.

B. **Children.** In general, newborns and infants more often present with a fulminant illness than older children (age greater than 2 years) and adults. While the most common symptoms are respiratory distress and lethargy, additional symptoms may include cough, chest pain, abdominal pain, fever, myalgia, fatigue, anorexia, malaise, and anxiousness.

V. **APPROACH TO THE PATIENT**

A. **History.** Myocarditis is a diagnosis often missed; therefore, this illness should always be included in the differential diagnosis when evaluating a patient with chest pain, heart failure, or cardiac arrhythmia. The history should focus on the timing of events, recent infections, vaccination history, comorbid illnesses, occupational or environmental exposures, medications, and recent travels.

B. **Physical Examination.** A complete examination should be performed in the evaluation of myocarditis; however, the examination should also emphasize:

1. **Cardiovascular examination** (to detect murmurs, S3 or S4 gallop, pericardial friction rub, tachycardia, or laterally displaced point of maximal impulse).

2. **Head, eyes, ears, nose, and throat (HEENT) examination.** *Parotid gland swelling* may indicate mumps, Chagas, or HIV. *Conjunctival erythema* may indicate adenovirus, enterovirus, Chagas, tuberculosis (TB; usually unilateral), or collagen vascular disorder. *Palatal petechiae* may indicate EBV, CMV, HSV, varicella-zoster virus (VZV), rubella, and HIV. *Palatal vesicles* are associated with HSV, VZV, and Coxsackie virus.

3. **Lymphatic system examination.** *Splenomegaly* may indicate EBV, CMV, or malaria. *Generalized lymphadenopathy* may indicate HIV, TB, HHV-6, CMV, rubella, *Trypanosoma cruzi,* or sarcoidosis.

4. **Pulmonary examination.** Inspiratory bibasilar rales may indicate heart failure, whereas diffuse expiratory wheezing may indicate influenza or hypereosinophilic syndrome (e.g., Churg–Strauss syndrome).

5. **Musculoskeletal examination.** Joint swelling and synovitis may indicate a collagen vascular disorder.

6. **Dermatologic examination.** A *petechial rash* involving the palms and soles may indicate RMSF or EBV. *Erythema nodosum* may indicate TB, EBV, histoplasmosis, or blastomycosis. *Erythema multiforme* may suggest HSV or Coxsackie virus. *Erythema migrans* may indicate Lyme disease. A *morbilliform rash* on the chest may signify acute HIV infection.

C. **Laboratory and Diagnostic Studies**

1. **Complete Blood Count (CBC).** Routinely ordered but usually nonspecific. *Leukopenia* may indicate TB, hepatitis C, EBV, CMV, HHV-6, or histoplasmosis. *Lymphocytosis or atypical lymphocytes* may suggest EBV, CMV, HHV-6, mumps, toxoplasmosis, RMSF, dengue, or rubella. *Monocytosis* may indicate TB, RMSF, syphilis, diphtheria, or histoplasmosis. *Eosinophilia* may suggest trichinosis, hypersensitivity or hypereosinophilic disease, strongyloidiasis, or histoplasmosis. *Anemia* may indicate malaria (*a thick and thin blood film may also indicate malaria*) or CMV. *Thrombocytopenia* may be associated with parvovirus B19, EBV, CMV, dengue, TB, HIV, histoplasmosis, trypanosomiasis, diphtheria, or RMSF.

2. **Complete metabolic profile (CMP).** Routinely ordered but usually nonspecific. Elevated hepatic transaminases, alkaline phosphatase, or total bilirubin may indicate EBV, CMV, HHV-6, HIV, tuberculosis, *N. gonorrhoeae,* syphilis, Q fever, histoplasmosis, or hepatitis C.

3. **Urinalysis.** Routinely ordered but nonspecific. Pyuria (greater than 5 white blood cells [WBCs] on microscopy) may be associated with TB, leptospirosis, gonorrhea, or diphtheria.

4. **Blood cultures.** Two sets should be ordered on all patients but rarely indicate a particular pathogen.

5. **Cardiac biomarkers.** Creatine kinase and troponins (i.e., troponin I and T) should be ordered in all patients. Troponin I and T are elevated more

frequently than creatine kinase in acute myocarditis. Troponin I has a low sensitivity (34%) but high specificity (89%) for acute myocarditis.

6. **Serum markers of inflammation.** Both the erythrocyte sedimentation rate (ESR) and C-reactive protein (CRP) are elevated in acute myocarditis but are nonspecific.

7. **Serology.** The utility of viral serology for the diagnosis of myocarditis remains unproven and should *not* be routinely performed; however, most patients should have an HIV enzyme-linked immunosorbent assay (ELISA), rapid plasma reagin (RPR), and viral hepatitis panel ordered. Serology may be helpful for EBV, CMV, dengue, Lyme disease, leptospirosis, toxoplasmosis, or RMSF in selected patients with a history or examination finding associated with these disorders.

8. **ECG.** Should be ordered in all patients but nonspecific and associated with a low sensitivity (47%) for acute myocarditis. Findings vary from ST-segment elevation or depression, PR-interval depression, Q-wave development, QRS complex prolongation, and QTc interval prolongation. Atrioventricular heart block may suggest Lyme disease, Chagas disease, or diphtheria. *The presence of pathologic Q waves, prolonged QRS complex (greater than 120 ms), new left bundle branch block, or prolonged QTc interval (greater than 440 ms) is associated with higher rates of cardiac death or need for cardiac transplantation.*

D. Radiology

1. **Echocardiography.** A *transthoracic echocardiogram* should be ordered for all patients to exclude other causes of heart failure; echocardiography findings suggestive of myocarditis are nonspecific but commonly may include left ventricular systolic dysfunction, restrictive diastolic filling, segmental or global myocardial wall motion abnormalities, and small pericardial effusion. *The presence of right ventricular systolic dysfunction is the most important predictor of cardiac death or need for cardiac transplantation in acute myocarditis.*

2. **Cardiac gallium-67 scintigraphy and 18-fluorodeoxyglucose PET.** These diagnostic studies are more useful in the evaluation of cardiac sarcoidosis.

3. **Cardiac MRI (cardiovascular magnetic resonance [CMR]).** A noninvasive imaging tool useful for diagnosing myocarditis. Early and late enhancement following gadolinium *contrast* administration is helpful for the differentiation of acute myocardial infarction from acute myocarditis. Common findings for acute myocarditis include nodular, patchy, and subepicardial late enhancement of the lateral or inferior walls of the myocardium.

   The diagnostic criteria for myocarditis by CMR include at least two or more of the following (Lake Louise Criteria):

   a. Regional or global myocardial signal intensity (SI) increase in T2-weighted images (SI ratio greater than 2.0)

   b. Increased global myocardial early gadolinium enhancement ratio (a score greater than 4.0) between myocardium and skeletal muscle in gadolinium-enhanced T1-weighted images

   c. At least one focal lesion with nonischemic regional distribution in inversion-recovery-prepared gadolinium-enhanced T1-weighted images (e.g., late gadolinium enhancement)

Acute myocardial infarction is more likely if myocyte edema is more suben-docardial or transmural in combination with a colocalized ischemic injury pattern of late gadolinium enhancement.

E. **Endomyocardial Biopsy (EMB).** At least three samples, 1 to 2 mm, should be taken from the right or left ventricle and immediately fixed in 10% buffered formalin at room temperature; additional samples should be snap-frozen in liquid nitrogen and stored at −80°C or stored in RNA tubes at room temperature for possible viral polymerase chain reaction (PCR) testing.

Defined by the *Dallas criteria* for histology, *EMB remains the gold standard for the diagnosis of myocarditis.* Based on these criteria, *acute myocarditis is defined as a lymphocytic infiltrate in association with myocardial necrosis.* The use of immunohistochemistry (e.g., monoclonal antibodies to T-lymphocytes and activated macrophages) has improved the detection of myocarditis and requires detection of a focal or diffuse inflammatory infiltrate of T-lymphocytes and macrophages with greater than 14 cells/mm^3. Additionally, molecular detection methods (e.g., PCR) can be performed on biopsy samples for the detection of viral pathogens.

While a number of recommendations exist for the indication of endomyocardial biopsy, the two most important recommendations are:

1. EMB should be performed in a patient with unexplained, new-onset heart failure of less than 2 weeks, duration with hemodynamic compromise, and echocardiographic findings of a normal-sized or dilated left ventricle.

2. EMB should be performed in a patient with unexplained, new-onset heart failure of 2 weeks' to 3 months' duration with echocardiographic evidence of a dilated left ventricle and ECG findings of a new ventricular arrhythmia, high-grade atrioventricular block (i.e., second- or third-degree block), and who fails to respond to the standard heart failure care within 1 to 2 weeks.

Recommended Diagnostic Criteria for Clinically Suspected Myocarditis*

Clinical criteria

1. Acute chest pain
2. New onset (less than 3 months' duration) or worsening of dyspnea at rest, dyspnea with exercise with or without findings of heart failure
3. Subacute to chronic (greater than 3 months' duration) or worsening of dyspnea at rest, dyspnea with exercise with or without findings of heart failure
4. Unexplained palpitations, cardiac arrhythmia, or syncope
5. Unexplained cardiogenic shock or aborted sudden cardiac death

Diagnostic criteria

1. New-onset abnormal 12-lead ECG in the absence of angiographically detectable coronary artery disease (e.g., coronary stenosis greater than or equal to 50%)
2. Elevated myocardial injury markers in the absence of angiographically detectable coronary artery disease (e.g., coronary stenosis greater than or equal to 50%)
3. New unexplained functional or structural myocardial abnormalities on cardiac imaging
4. CMR findings consistent with myocarditis

(continued)

(continued)

Recommended Diagnostic Criteria for Clinically Suspected Myocarditis*

Myocarditis should be suspected in the presence of:
one or more of the clinical criteria
AND
one or more of the diagnostic criteria

---

*The aforementioned diagnostic criteria endorse the concept that endomyocardial biopsy should be the gold standard for the definitive diagnosis of myocarditis. Additionally, these diagnostic criteria should be applied to cases in the absence of angiographically detectable coronary artery disease (e.g., coronary stenosis greater than or equal to 50%) or known preexisting cardiovascular diseases (e.g., valvular heart disease, congenital heart disease, hyperthyroidism) that could otherwise better explain the clinical findings.

CMR, cardiovascular magnetic resonance.

VI. TREATMENT

A. **Medical Treatment.** The mainstay of treatment is standard supportive care for heart failure and arrhythmias.

1. **Antiviral therapy.** Specific antiviral therapy is usually not provided early enough to benefit patients with acute viral myocarditis; therefore, routine antiviral therapy is not recommended. Interferon-beta may provide benefit to adults with chronic viral myocarditis with stable cardiomyopathy.

2. **Intravenous immunoglobulin (IVIG).** While IVIG has both antiviral and immunomodulation effects, routine use in adults with acute myocarditis failed to show any benefit and is not recommended. High-dose IVIG has shown benefit in pediatric groups and may be considered in select cases with acute myocarditis.

3. **Immunosuppressive or anti-inflammatory agents.** Immunosuppressants (e.g., prednisone, cyclosporine, and azathioprine) have provided no treatment benefit in both adults and children with acute viral myocarditis but may improve the quality of life and improve left ventricular dysfunction in chronic autoimmune cardiomyopathy. *Nonsteroidal anti-inflammatory drugs (NSAIDs; e.g., indomethacin or ibuprofen) may worsen myocarditis and are generally reserved for patients with a preserved or normal ventricular function.*

4. **Physical activity.** Based on the risk of sudden cardiac death, all patients with proven or suspected myocarditis are advised to refrain from competitive athletic activity or vigorous exercise for **6 months** after the onset of symptoms. Patients may return to normal activity with:

   a. Normalization of left ventricular function

   b. Resolution of serum inflammatory markers (such as ESR or CRP)

   c. Normalization of ECG

   d. Absence of arrhythmias

B. **Surgical Treatment.** Patients may require cardiac transplantation if there are findings of:

1. Right ventricular systolic dysfunction on echocardiography and/or

2. The presence of pathologic Q waves, prolonged QRS complex (greater than 120 ms), new left bundle branch block, or prolonged QTc interval (greater than 440 ms) on ECG

BIBLIOGRAPHY

Caforio AL, Pankuweit S, Arbustini E, et al. Current state of knowledge on aetiology, diagnosis, management, and therapy of myocarditis: a position statement of the European Society of Cardiology Working Group on Myocardial and Pericardial Diseases. *Eur Heart J.* 2013;34(33):2636–2648.

Cooper LT Jr. Myocarditis. *N Engl J Med.* 2009;360(15):1526–1538.

Ellis CR, Di Salvo T. Myocarditis: basic and clinical aspects. *Cardiol Rev.* 2007;15(4):170–177.

Kindermann I, Barth C, Mahfoud F, et al. Update on myocarditis. *J Am Coll Cardiol.* 2012;59(9): 779–792.

Sagar S, Liu PP, Cooper LT Jr. Myocarditis. *Lancet.* 2012;379(9817):738–747.

Schultz JC, Hilliard AA, Cooper LT Jr, Rihal CS. Diagnosis and treatment of viral myocarditis. *Mayo Clin Proc.* 2009;84(11):1001–1009.

CARDIOVASCULAR IMPLANTABLE PROSTHETIC DEVICE INFECTIONS

William F. Wright

I. **INTRODUCTION.** Certain intravascular cardiac devices are life-saving therapies for patients with arrhythmias, coronary artery disease, heart failure, and occlusive vascular disease but can be associated with the complication of infection. The intravascular devices that carry the most risk of infection include:

A. **Pacemakers and Implantable Cardioverter Defibrillators (ICDs).** These implantable electronic devices help provide hemodynamic stability and prevent potentially fatal arrhythmias. Devices are usually placed under the skin of the chest wall by a surgically created pulse-generator pocket that is then connected transvenously (nonthoracotomy) to leads that terminate in the right atrial and/or ventricular endocardium.

B. **Left Ventricular Assist Devices (LVADs).** These devices usually provide cardiovascular support to patients awaiting cardiac transplantation. Devices typically have the components of an external generator, driveline and cutaneous exit site, cutaneous pocket with pump, and an inflow/outflow conduit with communication to the left ventricle.

C. **Vascular Grafts.** These devices include central (aortic), peripheral, and hemodialysis-related vascular grafts that are surgically placed and typically consist of prosthetic material (e.g., Dacron; *polyethylene terephthalate*).

D. Other devices rarely associated with infections **include** coronary artery stents, peripheral vascular stents, and intra-aortic balloon pumps.

II. **EPIDEMIOLOGY**

A. **Pacemaker and ICD.** Infections can range from a superficial localized incision site infection (e.g., cellulitis) to deeper pocket-site infections (e.g., cellulitis and abscess) or an intravascular infection (e.g., endocarditis). Pacemaker infection rates are estimated to range from 1% to 20% with 10% of those infections classified as endocarditis. ICD infection rates range from 0.5% to 3.2%. Intra-abdominal ICD implantation is associated with higher rates than pectoral implantations.

B. **LVAD.** Infection can involve any component of the device but more commonly involves the driveline or pocket site. Infections are higher within the first 90 days following initial placement of the device.

C. **Vascular Grafts.** Infections can range from a superficial localized incision site infection (e.g., cellulitis), to deeper perivascular infections (e.g., cellulitis and abscess), or intravascular infection (e.g., endocarditis) resulting from bacteremia.

In general, peripheral and hemodialysis grafts, especially infrainguinal (i.e., inguinal sites and below), are associated with more infections than centrally placed vascular grafts.

III. RISK FACTORS AND PATHOGENESIS

A. Risk Factors. While conditions predisposing to intravascular device infections are common to many devices, some unique risks are associated with certain ones.

1. **Pacemaker and ICD.** Risk factors are mainly related to poor wound healing and altered immune status and include:

   a. Diabetes mellitus

   b. Heart failure (altered cell-mediated immunity)

   c. Chronic kidney disease (CrCl less than 60 mL/min)

   d. Chronic obstructive pulmonary disease (COPD; usually advanced disease in association with corticosteroids)

   e. Corticosteroid use

   f. Anticoagulation or pocket hematoma

   g. Dermatologic condition (e.g., psoriasis)

   h. Emergent procedure, multiple surgical revisions, or prolonged hospitalization

2. **LVAD.** Risk factors include:

   a. Diabetes mellitus, heart failure, chronic kidney disease, COPD, corticosteroid use (associated with altered immune status)

   b. Anticoagulation or pocket hematoma

   c. Emergent procedure, multiple surgical revisions, or prolonged hospitalization

   d. Dermatologic condition or site of device placement (e.g., preperitoneal site vs. abdominal cavity)

   e. Surgical-site infection (e.g., cellulitis)

   f. Hematogenous source infection (e.g., dialysis catheter or central venous catheter bloodstream infection)

3. **Vascular grafts.** Same risk factors as pacemaker and ICD but mainly associated with poor wound healing risks.

B. Pathogenesis. In general, the pathogenesis can be summarized by three basic mechanisms:

1. Bacterial contamination at the time of initial surgery or during subsequent surgical revisions (most common)

2. Contiguous spread from an adjacent site of infection (e.g., surgical incision site cellulitis)

3. Hematogenous seeding from a distant source infection (e.g., dialysis or central venous catheter associated bacteremia)

   A unique aspect involving the pathogenesis of intravascular device infections is the ability of certain bacteria to bind to the device and develop a biofilm. A biofilm, also known as glycocalyx or slime, increases bacterial resistance to the host immune response and antibiotics. The type of plastic polymer, surface irregularity, and shape can affect the ability of bacterial adherence. In general, polyvinyl chloride favors the most adherence when compared to Teflon followed by polyethylene greater than polyurethane, then silicone more than polytetrafluoroethylene, and then latex is more conducive to adherence than silicone. Finally, stainless steel promotes bacterial adherence more than titanium.

IV. **MICROBIOLOGY.** For the majority of intravascular device infections, the most common pathogens are coagulase-negative staphylococci (*Staphylococcus epidermidis*) and *Staphylococcus aureus*. Pathogens most commonly related to each device include:

A. **Pacemaker and ICD**

1. *Staphylococcus epidermidis* and other coagulase-negative *Staphylococcus* spp; account for approximately 42% of cases

2. *Staphylococcus aureus;* account for approximately 29% of cases

3. *Enterococcus* spp (e.g., *E. faecalis* and *E. faecium*)

4. *Pseudomonas aeruginosa*

5. *Corynebacterium* spp (e.g., *C. jeikeium* and *C. amycolatum*)

6. Enteric gram-negative bacteria (e.g., *Enterobacter* spp, *Klebsiella* spp, *Acinetobacter* spp, *Serratia* spp, *Citrobacter* spp, and *Proteus* spp); account for approximately 9% of cases

7. Fungi (e.g., *Candida* spp and *Aspergillus* spp); account for approximately 2% of cases

B. **LVAD.** Same as the preceding.

C. **Vascular Grafts.** Same as the preceding.

V. **CLINICAL MANIFESTATIONS.** The clinical manifestations of intravascular device infections are variable and can range from an uncomplicated localized skin and soft-tissue infection to systemic involvement associated with shock and multiorgan dysfunction. These manifestations depend on the duration between the device placement and onset of infection, the type of device and location of placement (e.g., Dacron device and infrainguinal location), microorganism, age of the patient, and underlying comorbid medical history. In general, the most common clinical manifestations include:

A. **Superficial Incision Site Infection.** Localized signs and symptoms include erythema, tenderness or pain, swelling or edema, warmth, and purulent drainage through a dehiscence, erosion, or poorly healed incision.

B. **Pocket-Site or Perivascular Space Infection.** These infections usually present with localized symptoms and signs of erythema, tenderness or pain, swelling or edema, warmth, and purulent drainage through a dehiscence, erosion, or sinus tract formation. The cellulitis or abscess associated with this type of infection can also include systemic symptoms (e.g., fever, chills, night sweats, weight loss, nausea, anorexia, or malaise).

C. **Bacteremia and Endocarditis.** This type of infection usually presents with systemic symptoms (e.g., fever and chills) but symptoms *typically do not include vascular embolic phenomena* (e.g., Janeway lesions, Osler nodes, or splenomegaly) as seen with prosthetic or native valve endocarditis (except endocarditis involving an LVAD device). Less commonly, this type of infection may present as a chronic fever, isolated bacteremia (without associated signs or symptoms), recurrent bronchitis or pneumonia, recurrent pocket or perivascular space infection, vascular obstruction with resultant ischemia or necrosis, or pulmonary embolization with or without a deep vein thrombosis.

VI. APPROACH TO THE PATIENT

A. **History.** Intravascular device infections should always be included in the differential diagnosis when evaluating a patient for an infection and a history of an intravascular device. *Nonspecific symptoms and signs of systemic infection may include fevers, chills, night sweats, malaise, and/or anorexia.* While a complete chronologically accurate history should be obtained, the history should also emphasize:

1. Dates involving the original and revision surgeries for the intravascular device

2. Risk factors for infection and comorbid medical history

3. Recent and remote infections as well as antibiotic use

B. **Physical Examination.** A complete physical examination should be performed; however, the examination should also focus on these areas:

1. **Dermatologic examination.** Inspection of the device pocket site or surgical incision for signs of cellulitis (e.g., erythema, warmth, and edema), abscess (may be indicated by an inflammatory fluctuant mass located near the pocket or surgical incision site), or draining sinus tract.

   Cutaneous ulcers located over the tips of the toes, malleoli, and heels that appear black, wrinkled, and dry (i.e., dry gangrene) may indicate vascular obstruction due to a vascular graft infection (VGI).

2. **Cardiovascular examination.** Auscultation may be helpful in the identification of a new or changing murmur that may suggest endocarditis. While not commonly associated with intravascular device infections, splenomegaly may suggest endocarditis. Diminished or absence of arterial pulsations in the radial, femoral, popliteal, dorsalis pedis, or posterior tibial arteries may suggest vascular graft occlusion due to infection.

3. **Pulmonary examination.** Examination findings of pulmonary infection (e.g., egophony, bronchial breath sounds, or percussion dullness) may suggest pacemaker or ICD endocarditis due to pulmonary septic emboli.

4. **Musculoskeletal examination.** New or changing bone pain or joint swelling and pain associated with a diminished range of motion may be a distant infection (e.g., osteomyelitis or septic arthritis) associated with an intravascular device infection.

C. **Laboratory and Radiologic Studies**

1. **Complete blood count (CBC).** Commonly ordered and may demonstrate anemia of chronic disease, leukocytosis, leukopenia, and/or thrombocytopenia or thrombocytosis.

2. **Complete metabolic profile (CMP).** Useful for calculating renal clearance for antimicrobial therapy.

3. **Blood cultures.** All patients should have two to three sets ordered prior to initiation of antimicrobial therapy. *Blood cultures should also be repeated 48 to 72 hours after device removal.*

4. **Erythrocyte sedimentation rate (ESR), C-reactive protein (CRP), and rheumatoid factor.** Useful in evaluating for endocarditis.

5. **Prothrombin time/partial thromboplastin time/international normalized ratio (PT/PTT/INR).** Useful for patients considered to undergo removal of the device.

6. **Culture.** Generator-pocket tissue (2 cm) or device lead tips should be submitted for Gram stain and culture.

7. **Echocardiography.** All patients should undergo transesophageal echocardiography (TEE). A mass adherent to an implantable lead is usually either a thrombus or infected vegetation. While the majority are vegetations (95%), it is impossible to distinguish the two by echocardiography alone.

8. **Chest imaging (e.g., plain-film or computed tomography).** May be helpful in the evaluation for the presence of septic pulmonary emboli.

VII. TREATMENT. Initial antimicrobial treatment of an intravascular device–related infection should initially involve empirical broad-spectrum antimicrobial therapy that is administered parenterally (i.e., intravenously) and is deemed bactericidal.

Complete removal of the infected medical device (e.g., generator, leads), if possible, is preferable as treatment success is greatly improved with minimal to no relapse.

Once a pathogen is identified, antimicrobial therapy should be guided by the in vitro antimicrobial susceptibility tests. Goal-directed therapy many involve the following:

A. *Staphylococcus aureus**

1. *Methicillin-susceptible Staphylococcus aureus (MSSA)*—nafcillin 2 g every 4 hours IV

2. *Methicillin-resistant Staphylococcus aureus (MRSA)*—vancomycin 15 mg/kg every 12 hours IV (presuming normal renal function)

B. *Staphylococcus epidermidis** (Coagulase-Negative *Staphylococcus*)

1. *Methicillin-susceptible Staphylococcus epidermidis (MSSE)*—nafcillin 2 g every 4 hours IV

2. *Methicillin-resistant Staphylococcus epidermidis (MRSE)*—vancomycin 15 mg/kg every 12 hours IV (presuming normal renal function)

C. *Corynebacterium* spp (e.g., *C. jeikeium* and *C. amycolatum*). Vancomycin 15 mg/kg every 12 hours IV (presuming normal renal function).

D. Enteric Gram-Negative Bacilli (e.g., *Enterobacter* spp, *Klebsiella* spp, *Acinetobacter* spp, *Serratia* spp, *Citrobacter* spp, and *Proteus* spp). Ceftriaxone 2 g daily, cefepime 2 g twice daily, meropenem 1 g every 8 hours or ertapenem 1 g daily (carbapenem antibiotics are typically reserved for infections with multidrug-resistant pathogens), or cipro 500 mg twice daily or moxifloxacin 400 mg daily.

E. *Pseudomonas aeruginosa.* Cefepime 2 g every 8 hours, meropenem 1 g every 8 hours, cipro 400 mg IV every 8 hours, or piperacillin/tazobactam 4.5 g IV every 6 hours.

---

*If the infected intravascular device was recently placed (less than 1 month) and cannot be removed, physicians may consider adding **rifampin** 300 mg three times daily or 450 mg twice daily for biofilm penetration.

F. Fungal. Amphotericin B (lipid 5 mg/kg/day; liposomal 3–5 mg/kg/day; colloidal 3–4 mg/kg/day) is used for molds such as *Aspergillus* spp. Fluconazole (used for fluconazole-susceptible *Candida* spp) 400 mg daily PO or micafungin 100 mg daily (IV; used for fluconazole-resistant *Candida* spp).

There are no clinical trial data to define the *optimal duration of therapy*. The following are general expert recommendations for prosthetic devices (e.g., pacemaker, ICD, or LVAD):

1. **Pocket-site limited erosion (e.g., no symptoms or signs of infection).** 7 to 10 days of therapy after device removal.

2. **Pocket-site limited infection (e.g., infection but no bloodstream or other complications).** 10 to 14 days of therapy after device removal.

3. **Device infection associated with bacteremia only.** 14 days of therapy after device removal and from the first set of negative blood cultures.

4. **Device infection associated with persistent bacteremia (greater than 24 hours after device removal) and no evidence of endocarditis.** 14 days of therapy from the first set of negative blood cultures for non–*Staphylococcus aureus* infection. 14 to 28 days of therapy from the first set of negative blood cultures for *Staphylococcus aureus*–related infections.

5. **Device infection associated with persistent bacteremia (greater than 24 hours after device removal) with evidence of endocarditis, septic venous thrombosis, and/or osteomyelitis.** Six weeks of antimicrobial therapy has been suggested from the first set of negative blood cultures.

6. **Device infection in which the device cannot be removed.** Long-term suppressive antimicrobial therapy (following standard antibiotic therapy as noted previously) is a useful treatment option for selected patients for whom removal of the device is not possible.

There are no clinical trial data to define the optimal duration of therapy for VGIs; however, Table 9.1 provides the general expert recommendations for VGIs.

TABLE 9.1 ■ Treatment Recommendations for Vascular Graft Infections

Infection Grade	Samson Classification	Duration of Antimicrobial Therapy
I and II	Infections extend no deeper than the dermis and do not directly come into contact with the vascular graft	2–4 weeks IV/PO
III and IV	Infections directly contact the vascular graft but not at the anastomosis site and are without bleeding and/or bacteremia	4–6 weeks IV followed by 3–6 months of PO
V	Infections involve the anastomosis site and are associated with bleeding, bacteremia, and/or sepsis	4–6 weeks IV followed by 6 months of PO

Note: Lifelong antimicrobial suppression therapy should be considered for patients who are poor candidates for reoperation, patients with multiple recurrent vascular graft infections, and infections involving MRSA/MSSA, *Pseudomonas* spp, multidrug-resistant pathogens, and *Candida* spp.

MRSA, methicillin-resistant *Staphylococcus aureus*; MSSA, methicillin-susceptible *Staphylococcus aureus*.

Source: Wilson WR, Bower TC, Creager MA, et al. Vascular Graft Infections, Mycotic Aneurysms, and Endovascular Infections: a scientific statement from the American Heart Association. *Circulation.* 2016;134(20):e412–e460.

Once an infected device is completely removed, patients should be reevaluated for the continued need of an implantable device. If the patient does have ongoing need for a device, then a new device should be placed at an alternative location to the original infected device. In general, blood cultures should be negative for a minimum of 72 hours prior to implantation of a new device. The exception to this rule is the delay of implantation for 14 days when there is valvular endocarditis and the need for new transvenous lead placement.

BIBLIOGRAPHY

Baddour LM, Bettmann MA, Bolger AF, et al. Nonvalvular cardiovascular device-related infections. *Circulation*, 2003;108(16):2015–2031.

Baddour LM, Epstein AE, Erickson CC, et al. Update on cardiovascular implantable electronic device infections and their management: a scientific statement from the American Heart Association. *Circulation*. 2010;121(3):458–477.

Gandelman G, Frishman WH, Wiese C, et al. Intravascular device infections: epidemiology, diagnosis, and management. *Cardiol Rev*. 2007;15(1):13–23.

Gandhi T, Crawford T, Riddell J IV. Cardiovascular implantable electronic device associated infections. *Infect Dis Clin North Am*. 2012;26(1):57–76.

Sandoe JA, Barlow G, Chambers JB, et al.. Guidelines for the diagnosis, prevention and management of implantable cardiac electronic device infection. Report of a joint Working Party project on behalf of the British Society for Antimicrobial Chemotherapy (BSAC, host organization), British Heart Rhythm Society (BHRS), British Cardiovascular Society (BCS), British Heart Valve Society (BHVS) and British Society for Echocardiography (BSE). *J Antimicrob Chemother*. 2015;70(2):325–359.

Wilson WR, Bower TC, Creager MA, et al. Vascular graft infections, mycotic aneurysms, and endovascular infections: a scientific statement from the American Heart Association. *Circulation*. 2016;134(20):e412–e460.

10

INFECTIONS INVOLVING INTRAVASCULAR CATHETERS AND SUPPURATIVE THROMBOPHLEBITIS

Eric Cox
Kerri A. Thom

I. INTRODUCTION

A. Definition and Classifications. Intravascular Catheter–Related Bloodstream Infections (CRBSIs) are defined as primary bloodstream infections (e.g., those not due to another identifiable source) that occur while a central catheter is in place (usually 48 hours after having the catheter).

1. **Types of Catheters.** Infections involving intravascular catheters are a diverse clinical entity involving peripheral, arterial, or central venous catheters and may include both temporary and tunneled catheters. Types of commonly used catheters include (from lowest to highest infection risk):

   a. **Peripheral venous or arterial catheter.** Usually placed in a peripheral vein of the hand or arm and intended for short-term (i.e., 3–5 days) use but does not enter the central vessels (i.e., superior vena cava).

   b. **Midline catheter.** Usually placed through the antecubital fossa into the proximal basilic or cephalic veins but does *not* enter the central vessels (i.e., superior vena cava).

   c. **Peripherally inserted central catheter (PICC line).** These catheters are becoming more widely used for home-infusion therapy (especially antibiotics) and are usually placed through the antecubital fossa into the basilic or cephalic veins to the superior vena cava.

   d. **Surgically implanted central venous catheters (CVCs; e.g., Hickman, Broviac, or Groshong).** Commonly used for chemotherapy and/or hemodialysis.

2. **Long-Term Versus Short-Term Catheter Criteria.** Classifying catheters as long term or short term is important for assessing the risk of infection and treatment recommendations. In general, long-term catheters have a higher risk of infection.

   a. **Long-term catheters** (e.g., those that have been indwelling for greater than or equal to 14 days). Typically are surgically implanted catheters (e.g., Hickman, Broviac, or Groshong catheter) with the tunneled portion exiting the skin and Dacron cuff just inside the exit site. They are used to provide vascular access to patients who require prolonged chemotherapy, home-infusion therapy, or hemodialysis.

b. **Short-term catheters**. Typically are nonsurgically implanted catheters (e.g., PICC, subclavian, or jugular vein catheters). They may be used to provide vascular access to patients who require intensive care unit care.

3. **Further Important Definitions.** Infections related to vascular catheters include phlebitis, exit- and tunnel-site infections, pocket infections of a totally implantable device (i.e., medical port), and bloodstream infections. Common definitions relating to these infections include:

   a. **Colonization.** Significant growth of a microorganism that is confined to the catheter and without symptoms or signs of infection.

   b. **Phlebitis.** Skin infection (e.g., erythema, warmth, tenderness, and swelling) along the tract of the catheterized vessel. Phlebitis involving short-term, peripheral intravenous catheters is typically not a result of catheter-related infections.

   c. **Exit-site infection.** Skin infection located within 2 cm at the exit site of the catheter (may or may not be associated with purulent drainage and fever).

   d. **Tunnel-site infection.** Skin infection that extends beyond 2 cm at the exit site of the catheter.

   e. **Infusate-related infection.** Concordant growth of a microorganism from infusate and cultures of percutaneously obtained blood cultures with no other identifiable source of infection.

B. Epidemiology and Risk Factors

1. More than 150 million intravascular catheters are used and as many as 250,000 bloodstream infections are occurring in U.S. hospitals each year (estimated incidence 0.1–2.7 per 1,000 line days), increasing the economic burden to our strained medical system. Catheter-related infections have been associated with an attributable mortality rate as high as 25% and thus may be responsible for nearly 20,000 deaths annually. Further, they lead to increased hospital length of stay and may cost an additional $4,000 to $56,000 per episode as these infections may also include endovascular or metastatic infections such as *suppurative thrombophlebitis, endocarditis*, and/or *osteomyelitis*.

2. **Risk factors** include: catheter type (see the preceding), catheter duration, breaks in aseptic techniques, anatomic location (e.g., groin/femoral [highest], neck/jugular [intermediate], and subclavian [lowest]), and patient-related factors (e.g., severity of illness, neutropenia, compromised skin integrity, and distant infection).

C. Pathogenesis. The four main routes of catheter contamination that can lead to infection include:

1. Migration of skin flora into insertion site and subsequent colonization of the tip of the catheter—the most common route of short-term catheter infections.

2. Direct contamination of the catheter hub by contact with healthcare worker hands or other contaminated fluids or devices.

3. Hematogenous spread from a distant site, leading to seeding of the catheter.

4. Rarely, infusion of contaminated products can lead to catheter infection.

II. MICROBIAL CAUSES OF CENTRAL CATHETER INFECTIONS

A. **Gram-Positive Cocci** including coagulase-negative *Staphylococcus* spp and *Staphylococcus aureus*—methicillin-sensitive (*methicillin-susceptible Staphylococcus aureus* [MSSA]) and methicillin-resistant strains (*methicillin-resistant Staphylococcus aureus* [MRSA])—are the most commonly identified pathogens. Other common gram-positive agents include: *Enterococcus* spp and *Streptococcus* spp.

B. **Gram-Negative Bacilli** comprise about 20% of catheter infections, including *Klebsiella* spp, *Enterobacter* spp, *Serratia* spp, *Pseudomonas* spp, *Proteus* spp, *Providencia* spp, *Acinetobacter* spp, and *Stenotrophomonas maltophilia* (usually associated with catheters used in the groin/femoral position, cancer patients, or rarely infusate contamination).

C. **Fungal** agents most commonly include *Candida* spp (usually associated with catheters in the groin/femoral position or catheters used for parenteral nutrition). Additionally, *Malassezia furfur* is commonly associated with infusion of intravenous lipid components.

III. CLINICAL MANIFESTATIONS OF CATHETER INFECTIONS

A. In cases of **local infection**, for example exit-site infection, tunnel infection, or pocket infection, clinical signs and symptoms including erythema, warmth, and tenderness over the area may be present. Purulence can be expressed from the exit site. If thrombophlebitis occurs, a palpable cord can be present. Purulence at the exit site or a palpable cord should raise suspicion for underlying septic thrombophlebitis.

B. In **CRBSI (e.g., bacteremia)**, often there are no physical examination findings at the catheter site. Patients may present primarily with nonspecific signs and symptoms such as fever, chills/rigors, tachycardia, tachypnea, or manifestations of sepsis (see Chapter 47). Catheter malfunction or systemic symptoms including rigors and fevers after catheter manipulation may raise suspicion of a catheter infection.

IV. APPROACH TO THE PATIENT

A. **History.** *A complete and chronologically accurate history should be obtained* as presenting symptoms may be nonspecific; therefore, any infectious workup in a patient with an intravascular catheter needs to consider catheter-related infections in the differential diagnosis. Rarely the patient or nursing staff will notify the clinician to a local-site infection. In dialysis patients, a thorough history spanning the last several sessions may reveal rigors, fever, low blood pressures, or malaise while the catheter is being manipulated by the technician. Fever may be the only presenting symptom in many cases.

B. **Physical Examination.** *A complete physical examination should be performed,* with a focus on all catheter devices and the skin surrounding the device as well as attempts to palpate for venous cords to evaluate for thrombophlebitis. Fever, tachycardia, and the patient's general appearance will also guide the clinician on the severity of the possible infection. In the majority of cases, the only sign or symptom that is present is fever.

V. LABORATORY STUDIES

A. **Complete Blood Count (CBC) With Differential.** Commonly ordered and may demonstrate leukocytosis with polymorphonuclear leukocyte predominance.

B. **Basic Metabolic Panel (BMP).** Commonly ordered and may be used for estimating the renal clearance for therapy.

C. **Blood Culture.** Most commonly ordered and any positive blood culture sample should raise concern for central line infection. ***Two sets of blood cultures (i.e., one set is defined as one aerobic bottle and one anaerobic bottle).***

Skin preparation for obtaining percutaneously drawn blood samples should be performed carefully, with use of either alcohol or tincture of iodine or alcoholic chlorhexidine; allow adequate skin contact and drying times to mitigate blood culture contamination. If a blood sample is obtained through a catheter, clean the catheter hub with either alcohol or tincture of iodine or alcoholic chlorhexidine, allowing adequate drying time to mitigate blood culture contamination.

Blood cultures should be repeated if they are initially positive to ensure that the bacteremia has resolved and to determine the duration of treatment.

The definitive diagnosis of a catheter-related bloodstream infection requires any one of the following:

1. ***That a peripheral percutaneous blood culture and a catheter-tip culture grow the same pathogen.***

2. ***That a peripheral percutaneous blood culture and a catheter-lumen culture grow the same pathogen, with culture growth detected 2 hours earlier from the catheter-lumen sample.***

3. ***That a peripheral percutaneous blood culture and a catheter-lumen culture grow the same pathogen, with culture growth detected at a quantity of threefold greater from the catheter-lumen sample.***

D. **Catheter-Tip Culture.** *In patients with sepsis* (see Chapter 47) *with suspected catheter-related infection, the device should be removed.* Consider culturing the catheter tip if the catheter is removed for suspected infection; bacterial growth of greater than 15 colony-forming units (CFUs) using the roll tip method or greater than 10^2 CFUs using quantitative broth culture is consistent with catheter colonization and suggestive of catheter-related infection in the appropriate clinical setting. *A positive catheter tip without other signs of infection is not necessarily indicative of a central-line infection.*

E. **Swab Microbiology Culture.** When there is a catheter-exit-site exudate, swab the drainage to collect specimens for Gram stain and culture.

F. **Erythrocyte Sedimentation Rate (ESR), C-Reactive Protein (CRP), and Rheumatoid Factor.** May be helpful in the evaluation of complications such as suppurative thrombophlebitis, endocarditis, or osteomyelitis.

G. **Prothrombin Time (PT)/Partial Thromboplastin Time (PTT)/International Normalized Ratio (INR).** Useful if a surgically implanted CVC needs to be removed.

VI. RADIOLOGIC STUDIES

A. **Ultrasound.** May be useful to evaluate for thrombophlebitis.

B. **Plain-Film Chest Imaging or CT.** Can aid in evaluating for septic emboli to the lungs.

C. **Echocardiography.** Should be obtained if concern for intracardiac focus of infection (e.g., if there is evidence for persistent bacteremia or embolic disease).

Transesophageal echocardiogram is preferred and should be performed for the following reasons:

1. Persistent bacteremia or fungemia with or without a fever more than 72 hours after catheter removal or appropriate antimicrobial therapy.

2. Patients with a prosthetic heart valve, pacemaker, or implantable defibrillator.

VII. PREVENTION.
As many *CVC infections are preventable,* a healthcare systemwide approach on prevention should be implemented. Many hospitals and medical centers are "bundling" some of the interventions described in the following; these strategies have been highly effective in reducing or, in some cases, nearly eliminating central-line-associated bloodstream infections.

A. Insertion

1. Review the risk and benefits of **CVC** placement, especially procedural complications.

2. **The preferred site for catheter placement is the subclavian vein.** *Femoral vein access should be avoided whenever possible, as it is associated with the highest rates of both mechanical and infectious complications.* Subclavian vein stenosis can occur from CVC placement and alternate sites should be sought in patients with end-stage renal disease. **PICCs** are not associated with reduced risk of infection among hospitalized patients.

3. **Tunneled lines have lower risks of infections** compared to temporary catheters and may be considered if the need for long-term access is anticipated.

4. Ultrasound guidance should be used when possible to reduce the risk of complications from multiple attempts.

5. *Proper handwashing with soap and water or an alcohol-based solution should be used before and after placement of a catheter.*

6. For placement of a new CVC or PICC as well as for guide wire exchanges, maximal barriers including mask, cap, sterile gown and gloves, and sterile drape should be used.

7. Chlorhexidine solutions have been shown to be more efficacious than other cleansers, and should be used primarily unless they are contraindicated.

8. Catheters with antimicrobial- or antiseptic-impregnated material can be used in institutions where the rate of CRBSI is not decreasing after a comprehensive strategy to reduce infection rates has been employed, including maximal sterile barrier precautions, use of greater than 0.5% chlorhexidine solution with alcohol, and provider education on insertion of catheters.

9. Use of **systemic antibiotics** is *not* recommended to *prevent* catheter-related infections.

10. **For arterial catheters, preferred sites include radial, brachial, or dorsalis pedis over femoral or axillary locations to reduce risk of infection.** During insertion, a cap, mask, and sterile gloves and a small drape should be used. If femoral or axillary sites are chosen, maximal sterile precautions are needed.

B. Catheter Maintenance

1. CVCs should be removed as soon as possible and when no longer clinically indicated.

2. If CVCs are placed during emergent situations (e.g., during cardiopulmonary resuscitation [CPR]) and sterile technique cannot be ensured, the catheter should be replaced as soon as possible and under sterile conditions.

3. *Daily inspection of catheters* should be performed to assess for induration or pain at insertion site, which might suggest infection.

4. *Whenever possible, sponge dressings impregnated with chlorhexidine gluconate should be used*; in cases where this is not indicated, sterile gauze or a transparent semipermeable dressing can cover the catheter. Dressings generally are not required for tunneled catheters once the insertion site has healed.

5. *Antibiotic ointments* can promote fungal infections and antimicrobial resistance and should *not* be used.

6. *Catheters should **not** be submerged in water.* For showering, the catheter should have a waterproof dressing applied.

7. Daily bathing of patients with a 2% chlorhexidine solution may prevent catheter infections in certain patient populations.

8. Replacement *of central catheters to prevent infection is not routinely recommended in asymptomatic patients.* In patients with fever, clinical judgment and physical examination findings should guide the need to remove the catheter but do not necessarily warrant removal.

9. *Guide wire exchanges are not recommended for routine exchange of nontunneled catheters to prevent infection or in cases of a suspected catheter infection.* It is reasonable to use a guide wire exchange approach when the catheter is malfunctioning when no signs of active infection are present; however, maximal sterile precautions should be taken with any guide wire exchange.

10. Replace arterial catheters only if they are malfunctioning and remove as soon as they are not needed. Manipulations and samplings from the system should be minimized.

VIII. TREATMENT. *Often, removal of the affected catheter is curative.*

A. Blood cultures should be obtained before antibiotics are administered.

B. Empiric antimicrobial therapy should have activity against common hospital-acquired pathogens, including MRSA and *Pseudomonas aeruginosa*, and should be guided by local epidemiology and antimicrobial susceptibility. Some possible regimens are outlined in the following.

1. *Empiric regimens.* Vancomycin 15 mg/kg IV q12–24 is preferred for MRSA and coagulase-negative *Staphylococcus plus* an anti-*Pseudomonas* agent, such as piperacillin–tazobactam 4.5 g IV q6, if there is concern for gram-negative pathogens.

   For vancomycin-resistant *Enterococcus*, we would recommend daptomycin 6 mg/kg IV q24–48 over linezolid 600 mg IV q12, as it is bactericidal.

Regarding fungal-related infections, we would recommend use of an echinocandin, such as micafungin 100 mg IV q24, initially to cover for fluconazole-resistant *Candida* spp, such as *C. glabrata*. Fluconazole can be used for patients without azole exposure in the previous 3 months and in healthcare settings where the risk of *Candida krusei* or *Candida glabrata* infection is very low.

2. **Suggested tailored regimens.** The empiric regimen should be tailored based on the culture data and the antibiotic susceptibility results once available; typically, an appropriate agent with the narrowest spectrum should be selected. A regimen commonly used for certain pathogens includes:

   a. **Staphylococcus spp**

      i. **MSSA.** Nafcillin 2 g IV q4, oxacillin 2 g IV q4, or cefazolin 2 g IV q8. For cefazolin and hemodialysis related infections, use a dosage of 20 mg/kg (actual body weight), rounded to the nearest 500-mg increment, after dialysis.

      ii. **MRSA.** Vancomycin 15 mg/kg IV q12–24 or daptomycin 6 mg/kg IV q24–48 (should be dosed after hemodialysis sessions).

   b. **Enterococcus spp**

      i. **Ampicillin-sensitive.** Ampicillin 2 g IV q4–6 plus gentamicin 1 mg/kg IV q8

      ii. **Ampicillin-resistant.** Vancomycin 15 mg/kg IV q12–24 plus gentamicin 1 mg/kg IV q8

      iii. **Vancomycin-resistant.** Daptomycin 6 mg/kg IV q24–28 or linezolid 600 mg IV q12

   c. **Pseudomonas aeruginosa.** Cefepime 2 g IV q8, piperacillin–tazobactam 4.5 g IV q6, meropenem 1 g IV q8, or imipenem–cilastatin 500 mg IV q6

   d. **Enteric gram-negative species (e.g., E coli, Klebsiella, Enterobacter).** Ceftriaxone 1–2 g IV q24 (if susceptible), ertapenem 1 g IV q24, meropenem 1 g IV q8, imipenem–cilastatin 500 mg IV q6, or doripenem 500 mg IV q8

   e. **Stenotrophomonas maltophilia.** Trimethoprim–sulfamethoxazole 3–5 mg/kg IV q8

   f. **Malassezia furfur.** Lipid-based or liposomal complex amphotericin B 3–5 mg/kg or voriconazole 6 mg/kg IV q12 for 2 doses, then 4 mg/kg IV q12

3. **Duration of antibiotic therapy.** This depends on the factors of long-term versus short-term catheter, complicated versus noncomplicated infection, and infecting pathogen. When denoting duration of antimicrobial therapy, day 1 is the first day on which negative blood culture results are obtained.

   a. **Short-term catheter infections**

      i. **Complicated infection** (i.e., patients with persistent fungemia or bacteremia after catheter removal [i.e., more than 72 hours], suppurative thrombophlebitis, endocarditis, and/or osteomyelitis). Remove CVC and treat with appropriate antimicrobial therapy and duration (endocarditis is treated for 4–6 weeks and osteomyelitis is treated for 6–8 weeks).

     ii. Uncomplicated **infection** (i.e., infection and fever resolve within 72 hours and no evidence of complicated infection). Catheter removal is recommended with appropriate systemic antimicrobial therapy. While coagulase-negative *Staphylococcus* species is managed with 5 to 7 days of antimicrobial therapy, *Staphylococcus aureus* and *Candida* species are treated for 14 days. *Enterococcus* species and gram-negative pathogens are managed with 7 to 14 days of systemic antimicrobial therapy.

  b. Long-term catheter infections

    i. Complicated infection (i.e., patients with persistent fungemia or bacteremia after catheter removal [i.e., more than 72 hours], suppurative thrombophlebitis, endocarditis, and/or osteomyelitis). Remove CVC and treat with appropriate antimicrobial therapy and duration (endocarditis is treated for 4–6 weeks and osteomyelitis is treated for 6–8 weeks). Tunnel-site infection and/or medical port site abscess is managed by removal of the catheter and 7 to 10 days of appropriate systemic antimicrobial therapy.

    ii. Uncomplicated infection (i.e., infection and fever resolve within 72 hours and no evidence of complicated infection). Catheter removal is generally recommended with appropriate systemic antimicrobial therapy. Recommendations by pathogen include the following:

- **Coagulase-negative *Staphylococcus*** species is managed with 10 to 14 days of antimicrobial therapy.

- ***Staphylococcus aureus*** species is managed with catheter removal and 4 to 6 weeks of antimicrobial therapy. A duration of 14 days may be considered if the patient DOES NOT have any of the following: diabetes mellitus, immunosuppression therapy (e.g., corticosteroids, chemotherapy, transplantation medications, chronic kidney disease, and chronic liver disease), neutropenia, or prosthetic intravascular device.

- ***Candida*** species are treated for 14 days with catheter removal.

- ***Enterococcus* species and gram-negative pathogens** are managed with catheter removal and 7 to 14 days of systemic antimicrobial therapy.

4. Hemodialysis catheter treatment considerations. The infected catheter should always be removed for patients with hemodialysis CRBSI due to *S. aureus, Pseudomonas* species, or *Candida* species and a temporary (non-tunneled) catheter should be inserted into another anatomical site. When a hemodialysis catheter is removed for CRBSI, a long-term hemodialysis catheter can be placed once blood cultures with negative results are obtained. For hemodialysis CRBSI due to other pathogens (e.g., gram-negative bacilli other than *Pseudomonas* species or coagulase-negative staphylococci), a patient can initiate empirical intravenous antibiotic therapy without immediate catheter removal. If the symptoms persist or if there is evidence of a metastatic infection, the catheter should be removed.

Surveillance blood cultures should be obtained 1 week after completion of an antibiotic course for CRBSI if the catheter has been retained.

5. **Suppurative thrombophlebitis** due to CRBSI should receive at least a minimum of 3 to 4 weeks of antimicrobial therapy. This complication should be suspected in patients with persistent bacteremia or fungemia (i.e., patients whose blood culture results remain positive after 3 days of adequate antimicrobial therapy) without another source of intravascular infection (e.g., endocarditis). A diagnosis of suppurative thrombophlebitis requires the presence of positive blood culture results *plus* the demonstration of a thrombus by radiographic testing (e.g., CT or ultrasonography). Surgical resection of the involved vein for patients with suppurative thrombophlebitis should be limited to patients with purulent superficial veins or patients in whom the infection extends beyond the vessel wall, as well as patients who experience failure of conservative therapy with an appropriate antimicrobial regimen.

BIBLIOGRAPHY

Blot SI, Depuydt P, Annemans L, et al. Clinical and economic outcomes in critically ill patients with nosocomial catheter-related bloodstream infections. *Clin Infect Dis*. 2005;41:1591–1598.

Mermel LA, Allon M, Bouza E, et al. Clinical practice guidelines for the diagnosis and management of intravascular catheter-related infection: 2009 Update by the Infectious Diseases Society of America. *Clin Infect Dis*. 2009;49:1–45.

O'Grady NP, Alexander M, Burns LA, et al. Guidelines for the prevention of intravascular catheter-related infections. *Clin Infect Dis*. 2011;52:e162–e193.

Walz JM, Memtsoudis SG, Heard SO. Prevention of central venous catheter bloodstream infections. *J Intensive Care Med*. 2010;25:131–138.

Weber DJ, Rutala WA. Central line-associated bloodstream infections: prevention and management. *Infect Dis Clin North Am*. 2011;25:77–102.

11

PNEUMONIA

Ulrike K. Buchwald
Devang M. Patel

I. INTRODUCTION

A. Definition. An acute or chronic inflammatory condition of the lower respiratory tract and lung parenchyma that is most commonly due to an infection and results in a clinical syndrome of respiratory symptoms such as cough, shortness of breath, and pleuritic chest pain associated with fever and malaise and accompanied by radiographic abnormalities.

B. Classification. Pneumonia is often classified by the setting, timing of infection, clinical presentation, infecting pathogen, radiographic pattern, or comorbid status of the patient.

1. **Place of acquisition of the infection.** This determines which pathogens are likely to cause the disease.

   a. **Community-acquired pneumonia (CAP)** occurs without prior contact to the healthcare system in the *outpatient setting or within 48 hours* of hospital admission.

   b. **Hospital-acquired pneumonia (HAP)** is defined as a pneumonia that occurs *48 hours after admission* and was not incubating at the time of admission (e.g., no signs of pulmonary infection on hospital admission).

   c. **Ventilator-associated pneumonia (VAP)** occurs greater than or equal to 48 to 72 hours after endotracheal intubation.

   d. **Healthcare-associated pneumonia (HCAP)** occurs in a patient who had been hospitalized for more than 2 days duration within the last 90 days; is residing in a nursing home or long-term care facility; received intravenous antibiotics, chemotherapy, or wound care in the last 30 days; and/or attended a hospital or hemodialysis clinic within 30 days.

2. **Typical versus atypical pneumonia syndrome.** This is a historical classification system that refers to the distinguishing clinical features of pneumonia syndromes that are often linked to particular pathogens. *Atypical pneumonia* syndromes are thought to have a less abrupt course than the *classic or typical lobar pneumonia* with constitutional and mild upper respiratory tract symptoms preceding the onset of pneumonia (which is often associated with a non-productive cough). The classic lobar pneumonia is associated with an acute respiratory illness characterized by prominent dyspnea and productive cough.

3. **Radiographic pattern**

   a. **Lobar pneumonia** is associated with a lobar pattern of opacity on the chest radiograph. It develops in the distal air spaces, spreads to the adjacent lung without primary involvement of the airways, and is classically associated with an air bronchogram.

b. **Bronchopneumonia** is often a nosocomial infection caused by aspiration of secretions from a colonized trachea. The chest radiograph commonly appears as multifocal opacities centered in the distal airways but without an air bronchogram.

c. **Interstitial pneumonia** is characterized by inflammation and edema within the pulmonary interstitium between alveolar walls and in peribronchovascular and perilymphatic tissue. It is most commonly associated with the atypical pneumonia syndrome; additional causes are respiratory viruses and *Pneumocystis jirovecii* in immunocompromised patients.

4. **Acute versus chronic pneumonia**

   a. **Acute pneumonia** has an abrupt onset, measured in days.

   b. **Chronic pneumonia** develops over weeks to months and can have an infectious or noninfectious etiology.

5. **Pneumonia in the immunocompromised patient.** The etiology depends on the nature of the immunosuppression (e.g., HIV infection, solid organ or stem cell transplantation, or corticosteroid therapy) and includes pathogens seen in the immunocompetent host but also other bacterial, viral, and fungal pathogens.

C. **Pathogenesis.** Pathogens enter the lower respiratory tract most commonly by *microaspiration* from a colonized oropharynx; however, *droplet inhalation of suspended aerosolized microorganisms* can play a role in the pathogenesis of certain infections (e.g., respiratory viruses, *Legionella* spp, and *Mycobacterium tuberculosis*). Additionally, in hospitalized patients (with or without mechanical ventilation), increased colonization of the lower airways precedes the development of pneumonia. Mechanical ventilation associated pneumonia is due to leakage of bacteria containing secretions around the endotracheal tube and/or embolization from infected biofilm on the tube, both of which allow entry of bacteria into the lower respiratory tract. *In general,* the development of pneumonia is due to a combination of a host defense defect, exposure to a virulent pathogen, and/or a high pathogen inoculum. Rarely, pneumonia can also result from a hematogenous or contiguous focus of infection (e.g., tricuspid valve endocarditis, Lemierre syndrome, hepatic abscess).

D. **Risk Factors**

1. **Community-acquired pneumonia.** Risk factors:

   a. Alcoholism and smoking; these are associated with a decreased cough and mucociliary clearance.

   b. Age greater than 65 years.

   c. Recent viral upper respiratory tract infection; influenza is classically followed by a bacterial pneumonia caused by *S. pneumoniae* or *S. aureus*.

   d. Underlying pulmonary diseases (e.g., chronic obstructive pulmonary disease [COPD], bronchiectasis, lung cancer).

   e. Immunosuppression (e.g., HIV infection, solid organ or stem cell transplantation, and chronic corticosteroid use).

f. Medical comorbid conditions (e.g., heart failure, chronic kidney disease, chronic liver disease, and diabetes mellitus); these are associated with altered immune defense and risk for increased colonization.

g. Proton-pump inhibitor therapy; initiation of treatment with these in the last 30 days might be associated with an increased risk of gastric bacterial colonization that can eventually be aspirated into the lungs.

h. Stroke or sedating medications; these are associated with altered levels of consciousness, decreased cough, and dysphagia (increases risk of aspiration).

2. **Hospital-acquired pneumonia/ventilator-associated pneumonia risk factors.** These risk factors often combine an increased aspiration risk, immunosuppression, colonization with more pathogenic microorganisms, and alteration of the respiratory tract:

   a. Severity of underlying illness (e.g., malnutrition, uremia, neutropenia)

   b. Prior surgery

   c. Prior and recent antibiotic administration

   d. Presence of invasive respiratory devices

   e. Supine positioning

   f. Enteral feeding with nasogastric or orogastric tubes

   g. Stress ulcer prophylaxis

   h. Blood transfusions

   i. Poor oral hygiene

II. MICROBIOLOGY OF PNEUMONIA

A. CAP-Related Microorganisms

1. *Streptococcus pneumoniae,* as the most common pathogen, accounts for 40% of all CAP in adults and is associated with bacteremia in 20% to 30% of cases. It is the prototype of acute lobar pneumonia and often follows a prior viral infection such as influenza. *Risk factors associated with drug-resistant* Streptococcus pneumoniae *(DRSP):*

   a. Age greater than 65 years

   b. History of alcoholism

   c. Antimicrobial therapy within 3 months

   d. Immunosuppression and/or significant comorbid medical conditions

   e. Exposure to children in daycare

2. *Staphylococcus aureus* is an uncommon cause of CAP in healthy adults but may occur following an influenza infection. It can cause a severe necrotizing pneumonia that often requires intensive care unit (ICU) admission.

3. *Klebsiella pneumoniae* can be seen in alcoholics or excessive smokers and in association with aspiration. It has a greater tendency for abscess formation.

4. Nontypeable *Haemophilus influenzae* and *Moraxella catarrhalis* can cause pneumonia in older adults and patients with COPD. The latter can also be a copathogen.

5. *Pseudomonas aeruginosa* is a rare pathogen in CAP except in patients with structural lung disease such as cystic fibrosis and bronchiectasis.

6. Atypical pneumonia microorganisms account for up to 60% and may be present as copathogens in 40% of cases. The most common microorganisms include:

    a. *Mycoplasma pneumoniae* is the most common pathogen and can be associated with pharyngitis and extrapulmonary manifestations (skin rashes, erythema multiforme, arthritis, and aseptic meningitis).

    b. *Chlamydophila pneumoniae* is the second most common pathogen and responsible for 10% of CAP, often as copathogen.

    c. *Legionella* spp may cause for 2% to 15% of CAP and is associated with outbreaks and travel. *L. pneumophila* serogroup 1 accounts for 70% to 80% of cases.

7. Respiratory viruses most commonly include influenza A and B (associated with upper respiratory tract infections that predispose to a secondary bacterial pneumonia; however, primary influenza pneumonia can be seen in patients at the extremes of age, with multiple comorbidities, and pregnant women), parainfluenza viruses, respiratory syncytial virus (RSV), adenovirus, coronaviruses, and human metapneumovirus (hMPV). Rare causes include hantavirus and avian influenza virus.

8. Fungal pathogens most commonly seen are *Cryptococcus neoformans* and the endemic mycoses *Histoplasma capsulatum*, *Blastomyces dermatitidis*, and *Coccidioides immitis*.

B. **Hospital-Acquired Pneumonia and Ventilatory-Associated Pneumonia Related Microorganisms.** Sources of microbes include healthcare devices, the hospital environment, and transfer of microorganisms between staff and patients. These microorganisms are increasingly associated with multidrug resistance. The risk of multidrug resistance is increased in patients who have been hospitalized for more than 5 days, had received antibiotics in the previous 90 days, are immunocompromised, and/or have risk factors associated with HCAP. Viral or fungal pathogens are uncommon immunocompetent hosts. The microbiology of both conditions is similar:

1. *Pseudomonas aeruginosa* (very common after more than 4 days of mechanical ventilation)

2. *Klebsiella pneumoniae*, *Escherichia coli*, *Enterobacter* spp, *Serratia* spp

3. *Acinetobacter baumannii* (commonly associated with prolonged mechanical ventilation and significant antimicrobial resistance)

4. *Stenotrophomonas maltophilia*

5. *Staphylococcus aureus*, especially methicillin-resistant *Staphylococcus aureus* (MRSA). Risk factors for this pathogen include prolonged hospitalization and mechanical ventilation, COPD, and prior corticosteroid use, diabetes mellitus, head trauma, hemodialysis, prior antimicrobial therapy, and/or ICU admission.

C. **Healthcare-Associated Pneumonia Related Microorganisms.** Microbial causes include most pathogens found in CAP, especially *S. pneumoniae*, *S. aureus*, and *P. aeruginosa*.

D. Pneumonia in the Immunocompromised Patient

1. *Pneumocystis jirovecii* remains one of the most important infections in HIV infected patients. The pneumonia is characterized by a subacute progressive exertional dyspnea and nonproductive cough. HIV-negative patients at risk are those with: lymphoma, systemic lupus erythematosus, solid organ or stem cell transplantation, and long-term corticosteroid therapy (equivalent of greater than 20 mg prednisone for more than 3 months).

2. *Mycobacterium tuberculosis* should be considered as a possible etiology of pneumonia and other pulmonary parenchymal abnormalities (most commonly a cavity lung lesion) in patients at risk (see Chapter 14, Tuberculosis).

3. *Nocardia* spp can cause localized infiltrates, nodules, and cavitary lung lesions in patients with lymphoma, solid organ or stem cell transplantation, long-term corticosteroid therapy, collagen vascular disease, COPD, and pulmonary alveolar proteinosis.

4. *Rhodococcus equi* is most commonly seen in AIDS patients with a presentation similar to tuberculosis.

5. *Aspergillus* spp and other opportunistic molds (such as Zygomycetes) can cause a bronchopneumonia in patients with neutropenia (following chemotherapy or hematopoietic stem cell transplantation). These infections can be associated with angioinvasion and pulmonary infarction.

6. Reactivation of *herpesviruses* (cytomegalovirus [CMV], herpes simplex virus [HSV], and varicella-zoster virus [VZV]) can lead to pneumonia in immunocompromised patients.

7. Endemic fungi such as *Histoplasma, Coccidioides,* and *Blastomyces* are of concern in patients treated with *tumor necrosis factor* (TNF) alpha antagonists.

8. Rare pathogens include *Toxoplasma gondii* and *Strongyloides stercoralis.*

III. CLINICAL MANIFESTATIONS

A. Community-Acquired Pneumonia

1. **Typical.** The classic pneumonia presentation is an acute onset of cough productive of purulent sputum, fever, chills, chest pain, and/or dyspnea. This is usually associated with a lobar pneumonia pattern on chest radiography. While hemoptysis is a nonspecific manifestation, it may suggest a necrotizing pneumonia.

2. **Atypical.** This is usually a subacute process associated with malaise, cough, and fever. *Mycoplasma pneumoniae* represents the classic "walking pneumonia" in a young, otherwise healthy individual.

   Elderly and immunocompromised patients may present with subtle and nonrespiratory symptoms such as lethargy or delirium, poor oral intake, and decompensation of other comorbid medical conditions.

B. Healthcare-Associated Pneumonia/Hospital-Acquired Pneumonia/Ventilator-Associated Pneumonia. These may present with a new onset of nosocomial fever, new or increasingly purulent pulmonary secretions, new or increased leukocytosis, and a decline in oxygenation. VAP may also manifest as an increased need for mechanical ventilator support and/or pulmonary suction requirements.

IV. APPROACH TO THE PATIENT

A. **History.** A complete and chronologically accurate history should be obtained in all patients suspected of pneumonia. The history should focus on the timing of events, risk factors, comorbid conditions, smoking status, travel history, medication allergies, recent pulmonary infections, and recent antimicrobial therapy. The vaccination status for influenza and *S. pneumoniae* should be assessed.

B. **Physical Examination.** While a complete physical examination should always be performed, the physical examination should emphasize these areas:

1. **Vital signs.** Tachypnea and hypoxemia are common with all types of pneumonia but most pronounced with *Pneumocystis jirovecii* pneumonia. A respiratory rate greater than 30 breaths per minute, hypotension requiring aggressive fluid resuscitation, fever greater than 40°C, or hypothermia less than 36°C indicate more severe disease with possible poor outcome.

2. **Head, eyes, ears, nose, and throat (HEENT) examination.** Bullous myringitis and cervical lymphadenopathy may be seen with *Mycoplasma pneumoniae* infection.

3. **Pulmonary examination.** Lung consolidation typically produces these findings on examination:

   a. **Inspection.** Nasal flaring, intercostal retractions, chest splinting, and cyanosis may be present and indicate respiratory distress.

   b. **Palpation and percussion.** Consolidation of the lung is associated with *normal or increased fremitus* (chest wall vibrations produced by sound generated in the larynx) and *dullness to percussion.*

   c. **Auscultation.** Consolidation of the lung is associated with *bronchial breath sounds, increased vocal resonance, bronchophony or egophony,* and *inspiratory crackles.*

Lobar pneumonia will have signs of consolidation (e.g., crackles, dullness to percussion, and egophony). **Atypical pneumonia** may only have crackles while an interstitial pneumonia may present without any lung abnormalities on physical examination.

C. **Laboratory Studies.** *Routine diagnostic tests to identify the etiologic pathogen of CAP may be optional in the management of outpatients with CAP if they would not significantly change therapeutic decisions but are recommended if the result would impact therapy.* The collection of sputum for Gram stain and culture and of blood cultures is recommended before treatment initiation for hospitalized patients with CAP, in the presence of comorbidities (e.g., alcohol abuse, liver disease, asplenia, COPD) or certain clinical findings (e.g., pleural effusion, cavitary lung disease), with a history of recent travel, or with any clinical or epidemiologic suspicion for unusual pathogens. Blood cultures and lower respiratory tract specimens should be obtained in all patients with suspicion for HAP/VAP/HCAP.

1. **Sputum Gram stain** is the most important initial step to sputum analysis. *A sputum sample of good quality should have less than 10 squamous epithelial cells; the presence of greater than 25 neutrophils per low-power microscopic field supports infection rather than airway colonization.* In general, gram-positive cocci arranged in pairs suggest *S. pneumoniae* while gram-positive

cocci arranged in clusters suggest *S. aureus*. While gram-negative rods may also be observed (especially in nosocomial infections), the Gram stain is negative in atypical pneumonia.

2. **Special sputum stains** may be required, such as Ziehl–Neelsen for acid-fast bacilli or silver stain for *Pneumocystis jirovecii* and fungal pathogens.

3. **Sputum cultures** are reported in a semiquantitative manner using standard microbiology methods; however, fungal and mycobacterial pathogens require special cultures.

4. **Lower respiratory tract secretion samples should be obtained from all patients with suspected hospital- or ventilator-associated pneumonia prior to initiating antimicrobial therapy**. Respiratory samples can be collected by one of three common techniques, which include: blind tracheobronchial aspiration, bronchoalveolar lavage (BAL), and protected specimen brush (PSB). Quantitative cultures are established for each method:

    a. **Blind tracheobronchial aspiration**. The quantitative culture criterion is growth of more than *10^5 colony-forming units per milliliter* of sample. While false-negative rates are increased due to the blind nature of the technique, false-positive rates can occur from bacterial colonization within the proximal airways (i.e., contamination).

    b. **Bronchoalveolar lavage**. The quantitative culture criterion is growth of more than *10^4 colony-forming units per milliliter* of sample (sensitivity 93%; specificity 91%). While false-negative rates are decreased due to the nonblinded nature of the technique, false-positive rates can still occur from bacterial colonization within the proximal airways (i.e., contamination).

    c. **Protected specimen brush**. The quantitative culture criterion is growth of more than *10^3 colony-forming units per milliliter* of sample. The technique can be performed blindly or with bronchoscopic guidance in which case upper airway contamination may be reduced.

5. **Blood cultures** are recommended in all hospitalized patients and may be positive in 10% to 20% of bacterial infections. The presence of bacteremia in pneumococcal pneumonia suggests more severe disease. In suspected nosocomial infections, blood cultures may also reveal an extrapulmonary source of infection.

6. Antigen **tests** can be performed on urine for *L. pneumophila* serogroup 1 (sensitivity 70%–90%; specificity 99%) *S. pneumoniae* (sensitivity 50%–80%; specificity 90%); both tests should always be performed in patients with severe CAP. Several diagnostic antigen tests are Food and Drug Administration (FDA) approved for the diagnosis of influenza A and B from upper respiratory tract samples such as a nasal wash or aspirate (sensitivities 50%–70%; specificities 90%–95%). Fluorescence-based antigen tests can be performed on sputum and lower respiratory tract specimens for the diagnosis of *Pneumocystis jirovecii*. Antigen tests are also available for *Cryptococcus neoformans* (serum) and *Histoplasma capsulatum* (serum and urine).

7. **Polymerase chain reaction (PCR) testing** for *M. pneumoniae* may be available in some laboratories and used in combination to also identify

Chlamydophila spp but is poorly validated. One commercially available PCR probe has been FDA approved for detection of all serotypes of *Legionella pneumophila*, but clinical experience is lacking.

8. **Respiratory viral panel** may be ordered from either nasopharyngeal or lower respiratory tract secretions and uses PCR to identify common respiratory viruses (e.g., influenza, adenovirus, parainfluenza, and RSV). Commercially available tests have a sensitivity of 90% to 100% and specificity of 87% to 100%.

9. **Immunohistochemistry** can be performed on BAL specimens to detect viral infection such as CMV, VZV, or HSV.

10. **Histology** from a transbronchial biopsy is useful for detecting endemic fungal and mycobacterial pathogens.

11. **Acute-phase serologic testing** for specific pathogens is rarely helpful for patient management as antibiotic therapy will be completed before the matching convalescent sample can be obtained.

12. **Nonspecific laboratory studies include:**

    a. **Complete blood count (CBC)** is routinely ordered, and an elevated white blood cell (WBC) count is commonly observed in the majority of patients; however, *leukopenia* may be associated with severe *Streptococcus pneumoniae* infection. Both *thrombocytosis* and *thrombocytopenia* have been associated with an increased mortality in patients with CAP.

    b. **Complete metabolic profile (CMP)** is routinely ordered but nonspecific; however, a sodium level less than 130 mmol/L, (i.e., *hyponatremia*) or an elevated blood urea nitrogen (BUN) may indicate severe infection.

    c. **Erythrocyte sedimentation rate (ESR), C-reactive protein (CRP), and procalcitonin (PCT) level** may be ordered but are nonspecific; however, significantly elevated levels may suggest severe illness and/or increased mortality risk.

    d. **Oxygen saturation and arterial blood gas analysis** are important for management decisions (see the following).

13. **Pleural fluid analysis** is obtained by thoracentesis and may be required if the patient has a large pleural effusion and/or does not respond to appropriate antimicrobial therapy (see Chapter 12, Empyema).

D. **Radiologic Studies.** Radiographic evidence in association with symptoms and signs of pneumonia are paramount to establishing the diagnosis.

1. The *posterior–anterior and lateral plain-film radiographic technique* is the classic imaging modality for outpatients with CAP. However, this technique may be falsely negative in patients with severe dehydration, neutropenia, emphysema, or obesity. A chest film may be repeated after 24 to 48 hours in patients with a suspicion for pneumonia but with an initially negative study. In bedridden hospitalized patients, the anterior–posterior plain-film radiographic technique may have to be used, which may be less sensitive.

2. *CT scans* have better sensitivity in diagnosing pulmonary infiltrates and may be helpful in certain cases, especially in hospitalized patients and in subtle or early disease.

Characteristics that may appear on imaging include: lobar consolidation (classic CAP), patchy bilateral infiltrates (atypical or viral etiology CAP), dense consolidation with hilar lymphadenopathy (fungal or mycobacterial pneumonia), and cavitary disease (lung abscess, necrotizing pneumonia, and/or *Mycobacterium tuberculosis*).

V. DIAGNOSTIC CRITERIA. Pneumonia remains a clinical diagnosis suggested by a combination of systemic (e.g., fever) and respiratory (e.g., cough and dyspnea) symptoms, abnormal findings on lung examination. The clinical diagnosis for CAP has a sensitivity of 70% to 90% and a specificity of 40% to 70% and hence should be corroborated by radiographic studies. In the absence of clear imaging findings, the distinction from tracheobronchitis may be difficult. A microbiological diagnosis may or may not be obtained.

The diagnosis of HAP and VAP may be even more difficult as clinical findings such as fever, leukocytosis, tachypnea and tachycardia are often associated with many other conditions in hospitalized patients. Diagnostic scoring systems such as the clinical pulmonary infection score (CPIS) or the criteria for nosocomial pneumonia by the Centers for Disease Control and Prevention (CDC) may aid in the diagnosis. Frequent reevaluation of the clinical status and adjustment of therapy are particularly important in the management of the critically ill patient with suspected VAP.

Criteria for nosocomial pneumonia suggested by the CDC:

A. Radiology. At least one of the following: new, progressive, or persistent consolidation or cavity *and*

B. Clinical/Laboratory. At least one of the following: fever (without another defined focus); leukopenia or leukocytosis; or delirium *and*

C. Pulmonary. At least two of the following: new, changing, or progressive sputum; worsening cough and/or dyspnea; crackles or bronchial breath sounds; or worsening hypoxemia (or increased ventilation requirements)

VI. MANAGEMENT. The most important aspect of managing pneumonia is determining the severity of illness and the setting for which to provide treatment (e.g., outpatient or hospital).

A. Outpatient Management. Preferable in patients with CAP who do not meet criteria for inpatient admission. The recommendation for using empiric antimicrobial therapy is based on likely pathogens to cause infection as outlined the following:

1. Previously healthy patient without DRSP risks (see Section II.A.1).

    a. Azithromycin 500 mg PO daily *or*

    b. Doxycycline 100 mg PO BID

2. Presence of comorbidities and/or DRSP risks.

    a. Moxifloxacin 400 mg PO daily *or*

    b. Levofloxacin 750 mg PO daily *or*

    c. Amoxicillin 1 g PO TID *plus* azithromycin 500 mg PO daily *or* doxycycline 100 mg PO BID

B. **Inpatient Management.** Recommended for more severe illness. CURB-65 and Pneumonia Severity Index (PSI) are two different scoring systems used to assess severity of illness. **CURB-65** is more commonly used and assigns 1 point for each of the following criteria: **C**onfusion, **U**remia, **R**espiratory rate greater than 30, **B**lood pressure with systolic less than 90 mmHg or diastolic less than 60 mmHg, and age **65** or older. A score greater than 2 is associated with an increased mortality risk and therefore hospitalization is recommended. Management should include both supportive care and antimicrobial therapy as outlined in the following. The first dose of the antibiotic drug should be administered without delay:

1. **Inpatient, non-ICU setting**

   a. Moxifloxacin 400 mg PO/IV daily *or*

   b. Levofloxacin 750 mg PO/IV daily *or*

   c. Ceftriaxone 1 g IV daily *plus* azithromycin 500 mg PO/IV daily

2. **Inpatient, ICU setting**

   a. Risk factors for *Pseudomonas;* consider the following (gentamicin 5 mg/kg IV q24 can be added to these regimens):

      i. Piperacillin–tazobactam 4.5 g IV q6 *or*

      ii. Meropenem 500 mg IV q8 *or*

      iii. Cefepime 2 g IV q8 *or*

      iv. Aztreonam 2 g IV q8 (patients allergic to penicillin)

      plus

      i. Moxifloxacin 400 mg PO/IV daily *or*

      ii. Levofloxacin 750 mg PO/IV daily *or*

      iii. Ciprofloxacin 400 mg IV q12 *or*

      iv. Azithromycin 500 mg PO/IV daily

   b. Risk factors for *MRSA*; add the following to the aforementioned regimens:

      i. Vancomycin 15 mg/kg IV q12–24 *or*

      ii. Linezolid 600 mg PO/IV q12

C. **HCAP/HAP/VAP.** Broad-spectrum antimicrobial therapy is recommended initially as empirical therapy for the most likely causative pathogen. Empirical therapy should be based on the local antibiotic susceptibility patterns. Suggested empirical regimens include:

1. **Healthcare-associated or hospital-acquired pneumonia**

   a. Early onset (less than 5 days of hospitalization) and no multidrug resistance microorganism risks.

      i. Ceftriaxone 1 to 2 g IV daily *or*

      ii. Moxifloxacin 400 mg IV daily *or*

      iii. Levofloxacin 750 mg IV daily

   b. Late onset and multidrug resistance microorganism risks.

      i. Piperacillin–tazobactam 3.375–4.5 g IV q6 *or*

    ii. Cefepime 1–2 g IV q8–12 *or*

    iii. Ciprofloxacin 400 mg IV q12. Add vancomycin 15 mg/kg IV q12–24 *or*

    iv. Linezolid 600 mg IV q12 if concern for MRSA infection

  2. Ventilator-associated pneumonia. The suggested empirical regimen is the same as the preceding for nosocomial infections.

D. Influenza Pneumonia. Oseltamivir 75 mg PO BID for 5 days. It should be started within 48 hours of symptoms onset.

E. Immunocompromised Patients. Therapy is targeted to the causative pathogen, which may be bacterial, viral, fungal, or parasitic.

F. Management of Antibiotic Therapy

  1. Pathogen-directed therapy. Once culture results or other reliable microbiological methods reveal a specific etiology of pneumonia, antimicrobial therapy can be directed against this pathogen.

  2. Intravenous to oral switch. This can be done with the equivalent oral therapy once the patient is hemodynamically stable, clinically improving, and able to ingest and absorb medications.

  3. Discharge from the hospital. Patients can be discharged into a safe environment once they are clinically stable and have no other active medical problems.

  4. Length of antimicrobial therapy

    a. *CAP.* The treatment recommendation is for a minimum of 5 days. At therapy discontinuation patients should be afebrile for 48 to 72 hours and have stable vital signs and a normal mental status.

    b. *HCAP/HAP/VAP.* Most patients are successfully treated within 8 days; *P. aeruginosa*, *Acinetobacter* spp, or MRSA may require longer therapy (e.g., 14–21 days).

VII. PREVENTION. The main preventive measures for pneumonia involve vaccination for influenza and *Streptococcus pneumoniae* and—if applicable—**smoking cessation**.

A. Influenza Virus Vaccination. To permit time for production of protective antibody levels, vaccination optimally should occur before onset of influenza activity in the community. Vaccination providers should offer vaccination as soon as vaccine is available and vaccination should be offered throughout the influenza season. Available vaccine formulations are an inactivated trivalent vaccine, which is given intramuscularly and an intranasally administered live-attenuated vaccine, which is an alternative vaccine for healthy nonpregnant persons 2 to 49 years of age.

B. Streptococcus pneumoniae Vaccination. For the prevention of invasive pneumococcal disease, the pneumococcal polysaccharide vaccine is recommended for persons at or above 65 years of age and for those aged 19 to 64 years with selected high-risk concurrent diseases, according to current Advisory Committee on Immunization Practices (ACIP) guidelines. A one-time revaccination should be given to immunocompromised patients or those vaccinated prior to the age of 65 years. A protein polysaccharide conjugate vaccine has recently been approved for adults at or above 50 years of age for the prevention of pneumonia and invasive pneumococcal disease. Regularly updated ACIP guidelines can be viewed on the CDC website (www.cdc.gov). Specific recommendations are available for the sequential use of polysaccharide and conjugate vaccines.

Additional measures to prevent HAP or VAP include: standard hospital infection control practices, alcohol-based hand hygiene, aspiration precautions (i.e., elevation of the head of the bed to 30–45 degrees), oral hygiene (e.g., standard dental care and/or chlorhexidine oral care during hospitalization), removal or limiting of invasive devices, and antibiotic stewardship.

BIBLIOGRAPHY

American Thoracic Society, Infectious Diseases Society of America. Guidelines for the management of adults with hospital-acquired, ventilator-associated, and health care-associated pneumonia. *Am J Respir Crit Care Med*. 2005;171(4):388–416.

Kieninger AN, Lipsett PA. Hospital-acquired pneumonia: pathophysiology, diagnosis, and treatment. *Surg Clin North Am*. 2009;89(2):439–461.

Labelle A, Kollef MH. Healthcare-associated pneumonia: approach to management. *Clin Chest Med*. 2011;32(3):507–515.

Mandell LA, Wunderink RG, Anzueto A, et al. Infectious Diseases Society of America/American Thoracic Society consensus guidelines on the management of community-acquired pneumonia in adults. *Clin Infect Dis*. 2007;44(suppl 2):S27–S72.

Nair GB, Niederman MS. Community-acquired pneumonia: an unfinished battle. *Med Clin North Am*. 2011;95(6):1143–1161.

Reynolds JH, McDonald G, Alton H, Gordon SB. Pneumonia in the immunocompetent patient. *Br J Radiol*. 2010;83(996):998–1009.

EMPYEMA

Gonzalo Luizaga
Luciano Kapelusznik
William F. Wright

I. INTRODUCTION

A. **Definition.** Empyema is a parapneumonic exudative effusion in the pleural space associated with culture of bacterial organisms, a positive Gram stain, or aspiration of pus on pleural fluid evaluation.

B. **Classification.** Normally, pleural fluid consists of less than 1 mL volume of fluid located between the visceral and parietal pleurae. Parapneumonic effusions may develop in 50% to 60% of bacterial pneumonia cases. There are three stages of parapneumonic effusions that are a continuum to the development of empyema.

1. **Simple or uncomplicated parapneumonic effusion (exudative phase).** Commonly, this is a sterile exudative pleural fluid that crosses the visceral pleura into the pleural space. Increased capillary vascular permeability and inflammatory cytokines lead to increased secretion of pleural fluid fulfilling *Light's criteria* (see Section V). Pleural fluid characteristics in this phase include:

   a. Clear fluid (normal pleural fluid contains a small number of mesothelial cells, macrophages, and lymphocytes)

   b. pH greater than 7.20 (normal pleural fluid pH is 7.6)

   c. Lactate dehydrogenase (LDH) less than 1,000 IU/L or half the normal serum value

   d. Glucose greater than 40 mg/dL or 2.2 mmol/L

   e. Culture and Gram stain are negative

2. **Complicated or fibrinopurulent parapneumonic effusion (fibrinopurulent phase).** Progression to this stage involves bacterial invasion of the pleural space with migration of neutrophils and activation of the coagulation cascade with fibrin deposition. Pleural fluid characteristics in this phase include:

   a. Clear fluid or cloudy

   b. pH less than 7.20 (this is due to increased pleural fluid acidosis from anaerobic fermentation of glucose by bacteria and neutrophils producing lactic acid and carbon dioxide)

   c. LDH greater than 1,000 IU/L (LDH is released owing to leukocyte death)

   d. Glucose less than 40 mg/dL or 2.2 mmol/L (increased glucose metabolism)

   e. Gram stain and/or culture may be positive

Empyema is characterized by pleural fluid with the aforementioned findings along with the presence of bacterial organisms, positive Gram stain, or frank pus.

3. **Organizing phase.** Progression to this phase involves the formation of a pleural fibrous layer (called a pleural peel) due to the predominance of fibroblast proliferation.

C. **Risk Factors.** Most risk factors for the development of an exudative pleural effusion and empyema are the same risk factors for pneumonia; however, additional risk factors include:

1. Diabetes mellitus
2. Immunosuppressed conditions (e.g., HIV) or chronic use of immunosuppressive medications (e.g., corticosteroids)
3. Gastroesophageal reflux disease
4. Alcohol and intravenous drug abuse
5. Thoracic or esophageal surgical procedures or trauma (e.g., esophageal rupture)
6. Delirium or dementia (increased risk of aspiration)
7. Gingivitis or periodontal disease

Chronic obstructive pulmonary disease (COPD) is associated with a reduced risk of progression to pleural space infections.

II. **MICROBIOLOGY OF EMPYEMA.** In general, microorganisms responsible for complicated parapneumonic effusions or empyema are the same pathogens associated with bacterial pneumonia. *While gram-positive aerobic bacteria are the most frequently identified microorganisms, mixed aerobic and anaerobic infections are more likely to produce empyema than monomicrobial infections.* The microbiology of empyema differs between infections acquired in the community and those acquired in hospital settings.

A. **Community-Acquired Microorganisms**

1. **Gram-positive microorganisms.** This group includes both *Streptococcus* species (*Streptococcus pneumoniae* and *S. anginosus* group) and *Staphylococcus aureus.* The latter is more commonly seen in association with nosocomial infections, immunocompromised conditions, or postoperative care.
2. **Gram-negative microorganisms.** This group includes *Escherichia coli, Pseudomonas* spp, *Haemophilus influenzae,* and *Klebsiella* spp (particularly in diabetic patients).
3. **Anaerobe microorganisms.** Anaerobic bacteria may be present in as many as 36% to 76% of cases. A putrid odor is characteristic of anaerobic infection. Examples include *Fusobacterium* spp, *Prevotella* spp, *Peptostreptococcus* spp, and *Bacteroides fragilis* group.
4. **Fungal microorganisms.** This group represents a very rare cause of empyema and infection is predominantly due to *Candida* species in association with immunocompromised conditions.

B. **Hospital-Acquired Microorganisms**

1. **Gram-positive microorganisms.** *Staphylococcus aureus* may account for as many as 50% to 66% of cases and is more commonly seen in association with immunocompromised conditions or postoperative care.

2. **Gram-negative microorganisms.** This group has higher rates of infections in association with admission to the intensive care unit and includes *Escherichia coli, Pseudomonas* spp, *Haemophilus influenzae*, and *Klebsiella* spp.

3. **Anaerobe microorganisms.** Anaerobic bacteria may be present in as many as 36% to 76% of cases. Examples include *Fusobacterium* spp, *Prevotella* spp, *Peptostreptococcus* spp, and *Bacteroides fragilis* group.

4. **Fungal microorganisms.** This group represents a very rare cause of empyema and is predominantly due to *Candida* spp in association with immunocompromised conditions or esophageal rupture.

Mycobacterium tuberculosis should be suspected if fluid has a lymphocytic predominance and in patients with epidemiologic risk factors (see Chapter 14).

III. **CLINICAL MANIFESTATIONS OF EMPYEMA.** The clinical manifestations are variable but depend on the duration of illness (acute vs. chronic), microorganism, age of the patient (young vs. old), pulmonary location and size, and underlying comorbid medical history (renal failure, diabetes, etc.).

A. **Uncomplicated/Complicated Parapneumonic Effusion.** Similar symptoms to pneumonia with cough, fever, pleurisy chest pain, sputum production, and dyspnea.

B. **Empyema.** Clinical features as mentioned earlier but with a longer course with several days of fever and cough associated with no clinical improvement of symptoms despite adequate medical treatment.

IV. **APPROACH TO THE PATIENT**

A. **History.** A complete and chronologically accurate history should be obtained in all patients suspected of a pleural space infection. *A complicated exudative parapneumonic effusion and empyema should be included in the differential diagnosis of any patient who fails to respond to appropriate pneumonia therapy within 3 to 5 days.* The history should focus on the timing of events, risk factors, comorbid conditions, medication allergies, recent pulmonary infections, and recent antimicrobial therapy.

B. **Physical Examination.** While a complete physical examination should always be performed, the physical examination should emphasize these areas:

1. **Head, eyes, ears, nose, and throat (HEENT) examination.** Trachea deviation may develop in the opposite direction of the fluid accumulation. Additionally, findings of gingival or odontogenic disease may suggest anaerobic infections.

2. **Pulmonary examination.** Pleural fluid accumulation typically produces these findings on examination:

a. *Auscultation.* Pleural fluid accumulation is associated with *reduced breath sounds, reduced vocal resonance, or bronchophony* (e.g., egophony; E to A changes), and *absent inspiratory crackles.*

   b. *Palpation and percussion.* Pleural fluid accumulation is associated with *diminished fremitus* (chest wall vibrations produced by sound generated in the larynx) and *dullness to percussion.*

Skodaic resonance is a hyperresonant note (i.e., louder pitch) on percussion that lies within the lung immediately above the fluid accumulation and is thought to be due to distention of the lung alveoli above the lung compressed by the fluid accumulation.

C. Laboratory Studies

1. **Complete blood count (CBC).** Elevation of the white blood cell (WBC) count is observed in the majority of patients; however, a platelet count greater than 400×10^3/L may also indicate a pleural space infection.

2. **Complete metabolic profile (CMP).** Routinely ordered but nonspecific; however, an albumin level less than 30 g/L and sodium level less than 130 mmol/L may indicate a pleural space infection.

3. **C-reactive protein (CRP)** and erythrocyte sedimentation rate (**ESR**). Values are commonly elevated but nonspecific; however, a CRP value greater than 100 mg/L may indicate a pleural space infection.

4. **Pleural fluid chemistry.** The identification of frank purulence requires no chemistry evaluation. The most important variables to measure include:

   a. **pH measurement.** *This is the most important variable that determines the need for chest drainage.* For improved accuracy the sample should be collected under anaerobic conditions (the presence of air falsely elevates the pH) in a heparinized blood gas syringe and measured on a blood gas analyzer immediately. Additionally, contamination of the pleural fluid sample with lidocaine can falsely reduce the pH value.

   b. **Glucose.** *This is the second most important variable that determines the need for chest drainage.* A pleural fluid glucose value less than 60 mg/dL or 3.4 mmol/L should indicate the need for chest drainage.

   c. **Cell count with differential.** Commonly ordered but specific values do not accurately predict the need for chest tube drainage.

   d. **Protein and LDH levels.** Commonly ordered but specific values do not accurately predict the need for chest tube drainage.

   e. **Amylase level.** An elevated level of salivary amylase usually indicates an esophageal leak or rupture

5. **Blood cultures.** Two sets of cultures should be obtained in all patients but are only positive in 12% to 14% of cases.

6. **Pleural fluid Gram stain and cultures.** Pleural fluid should be sent for routine Gram stain and aerobic and anaerobic cultures. Evaluation for atypical organisms such as *Mycobacterium tuberculosis* and fungal pathogens should be decided on a case-by-case basis. Acid-fast bacillus (AFB) and fungal stains (e.g., calcofluor white) as well as cultures should be obtained in patients with immunosuppressed conditions or epidemiologically associated risk factors. Pleural fluid cultures are positive in about 50% of cases.

D. Radiologic Studies

1. **Plain-film radiology.** Posterior–anterior and lateral images may be performed in conjunction with lateral decubiti films. *A pleural effusion in association with image findings consistent with bacterial pneumonia may indicate a pleural space infection.* Complicated effusions and empyema might have an abnormal contour and not flow freely on decubitus examination.

2. **Ultrasonography.** This image modality is considered the most practical method in the evaluation and management of parapneumonic effusions and empyema. An echogenic pleural effusion is strongly associated with an exudative process (e.g., complicated parapneumonic effusion or empyema). Advantages of ultrasonography include:

   a. Ease of operation

   b. Guidance for thoracentesis

   c. No exposure to ionizing radiation

   d. Wide availability

3. **CT.** This is considered the gold standard test for evaluation of pleural effusions as it can identify other lung infections (e.g., lung abscess) as well as assist with management decisions (e.g., chest tube drainage vs. surgical drainage procedures). Classic findings suggestive of empyema include:

   a. Thickened parietal pleura (present in 86%–100% of cases)

   b. Lenticular-shaped effusion that compresses lung parenchyma

   c. The *split pleura* sign (caused by enhancement of both parietal and visceral pleura surfaces)

V. DIAGNOSTIC CRITERIA FOR EMPYEMA. All patients with suspected empyema require pleural fluid sampling by thoracentesis. Complications include pneumothorax, hemothorax, reexpansion pulmonary edema, and organ laceration.

According to Light's criteria, the pleural fluid is exudative if:

- Pleural fluid protein/serum protein ratio is greater than 0.5 *or*
- Pleural fluid LDH/serum LDH ratio is greater than 0.6 *or*
- Pleural fluid LDH is greater than two thirds the upper limits of the laboratory's normal serum LDH

Exudative effusions can be uncomplicated, complicated, or organizing (see Section I.B). **Empyema** should fulfill Light's criteria for an exudative pleural fluid and be associated with culture of bacterial organisms, a positive Gram stain, or aspiration of pus on thoracentesis.

VI. MANAGEMENT OF EMPYEMA. Inadequate treatment can result in prolonged hospitalization, systemic toxicity, residual ventilator impairment, spread of local inflammatory reaction, and increased mortality risk. Factors that contribute to morbidity and mortality include misdiagnosis, inappropriate antibiotics, and inappropriate delay in chest tube placement. *In general, if an effusion is less than 10 mm thick, it can typically be followed with clinical observation and/or antimicrobial therapy alone; however, if a pleural effusion is greater than 10 mm* *thick, or enlarges with time, it commonly necessitates pleural fluid analysis and/or drainage.*

A. **Medical Management.** All patients should receive appropriate antibiotic therapy for the underlying pneumonia. When cultures are unable to provide antimicrobial guidance, coverage for community-acquired pathogens and anaerobic organisms is suggested; however, hospital-acquired infections require broader-spectrum antimicrobial coverage. Penicillin and cephalosporin-class antimicrobial agents demonstrate good penetration into the pleural space; however, aminoglycoside agents should be avoided as they have a poor pleural penetration and may be inactive in the presence of pleural fluid acidosis.

Suggested empirical antimicrobial regimens include (listed agents are based on normal renal function):

1. Piperacillin–tazobactam 3.375 to 4.5 g IV q6 *or*

2. Ceftazidime 2 g IV q8–12 or cefepime 2 g IV q8–12 *plus* clindamycin 600–900 mg IV q8 *or*

3. Moxifloxacin 400 mg IV q24 *or*

4. Doripenem 500 mg IV q8 *or* imipenem–cilastatin 500 to 1000 mg IV q6 *or* meropenem 1 g IV q8 (these agents are commonly reserved for infections against multidrug-resistant pathogens)

Vancomycin 15 mg/kg IV q12–24 can be added to all the preceding listed options to provide methicillin-resistant *Staphylococcus aureus* (MRSA) coverage. Dosing adjustment may be required to maintain a serum trough level of 20 mcg/mL.

While duration of antibiotic therapy is not well established, it is usually given for at **least 3 weeks** but depends on resolution of clinical symptoms, normalization of vital signs, and laboratory parameters as well as adequate drainage of infected pleural fluid.

B. **Surgical and Chest Tube Management in Pleural Infection.** The optimal chest tube size for drainage has not been established; however, if a small-bore catheter (e.g., 10–14 French gauge) is to be used, regular saline flushing and suction is recommended to avoid blockage. Indications for chest tube placement include:

1. Complicated effusion with pleural fluid pH less than 7.20

2. Frank pus or turbid/cloudy pleural fluid on aspiration

3. Organisms seen on Gram stain or culture

4. Poor clinical response to antibiotics alone

5. Loculated collection

Chest tube placement can be guided either by ultrasonography or CT. Small-bore catheters can be used for multiloculated effusions and nonviscous fluid, while large-bore catheters are required for thick and purulent fluid. If the chest tube does not provide the expected amount of drainage despite flushing with normal saline, imaging such as contrast-enhanced CT can verify accurate tube location. Additional measures to ensure adequate pleural fluid drainage include:

a. ***Fibrinolysis agents.*** While not routinely performed, intrapleural fibrinolysis agents (streptokinase 250,000 IU given twice a day × 3 days or urokinase

100,000 daily × 3 days, tissue plasminogen activator (TPA) 10–100 mg daily) can improve drainage and radiologic features; however, data on potential short- and long-term outcomes are conflicting. Major adverse reactions associated with this therapy include fever, leukocytosis, and malaise.

b. *Mucolytic agents.* Intrapleural agents such as deoxyribonuclease (DNase) in combination with fibrinolysis agents (e.g., streptokinase) may decrease hospital stay, surgical need, and radiographic pleural opacity.

c. *Surgical treatment.* Patients who fail to improve despite antibiotic therapy and adequate drainage as well as have persistent signs of uncontrolled infection (e.g., systemic inflammatory response syndrome [SIRS]/sepsis) should be evaluated by a thoracic surgeon. Treatment options may include video-assisted thoracoscopic surgery (VATS) or open thoracotomy with decortication and drainage.

BIBLIOGRAPHY

Colice GL, Curtis A, Deslauriers J, et al. Medical and surgical treatment of parapneumonic effusions: an evidence-based guideline. *Chest*. 2000;118(4):1158–1171.

Davies HE, Davies RJ, Davies CW, BTS Pleural Disease Guideline Group. Management of pleural infection in adults: British Thoracic Society Pleural Disease Guideline 2010. *Thorax*. 2010;65(suppl 2):S41–S53.

Lee SF, Lawrence D, Booth H, et al. Thoracic empyema: current opinions in medical and surgical management. *Curr Opin Pulm Med*. 2010;16(3):194–200.

Light RW. Clinical practice. Pleural effusion. *N Engl J Med*. 2002;346(25):1971–1977.

Sahn SA. Diagnosis and management of parapneumonic effusions and empyema. *Clin Infect Dis*. 2007;45(11):1480–1486.

13

LUNG ABSCESS

Adrian Majid
Ulrike K. Buchwald
Devang M. Patel

I. INTRODUCTION

A. Definition. A local circumscribed collection of pus produced by liquefactive necrotic inflammation of the pulmonary parenchyma secondary to infection.

1. Often communicates with airways producing putrid purulent sputum.

2. Exists on a continuum with *necrotizing pneumonia* in which small cavities (usually less than 1 cm) form in contiguous areas of the lung.

B. Classification.

1. **Acute versus chronic.** An acute abscess is an infection of less than 4 to 6 weeks' duration. A chronic abscess has infection duration greater than 4 to 6 weeks' duration.

2. **Primary versus secondary.** Primary lung abscesses account for the majority of cases (80%) and usually occur in patients prone to aspiration with normal systemic but poor gingival dental health (e.g., alcoholism, substance abuse, and patients with a reduced level of consciousness, coma, or epileptic seizures). Secondary lung abscesses are associated with predisposing conditions that include:

   a. Congenital lung abnormalities

   b. Obstructing neoplasms

   c. Foreign body devices

   d. Bronchiectasis or contaminated pulmonary bulla

   e. Systemic infection (e.g., tricuspid valve endocarditis with septic pulmonary emboli)

   f. Immunocompromised states (e.g., HIV, immunosuppression related to malignancy, solid organ or stem cell transplantation)

3. **Microbiological classification.** The abscess is classified by the predominant causative organism (see the following).

II. PATHOGENESIS

A. Aspiration. This mechanism most commonly involves aspiration of anaerobic bacteria that originate from the oral cavity (especially the gingival crevice) and accounts for most primary lung abscesses. Aspiration may then lead to chemical injury (e.g., pneumonitis) or obstruction, predisposing to secondary bacterial superinfection with tissue necrosis and abscess formation. Abscesses may take 1 to 2 weeks to develop after aspiration. Alternatively, with a large aspiration event or smaller aspiration events in cases of compromised immunity, bacteria can be directly inoculated into the lung and cause infection. Certain conditions (e.g., **risk factors**) of altered consciousness (e.g., alcoholism, anesthesia, illicit drug use, seizures, stroke) or dysphagia (e.g., scleroderma) can predispose to aspiration and lung abscess formation.

B. **Hematogenous Spread.** This can include pulmonary septic emboli from tricuspid valve endocarditis (e.g., *Staphylococcus aureus* in intravenous drug abuse) or suppurative phlebitis. One unique scenario for embolic spread is *Lemierre syndrome*, characterized by septic phlebitis of the neck veins due to direct spread from an oropharyngeal infection, classically described with the anaerobic gram-negative bacterium *Fusobacterium necrophorum.*

C. **Transdiaphragmatic Spread.** This spread of bacteria from subphrenic infections (e.g., liver abscesses) may result in lung abscess formation.

D. **Impaired Mucus Clearance,** such as with bronchiectasis, or obstruction from bronchogenic neoplasms, can increase the risk of lung abscess formation.

III. MICROBIOLOGY OF LUNG ABSCESS

A. **Oral Anaerobic Bacteria** (traditionally associated with 60% to 80% of primary lungs abscesses). Most common isolated anaerobes include:

1. *Finegoldia magna* (formerly *Peptostreptococcus* spp)

2. *Fusobacterium nucleatum*

3. *Prevotella melaninogenica ureolyticus*

4. *Bacteroides* spp (more commonly *B. melaninogenicus, B. intermedius,* and *B. ureolyticus*)

B. *Streptococcus pyogenes* **(Group A),** *Streptococcus milleri,* and other micro-aerophilic streptococci (e.g., *S. intermedia*) may accompany anaerobic flora in mixed infections.

1. *Streptococcus pneumoniae* is usually *not* associated with lung abscess formation.

C. *Staphylococcus aureus* is usually associated with a severe, monomicrobial, and necrotizing pneumonia.

D. **Gram-Negative Rods** such as *Klebsiella pneumoniae* (especially patients with diabetes mellitus), *Pseudomonas aeruginosa, Burkholderia cepacia, Legionella* spp (e.g., *L. pneumophila* serotype 1 and *L. micdadei*)

E. **Mycobacterial Infections** include *Mycobacterium tuberculosis* and nontuberculous mycobacteria (e.g., *M. avium* complex)

F. **Fungal Pathogens** include *Aspergillus* spp and endemic mycoses such as *Histoplasma capsulatum, Blastomyces dermatitis,* and *Coccidioides immitis*

G. **Immunocompromised Hosts With Cell-Mediated Immune Defects.** *Pseudomonas aeruginosa* and *Staphylococcus aureus* can cause lung abscesses. Opportunistic pathogens, such as *Nocardia* spp (e.g., *N. asteroides*) and *Rhodococcus* spp, in addition to mycobacterial and fungal organisms, should also be included in the differential diagnosis.

IV. CLINICAL MANIFESTATIONS OF LUNG ABSCESS

A. **Symptoms Usually Manifest Over Weeks to Months** (most commonly within 2 weeks) in patients with anaerobic infections. Common symptoms include cough with purulent putrid (foul-smelling) sputum, fever, malaise, night sweats, and pleuritic chest pain. Patients often present with a persistent pneumonia.

B. **More Rapid Clinical Progression** can be seen with lung abscesses caused by aerobic bacteria such as *Staphylococcus aureus* or *Klebsiella pneumoniae*.

V. APPROACH TO THE PATIENT

A. **History.** A complete and chronologically accurate history should be obtained in all suspected cases of lung abscess. The history should focus on the timing of events, risk factors (see the preceding), comorbid conditions, medication allergies, recent pulmonary infections, and recent antimicrobial therapy. *A lung abscess should be included in the differential diagnosis of any patient who fails to respond to appropriate pneumonia therapy.* The history usually suggests an indolent and prolonged course with fever, productive cough (putrid sputum with foul-smelling breath is estimated to occur in 50% of cases), malaise, night sweats, and/or significant weight loss. Shaking chills or rigors (indicative of bacteremia) are unusual symptoms.

B. **Physical Examination.** A complete physical examination should be performed, but areas of focus include:

1. **Vital signs.** Fever is common; however, patients may or may not demonstrate tachypnea.

2. **Head, eyes, ears, nose, and throat (HEENT) examination.** Most patients with primary lung abscesses will have findings of dental disease (e.g., caries, gingivitis). Assess for the presence of a gag reflex.

3. **Pulmonary examination.** Lung abscesses can be associated with dullness to percussion, increased fremitus, inspiratory crackles, and bronchovesicular and/or amphoric (*resembling the sound produced by blowing into a bottle*) sounds on auscultation of the peripheral lung.

4. **Musculoskeletal examination.** Digital clubbing is associated with chronic lung abscesses.

C. **Laboratory Studies**

1. **Complete blood count (CBC).** Routinely ordered and may reveal leukocytosis and anemia of chronic disease.

2. **Basic metabolic panel (BMP).** Routinely ordered but nonspecific for lung abscess infections.

3. **Blood cultures.** Commonly two sets are ordered but are of low yield; however, blood cultures are more likely to provide a pathogen in the setting of secondary lung abscesses (see the preceding).

4. **Sputum culture and pleural fluid culture.** A sputum sample for Gram stain and culture can be collected. If a pleural effusion is present, pleural fluid should be sent for routine Gram stain and aerobic and anaerobic cultures. Evaluation for atypical organisms such as *Mycobacterium tuberculosis* and fungal pathogens should be decided on a case-by-case basis. Acid-fast bacillus (AFB) and fungal stains (e.g., calcofluor white) as well as cultures should

be obtained in patients with immunosuppressed conditions or epidemiologically associated risk factors.

5. **Bronchoalveolar lavage (BAL) cultures and routine sputum cultures** are more likely to yield aerobic organisms. Anaerobic bacteria are difficult to isolate and are extremely sensitive to antibiotics, which may have been administered prior to collection. In typical cases of lung abscess, BAL/sputum cultures are *not* routinely recommended.

D. **Radiologic Studies**

Radiologic findings consist of solitary or multiple thick-walled cavities within the lung parenchyma, without pressing on the adjacent bronchi, and forming a sharp angle with the thoracic wall. Cavitation occurs when erosion of the lung parenchyma leads to communication with a bronchus resulting in drainage of the necrotic material, entry of air, and creation of an air-fluid level.

1. **Plain-film chest x-ray (CXR).** Imaging typically demonstrates a lung cavity with irregular thick or thin walls and an air-fluid level surrounded by a pulmonary infiltrate that is usually localized to one pulmonary segment. Primary lung abscess from aspiration may locate to the posterior segments of the upper lobes and the superior segments of the lower lobes. Multiple cavities located in the lower pulmonary segments may suggest a hematogenous (e.g., embolic abscess) source of infection.

2. **Chest CT.** More useful for identifying smaller abscesses, evaluating for endobronchial lesions, and distinguishing between lung abscess and empyema with air-fluid levels.

VI. MANAGEMENT OF LUNG ABSCESS

A. **Medical Management.** Appropriate antimicrobial therapy is the mainstay of treatment. Though initially with favorable response rates for decades after its discovery in the 1950s, *penicillin does not currently offer adequate coverage for lung abscesses*, especially with increased anaerobic beta-lactamase activity. General antimicrobial therapy recommendations for the treatment of lung abscesses include (dosing assumes normal renal function):

1. Clindamycin has shown superior efficacy to penicillin with faster resolution of fever and putrid sputum, better efficacy at clinical cure, and fewer relapses in randomized trials.

    a. The standard dose is **clindamycin 600 mg intravenous (IV) q8** followed by clindamycin 150–300 mg PO four times daily.

    b. If there is suspicion for polymicrobial infection, the addition of gram-negative coverage should be considered with **ceftriaxone 1 to 2 g IV daily**.

2. Metronidazole should *not* be used as monotherapy given high rates of treatment failure and inadequate activity against microaerophilic streptococci; however, this agent may be used in selected cases in conjunction with a beta-lactam antibiotic such as ceftriaxone. The standard dose is **metronidazole 500 mg IV/PO q6–8**.

3. A beta-lactam–beta-lactamase inhibitor, potentially in combination with an antibiotic with methicillin-resistant *Staphylococcus aureus* (MRSA) coverage (e.g., vancomycin), is also an empirical treatment option.

a. **Ampicillin–sulbactam 3 g IV q8** (q6 dosing also possible) has shown similar efficacy to clindamycin (with or without cephalosporin) for significant aspiration events leading to bacterial infection and/or lung abscesses.

b. Some data support the use of a fluoroquinolone antibiotic (e.g., moxifloxacin or levofloxacin) with anaerobic activity due to similar cure rates reported with **moxifloxacin 400 mg PO daily** as compared to ampicillin–sulbactam.

c. Carbapenem antimicrobial options include **ertapenem 1 g IV q24 , imipenem–cilastatin 500–1000 mg IV q6, or meropenem 1 g IV q8**.

In the absence of strong evidence to support a definitive length of treatment, antimicrobials are typically administered for at least *3 to 6 weeks* up to *8 weeks*.

Clinical improvement is reflected in the subsidence of fever (within the first 3–4 days) and complete defervescence within 7 to 10 days. Persistent fever can be explained by treatment failure due to uncommon pathogens (e.g., multidrug-resistant bacteria, mycobacteria, fungi) or by the presence of an alternative diagnosis.

B. Surgical Management

1. Most lung abscesses can drain themselves through the tracheobronchial tree; therefore, if the patient is clinically improving with adequate sputum production, no surgical management should be required.

2. **Drainage procedures** are reserved for cases failing antimicrobial therapy (about 10%–15% of patients) and are performed under fluoroscopic, ultrasound, or CT guidance. CT is usually the preferred modality owing to additional information provided about location, content, and wall thickness of the abscess. In addition, it has been proved useful in differentiation between empyema and abscess and in exclusion of endobronchial lesions. Drainage procedures, such as by either percutaneous or endoscopic methods, are *not* routinely done as they may lead to rapid unloading of pus into other segments of the lung or pleural space, resulting in further pulmonary complications.

   a. *Percutaneous drainage of lung abscesses* has been established as the treatment of choice for patients who have failed to respond to antibiotic therapy, have an impaired cough reflex, and/or are unsuitable for surgical intervention. The percutaneous procedure is also usually selected for lung abscesses with diameters greater than 4 to 8 cm. The Seldinger technique is considered to be safe when placing a drainage tube. The duration of the drainage tube varies but 4 to 5 weeks may be required.

   b. *Endoscopic drainage of the cavity* is an alternative therapeutic approach. This method should be considered in cases of coagulation disorders, when a large amount of lung tissue must be traversed or when adjacent anatomic areas hinder direct access to the cavity. The procedure involves insertion of a guidewire into the cavity through the working channel of a flexible bronchoscope followed by a fluoroscopically based placed drainage catheter. The cavity is flushed daily with normal saline solution through the catheter, with or without antibiotic infusions. The catheter is typically removed after 4 to 6 days with immediate improvement of clinical and radiologic imaging status.

3. Indications for *surgical resection* of the involved part of the lung (e.g., seg-
mentectomy, lobectomy, or rarely pneumonectomy) due to potential failure
of medical treatment either alone or combined with transcutaneous drainage include large cavities (greater than 6–8 cm), abscesses caused by resistant organisms (e.g., MRSA, multidrug-resistant *Pseudomonas aeruginosa*),
an obstructing neoplasm, associated bronchopleural fistula with or without
empyema, massive hemoptysis, and/or extensive necrosis.

VII. PROGNOSIS

A. In the antibiotic era, mortality rates are currently estimated between 10% and
20%.

B. Clinically, patients on antibiotic treatment typically report improvement in symptoms within 7 to 10 days. Imaging may lag behind clinical symptom **improvement** and should *not* be repeated within this time frame.

C. Further imaging should be performed in patients *not* responding beyond
2 weeks of treatment. Examples **include** CT scan and bronchoscopy to evaluate
for endobronchial lesions and/or BAL to evaluate for an atypical or opportunistic pathogen.

D. Increased mortality **rate has** been reported in lung abscess patients with a
higher number of predisposing factors (e.g., malignancy, altered consciousness),
anemia (hemoglobin less than 10 g/dL), and infection with certain microorganisms such as *Pseudomonas aeruginosa, Staphylococcus aureus,* or *Klebsiella
pneumoniae.*

BIBLIOGRAPHY

Allewelt M, Schüler P, Bölcskei PL, et al. Ampicillin + sulbactam vs. clindamycin +/– cephalosporin
for the treatment of aspiration pneumonia and primary lung abscess. *Clin Microbiol Infect.*
2004;10(2):163–170.
Bartlett JG. The role of anaerobic bacteria in lung abscess. *Clin Infect Dis.* 2005;40(7):923–925.
Hirshberg B, Sklair-Levi M, Nir-Paz R, et al. Factors predicting mortality of patients with lung
abscess. *Chest.* 1999;115(3):746–750.
Kuhajda I, Zarogoulidis K, Tsirgogianni K, et al. Lung abscess-etiology, diagnostic and treatment
options. *Ann Transl Med.* 2015;3(13):183. doi:10.3978/j.issn.2305-5839.2015.07.08
Levison ME, Mangura CT, Lorber B, et al. Clindamycin compared with penicillin for the treatment
of anaerobic lung abscess. *Ann Intern Med.* 1983;98(4):466–471.
Lorber B. Bacterial lung abscess. In: Mandell G, Bennett J, Dolin R, eds. *Principles and Practice of
Infectious Diseases.* 7th ed. Philadelphia, PA: Churchill Livingstone Elsevier; 2010: 925–929.
Ott SR, Allewelt M, Lorenz J, et al. Moxifloxacin vs. ampicillin/sulbactam in aspiration pneumonia
and primary lung abscess. *Infection.* 2008;36(1):23–30.

14

TUBERCULOSIS

David W. Keckich
Ulrike K. Buchwald

I. INTRODUCTION

A. Definition. Tuberculosis (TB) is an acute or chronic infection associated with the bacterium *Mycobacterium tuberculosis,* which can present with a wide range of clinical manifestations.

B. Classification

1. **Infection stage.** Exposure to *M. tuberculosis* (MTB) results in infection as defined by transient or ongoing multiplication of bacteria in about 30% of exposed individuals.

   a. **Primary tuberculosis** defines the events following the initial infection with tubercle bacterium.

   b. **Latent tuberculosis infection (LTBI)** is a *persistent asymptomatic infection* following primary TB that is contained by host defenses. Dormant bacteria are contained in granulomata, are not detectable by smear or culture, and can persist throughout a patient's lifetime without causing further illness.

   c. **Postprimary or reactivation tuberculosis** occurs when immune control of latent infection is lost, and dormant bacteria reemerge. *The most common site of reactivation is the lungs.* Persons with LTBI have a lifetime risk of reactivation TB of 5% to 10% if they are HIV uninfected, but this risk increases to 5% to 10% per year with HIV infection.

      The terms *active tuberculosis* and *tuberculosis disease* are used commonly to describe stages of the infection in which the bacterium can be identified and/or clinical symptoms and findings are present.

2. **Localization of tuberculosis disease**

   a. **Pulmonary tuberculosis** is infection confined to the lungs and represents 85% of TB cases in the United States. It is most commonly due to reactivation.

   b. **Extrapulmonary tuberculosis** refers to disease in any site outside the lung. It is due to systemic dissemination of bacterium, usually during primary infection.

C. Epidemiology. One third of the world's population has LTBI. There are 9 million cases of active TB and 2 million deaths per year. The incidence per 100,000 population ranges from 3.6 (United States) to 981 (South Africa) cases. The case rate in the United States is 11 times higher in foreign-born than in U.S.-born persons. TB and HIV act synergistically to cause severe disease in coinfected patients.

D. Transmission. The predominant mode is via *inhalation of droplet nuclei* that contain viable bacteria and that are aerosolized by coughing, sneezing, or talking. Patients with pulmonary or laryngeal TB, a positive sputum acid-fast bacillus (AFB) smear (see the following), and/or cavitary lung disease are more likely to transmit by this route. HIV coinfection increases organism burden and infectiousness, even in the absence of cavitary disease. Rare modes of transmission include direct skin inoculation and/or oral ingestion.

E. Risk Factors for Development of Tuberculosis Disease. These factors can be categorized into those that *increase the likelihood of exposure to individuals with infectious TB* and *those that increase the risk of progressive or reactivation disease*. Persons with any of these risk factors should be tested for LTBI (see Section VI.A). Risk factors for TB include:

1. Recent contact of a person with infectious TB

2. Recent migration from TB endemic country (less than 5 years)

3. Work or residency at homeless shelters, correctional facilities, and health-care facilities

4. Radiographic evidence of prior-healed TB

5. Recent conversion in the tuberculin skin test (TST) as defined by an increase of the induration greater than 10 mm within a 2-year period

6. HIV infection

7. Immunosuppressive therapy (equivalent of greater than or equal to 15 mg/day prednisone for greater than or equal to 4 weeks or long-term use of tumor necrosis factor [TNF] alpha antagonists)

8. Drug and tobacco abuse

9. Underlying diseases such as diabetes mellitus, silicosis, gastric bypass, end-stage renal disease, cancer, solid organ transplant, malnutrition

10. Children less than 5 years of age with recent exposure or persons at advanced age

11. Inherited or acquired immune defects in the interferon-gamma/interleukin-12 (IFN-gamma/IL-12) pathway (i.e., immunomodulation medications)

II. MICROBIOLOGY. Members of the *Mycobacterium tuberculosis* group (mainly *M. tuberculosis, M. africanum, M. bovis*) are characterized as aerobic, nonmotile, and nonspore-forming bacilli. The cell walls of these bacteria are rich in ***mycolic acids***, which confers resistance to antibiotics, environmental stress, and intracellular killing, and renders bacilli acid-fast (retention of dye upon acid alcohol based decolorization). Bacterial growth is slow with a generation time of 15 to 24 hours.

III. CLINICAL MANIFESTATIONS OF TUBERCULOSIS DISEASE

A. Pulmonary Tuberculosis

1. **Primary tuberculosis** is often subclinical or asymptomatic and may occur silently during childhood in endemic areas. Fever can occur in as many as 70% of cases. Pulmonary hilar lymphadenopathy, pleural effusion, and infiltrates may also occur.

2. **Primary progressive tuberculosis** is a severe progressive primary infection in 5% to 10% of patients, mainly those with immunosuppression. In the lung, consolidation with lymphadenopathy, cavitation, endobronchial spread, and airway compromise can be seen. Extrapulmonary dissemination can occur.

3. **Postprimary or reactivation tuberculosis** in the lung is characterized by parenchymal infiltrates with cavitation, most commonly in the apical lung zones. Severe lung destruction may occur. Hilar lymphadenopathy is rare.

B. **Extrapulmonary Tuberculosis.** The most commonly affected sites are:

1. **Tuberculosis lymphadenitis** is the most common site of dissemination. Indolent cervical, axillary, or mediastinal lymphadenopathy is typical.

2. **Pleural tuberculosis** can be divided into two categories.

   a. ***Tuberculosis pleural effusion*** may occur with pulmonary TB. Generally the organism burden is low, and effusion is self-limited. *The diagnosis is usually made by pleural biopsy.*

   b. ***Tuberculosis empyema*** is the result of a cavitary lung lesion that ruptures into the pleural space releasing a high number of organisms. Scarring and calcification of the pleura may then result.

3. **Pericardial tuberculosis** can present clinically with chest pain and dyspnea; however, a pericardial effusion may or may not be present. It may also present as a large effusion with cardiac tamponade, as a calcified constrictive pericarditis, or as a mixture of an effusion with cardiac constriction. *Diagnosis can be made by pericardial biopsy.*

4. **Tuberculosis meningitis** presents subacutely with malaise, headache, and fever but can progress to a debilitating disease with coma. It is a basilar brain infection involving the pons and optic chiasm. Caseating granulomata in the brain parenchyma (i.e., **central nervous system [CNS] tuberculoma**) occasionally develop, causing focal neurologic signs and hydrocephalus.

5. **Skeletal tuberculosis** most often develops in the spine (**Pott's disease**), and patients usually experience bony pain of the affected area. Unlike other forms of extrapulmonary TB, systemic signs and symptoms are often absent. *Bone biopsy is the diagnostic test of choice.*

6. **Miliary tuberculosis** is a life-threatening disseminated infection in severely immunocompromised patients. It may be acute, subacute, or chronic and involve all organ systems. Small, millet-seed-like nodules may be seen on the chest x-ray (CXR). Hepatosplenomegaly, lymphadenopathy, meningismus, and choroid tubercles may be present with this form of disease.

IV. APPROACH TO THE PATIENT

A. **History.** A complete and accurate history should be performed. Providers should pay attention to prior TB exposure and risk factors for disease (see Section I.E). *The presence of fever, night sweats, or weight loss, while nonspecific, should raise suspicion for TB.* Chronic cough and hemoptysis suggest pulmonary TB, while extrapulmonary TB may have a protean presentation, depending on the site of infection.

B. **Physical Examination.** A complete physical examination should be performed in *all* cases. The physical examination should focus on the following:

1. **General appearance.** Cachexia and malnutrition may indicate long-standing infection.

2. **Lymphatic examination.** The presence of lymphadenopathy should be assessed.

3. **Pulmonary examination.** Pleural effusion with signs of consolidation, rales, or egophony can be found on examination of patients with pulmonary TB.

4. **Musculoskeletal and neurologic examination.** Pott's disease is associated with gibbus formation, direct bone pain on palpation, and *tuberculous meningitis* with deficits of cranial nerves III, IV, and VI.

5. **Gastrointestinal examination.** Gastrointestinal TB may be associated with ascites and/or an abdominal mass.

C. Laboratory Studies

1. **AFB smear.** The Ziehl–Neelsen stain is a rapid, inexpensive method to diagnose mycobacterial infection on specimens from all sites. It does not distinguish live from dead bacilli or *M. tuberculosis* from nontuberculous mycobacteria. Sensitivity of a single sputum sample is 50% to 60% but is improved by collecting two to three early morning *sputum samples*. Sputum induction or bronchoalveolar lavage (BAL) facilitates specimen collection.

2. **Mycobacterial cultures.** These remain the gold standard for diagnosis. Solid media require 4 to 8 weeks for results and liquid media 7 to 20 days. They are used in conjunction and can be done on specimens from all sites.

3. **Nucleic acid amplification tests (NAATs).** These assays allow identification of *M. tuberculosis* within a few hours with high specificity but varying sensitivity. Sensitivity is 95% on AFB smear–positive sputum samples and 50% to 85% on AFB smear–negative. Performance on nonrespiratory samples is less reliable and remains mostly investigational. NAATs do not distinguish live from dead bacilli.

4. **Drug susceptibility tests (DSTs).** This is done by observing growth in solid or liquid media containing antituberculosis medications. Drug susceptibility testing should be performed at least for first-line antituberculosis drugs on all cultures. The role of molecular tests that identify genetic mutations associated with resistance to antituberculosis drugs is currently being evaluated.

5. **Histology.** Biopsy specimens (see Section III.B) can detect caseating granulomata. AFB smear and mycobacterial culture should be performed on the biopsy specimen.

6. **Tests for the detection of an immune response.** These tests reveal prior exposure to TB but *do not distinguish between latent and active infection*. The results must be interpreted in the clinical context of the patient. For the diagnosis of LTBI, a positive test is followed by a clinical and radiographic evaluation (see Section VI). The role of these tests in the diagnosis of active TB is limited as they may also be falsely negative in patients with immunosuppression or with severe disease.

   a. **Tuberculin skin test.** This requires the intradermal injection of 0.1 mL of purified protein derivative (PPD) into the skin of the forearm. *Only the induration (not the erythema) is measured after 48 to 72 hours.* Prior vaccination with bacillus Calmette-Guérin (BCG) and exposure to nontuberculous mycobacteria can give false positive results.

Two-step TST testing. Immune responses may wane in long-standing latent infection and an initial TST may be negative; however, this initial TST may "boost" the immune response, resulting in a subsequently positive test that would be erroneously interpreted as conversion. Hence, in settings where serial testing is expected (e.g., in healthcare workers), an initial negative TST should be repeated within 1 to 3 weeks. If this second test is positive ("booster phenomenon"), the patient should be evaluated for LTBI (see Section VI). If the second test is negative, the person does not have LTBI.

b. **Interferon-gamma release assays (IGRAs).** These blood tests measure IFN-gamma released by T cells after incubation with antigens specific to *M. tuberculosis*. Food and Drug Administration (FDA) approved tests are the QuantiFERON-TB Gold In-Tube test (enzyme-linked immunosorbent assay [ELISA] based) and the T-SPOT TB test (based on the Elispot technique). Advantages to IGRAs over the TST are that they are practitioner independent, do not require patient return for reading, and do not cross-react with previous BCG vaccination. The disadvantages are mainly high costs and time of test result. According to Centers for Disease Control and Prevention (CDC) recommendations, either test may be used for the diagnosis of LTBI, but IGRAs may be preferred in patients with a history of BCG vaccination or those who are not likely to return for TST reading. *The combination of both tests* (i.e., TST and IGRA) *for the diagnosis of LTBI is* currently not *recommended in the United States.*

7. **Nonspecific laboratory studies**

   a. *Complete blood count (CBC).* May show leukocytosis or leukopenia with a relative lymphocytosis. Anemia suggestive of chronic disease may indicate long-standing disease.

   b. *Erythrocyte sedimentation rate (ESR) and C-reactive protein (CRP).* May be elevated but are nonspecific.

   c. *Pleural fluid analysis.* Usually reveals an exudate process; adenosine deaminase (ADA), a marker of T-cell activation, can be elevated. Pleural biopsy is often necessary to confirm the diagnosis, as AFB smear and culture are insensitive in cases of pleural effusions.

   d. *Cerebrospinal fluid (CSF).* TB meningitis shows a monocytic pleocytosis (100–500 cells/mcL), protein elevation (100–500 mg/dL), and hypoglycorrhachia (glucose less than 45 mg/dL).

   e. *Complete metabolic profile (CMP).* Hyponatremia may be associated with TB-related syndrome of inappropriate antidiuretic hormone secretion (SIADH) or adrenal insufficiency.

   f. *Urinalysis.* Genitourinary TB may *be associated* with pyuria and recurrent negative urine cultures.

8. **Evaluation for HIV infection.** All patients diagnosed with TB should be tested for HIV infection (see Chapter 43, HIV and AIDS).

D. Radiologic Studies

1. **CXR and chest CT** typically show apical or posterior lung infiltrates. Cavities and air-fluid levels may be present in 20% of cases. Chest imaging with a CT scan may also show a nonspecific *tree in bud pattern* in some cases. Nodules, effusions, or a miliary pattern may be present; however, 5% of cases have normal chest imaging.

2. **Imaging studies for extrapulmonary tuberculosis** depend on the site of infection. CT scan of the chest may show hilar or cervical adenopathy as well as pericardial effusions or calcification. Echocardiography may also show pericardial effusion. Conventional x-ray, CT, and MRI may diagnose skeletal TB disease.

V. **DIAGNOSIS OF TUBERCULOSIS DISEASE.** The diagnosis of TB is based on a combination of exposure history, clinical findings, laboratory testing, and radiographic data.

A. **Pulmonary Tuberculosis.** This infection can be AFB smear-positive or smear-negative.

1. **Smear-positive disease.** The rapid identification of *M. tuberculosis* should be sought with NAATs to distinguish MTB from nontuberculous mycobacteria for treatment initiation; however, culture is required to confirm the diagnosis and to establish *sensitivities to antituberculosis drugs.*

2. **Smear-negative disease.** The results of NAATs and/or culture may establish the diagnosis. Treatment should be initiated prior to microbiological confirmation if TB is suspected and the patient is seriously ill and/or there is a high risk to transmit disease. If empiric therapy is initiated, patients should show signs of clinical response within 2 to 3 weeks (all patients should respond by 8 weeks).

B. **Extrapulmonary Tuberculosis.** These manifestations are often more difficult to diagnose as AFB smears and cultures are less sensitive. Whenever possible, tissue should be collected for histology, smear, and culture. The diagnosis may eventually be made on clinical grounds with the support of a positive TST or IGRA.

VI. **SCREENING AND DIAGNOSIS OF LATENT TUBERCULOSIS INFECTION**

A. **Screening.** *The goal of screening for LTBI is to identify persons who are at increased risk for developing active TB disease and would benefit from treatment of LTBI.* Hence a decision to test presupposes a decision to treat. Screening for LTBI starts with a careful medical and social history that identifies risks for exposure or development of disease. The CDC recommends "targeted testing" with TST or IGRA of persons with recent exposure or at high risk for reactivation disease (see Section I.E).

Persons with a known history of a positive TST or IGRA, a history of treatment for LTBI, or active TB should *not* undergo repeated testing.

B. **Diagnosis.** A TST or IGRA can provide the initial step for the diagnosis of LTBI (see Section IV.C.6). If the test result is positive, it is followed by clinical and laboratory assessment to rule out active TB. The diagnosis of LTBI can be made in the absence of clinical symptoms, physical examination, and laboratory or radiographic findings suggestive of active TB disease. Sputum smears and cultures should be sent for patients with respiratory symptoms or an abnormal CXR (i.e., infiltrate or cavitary lung lesion). If a patient is referred with a positive TST or IGRA, the assessment follows the same steps, and a diagnosis of LTBI is made if active TB disease is not confirmed.

C. **Guidelines for the Interpretation of the TST.** These guidelines are proposed by the American Thoracic Society (ATS). Diameter refers to the horizontal *induration* measured at 48 to 72 hours. *A positive TST is defined as an induration diameter of:*

1. **Greater than or equal to 5 mm.** In patients with the following characteristics: HIV-positive, recent contacts of known TB cases, CXR consistent with prior TB, and immunosuppressed patients (see Section I.E).

2. **Greater than or equal to 10 mm.** In patients with the following characteristics: recent arrival (less than 5 years) from endemic countries, injection drug users, residents and employees of high-risk settings (e.g., prisons, healthcare facilities, and homeless shelters), high-risk comorbid conditions (e.g., silicosis, diabetes mellitus, chronic kidney disease, and malignancy), weight loss of greater than 10% ideal body weight, gastrectomy, jejunoileal bypass, children less than 4 years of age, and/or infants, children, or adolescents exposed to adults in high-risk categories.

3. **Greater than or equal to 15 mm.** Persons with *no* risk factors for TB.

VII. MANAGEMENT OF TUBERCULOSIS

A. **Goals and Principles of TB Treatment.** Goals of treatment are to cure the patient and to prevent transmission. Treatment should also aim to reduce the development of resistance to antituberculosis drugs; therefore, multidrug-combination therapy is always used to prevent drug resistance. Several months of treatment are necessary to target slow-growing bacteria.

Treatment is divided into an **initial phase** that contains greater than or equal to three drugs and a **continuation phase** with fewer drugs. Directly observed therapy (DOT) should be practiced whenever possible with treatment provided in a private clinic, at an academic center, or at a designated Department of Health (DOH) facility. The DOH is ultimately responsible for access to diagnostic and treatment services and monitoring of treatment outcome.

B. **Antituberculosis Drugs**

1. **First-line drugs.** *These are isoniazid (INH), rifampin (RIF), ethambutol (EMB, E), pyrazinamide (PZA), and streptomycin (SM).* INH, RIF, EMB, and PZA form the standard treatment for drug-sensitive TB (see Section VII.E). First-line drugs are more effective and less toxic than other drugs.

Characteristics of first-line drugs: INH has profound early bactericidal activity against rapidly dividing TB bacilli; RIF is active against rapidly dividing and semidormant bacilli; PZA acts against semidormant bacilli in the acidic environment of caseous foci; EMB is bacteriostatic; and SM has to be given intravenously or intramuscularly.

RIF can be substituted with other rifamycins such as rifabutin and rifapentine in special circumstances (see Section VII.C and J).

2. **Second-line drugs.** These drugs include fluoroquinolones (preferred are moxifloxacin and levofloxacin), aminoglycosides (amikacin, kanamycin, cap-

reomycin), and oral bacteriostatic drugs such as ethionamide, prothionamide, cycloserine, terizidone, and *p*-aminosalicylic acid.

C. **Side Effects of Drugs and Monitoring**

1. **Hepatotoxicity.** INH, RIF, and PZA are *all* associated with liver function test (LFT) abnormalities and hepatitis. The risk is elevated in patients with chronic hepatitis B, hepatitis C, and with concomitant alcohol consumption. Additionally, INH hepatotoxicity is associated with increasing age. *An asymptomatic, self-limited elevation of aspartate aminotransferase (AST) occurs in 20% of patients; however, discontinuation of drugs is recommended for symptomatic patients with LFT elevation greater than thrice normal and for asymptomatic patients greater than five times normal.* Second-line agents can be substituted temporarily and the first-line agents stepwise reintroduced under careful monitoring of the LFTs. Monthly monitoring of the hepatic enzymes is recommended for patients with abnormal baseline LFTs, preexisting liver disease, alcohol use, pregnancy, and suspected drug reaction.

2. **Peripheral neuropathy.** This can be caused by INH due to interference with pyridoxine metabolism. The risk is increased in patients with other risk factors for neuropathy such as diabetes, HIV infection, nutritional deficiencies, renal failure, and pregnancy. Daily pyridoxine supplementation with 25 to 50 mg can prevent this complication.

3. **Optic neuritis.** This is associated with EMB; therefore, patients taking EMB should be questioned at monthly visits for visual problems such as blurry vision and scotomata. An ophthalmologic examination for visual acuity and color discrimination is recommended at baseline and monthly for patients who continue to take EMB for more than 2 months.

4. **Rash.** This can be caused by all *antituberculosis* drugs and if mild can be managed symptomatically. A general erythematous rash should prompt discontinuation of drugs and stepwise reintroduction.

5. **Arthralgias, gouty flares, and asymptomatic hyperuricemia.** This may occur with PZA.

6. **Ototoxicity.** Occurs mainly with SM and can adversely affect auditory or vestibular function.

7. **Urine and bodily fluid discoloration.** RIF leads to orange discoloration of bodily secretions, and permanent staining of contact lenses may occur.

D. **Baseline Evaluation and Monitoring for Side Effects.** At baseline, a CBC, CMP, and uric acid level should be measured. Serology for hepatitis B and C should be obtained in patients with epidemiologic risk factors. Patients should be educated about clinical symptoms of hepatic dysfunction such as anorexia, nausea, vomiting, dark urine, abdominal pain, arthralgias, or easy bruising. Patients should be evaluated at monthly intervals for treatment response and any side effects.

E. **Pulmonary Tuberculosis Treatment.** The following regimen is for patients with a new diagnosis of TB disease and low likelihood of harboring bacilli with resistance to first-line agents.

1. **Initial Phase** (2 months):
   INH 5 mg/kg (up to 300 mg) PO daily *plus*

RIF 10 mg/kg (up to 600 mg) PO daily *plus*
PZA 15 to 30 mg/kg (up to 2,000 mg) PO daily *plus*
EMB 15 to 20 mg/kg (up to 1,000 mg) PO daily.
EMB may be dropped if the strain is susceptible to all first-line drugs.
Pyridoxine is also given to prevent neuropathy (see Section VII.C.2).

2. **Continuation Phase** (4–7 months' duration):
INH 5 mg/kg (up to 300 mg) PO daily *plus*
RIF 10 mg/kg (up to 600 mg) PO daily.

Alternative treatment regimens allow intermittent drug dosing and can be used in selected cases. Follow-up smear and cultures are taken at least monthly until two consecutive are culture-negative. Reevaluation is required if cultures are positive after the initial treatment phase.

Respiratory isolation in a negative-pressure room is required while hospitalized if smears are positive; healthcare workers should wear fit-tested N95-type masks or powered-air-purifying respirators (PAPRs). Removal from respiratory isolation may depend on local hospital policy, but typically requires three negative AFB smears obtained on different days.

F. **Extrapulmonary Tuberculosis.** This is treated with the same regimen and schedule as pulmonary TB, with the following additions:

1. Tuberculosis meningitis should be treated for a minimum of 9 to 12 months

2. Tuberculosis meningitis and pericarditis should receive corticosteroid therapy in addition to antituberculosis therapy: prednisone 60 mg/day PO for 4 weeks, followed by 30 mg/day for 4 weeks, 15 mg/day for 2 weeks, and 5 mg/day for 1 week.

G. **Management of Tuberculosis in HIV-Infected Persons.** This follows the same principles as in HIV-negative patients. RIF interacts with many antiretroviral drugs and may have to be substituted with rifabutin. Regimens using once or twice weekly treatment should be avoided in most HIV infected patients. Treatment should be done by clinicians with experience in managing both infections.

H. **Pregnancy.** Active TB disease should be treated using a regimen of INH, RIF, and EMB for 9 months. LTBI should be treated in recent contacts or HIV-infected patients.

I. **Cases of Relapse, Treatment Failure, Drug Resistance, and Use of Second-Line Drugs.** Should be managed by specialists. In the United States, primary INH resistance is found in 8.2% of cases (2008) and multidrug resistance (resistance to INH and RIF) in about 1.2% (2010).

J. **Latent Tuberculosis Infection.** This is treated with 9 months of daily INH 5 mg/kg (up to 300 mg) PO daily (*plus* pyridoxine) if no contraindications exist. A new regimen consists of weekly INH 15 mg/kg (up to 900 mg) *plus* weight-based rifapentine (greater than 50 kg, 900 mg) given under DOT for 3 months. An alternative is RIF 10 to 20 mg/kg daily (up to 600 mg) given daily for 4 months for patients unable to tolerate INH or presumed to have INH-resistant TB. Baseline evaluation should include LFTs. Periodic assessment is done to assess adherence and side effects (see Section VII.C and D).

VIII. PREVENTION OF TUBERCULOSIS. The most important prevention measure for TB involves the identification and treatment of those who have LTBI; however, additional measures include:

A. **Airborne Isolation.** This is used for *all* patients suspected of pulmonary TB, including HIV-positive patients with pneumonia, until lack of infectivity is documented by three separate negative AFB smears from sputum or one BAL specimen (usually collected on three separate days).

B. **Vaccines.** BCG vaccine is given at birth in most endemic countries to protect children from disseminated infection; however, it is not effective to prevent reactivation disease.

BIBLIOGRAPHY

Blumberg HM, Burman WJ, Chaisson RE, et al. American Thoracic Society/Centers for Disease Control and Prevention/Infectious Diseases Society of America: treatment of tuberculosis. *Am J Respir Crit Care Med.* 2003;167:603–662.

Centers for Disease Control and Prevention. Latent tuberculosis infection: a guide for primary health care providers. http://www.cdc.gov/tb/publications/LTBI/diagnosis.htm

Escalante P. Tuberculosis. *Ann Intern Med.* 2009;150(11):ITC6-1–ITC6-16.

Hauck FR, Neese BH, Panchal AS, et al. Identification and management of latent tuberculosis infection. *Am Fam Physician.* 2009;79(10):879–886.

Jasmer RM, Nahid P, Hopewell PC. Latent tuberculosis infection. *N Engl J Med.* 2002;347:1860–1866.

Sia IG, Wieland ML. Current concepts in the management of tuberculosis. *Mayo Clin Proc.* 2011;86(4):348–361.

15

DIVERTICULITIS

William F. Wright

I. INTRODUCTION

A. Classification, Definition, and Pathophysiology. Diverticula are outpouchings of the colon wall. While true diverticula involve all layers of the colonic wall, pseudodiverticula (false diverticula) typically are more common and involve only colonic mucosa and submucosa layers (lack muscular coat). Pseudodiverticula develop in areas of weakness where the vasa recta arteries penetrate the muscularis layer as a result of colonic hypermotility and a low-fiber diet. They are most commonly found in the sigmoid colon where the colon has both a small caliber and high intraluminal pressures due to contractions (e.g., Laplace's law).

Diverticulosis also develops as a result of aging (colonic muscular weakness) and connective tissue diseases (e.g., Ehlers–Danlos and Marfan's syndromes).

Diverticulitis is an infectious complication of colonic diverticula that is associated with macro- or microscopic perforation. Of those who have diverticulosis, the lifetime prevalence of developing acute diverticulitis is approximately 25% (e.g., pretesting probability of disease), 13% to 36% will experience recurrence within 5 years, and the risk of future emergency surgery is approximately 4% to 7%.

B. Epidemiology. Diverticulitis is almost exclusively a disease of industrialized societies.

1. Prevalence increases with age. Diverticulosis occurs in 5% to 10% of persons older than 45 years and approximately 80% of those older than 85 years.

2. Disease is similar in men and women.

3. Cecal diverticula are more common in Asians and patients less than 60 years; however, diverticulitis isolated to the right colon is uncommon and usually occurs with left-sided disease.

C. Risk Factors

1. *Diets low in dietary fiber and high in red meat* (most important association for development of diverticula). Diverticulitis has not been associated with nut, corn, or popcorn ingestion.

2. Treatment with *nonsteroidal anti-inflammatory drugs (NSAIDs), opioids, and corticosteroids* on a long-term basis has been convincingly associated with increased risk of perforated diverticulitis.

3. *Smoking* (controversial risk factor).

4. *Obesity and physical inactivity* (considered risk factors that are not supported by much data).

5. *Constipation* (considered a risk factor but not supported by much data).

6. *Genetic susceptibility.* Monozygotic twins are twice as likely as dizygotic twins to develop diverticulosis.

II. CLASSIFICATION OF DIVERTICULITIS

A. Most Commonly Classified as Noninflammatory, Acute (Simple or Complicated), or Chronic.

1. **Noninflammatory.** Patients have symptoms of diverticulitis without associated inflammation.

2. **Acute, uncomplicated.** Patients have signs and symptoms of acute inflammation, but do not have complications. Inflammation is limited to the colonic wall and adjacent tissues.

3. **Acute, complicated.** Patients have signs and symptoms of acute inflammation with a complication (see the following).

4. **Chronic.** Patients have symptoms (either intermittently or persistently) despite standard treatment.

B. Hinchey Classification of Acute, Complicated Diverticulitis

1. **Class I.** Small, confined pericolic or mesenteric abscess.

2. **Class II.** Larger abscess but confined to pelvis, intra-abdominal cavity, or retroperitoneal space.

3. **Class III.** Ruptured peridiverticular abscess causing generalized purulent peritonitis.

4. **Class IV.** Direct rupture of diverticula with generalized fecal peritonitis.

III. MICROBIOLOGY OF DIVERTICULITIS

A. Gram-Negative Rods. Most common enteric pathogens.

1. *Escherichia coli*

2. *Klebsiella* spp

3. *Enterobacter* spp

4. *Proteus* spp

5. *Citrobacter* spp

6. *Fusobacterium* spp (anaerobe)

7. *Bacteroides* spp (anaerobe)

B. Gram-Positive Cocci

1. *Enterococcus* spp

2. *Peptostreptococcus* spp (anaerobe)

C. **Gram-Positive Rods**

1. *Clostridium* spp (anaerobe)

IV. CLINICAL MANIFESTATIONS OF DIVERTICULITIS

A. **Classic Manifestations.** Characterized by **acute abdominal pain that localizes to the left lower quadrant** (location varies depending on diverticula site) and **fever.**

B. **Additional Manifestations**

1. Nausea and vomiting

2. Constipation or diarrhea

3. Dysuria and urinary frequency

4. Anorexia

C. **Clinical Complications of Diverticulitis.** May be more frequent and/or severe in patients with an immunocompromised condition (e.g., diabetes, renal failure, cirrhosis, and malignancy), hematopoietic or solid organ transplant, HIV/AIDS, and/or patients taking chronic corticosteroids or NSAIDs. Complications include:

1. **Intra-abdominal abscesses and/or hepatic abscesses.** Abscess formation is probably the result of a contained perforation.

2. **Fistulas.** Most frequently involves the bladder. Other relatively common fistulas associated with diverticular disease are colocutaneous, colovaginal, and coloenteric.

3. **Peritonitis.** Generally, a secondary peritonitis as a result of a ruptured abscess. Use of NSAIDs and corticosteroids may increase the risk of perforation and peritonitis.

   Peritonitis is an indication for emergency surgical consultation.

4. **Stricture.** May lead to obstruction.

   Hemorrhage is a feature of diverticulosis, but not diverticulitis. It is usually arterial in nature and is the most common cause of major lower gastrointestinal bleeding attributed to medial thinning of the vasa recta arteries. Most cases are self-limited but some may require colonoscopy with therapeutic intervention or angiographic embolization.

V. APPROACH TO THE PATIENT

A. **History.** Diverticulitis is most often considered on the basis of clinical history and examination. *It should be included in the differential diagnosis for patients being evaluated for fever and abdominal pain.* The history should focus on the timing and location of abdominal pain, prior history of colonic diverticular disease, comorbid illnesses, and risk factors. The history should also attempt to identify other possible etiologies such as:

1. Inflammatory bowel disease (IBD; e.g., Crohn disease and ulcerative colitis)

2. Cystitis

3. Pelvic inflammatory disease (PID)

4. Ectopic pregnancy

5. Ovarian torsion/abscess

6. Colonic or mesenteric ischemia

7. Colorectal cancer

A family history of diverticulitis may predict recurrence.

B. **Physical Examination.** A complete physical examination should be performed, but examination areas to focus attention include:

1. **Vital signs.** Patients with diverticulitis typically have a fever. Tachycardia and hypotension may occur and should raise suspicion for complicated diverticulitis.

2. **Oral–pharyngeal examination** (oral ulcers may suggest IBD).

3. **Cardiovascular examination** (tachycardia and/or hypotension may suggest sepsis or bleeding).

4. **Abdominal examination.** Tenderness on palpation in the left lower quadrant significantly increases the likelihood of acute diverticulitis (positive likelihood ratio = 10.4). Rebound tenderness, rigidity, and the absence of bowel sounds are not accurate for diagnosis of acute diverticulitis, but may suggest peritonitis (positive likelihood ratio = 1.6; negative likelihood ratio = 0.4).

5. **Rectal examination** (a positive stool for occult blood may suggest a diverticular hemorrhage).

C. **Laboratory Studies**

1. **Complete blood count (CBC).** Most patients have leukocytosis (55%) and thrombocytopenia. Anemia may suggest a diverticular bleed.

2. **Basic metabolic panel (BMP).** Nonspecific but a low serum HCO_3 may suggest metabolic acidosis and sepsis. A serum amylase elevation may suggest perforation.

3. **Liver function tests (LFTs).** Routinely ordered, but commonly normal. Elevated values may signify biliary tract disease (e.g., hepatic abscess).

4. C-reactive **protein (CRP)/erythrocyte sedimentation rate (ESR).** Nonspecific but commonly elevated. CRP level greater than 50 mg/L, in the absence of vomiting, the likelihood of acute diverticulitis is significantly increased (positive likelihood ratio = 18).

5. **Urinalysis.** May be helpful in cases of colovesical fistulas and also when a urinary source is suspected (e.g., cystitis, pyelonephritis).

6. Serum **beta human chorionic gonadotropin (beta-HCG).** Helpful to rule out ectopic pregnancy in younger women presenting with abdominal pain.

7. **Lactate dehydrogenase (LDH).** May be elevated in cases of ischemic disease (e.g., ischemic colitis, mesenteric ischemia).

8. **Blood cultures.** Two sets are routinely ordered and more likely to yield a pathogen prior to the administration of antibiotics and/or more severe disease/complications.

9. **Cultures.** Aspirated contents should be routinely sent for Gram stain and culture.

10. **Prothrombin time (PT)/partial thromboplastin time (PTT).** May be helpful prior to drainage or surgical procedure.

D. **Radiography Studies**

1. **Plain films.** Acute abdominal series (AAS) are routinely ordered, but are mainly helpful in identifying perforation with pneumoperitoneum and obstruction.

2. **Ultrasound.** Transabdominal, high-resolution ultrasound is an alternative imaging modality that may be useful in patients with relative contraindications to CT scanning (pregnancy, renal insufficiency, and contrast allergy). Usually difficult to evaluate diverticulitis (seen as colonic thickening, pericolic inflammation, and visualization of diverticula) with an overall sensitivity of 77%.

3. **CT.** Considered the imaging modality of choice with oral contrast (or water-soluble contrast enema) and intravenous (IV) contrast (if no contraindications such as renal failure) to aid in the diagnosis and Hinchey staging of patients with suspected diverticulitis, to assess disease severity, and to help plan treatment. Sensitivity ranges from 85% to 97%, and CT scan can classify the severity of disease.

4. **Contrast enema.** Rarely used, contrast enemas are most helpful in identifying colovaginal and coloenteric fistulas.

5. **Magnetic resonance (MR) colonography.** May be an additional image test that does not expose the patient to ionizing radiation. Sensitivity is 86% for diverticulitis. The disadvantage is that the procedure requires colonoscopy bowel prep followed by filling the colon with 2 to 2.5 L water prior to MRI with gadolinium.

VI. **TREATMENT.** Most patients who can tolerate oral intake, are immunocompetent, have mild, uncomplicated disease and can be successfully treated on an outpatient basis.

A. **Indications for Hospitalization**

1. Failure to improve within 48 to 72 hours despite adequate outpatient therapy

2. Patients who present with complicated diverticulitis

3. Age older than 85 years

4. Significant comorbid illnesses

5. Inability to tolerate oral intake

6. Pain management

7. Further diagnostic evaluation

B. **Percutaneous Drainage.** Image-guided percutaneous drainage is usually the most appropriate treatment for stable patients with large diverticular abscesses. In patients with diverticular **abscesses larger than 3 cm,** image-guided percutaneous drainage is indicated in order to convert emergent operations into less morbid elective procedures. **Small pericolic abscesses smaller than 3 cm** may be treated with bowel rest and empirical antibiotics.

C. **Antibiotic Treatment.** Antibiotics should be used selectively, rather than routinely, in patients with acute uncomplicated diverticulitis based on the emerging belief that acute diverticulitis may be more inflammatory than infectious. Studies have found that antibiotic therapy did not prevent complications, accelerate recovery, or prevent recurrences.

Traditionally, most patients have been treated for 7 to 10 days; however, 5 to 7 days may be adequate in some cases. Recommended therapeutic regimens may include:

1. **Outpatient treatment**

   a. Metronidazole 500 mg PO q8 *plus* ciprofloxacin 500 to 750 mg PO q12

   b. Amoxicillin–clavulanate 875 mg PO q12

   c. Metronidazole 500 mg PO q8 *plus* trimethoprim–sulfamethoxazole 160 mg/800 mg PO q12

2. **Inpatient treatment.** Patients can be switched to oral antibiotics with improvement in vital signs, abdominal examination, and laboratory values as well as ability to tolerate oral intake.

   a. Ampicillin–sulbactam 3 g IV q6

   b. Ceftriaxone 2 g IV q24 *plus* metronidazole 500 mg IV q8

   c. Meropenem or doripenem 500 mg IV q8

   d. Ciprofloxacin 400 mg IV q12 *plus* metronidazole 500 mg IV q8

D. Surgical Management. Indications for surgical interventions are dependent on the severity of disease, number of recurrent episodes (increases approximately twofold with each episode), age, and comorbid illnesses.

1. **Indications for emergency surgical therapy**

   a. Failure to respond to nonoperative management

   b. Generalized peritonitis

   c. Signs of sepsis

   d. Undrainable or inaccessible abscess

   e. Obstruction that does not resolve with conservative management

2. **Indications for elective surgical therapy.** Elective colonic resection in patients with an initial episode of acute uncomplicated diverticulitis should be individualized as approximately 10% of patients managed with elective sigmoid resection may experience short-term complications of surgery such as wound infection, anastomotic leak, and/or cardiovascular/thrombotic events. Long-term complications may include abdominal distention, cramping, altered defecation, and fecal incontinence in approximately 25% of patients. Some indications for elective surgery may include the following:

   a. Recurrent episodes of acute, uncomplicated diverticulitis (traditionally has been defined as greater than two episodes)

   b. History of acute diverticulitis with abscess or fistula

   c. Chronic diverticulitis

   d. Diverticular stricture causing obstructive symptoms

3. **Surgical procedures.** The choice of procedure depends on the disease presentation and comorbid illnesses of the patient.

    a. **One-stage procedure.** Disease colonic segment is resected with immediate reanastomosis. Typically used for Hinchey class I and II disease.

    b. **Two-stage procedure.** Disease colonic segment is resected with end colostomy and distal rectal stump (Hartmann's procedure). Later-stage colonic reanastomosis. Required for most cases of Hinchey class III and IV disease.

    c. **Three-stage procedure.** Largely abandoned. The first stage includes operative drainage and creation of a diverting stoma. The diseased segment is removed and a primary anastomosis performed during the second stage. The colostomy is reversed during the third stage.

    d. **Laparoscopic colectomy.** Safe, and associated with decreased length of hospital stay, less pain and narcotic use, quicker return of bowel function, quicker return to work, and better cosmetics.

The laparoscopic approach is preferred with elective colectomy and resection should include the entire sigmoid colon with margins of healthy colon and rectum. A leak test of the colorectal anastomosis should be performed during surgery.

E. Management Following Resolution of Acute Diverticulitis

    1. **Colonoscopy.** Observational studies of patients with imaging-proven diverticulitis suggest that colonoscopy be performed approximately 6 to 8 weeks after resolution of acute diverticulitis in appropriate candidates to exclude the misdiagnosis of a colonic neoplasm and confirm the diagnosis of diverticulitis suspected on imaging.

    2. **Diet.** A fiber-rich diet or fiber supplementation may be helpful in patients with a history of acute diverticulitis. There is no evidence to routinely advise patients to avoid consumption of nuts and popcorn.

BIBLIOGRAPHY

Feingold D, Steele SR, Lee S, et al. Practice parameters for the treatment of sigmoid diverticulitis. Prepared by the Clinical Practice Guideline Task Force of the American Society of Colon and Rectal Surgeons. *Dis Colon Rectum.* 2014;57:284–294.

Jacobs DO. Clinical practice. Diverticulitis. *N Engl J Med.* 2007;357(20):2057–2066.

Morris AM, Regenbogen SE, Hardiman KM, et al. Sigmoid diverticulitis: a systematic review. *JAMA.* 2014;311(3):287–297.

Stollman N, Smalley W, Hirano I, et al. American Gastroenterologic Association Institute Guideline on the management of acute diverticulitis. *Gastroenterology.* 2015;149:1944–1949.

Wilkins T, Embry K, George R. Diagnosis and management of acute diverticulitis. *Am Fam Physician.* 2013;87(9):612–620.

16

APPENDICITIS

William F. Wright

I. INTRODUCTION

A. Definition. An acute inflammatory process involving the tubular structure, usually 8 to 10 cm in length, attached to the base of the cecum called the appendix.

1. **Simple appendicitis.** Not associated with perforation or abscess.

2. **Complicated appendicitis.** Associated with perforation or abscess.

   *Appendicitis has also been described as **early** (inflammation and symptoms intensify within 24 hours) or **late** (inflammation and symptoms develop over a period of greater than 24 hours) appendicitis.*

B. Pathogenesis. The prevailing hypothesis in approximately 70% of cases is luminal obstruction by fecaliths (fecal stone), lymphatic hypertrophy, tumor (primary or secondary), or foreign bodies, leading to increased intraluminal pressure and distention with vascular compromise. This is followed by an inflammatory reaction associated with a secondary infection. In approximately 30% of cases there is no direct luminal obstruction but rather hyperplasia of the submucosal lymphoid tissue related to a recent upper respiratory or gastrointestinal (GI) tract viral infection that secondarily compromises the appendiceal lumen.

C. Epidemiology

1. Appendicitis is the most common indication for emergent surgery performed worldwide.

2. Most commonly presents between the ages of 10 to 20 years, but can occur at any age.

3. More common in men.

4. Complicates 1 in 1,500 pregnancies and is the most common nonobstetrical operation performed during pregnancy.

II. MICROBIOLOGY OF APPENDICITIS.
A wide variety of microorganisms have been identified from appendectomy specimens. Bacterial pathogens are most common; however, unusual microorganisms have also been identified and cause infection by either direct invasion or secondary infection.

A. Bacteria

1. **Early appendicitis.** Typically involves facultative aerobic gram-negative enteric pathogens (Enterobacteriaceae).

   a. *Escherichia coli*

   b. *Klebsiella* spp

    c. *Enterobacter* spp

    d. *Proteus* spp

2. Late appendicitis. Usually involves a mixed infection, including anaerobes.

    a. *Bacteroides* spp (*B. fragilis*)

3. Additional bacterial pathogens

    a. *Yersinia enterocolitica* and *Y. pseudotuberculosis* (gram-negative coccobacilli). Can cause appendicitis, but more often causes inflammation of the terminal ileum (ileitis) that mimics appendicitis.

    b. *Actinomyces israelii* (anaerobic gram-positive bacteria) is a normal oral cavity bacterium but can sometimes produce a chronic granulomatous appendicitis (can mimic Crohn disease).

    c. *Campylobacter jejuni* (anaerobic gram-positive rod).

    d. *Salmonella* (**typhoid** and **nontyphoid**) and *Shigella* **spp** (gram-negative rod).

    e. *Mycobacterium tuberculosis* and *M. avium-intracellulare*. Usually associated with infection elsewhere in the abdomen in immunocompromised patients.

B. Parasitic Pathogens. Rare etiologies of appendicitis and are usually associated with a travel or exposure history.

    1. *Enterobius vermicularis* **(pinworm).** Most common parasite related to appendicitis.

    2. *Strongyloides stercoralis.* Endemic to southeast United States and tropics.

    3. *Trichuris trichiura* **(whipworm).**

    4. *Ascaris lumbricoides.*

    5. *Schistosoma* **spp** (particularly *S. haematobium*).

    6. *Entamoeba histolytica.*

    7. *Cryptosporidium* **spp.** More common with immunocompromised patients (e.g., HIV/AIDS).

C. Fungal Pathogens. Rare cause of appendicitis in immunocompromised patients (e.g., patients receiving chemotherapy).

    1. Zygomycetes (e.g., *Rhizopus* or *Mucor*).

    2. *Histoplasma capsulatum.* May cause appendicitis with disseminated infection in immunocompromised patients (e.g., HIV/AIDS).

D. Viral Pathogens. Rare etiologies of appendicitis associated with lymphoid hyperplasia.

    1. Cytomegalovirus (CMV). May be associated with appendicitis in patients with HIV/AIDS-related CMV colitis.

    2. Epstein–Barr virus (EBV). May cause appendicitis in the setting of infectious mononucleosis.

    3. Measles. May be associated with appendicitis in persons not vaccinated.

III. CLINICAL MANIFESTATION OF APPENDICITIS. Distention of an inflamed or infected appendix initially causes periumbilical dull pain due to visceral afferent nerves. The onset of pain is usually short in duration (24 hours or less). As the process continues, inflammation and infection of the serosal layer cause localized parietal peritoneal inflammation and pain (most commonly in the right lower quadrant).

A. **Classic Findings.** The classic presentation of appendicitis includes the following: short duration of pain, abdominal rigidity, migration of pain to the right lower quadrant, pain centered in the right lower quadrant, right lower quadrant tenderness, and anorexia. Clinically the progression of events may be acute, colicky, periumbilical abdominal pain, possibly followed by nausea and vomiting, with subsequent localization of pain to the right lower quadrant. This series of events occurs in about one half of cases over several hours.

B. **Abdominal Pain.** Can vary based on **age of the patient** (subtle and variable pain may occur in young children or elderly patients) and **location of appendix.**

1. **Retrocecal/retrocolic appendix (75%).** Right flank or side pain.

2. **Subcecal appendix (20%).** Right lower quadrant or suprapubic pain.

3. **Ileal appendix (5%).** May present with only vomiting or diarrhea.

C. **Nausea, Vomiting, and Anorexia.** Occur in the majority of patients following the progression of pain.

D. **Fever.** Occurs in about one half of cases.

E. **Confusion/Delirium.** This may be the only manifestation in older adults.

IV. DIFFERENTIAL DIAGNOSIS IN PATIENTS SUSPECTED OF APPENDICITIS

A. **Gynecologic Etiology.** Ectopic pregnancy, ovarian torsion, ruptured ovarian follicle, pelvic inflammatory disease (PID), or endometriosis.

B. **Urologic Etiology.** Cystitis, pyelonephritis, or urinary tract stones.

C. **Porphyria.** The human porphyrias are clinical disorders reflecting defects in heme biosynthesis and acute attacks are triggered by certain drugs, sex steroid hormones, reduced intake of calories and carbohydrate, alcohol, and unknown factors. Acute abdominal pain occurs in about 85% to 90% of attacks and is neurologic in origin. The pain is usually severe, diffuse, unremitting for hours and poorly localized, but is sometimes colicky. Nausea, vomiting, and constipation are common, but diarrhea is sometimes noted.

D. **Other GI Pathology.** Pancreatitis, acute cholecystitis, peptic ulcer disease, intestinal perforation, peritonitis, or intestinal obstruction (e.g., malignancy).

E. **Community-Acquired Pneumonia**

F. **Herpes Zoster (Varicella-Zoster Virus [VZV]).** Flank pain can precede the onset of the vesicular rash.

G. **Diabetic Ketoacidosis**

H. **Inflammatory Bowel Disease** (e.g., Crohn disease or ulcerative colitis).

I. **Vertebral Osteomyelitis or Osteoporosis-Related Fracture.** Patients usually have localized back pain that can mimic symptoms similar to acute appendicitis; especially older adults.

V. APPROACH TO THE PATIENT. The approach to the patient suspected of appendicitis is predominantly clinical; therefore, the history and physical examination remain most important to the diagnosis of appendicitis.

A. History. Appendicitis should be included in the differential diagnosis of any patient being evaluated for abdominal pain. **The most predictive history for appendicitis is the migration of pain from the periumbilical region to the right lower quadrant, abdominal rigidity, and right lower quadrant abdominal pain.** A history of **vaginal discharge** and/or **dysuria** or **urinary frequency** suggests an alternate diagnosis. The history should include a complete evaluation of comorbid illnesses that may suggest other etiologies for abdominal pain.

B. Physical Examination. A complete physical examination should be performed with focused attention on:

1. **Vital signs.** Fever, defined as greater than 38.3°C, has a reported sensitivity of 67% and specificity of 69% in a patient suspected of having acute appendicitis.

2. **General appearance** (patients with appendicitis may be lying motionless with the right thigh flexed at the hip to relieve pain and pressure).

3. **Cardiovascular examination** (tachycardia is nonspecific but may indicate pain or infection).

4. **Pulmonary examination** (to detect egophony or inspiratory rales/rhonchi that may indicate pneumonia).

5. **Dermatologic examination** (to detect a vesicular flank rash that may suggest VZV).

6. **Pelvic examination—women** (to detect vaginal discharge or cervical motion tenderness, suggestive of PID).

7. **Back examination** (to detect flank pain that may suggest pyelonephritis or spinal tenderness that may be associated with spinal infection or compression fracture).

8. **Abdominal examination** (most important component of physical examination).

   a. Bowel sounds may be absent.

   b. **Direct palpation** or asking the patient to **cough** often elicits pain at the **McBurney point** (2/3 along a straight line from the umbilicus to the anterior superior iliac spine).

   c. **Involuntary guarding** (involuntary muscle contraction in response to parietal peritoneal inflammation, sensitivity 39%–74%; specificity 57%–84%).

   d. **Rovsing's sign.** Right lower quadrant pain elicited with left lower quadrant palpation (sensitivity 68%; specificity 58%).

   e. **Psoas signs.** Right lower quadrant pain elicited with extension of the right thigh. More commonly positive with a retrocecal/retrocolic appendix (sensitivity 16%; specificity 95%).

    f. Obturator signs. Pain elicited with internal rotation of a flexed right thigh. May be more commonly positive with a subcecal or pelvic appendix.

C. Laboratory Studies

1. **Complete blood count (CBC).** The majority of patients (70%–90%) will have a neutrophilia leukocytosis. A white blood cell (WBC) count greater than or equal to 18,000/mL may suggest a ruptured appendix. Eosinophilia may indicate a parasitic etiology.

2. **Basic metabolic panel (BMP).** Routinely ordered, but nonspecific. Abnormalities may be helpful to identify other etiologies. A low serum HCO_3 may suggest sepsis from a ruptured appendix.

3. **C-reactive protein (CRP)/erythrocyte sedimentation rate (ESR).** Commonly elevated, but nonspecific. A normal CRP and WBC has been associated with a 100% negative predictive value (NPV) for appendicitis.

4. **Prothrombin time (PT)/partial thromboplastin time (PTT).** Useful tests for operative management.

5. **Beta human chorionic gonadotropin (beta-HCG).** Should be ordered for ALL females of reproductive age to rule out ectopic pregnancy.

6. **Liver function tests (LFTs).** May be helpful in identifying biliary tract disease as an alternative diagnosis.

7. **Amylase/lipase.** Usually performed to rule out pancreatitis.

8. **Urinalysis.** Typically shows mild hematuria or bacteriuria in appendicitis. A urinary red blood cell (RBC) count greater than or equal to 30 cells/hpf or WBC greater than or equal to 20 cells/hpf is more suggestive of a urinary tract infection.

9. **Blood cultures.** More likely to yield a pathogen in more severe cases. Usually, two sets of cultures are ordered.

10. **Appendix fluid culture.** Samples are routinely sent for Gram stain and culture following removal of the infected or inflamed appendix.

11. **Stool cultures and ova/parasites.** Not routinely ordered, but may be helpful in cases of suspected parasitic disease.

D. Radiography Studies

1. **Kidney, ureter, and bladder (KUB)/acute abdominal series (AAS).** Associated with a low sensitivity and specificity; therefore, these tests are not recommended.

2. **Ultrasound.** Has a reported sensitivity of 75% to 90% and specificity of 86% to 100%. It is a rapid and noninvasive test that is safe in pregnancy. Findings that support the diagnosis include:

    a. Appendix wall thickening greater than or equal to 6 mm in diameter

    b. Absence of appendix lumen gas

    c. Increased blood flow in the appendix wall

3. **CT.** Helical multislice spiral CT scan with slice thickness of no more than 5 mm has a sensitivity of 90% to 100%, specificity of 91% to 99%, and positive

predictive value of 95% to 97%. Among patients suspected of having appendicitis, alternative diagnoses or abscesses are detected more often with CT. Findings that support the diagnosis of appendicitis include:

a. Enlarged appendix; greater than or equal to 6 mm

b. Appendix wall thickening

c. Right lower quadrant fat stranding, free fluid, bowel wall thickening, and free air

VI. TREATMENT. The treatment of choice is timely appendectomy with appropriate medical care, fluid resuscitation, and antimicrobial therapy.

A. Medical Treatment. Medical therapy alone is successful in the initial management of most patients; however, the high rate of recurrence and risk for progression to appendiceal rupture leading to higher morbidity and mortality makes surgical therapy warranted. Suggested antibiotic regimens include (antimicrobial agents listed presume normal renal function):

1. Ampicillin/sulbactam 3 g intravenous (IV) q6

2. Piperacillin/tazobactam 3.375 g IV q6

3. Moxifloxacin 400 mg IV q24

4. Ceftriaxone 1 to 2 g IV q24 plus metronidazole 500 mg PO/IV q6–8

5. Meropenem 1,000 mg or doripenem 500 mg IV q8

The typical duration of antibiotic therapy has been 7 to 10 days without surgical intervention; however, antibiotics should be discontinued within 24 hours after appendectomy.

B. Surgical Treatment. Nonoperative management of selected patients with acute, nonperforated appendicitis may be considered if there is a marked improvement in the patient's clinical and laboratory condition prior to operative consideration.

The most important aspect of surgical therapy is the **timing of operation**. The risk of appendix **perforation increases following the onset of symptoms and is estimated at 20% to 40% by 48 hours, followed by 5% increases for every additional 12 hours**. Therefore, appendectomy should be performed with minimal delay if there is persistent or worsening clinical and/or laboratory findings or documented perforation so as to provide adequate infection source control. No significant differences are noted with the type of operation; thus, the choice of surgery depends on the surgeon. There is some data suggesting a lower wound-infection rate after laparoscopic compared to open appendectomy.

1. Open appendectomy. Traditional surgery performed through an incision (e.g., Rockey–Davis or McBurney incision) made perpendicular to the line from the umbilicus to the anterior superior iliac spine. The infected or inflamed appendix is removed either using a GI stapler or via simple ligation. If perforation has occurred, the wound is typically left open and allowed to heal by secondary intention. This minimizes the risk of wound infection.

2. Laparoscopic appendectomy. A minimally invasive technique, which utilizes a camera and long instruments inserted through 5 to 10 mm operation trocars, to resect and remove the inflamed appendix.

The laparoscopic approach is advocated to clarify the diagnosis in equivocal cases and to allow a more complete abdominal cavity visualization should the appendix be normal.

BIBLIOGRAPHY

Dominguez EP, Sweeney JF, Choi YU. Diagnosis and management of diverticulitis and appendicitis. *Gastroenterol Clin North Am.* 2006;35(2):367–391.

Humes DJ, Simpson J. Acute appendicitis. *BMJ.* 2006;333(7567):530–534.

Lamps LW. Infectious causes of appendicitis. *Infect Dis Clin North Am.* 2010;24(4):995–1018.

Paulson EK, Kalady MF, Pappas TN. Clinical practice. Suspected appendicitis. *N Engl J Med.* 2003;348(3):236–242.

Solomkin JS, Mazuski JE, Bradley JS, et al. Diagnosis and management of complicated intra-abdominal infection in adults and children: guidelines by the Surgical Infection Society and Infectious Diseases Society of America. *Clin Infect Dis.* 2010;50:133–164.

Wagner JM, McKinney WP, Carpenter JL. Does this patient have appendicitis? *JAMA.* 1996; 276(19):1589–1594.

17

PANCREATIC INFECTIONS

William F. Wright

I. INTRODUCTION

A. **Acute Pancreatitis: Definition, Staging, and Pathophysiology.** Acute pancreatitis is defined as two out of three of the following criteria:

1. **Clinical.** Upper abdominal epigastric pain

2. **Laboratory.** Serum amylase or lipase greater than thrice the upper limit of normal (sensitivity and specificity of 95%–96%) and/or

3. **Imaging.** Evidence of pancreatic inflammation

   The severity of acute pancreatitis has traditionally been determined by the following (known as the Atlanta Criteria):

   a. **Mild acute pancreatitis.** Absence of organ failure or local complications

   b. **Moderate acute pancreatitis.** Local complications (e.g., necrosis or fluid collection) and/or transient organ failure of less than 48 hours

   c. **Severe acute pancreatitis.** Local complications (e.g., necrosis of fluid collection) and/or persistent organ failure of greater than 48 hours. Usually further defined as two or more of the following: systolic blood pressure less than 90 mmHg, pulmonary insufficiency with PaO_2 less than 60 mmHg, acute kidney injury with serum creatinine greater than 2 mg/dL, and/or gastrointestinal bleeding of greater than 500 mL per 24 hours.

   Acute pancreatitis is a disorder that is most commonly due to the migration of small gallstones (less than or equal to 5 mm) that obstruct the pancreatic duct or by chronic alcohol consumption.

   Common noninfection causes of acute pancreatitis include:

   a. *Biliary stones (or biliary tract tumors)*

   b. *Alcohol abuse (a serum lipase-to-amylase ratio of greater than 4 or 5 strongly suggests an alcoholic cause)*

   c. *Hyperlipidemia (especially elevated triglyceride levels greater than 1,000 mg/dL) and hypercalcemia*

   d. *Trauma*

   e. *Post–endoscopic retrograde cholangiopancreatography (ERCP) or endoscopic sphincterotomy*

   f. *Congenital defects (i.e., pancreatic divisum and sphincter of Oddi dysfunction) are reported to occur in approximately 10% to 15% of cases*

   g. *Systemic illness (e.g., vasculitis)*

h. *Medications (e.g., sulfonamides, nitrofurantoin, metronidazole, tetracy-cline, furosemide, ranitidine, estrogens, valproic acid, azathioprine, and pentamidine)*

B. Acute pancreatitis, however, can rarely (less than 1% of cases) be associated with an infectious process that may include:

1. *Ascaris lumbricoides* (second most common cause in India; due to migration up the common bile duct)

2. *Echinococcus granulosus* (due to pancreatic duct obstruction)

3. *Aspergillus* spp (due to pancreatic thrombotic infarct)

4. **Acute HIV infection**

5. **Cytomegalovirus (CMV), herpes simplex virus (HSV), Epstein–Barr virus (EBV), and varicella-zoster virus (VZV)**

6. **Hepatitis B**

7. **Coxsackie B virus, measles, rubella, and rubeola virus**

8. **Adenovirus**

9. *Mycoplasma pneumonia, Yersinia* spp, *Salmonella typhi, Campylobacter jejuni, Mycobacterium tuberculosis,* and *M. avium* (usually in the setting of other infections)

C. Severe Acute Pancreatitis. Observed in about 15% of patients with acute pancreatitis and characterized as pancreatitis with multiorgan failure that persists for greater than 48 hours. *Pancreatic necrosis can develop in the course of severe acute pancreatitis and is defined as diffuse or focal areas of nonviable pancreatic tissue greater than 3 cm or greater than 30% of pancreatic tissue.* Pancreatic necrosis can then become infected (usually week 2 or 3 of disease or as long as 4 to 5 weeks) with two distinct forms:

1. **Infected pancreatic necrosis** (most common form; usually occurs during the second week of illness).

2. **Pancreatic abscess** (usually develops after 4 weeks of illness). *Current opinion suggests that a pancreatic abscess represents what was previously infected pancreatic necrosis that the host is able to handle without becoming so ill as to require early surgical debridement. As the pancreatic necrosis matures it becomes an abscess.*

II. PATHOPHYSIOLOGY OF PANCREATIC INFECTIONS

A. Two Clinical Phases of Severe Pancreatitis

1. **Early phase (first week).** Associated with inflammatory response with systemic inflammatory response syndrome (SIRS) and usually is not associated with any significant necrosis but organ failure.

2. **Late phase (2 weeks or more).** Associated with progressive disease and necrosis with eventual infection of the pancreatic necrosis (usually greater than or equal to 30% necrosis).

B. Microbiology of Pancreatic Infection. Bacteria that compose the gastrointestinal flora are the main pathogens. While lymphatic or hematogenous spread may occur, bacterial translocation from the colon is the main mode of infection. Pathogens include:

1. **Gram-negative organisms.** *Escherichia coli, Enterobacter* spp, *Proteus* spp, *Klebsiella* spp, *Citrobacter* spp, and *Pseudomonas.*

2. **Gram-positive organisms.** Viridans streptococci, *Staphylococcus* spp, *Enterococcus* spp, and beta-hemolytic streptococci.

3. **Anaerobes.** *Bacteroides* spp and *Clostridium* spp.

4. **Fungi.** *Candida* spp.

III. CLINICAL MANIFESTATIONS OF PANCREATIC INFECTIONS

A. Patients already have an established diagnosis of acute pancreatitis but may experience the additional following symptoms:

1. Persistent abdominal pain

2. Anorexia

3. Fevers

4. Malaise

B. Multiorgan failure is more common in association with pancreatic infections than with noninfected pancreatic necrosis.

C. *Pancreatic infections should be suspected in any patient with fever, multiorgan failure, and increased white blood cell (WBC) **count for** 7 to 10 days following hospitalization for acute pancreatitis.*

D. *In critically ill patients, infection of preexisting pancreatic necrosis should be suspected in patients with persistent or worsening symptoms consistent with infection after 7 to 10 days of illness.*

IV. APPROACH TO THE PATIENT

A. **History.** A complete and chronologically accurate medical history should be performed. Usually pancreatic infections are suspected in patients with persistent abdominal pain and fevers for 7 to 10 days after being diagnosed with acute pancreatitis. (Most patients are still in the hospital from their initial acute pancreatitis episode.)

B. **Physical Examination.** A complete examination should be performed but areas to focus attention include:

1. **Neurologic examination** (to detect mental status changes as a decrease in Glasgow coma scale score can be associated with severe pancreatitis).

2. **Abdominal examination** (flank ecchymosis [Grey Turner sign] and paraumbilical ecchymosis [Cullen sign] may suggest severe pancreatitis). Additionally, the new onset of peritoneal signs may be indicative of new onset of infection.

C. **Laboratory Studies.** Serum amylase and lipase are usually ordered to establish the diagnosis of acute pancreatitis, and additional testing is nonspecific and provides no prediction to pancreatic infections. Lipase level testing is considered more sensitive and specific than measuring amylase levels.

1. Complete **blood count (CBC).** Routinely elevated leukocyte count with a WBC count greater than or equal to 15,000 cells suggesting severe pancreatitis. A hematocrit greater than or equal to 44 mg/dL also suggests severe pancreatitis.

2. Basic **metabolic panel (BMP).** A serum blood *urea* nitrogen (BUN) greater than or equal to 5 mg/dL, calcium less than or equal to 8 mg/dL, HCO_3 deficit greater than or equal to 4 mEq/L, and glucose greater than or equal to 10 mmol/L may suggest severe pancreatitis. An elevated serum creatinine may suggest organ failure.

3. **Liver function tests (LFTs).** A low albumin and elevated *aspartate aminotransferase* (AST) may be associated with severe pancreatitis.

4. **Blood gas analysis.** PaO_2 less than 60 mmHg may suggest respiratory failure.

5. **Lactate dehydrogenase (LDH).** An elevated value may suggest severe pancreatitis.

6. **C-reactive protein (CRP)/erythrocyte sedimentation rate (ESR).** While these are nonspecific markers of inflammation and not routinely recommended, a CRP value greater than 150 mg/L may suggest pancreatic necrosis (sensitivity 80%).

7. **Procalcitonin.** While not routinely recommended, a level greater than or equal to 1.8 ng/mL may be a marker of infection with pancreatic necrosis (sensitivity 75%–94%).

8. **Blood cultures.** Routinely ordered but may be more helpful to identify other infections (e.g., catheter bloodstream infection).

9. **Urinary trypsinogen-2 (UT-2).** Trypsinogen is a 25-kDa pancreatic proteinase. The two main isoenzymes, (cationic) trypsinogen-1 and (anionic) trypsinogen-2, are secreted at high concentrations into pancreatic fluid, but a small proportion escapes into the circulation. Because of their relatively small size, trypsinogens are readily filtered through the glomeruli. For unknown reasons, the tubular reabsorption of trypsinogen-2 is lower than that of trypsinogen-1, and consequently, the urinary concentration of trypsinogen-2 is higher.

   The pooled sensitivity and specificity of UT-2 for the diagnosis of acute pancreatitis are 80% and 92%, respectively. The pooled sensitivity and specificity for the diagnosis of post-ERCP pancreatitis are 86% and 94%, respectively.

10. **Cultures.** Patients suspected of pancreatic necrosis and infection may undergo fine needle aspiration (FNA) with samples sent for Gram stain and culture (sensitivity 88%; specificity 90%) to confirm infection (false-negative results can occur in 15%–25% of the cases). *Routine percutaneous FNA of peripancreatic collections to detect bacteria is not indicated, because clinical signs such as persistent fevers, increasing inflammatory markers (e.g., ESR and CRP), and imaging studies demonstrating gas in peripancreatic collections are accurate predictors of infected necrosis in the majority of patients.*

D. **Radiography Studies.** Evidence-based guidelines recommendations suggest an initial transabdominal ultrasound should be performed first and that contrast-enhanced CT imaging be performed for patients in which the diagnosis is unclear or who fail to improve clinically within the first 48 to 72 hours following hospital admission.

1. **Nonionic intravenous (IV) contrast (100–150 mL at a rate of 3 mL/sec) enhanced multidetector CT (slice thickness 5 mm or less).** Diagnostic imaging test of choice during the pancreatic and/or portal venous phase (50–70 second contrast delay) to demonstrate:

   a. Pancreatic necrosis (nonenhancing areas)

   b. Pancreatic infection (seen as cysts, abscesses, or gas bubbles)

   c. Pancreatic anatomic abnormalities

   In the absence of an abscess the most reliable finding for pancreatic infection on CT is **multiloculated gas bubbles in the area of necrosis.** Additionally, the finding of **greater than or equal to 50% of pancreatic** necrosis is associated with an **80% chance of subsequent pancreatic infection.**

V. **TREATMENT.** Uncontrolled pancreatic infections that are not treated with surgical intervention are associated with greater than or equal to 90% mortality rate; however, surgery should be delayed in a physiologically stable patient until the pancreatic necrosis walls off and becomes a well-defined abscess. Uncontrolled septic shock secondary to an infected pancreatic necrosis requires immediate surgical intervention. Thus, the diagnosis of an infected pancreas requires immediate surgical consultation along with the initiation of appropriate supportive medical therapy.

A. **Antibiotic Therapy.** Primarily used as an adjunct to surgical treatment. *The administration of prophylactic antibiotics to patients with severe necrotizing pancreatitis prior to the diagnosis of pancreatic infection is not recommended.* Recommended antibiotic regimens for documented pancreatic infections may include any of the following:

   1. Imipenem 500 mg IV q6 (traditionally the antibiotic of choice)

   2. Ciprofloxacin 500 mg IV q12 *plus* metronidazole 500 mg IV q6–8

   3. Meropenem 1,000 mg or doripenem 500 mg IV q8

   4. Ampicillin/sulbactam 1.5–3.0 g IV q6

   5. Piperacillin/tazobactam 3.375 g IV q6

   *The typical **duration** of antibiotics may range from 14 to 28 days but is individualized to each patient's condition and the timing/completeness of source control. Because of the difficulty of achieving adequate source control in patients with infected pancreatic and peripancreatic tissue, a longer duration of therapy may be required.*

B. **Surgical Treatment.** Once pancreatic necrosis has been documented, surgical drainage or debridement is indicated. The optimal intervention strategy for patients with suspected or confirmed infected necrotizing pancreatitis is initial image-guided percutaneous (retroperitoneal) catheter drainage or endoscopic transluminal drainage, followed, if necessary, by endoscopic or surgical necrosectomy. However, the timing of invasive intervention for infected pancreatic or peripancreatic tissue should be delayed where possible until at least 4 to

8 weeks after initial presentation to allow the infected collection to become "walled-off."

1. **Percutaneous, CT-guided drainage.** This option is reserved for draining pancreatic abscesses but can be used in unstable patients with pancreatic necrosis infection as a bridging procedure for surgical debridement.

2. **Surgical debridement.** Currently, these procedures are best delayed until at least 4 to 8 weeks after the onset of illness as delay allows clear demarcation of infected necrosis and viable tissue with lower surgical mortality risk. Procedures or techniques are varied and aim to remove infected tissue while preserving live tissue and ensuring continuity or appropriate drainage of the pancreatic duct. Procedures include:

   a. **Open necrosectomy with or without open packing with planned relaparotomy** (usually every 48 hours) until all necrotic tissue is removed and infection controlled.

   b. **Open necrosectomy with continuous lavage of the lesser sac and retroperitoneum,** and two to four flushing drains with 10 to 15 L/24 hours are associated with the lowest mortality of the open procedures.

   c. **Open necrosectomy with closed packing and placement of a drain** (e.g., Penrose drain). Drains can usually be removed as the necrotic process resolves and is removed.

   d. **Hand-assisted laparoscopic necrosectomy with drain placement.** A retroperitoneal approach reduces bacterial contamination but laparoscopic methods are associated with more complications and incomplete debridement.

   e. **Open, laparoscopic, or totally endoscopic transgastric debridement with cyst gastrostomy**

   f. **Video-assisted laparoscopic retroperitoneal debridement**

VI. **PANCREATIC PSEUDOCYST.** Pancreatic pseudocysts are well-defined encapsulated fluid collections within the pancreatic tissue or adjacent peripancreatic tissue that occur most commonly as a consequence of acute pancreatitis associated with loss of integrity of a pancreatic duct (occurs in an estimated 5% to 15% of acute pancreatitis cases). Pseudocysts are considered a chronic pancreatic and/or peripancreatic fluid collection (without the presence of solid debris) that typically develops a minimum of 4 weeks after the initial acute pancreatitis injury. Most pseudocysts resolve spontaneously. Indications for intervention include the following: rapid enlargement of 6 cm or more in association with abdominal symptoms, a pseudocyst of 6 cm or more that persists for longer than 8 weeks (especially in association with symptoms), an infected pseudocyst that is distinguished from a pancreatic abscess, and/or pseudocyst-related hemorrhage or obstruction (e.g., duodenal or common bile duct). Intervention techniques may involve any of the following procedures:

A. **Surgical Cystogastrostomy.** Involves an open or laparoscopic procedure in which an anastomosis is created between the lumen of the cyst cavity and the stomach or small bowel using suturing or stapling devices.

B. **Percutaneous Drainage.** Involves placement of an external drainage catheter into the pseudocyst using real-time imaging guidance, usually with CT or ultrasound with fluoroscopy.

C. **Endoscopic Drainage.** Involves endoscopically creating a fistulous tract between the pseudocyst cavity and the gastric lumen using a Seldinger technique, advancing a guidewire into the pseudocyst cavity, dilating the tract, and finally deploying one or more plastic stents to secure apposition and allow for continuous drainage.

BIBLIOGRAPHY

Besselink M, van Santvoort H, Freeman M, et al. IAP/APA evidence-based guideline for the management of acute pancreatitis. Working group IAP/APA acute pancreatitis guidelines. *Pancreatology*. 2013;13(4 Suppl 2):e1–e15.

Hartwig W, Werner J, Muller CA, et al. Surgical management of severe pancreatitis including sterile necrosis. *J Hepatobiliary Pancreat Surg*. 2002;9(4):429–435.

Hartwig W, Werner J, Uhl W, et al. Management of infection in acute pancreatitis. *J Hepatobiliary Pancreat Surg*. 2002;9(4):423–428.

Mishra G, Pineau BC. Infectious complications of pancreatitis: diagnosis and management. *Curr Gastroenterol Rep*. 2004;6(4):280–286.

Sakorafas GH, Lappas C, Mastoraki A, et al. Current trends in the management of infected necrotizing pancreatitis. *Infect Disord Drug Targets*. 2010;10(1):9–14.

Schneider L, Buchler MW, Werner J. Acute pancreatitis with an emphasis on infection. *Infect Dis Clin North Am*. 2010;24(4):921–941.

Solomkin JS, Mazuski JE, Bradley JS, et al. Diagnosis and management of complicated intra-abdominal infection in adults and children: guidelines by the Surgical Infection Society and the Infectious Diseases Society of America. *Clin Infect Dis*. 2010;50:133–164.

Tenner S, Baillie J, DeWitt J, et al. American College of Gastroenterology guideline: management of acute pancreatitis. *Am J Gastroenterol*. 2013;108(9):1400–1415.

INFECTIOUS PERITONITIS

William F. Wright

I. INTRODUCTION

A. Definition. An acute or chronic inflammatory process of the peritoneum (a membrane that lines the inside of the abdominal cavity) that is most commonly due to a bacterial or fungal infection

B. Classification. While peritonitis can be acute or chronic, classification is based on the mechanism of infection and includes the following:

1. **Primary peritonitis.** Commonly known as *spontaneous bacterial peritonitis* **(SBP).** It most commonly occurs in the setting of **ascites** and is not directly related to any other intra-abdominal infection.

2. **Secondary peritonitis**. A peritonitis that is due to a secondary abdominal infection and/or abnormality (e.g., perforated appendicitis, perforated colon, diverticulitis). This form of peritonitis manifests as either *generalized peritonitis* or a *localized abscess*.

3. **Tertiary peritonitis**. Patients with a secondary-peritonitis process continue with persistent peritonitis and/or sepsis despite appropriate therapy (usually greater than or equal to 48 hours after initiation of therapy).

*Peritonitis related to **continuous ambulatory peritoneal dialysis (CAPD)** is a secondary-peritonitis process that can be due to bacterial or fungal pathogens.*

II. PATHOGENESIS AND CAUSES OF PERITONITIS

A. Primary Peritonitis. Normally the liver functions to remove bacteria from the blood as well as the intrinsic bacteriostatic activity of peritoneal fluid. These processes are impaired with liver disease and/or ascites fluid accumulation (e.g., decreased ascitic complement and protein levels). Additionally, portal hypertension increases bacterial translocation of the lymphatic system and portal vein with resultant seeding of ascites fluid; therefore, the routes of infection can be **hematogenous** (dysfunction of hepatic reticuloendothelial function), **lymphogenous** (increased portal hypertension), or **transmural bacterial migration**. Therefore, the most common organisms include:

1. **Enteric gram-negative bacilli**

   a. *Escherichia coli*

   b. *Klebsiella* spp

2. **Gram-positive cocci**

   a. *Streptococcus* spp

      b. *Staphylococcus aureus* **(usually a rare cause)**

      c. *Enterococcus* spp. (more commonly associated with healthcare-associated intra-abdominal infections)

   3. Anaerobic bacteria

      a. *Bacteroides* spp

Other unusual organisms associated with primary peritonitis include:

   4. *Mycobacterium tuberculosis.* Most commonly disseminated from a remote infection

   5. *Neisseria gonorrhoeae* and *Chlamydia trachomatis.* Most likely a transfallopian spread in women from a primary genital infection

   6. *Coccidioides immitis.* Most likely secondary to a disseminated infection

  B. Secondary Peritonitis. Normally the stomach, duodenum, and proximal small intestine contain minimal bacteria or microflora; however, intestinal obstruction and/or stomach acid reduction result in an increased colonization from oral bacteria. The distal small intestine and colon contain a much greater microbial flora; therefore, gastrointestinal infections with either perforation and/or resultant spillage of microorganisms into the peritoneal space will result in the process and may include any of the following microorganisms:

   1. *Escherichia coli.* Most frequently isolated facultative anaerobe

   2. *Bacteroides fragilis* **group.** Most frequently isolated anaerobe

   3. *Enterobacter* spp

   4. *Klebsiella* spp

   5. *Serratia* spp

   6. *Citrobacter* spp

   7. *Morganella* spp

   8. *Acinetobacter* spp

   9. *Pseudomonas* spp

  10. Viridans streptococci

  11. *Candida* **spp.** Most common cause of CAPD peritonitis.

  C. Tertiary Peritonitis. Microorganisms are similar to those isolated in secondary peritonitis but gain access to the peritoneal cavity by:

   1. Contamination during operative interventions

   2. Translocation of intestinal microflora

   3. Selection of multidrug-resistant pathogens by antimicrobial therapy

III. RISK FACTORS FOR PERITONITIS

  A. Primary Peritonitis. The presence of **ascites** is the most important factor.

   1. Alcoholic cirrhosis

   2. Chronic hepatitis

   3. Heart failure

    4. Metastatic malignant disease

    5. Systemic lupus erythematosus (SLE)

    6. Intrauterine devices

    7. Fitz-Hugh and Curtis syndrome

    8. Lymphedema and malnutrition

    9. Renal failure and/or nephritic syndrome

B. Secondary Peritonitis. Penetrating bowel wound or perforation is the most important factor.

    1. Intra-abdominal infection (e.g., appendicitis, diverticulitis, cholecystitis)

    2. Intra-abdominal surgery or trauma

    3. Gastric or duodenal ulcer

    4. Nonsteroidal anti-inflammatory drug (NSAID) or corticosteroid use (can result in ulcer development)

    5. Small-bowel obstruction, megacolon, or sigmoid volvulus

    6. Intestinal ischemia

    7. Cytomegalovirus (CMV) colitis (e.g., HIV/AIDS)

    8. Inflammatory bowel disease (e.g., Crohn disease or ulcerative colitis)

    9. Chemotherapy

    10. CAPD; usually as a result of a break in sterile technique during dialysate exchange or catheter/catheter-site maintenance

IV. CLINICAL MANIFESTATIONS OF PERITONITIS. Many of the clinical manifestations, systemic and abdominal, are thought to be mediated by the production of cytokines (e.g., tumor necrosis factor [TNF], interleukin 1 [IL-1], interleukin 6 [IL-6], interferon-gamma [IFN-gamma]) in response to infection.

    A. Abdominal Manifestations. Usually diffuse abdominal tenderness associated with nausea, vomiting, and/or diarrhea. Peritoneal signs (rebound tenderness and/or involuntary guarding) are often elicited on physical examination in the reliable patient.

    B. Systemic Manifestations

        1. Fever (greater than or equal to 100°F). The most common manifestation.

        2. Hepatic encephalopathy

        3. Weight loss, malaise, and night sweats. May indicate peritonitis due to tuberculosis.

The clinical manifestations of peritonitis may be **atypical** *with elderly or immunocompromised patients. Additionally, a* **turbid dialysate** *may be the first manifestation of CAPD peritonitis.*

V. APPROACH TO THE PATIENT

    A. History. A complete clinical history should be obtained, but peritonitis should be considered in the differential diagnosis of a patient being evaluated for fever and diffuse abdominal pain as well as decompensation (e.g., worsening hepatic encephalopathy) of a previously stable chronic liver disease patient. The history should focus on risk factors for peritonitis.

B. **Physical Examination.** In addition to performing a complete physical examination, areas to focus attention include:

1. **Neurologic examination** (to detect evidence of encephalopathy with mental status changes and search for asterixis)

2. **Abdominal examination** (to detect rebound tenderness/involuntary guarding or changes with bowel sounds; the finding of a "doughy abdomen" on palpation suggests tuberculous peritonitis)

3. **Cardiovascular examination** (to detect heart failure or lymphedema)

4. **Dermatologic examination** (to search for signs of hyperbilirubinemia [e.g., jaundice, sclera icterus])

C. **Laboratory Studies**

1. **Complete blood count (CBC).** Routinely ordered but nonspecific. Thrombocytopenia may occur with chronic liver disease.

2. **Basic metabolic panel (BMP).** Routinely ordered but nonspecific. May show renal insufficiency or hyponatremia associated with chronic liver disease.

3. **Liver function tests (LFTs).** Routinely ordered but may show low albuminemia with chronic liver disease or hyperbilirubinemia with peritonitis.

4. **Prothrombin time (PT)/partial thromboplastin time (PTT).** Routinely ordered for intra-abdominal surgeries or paracentesis and may be prolonged with chronic liver disease.

5. **Bacterial cultures.** Bacteremia occurs in up to 75% of patients. Serum beta-D glucan and/or serum galactomannan may be helpful in cases of fungal peritonitis. Ascitic fluid should be inoculated into blood culture bottles at the bedside.

6. **Peritoneal fluid analysis.** The diagnostic gold standard for peritonitis and should be sent for:

   a. **Cell count and differential.** The white blood cell (WBC) count is typically greater than or equal to 1,000/mm^3 with a predominance of polymorphonuclear leukocytes (PMNs). The PMN count is the single best predictor of SBP with a PMN count greater than or equal to 250/mm^3 having an 85% sensitivity and 93% specificity (PMN greater than or equal to 500/mm^3; sensitivity 80%, specificity 98%). **Peritoneal eosinophilia** may indicate either fungal peritonitis or intraperitoneal antibiotics. **A lymphocytic peritonitis** may indicate tuberculosis.

   The follow-up PMN count after 48 hours of treatment assists in detecting perforated versus nonperforated patients. The 48-hour PMN count is essentially always below the pretreatment value in SBP when an appropriate antibiotic is used; in contrast, the PMN count rises despite treatment in perforation and nonperforation secondary peritonitis.

   b. **Gram stain.** Diagnostic of peritonitis when positive but is more commonly negative. Direct smears of ascitic fluid for tuberculosis (e.g., acid-fast bacillus [AFB]) have 6% sensitivity and 20% specificity. Biopsy and/or culture are preferred for tuberculous peritonitis.

    c. **Ascites culture**. Specimens should be obtained by sterile methods and should be greater than or equal to 10 mL with direct inoculation into aerobic and anaerobic broth media. *Even a single dose of an effective broad-spectrum antimicrobial agent causes the culture to produce no growth if paracentesis is repeated 6 hours after the empirical antimicrobial dose is given in 86% of cases; only resistant flora would be detected.* Therefore, culture samples should be obtained prior to initiation of empirical antimicrobial therapy.

    d. **Ascites pH, protein, and lactate dehydrogenase (LDH) concentration.** A pH less than or equal to 7.35 with an LDH concentration greater than or equal to 25 mg/dL may support the diagnosis of SBP. Ascitic fluid protein may be low in concentration (less than or equal to 3.5 g/L) with primary and tuberculous peritonitis because of hypoalbuminemia and transudative ascitic fluid. The total protein, LDH, and glucose criteria are only 50% sensitive in detecting nonperforation secondary peritonitis.

    e. **Adenosine deaminase (ADA).** A level greater than or equal to 33 mcL has 97% sensitivity and 100% specificity for tuberculous peritonitis.

    f. An ascitic fluid **carcinoembryonic antigen (CEA)** greater than 5 ng/mL or ascitic fluid **alkaline phosphatase** greater than 240 units/L has also been shown to be accurate in detecting gut perforation into ascitic fluid with a sensitivity of 92% and specificity of 88%.

D. Radiography Studies. There is a minimal role for imaging in peritonitis but it may be useful to document ascites and for detecting an infected fluid collection. The two most common tests include:

  1. Ultrasonography. Rarely used as gas causes artifacts and leads to a poor study as well as gas outside the bowel is almost never identified in this manner and is limited by operator dependence; however, this method has the advantage of no exposure to ionizing radiation or contrast dye. Findings may include:

    a. **Bacterial and fungal peritonitis**. Infected fluids have an abnormal internal echogenicity, and the observation of gas within a fluid almost always suggests infection.

    b. **Tuberculous peritonitis**. The predominant finding is thickening of the small-bowel mesentery to more than 15 mm in association with enlargement of the mesenteric lymph nodes.

  2. CT. Has the disadvantage of exposure to ionizing radiation and iodinated contrast medium but is particularly useful for the detection of abscesses or loculated fluid collections and numerous other diagnoses (e.g., gastrointestinal perforations or fistulas and biliary causes of peritonitis). Findings include:

    a. **Bacterial and fungal peritonitis**. Gas, fat stranding, and/or peritoneal wall enhancement following intravenous (IV) contrast administration. Abscesses may appear as loculated fluid collections.

    b. **Tuberculous peritonitis.** The combined findings of highly attenuated (20–45 HU) ascites, enlarged lymph nodes with caseation (seen as low central area of attenuation), peritoneal wall enhancement, and mesenteric inflammatory changes suggest tuberculous peritonitis.

VI. DIAGNOSIS OF PERITONITIS

The diagnosis of SBP is made in the presence of an elevated ascitic fluid absolute PMN count (e.g., ≥250 cells/mm^3) without an evident intra-abdominal, surgically treatable source of infection. An abdominal paracentesis must be performed and ascitic fluid must be analyzed before a confident diagnosis of ascitic fluid infection can be made. A "clinical diagnosis" of infected ascitic fluid without a paracentesis is not adequate; the clinician's clinical impression that infection is unlikely does not rule out infection.

The characteristic analysis and diagnosis in the setting of free perforation, or secondary bacterial peritonitis, is a PMN count greater than or equal to 250 cells/mm^3 (usually many thousands), multiple organisms (frequently including fungi and enterococcus) on Gram stain and culture, and at least two of the following criteria: total protein greater than 1 g/dL, LDH greater than the upper limit of normal for serum, and glucose less than 50 mg/dL.

VII. TREATMENT OF PERITONITIS

A. **Primary Peritonitis/SBP.** The initiation of antibiotics is most often empirical and for a duration of 5 days. Antibiotic regimens are based on the most likely pathogen and some suggested regimens include (*listed agents are standard dosing with normal renal function, and agents should be adjusted to renal clearance*):

1. Ceftriaxone 1 to 2 g IV q24, cefepime 2 g IV q8–12, *cefotaxime 2 g IV q 8 or* ceftazidime 2 g IV q8 *plus* metronidazole 500 mg IV q6–8. ***Cefotaxime, a third-generation cephalosporin, has been shown to be superior to ampicillin plus tobramycin in a controlled trial; therefore, cefotaxime 2 g intravenously every 8 hours for 5 days is the PREFERRED treatment. An uncontrolled study demonstrated that 5 days of ceftriaxone 1 g intravenously twice a day was effective in treating culture-negative neutrocytic ascites.***

2. Piperacillin–tazobactam 3.375 g IV q6 (*for* Pseudomonas *the dose should be 4.5 g IV q6*) *or* ticarcillin–clavulanic acid 3.1 g IV q6 *or* ampicillin–sulbactam 3 g IV q6.

3. Meropenem 500 mg IV q8, doripenem 500 mg IV q8, ertapenem 1 g VI q24, *or* imipenem–cilastatin 500 mg IV q6 (or 1 g IV q8).

4. Moxifloxacin 400 mg PO/IV q24, ciprofloxacin 400 mg IV q12, *or* levofloxacin 500 mg PO/IV q24 *plus* metronidazole 500 mg IV q6–8.

5. Aztreonam 1 to 2 g IV q6–8 *plus* metronidazole 500 mg IV q6–8.

6. Tigecycline 100 mg loading dose, then 50 mg IV q12.

7. Vancomycin 15 to 20 mg/kg IV q8–24 *or* gentamicin 5 to 7 mg/kg IV q24 can be added to the preceding regimens (except tigecycline) for additional coverage or penicillin (PCN) allergic patients.

   A beta-lactam antibiotic (e.g., carbapenem) with metronidazole or a beta-lactam/beta-lactamase (e.g., piperacillin–tazobactam) antibiotic combination should typically be used in infections suspected of being associated with multidrug-resistant organisms until microbial identification and antibiotic sensitivity testing is performed; then antibiotics should be tailored to the particular pathogen.

B. **Secondary Peritonitis.** Management of secondary peritonitis includes surgical corrective therapy for the underlying abnormality, antimicrobial therapy, and supportive medical management. Antimicrobial agents are similar to primary peritonitis treatment (see the preceding) and usually for duration of 1 to 2 weeks following corrective surgery.

C. **Tuberculous Peritonitis.** Consists of the same standard therapy as pulmonary tuberculosis.

D. **CAPD Peritonitis.** The most important aspect of treatment involves immediate catheter removal. Antimicrobial therapy is based on the likely pathogen and usually with 1- to 2-week duration.

1. **Bacterial**

   a. **Empirical therapy or coagulase-negative *Staphylococcus*.** Vancomycin 15 mg/kg IV *plus* gentamicin 5 mg/kg IV followed by renal maintenance dosing.

   b. **Methicillin-susceptible *Staphylococcus aureus* (MSSA).** Nafcillin 2 g IV q4, cefazolin 2 g IV (renally adjusted), *or* ceftriaxone 1 to 2 g IV q24.

   c. **Enterobacteriaceae.** Same coverage as for primary peritonitis (see the preceding).

   d. **Methicillin-resistant *Staphylococcus aureus* (MRSA).** Vancomycin 15 mg/kg or linezolid 600 mg IV followed by renal maintenance dosing.

   Certain patient groups at particularly high risk of a poor outcome due to *Enterococcus* species infection include (a) immunocompromised patients; (b) patients with healthcare–associated postoperative peritonitis; (c) patients with severe sepsis of abdominal origin who have previously received cephalosporins and other broad-spectrum antibiotics selecting for *Enterococcus* species; and (d) patients with peritonitis and valvular heart disease or prosthetic intravascular material, which place them at high risk of endocarditis. Therefore, in patients with healthcare-associated intra-abdominal infection, including those with postoperative infection, a reasonable option would be to include coverage of *Enterococcus* species in the empiric regimen until definitive culture results are available. Ampicillin and vancomycin are agents that have activity against this organism and could be added to a regimen lacking antienterococcal activity.

2. **Fungal**. *Candida albicans* or other fungi are cultured from approximately 20% of patients with acute perforations of the gastrointestinal tract. Even when fungi are recovered, antifungal agents are usually unnecessary in adults unless the patient has recently received immunosuppressive therapy for neoplasm or has a perforation of a gastric ulcer on acid suppression or malignancy, transplantation, or inflammatory disease or has postoperative or recurrent intra-abdominal infection. Patients with healthcare-associated intra-abdominal infection are at higher risk of *Candida* species peritonitis, particularly patients with recurrent gastrointestinal perforations and surgically treated pancreatic infection. Most cases are due to *Candida albicans* or nonalbicans *Candida* species; therefore, empirical antifungal treatment is recommended with initiation of empirical antimicrobial therapy:

   a. **Fluconazole.** Typically used for *C. albicans* and given intraperitoneally as 200 mg in one exchange daily or intravenously or orally as 100 to 200 mg daily.

    b. Echinocandins (e.g., caspofungin, micafungin). Typically used for empirical therapy and isolation of a nonalbicans *Candida* species.

        i. Caspofungin 70 mg loading dose, then 50 mg IV q24

        ii. Micafungin 100 mg IV q24

VIII. FOLLOW-UP PARACENTESIS, PREVENTION OF SBP, AND HEPATORENAL SYNDROME PREVENTION. A follow-up ascitic fluid analysis is not needed in many patients with infected ascites. The majority of patients have SBP in the typical setting (e.g., advanced cirrhosis) with typical symptoms, typical ascitic fluid analysis (total protein ≤1 g/dL, LDH less than the upper limit of normal for serum, and glucose greater than or equal to 50 mg/dL), a single organism, and a dramatic clinical response. Repeat paracentesis can be performed to document sterility of culture and dramatic decrease in PMN count in patients with SBP; however, it is not necessary. In contrast, if the setting, symptoms, analysis, organism(s), or response are atypical, repeat paracentesis can be helpful in raising the suspicion of secondary peritonitis and prompting further evaluation and surgical intervention when appropriate. *Patients with ascitic fluid PMN counts greater than or equal to 250 cells/mm³ in a nosocomial setting and/or in the presence of recent beta-lactam antibiotic exposure and/or culture of an atypical organism(s) or who have an atypical clinical response to treatment should undergo a follow-up paracentesis after 48 hours of treatment to assess the response in PMN count and culture.*

    IV ceftriaxone for 7 days or twice daily norfloxacin for 7 days should be given to prevent bacterial infections in patients with cirrhosis and gastrointestinal hemorrhage.

    Patients with ascitic fluid PMN counts greater than or equal to 250 cells/mm³ and clinical suspicion of SBP, who also have a serum creatinine >1 mg/dL, blood urea nitrogen >30 mg/dL, or total bilirubin >4 mg/dL, should receive 1.5 g albumin per kilogram of body weight within 6 hours of detection and 1.0 g/kg on day 3 to prevent hepatorenal syndrome.

BIBLIOGRAPHY

Gilbert JA, Kamath PS. Spontaneous bacterial peritonitis: an update. *Mayo Clin Proc.* 1995;70(4):365–370.

Johnson CC, Baldessarre J, Levison ME. Peritonitis: update on pathophysiology, clinical manifestations, and management. *Clin Infect Dis.* 1997;24(6):1035–1045.

Kosseifi S, Hoskere G, Roy TM, et al. Peritoneal tuberculosis: modern peril for an ancient disease. *South Med J.* 2009;102(1):57–59.

Matuszkiewicz-Rowinska J. Update on fungal peritonitis and its treatment. *Perit Dial Int.* 2009;29(suppl 2):S161–S165.

Runyon BA. Management of adult patient with ascites due to cirrhosis: update 2012. AASLD practice guideline. *Hepatology.* 2013;57(4):1–96.

Solomkin JS, Mazuski JE, Bradley JS, et al. Diagnosis and management of complicated intra-abdominal infection in adults and children: guidelines by the Surgical Infection Society and the Infectious Diseases Society of America. *Clin Infect Dis.* 2010;50:133–164.

Wong CL, Holroyd-Leduc J, Thorpe KE, et al. Does this patient have bacterial peritonitis or portal hypertension? How do I perform a paracentesis and analyse the results? *JAMA.* 2008;299(10):1166–1178.

INFECTIOUS DIARRHEA

William F. Wright

I. INTRODUCTION

A. Definition. An increased frequency of defecation due to a microbial pathogen and defined as greater than three stools per day or greater than 200 g of stool per day *plus* an enteric symptom such as nausea, vomiting, abdominal pain/cramps, tenesmus, fecal urgency, or moderate–severe flatulence.

B. Epidemiology

1. Infectious diarrhea is the most common cause of diarrhea worldwide.

2. It is the second most common cause of death worldwide but the leading cause of childhood death worldwide.

3. In the United States, most episodes occur during the winter months and are due to viral pathogens (e.g., noroviruses, rotaviruses).

C. Diarrhea Syndromes

1. **Acute infectious diarrhea.** Lasting *less* than 14 days.

    a. Acute watery diarrhea (passage of stools without blood)

    b. Acute dysentery (passage of grossly bloody stools with or without fever)

2. **Chronic or persistent diarrhea.** Lasting *more* than 14 days.

D. Pathogenesis. Pathogens are transmitted through contaminated water or foods/food products and reach the gastrointestinal tract to cause:

1. **Increased intestinal secretion of fluid and electrolytes**, most commonly in the small intestine, through the production of **enterotoxins** (e.g., cholera toxin, *Escherichia coli* heat labile and heat stable toxins) that may mediate secretagogues (e.g., 5-hydroxytryptamine [5-HT]).

2. **Decreased intestinal absorption of fluid and electrolytes** in the small and large intestine through intestinal mucosal damage. Severe villous atrophy can occur with infection due to *Giardia, Cryptosporidium, Cyclospora,* and *Microsporidium* (intestinal protozoa). An alternative cause of villous atrophy is **celiac disease** (an autoimmune disorder due to gluten intolerance).

II. CAUSES OF INFECTIOUS DIARRHEA

A. Bacterial

1. ***Campylobacter jejuni.*** Most commonly from a foodborne exposure to poultry.

2. ***Salmonella* spp**

      a. Nontyphoid. Most commonly from a foodborne exposure to poultry or eggs.

      b. Typhoid and paratyphoid. Person-to-person contact during international travel.

    3. *Shigella* spp. Person-to-person contact.

    4. Shiga toxin—*E. coli* (0157:H7). Most commonly a foodborne exposure to undercooked beef or raw seed sprouts.

    5. *Vibrio* spp

      a. Cholera. Low level of endemicity in U.S. Gulf Coast states with transmission by water exposure or seafood exposure.

      b. Noncholera. Most commonly foodborne exposure to shellfish and seafood.

    6. *Yersinia enterocolitica*. Can be associated with swine and cattle exposure.

    7. *Aeromonas* spp. International travel to tropical regions.

    8. *Plesiomonas shigelloides*. International travel and ingestion of seafood.

    9. *Staphylococcus aureus*. Foodborne exposure (e.g., potato salad) due to preformed toxin.

    10. *Clostridium perfringens*. Contaminated meat, vegetables, or poultry with bacterial spores.

    11. *Bacillus cereus*. Contaminated rice (reheated rice) and vegetable sprouts with bacterial spores.

    12. *Clostridium difficile* (see Chapter 20).

B. Viruses. Most commonly occur during the winter months and are typically due to outbreaks in families, nursing homes, or day care centers (usually self-limiting and less than 1 day).

    1. Noroviruses.

    2. Rotavirus.

    3. Enteric adenoviruses (types 40 and 41).

    4. Cytomegalovirus (CMV). More common in immunocompromised patients.

C. Parasites. Most commonly related to international travel and/or contaminated water. Diarrhea usually persists for greater than 7 to 10 days.

    1. *Giardia intestinalis*

    2. *Cryptosporidium parvum*

    3. *Cyclospora cayetanensis*

    4. *Microsporidia* spp

    5. *Entamoeba histolytica*. (Africa, Asia, Latin America)

    6. *Balantidium coli*. (Asia)

III. CLINICAL MANIFESTATIONS OF INFECTIOUS DIARRHEA

A. Diarrhea. Usually one of two forms, but there can be considerable overlap.

    1. Watery diarrhea *without* blood. Usually self-limiting and clinically nonspecific to etiology.

2. **Diarrhea *with* blood (dysentery).** Usually indicates colitis (i.e., inflammatory diarrhea). Associated with fever, nausea, and abdominal pain and cramps. Most commonly due to *Shigella, Campylobacter,* nontyphoid *Salmonella,* and Shiga toxin—*E. coli.* Also, can be associated with *Aeromonas* spp, *Yersinia* spp, noncholeraic *Vibrio,* and *E. histolytica.*

B. **Abdominal Pain and Cramps.** Usually associated with dysentery but can also occur without dysentery.

C. **Nausea and Vomiting.** May be associated with abdominal pain and cramps but is typically due to viral illnesses.

D. **Fever.** Usually occurs with acute dysentery (i.e., inflammatory diarrhea) or bacteremia from salmonella.

E. **Tenesmus.** Defined as a clinical symptom, where there is a feeling of constantly needing to pass stools, despite an empty colon. This symptom may indicate inflammatory diarrhea.

F. **Delirium or Altered Mental Status.** Usually indicates dehydration and is usually associated with other findings such as tachycardia, dry mucous membranes, and poor skin turgor.

IV. APPROACH TO THE PATIENT

A. **History.** A complete history should be performed with attention to exposures or risk factors associated with infectious diarrhea, comorbid illnesses (*immunocompromised or pregnant patients may be at risk for certain infections*), medications, recent travel history, and occupation (e.g., day care or nursing home worker). Additionally, diarrhea in family members and the timing of diarrhea onset may be helpful:

1. **Incubation period less than 6 hours** (*S. aureus* or *B. cereus*).

2. **Incubation period 6 to 24 hours** (*C. perfringens* or *B. cereus*).

3. **Incubation period 16 to 72 hours** (all other causes).

B. **Physical Examination.** A complete physical examination should be performed with focused attention on:

1. **Neurologic examination** (to assess mental status by the Glasgow coma scale).

2. **Head, eyes, ears, nose, and throat (HEENT) examination** (dry mucous membranes can suggest dehydration).

3. **Cardiovascular examination** (resting tachycardia or orthostatic hypotension may suggest dehydration).

4. **Musculoskeletal examination** (joint pain may suggest *Yersinia* spp or *C. jejuni* as Reiter syndrome).

5. **Rectal examination** (to detect blood in the stool that may indicate dysentery).

C. **Clinical Evaluation.** Because the most feared complication of infectious diarrhea is *dehydration*, the clinical evaluation of the *degree of dehydration* remains important. (*The following are general considerations that would vary among different patients.*)

1. **Mild-to-moderate dehydration (3%–9% fluidlLoss)**

   a. Fatigue and restlessness

   b. Dry mucous membranes and thirst sensation

      c. Weak pulses and cool extremities

      d. Decreased urine output (may be indicated by a dark-concentrated urine and with less than 800 mL per day)

  2. Severe dehydration (greater than 10% fluid loss)

      a. Apathy and lethargy

      b. Dry mucous membranes, sunken eyes, and extreme thirst sensation

      c. Deep breaths and tachycardia

      d. Skin tenting, poor capillary refill, weak pulses, and cool extremities

      e. Minimal urine output (less than 500 mL dark-concentrated urine per day)

D. Laboratory Studies

  1. Complete blood count (CBC). Nonspecific. An elevated hematocrit may suggest dehydration.

  2. Basic metabolic panel (BMP). Infectious diarrhea may produce a non–gap metabolic acidosis in association with electrolyte abnormalities (e.g., hypernatremia, hypokalemia). An elevated blood urea nitrogen (BUN), creatinine, and metabolic alkalosis may suggest dehydration.

  3. Blood cultures. Usually *not* ordered and of low yield; however, bacteremia may occur with *Salmonella* spp–related infections.

  4. Stool leukocytes and/or lactoferrin. May be helpful for inflammatory diarrhea, but nonspecific.

      a. Stool leukocytes. Sensitivity 73% and specificity 84% for bacterial infectious diarrhea. A small content of stool mucus or liquid stool is stained with methylene blue stain or Wright stain and then examined for leukocytes. A false-negative test may occur with cytotoxigenic *C. difficile* or *E. histolytica* infection due to destruction of leukocytes.

      b. Stool lactoferrin. Sensitivity 92% and specificity 79% for bacterial infectious diarrhea. Lactoferrin is a glycoprotein found in neutrophil granules and is detected by a rapid immunologic latex agglutination method. The test performance is not altered by the destruction of leukocytes.

  5. Stool cultures. The diagnostic yield is estimated from 1% to 5%. Indicated when patients have any of the following:

      a. Severe diarrhea (greater than 6 stools per day)

      b. Dysentery

      c. Diarrhea associated with fever

      d. Persistent diarrhea (over more than 7 days)

      e. Multiple cases of diarrhea

  6. Serology. Serum polymerase chain reaction (PCR) is the preferred test for diagnosing CMV. Serum antibody testing may also be helpful.

  7. Stool antigen testing. Antigen testing (sensitivity 95%) may be useful for *Giardia intestinalis, Cryptosporidium parvum,* and rotavirus.

  8. Stool acid-fast stain. Useful for identification of *Cyclospora cayetanensis, Isospora belli,* and *Microsporidium.*

9. Stool ova and parasite exam. Should be ordered in patients with:

  a. International travel

  b. Exposure to untreated water (e.g., a hiker)

  c. Persistent diarrhea (over more than 7 days).

  d. Immunocompromised patients (e.g., HIV/AIDS and CD4 less than 50 cells/mm^3).

10. Stool Shiga toxin testing. Should be performed in patients with dysentery and include enzyme immunoassay (EIA) tests for Shiga toxin 1 and Shiga toxin 2. (Shiga toxin 2 is more important in the pathogenesis of hemolytic uremic syndrome [HUS]).

V. TREATMENT

  A. Supportive Care. Should be provided in *all* cases and can consist of **fluid and electrolyte replacement**, a **diet of easily digestible foods** (e.g., BRAT diet: bananas, rice, applesauce, and toast), and/or **antimotility medications** (e.g., loperamide). Adjunctive loperamide therapy can be administered to patients with traveler's diarrhea to decrease duration of diarrhea and increase chance for a cure; however, antimotility medications should be *avoided* in patients with dysentery or suspected inflammatory diarrhea. The recommended dose of loperamide for therapy for adults with diarrhea is 4 mg initially followed by 2 mg after subsequently passed watery stools not to exceed 8 mg per day. Loperamide is not given for more than 48 hours.

  Bismuth subsalicylates (BSSs) can be administered to control rates of passage of stool and may help travelers function better during bouts of mild-to-moderate illness. The recommended dose of BSS for therapy of acute diarrhea is 30 mL (525 mg) of liquid formulation or two tablets (263 mg per tablet) chewed well each 30 to 60 minutes, not to exceed eight doses in 24 hours. The drug will produce black stools and black tongues from harmless bismuth sulfide salt.

  Patients should **avoid milk or other dairy products** due to the development of transient lactose intolerance.

  B. Oral Rehydration Therapy. The initial treatment of infectious diarrhea should focus on the prevention of dehydration with rehydration efforts. Commercial formulations (e.g., Pedialyte) can be obtained and used according to the listed directions; however, as a general rule, a homemade oral rehydration solution can be produced by the following formula: *add 1 tablespoon of salt and 2 tablespoons of sugar to 1 liter of water.*

  Treatment recommendations according to the degree of dehydration include the following. (*These are general rules to the approach to rehydration and may not apply to all patients.*)

  1. Minimal dehydration (less than 3% fluid loss)

  a. Less than 10 kg weight: 60 to 120 mL of oral rehydration solution per diarrhea stool

  b. Greater than 10 kg weight: 120 to 240 mL of oral rehydration solution per diarrhea stool

  2. Mild-to-moderate dehydration (3% to 9% fluid loss)

  a. May be treated as an outpatient

   b. 50 to 100 mL per kg of body weight replaced over a 3- to 4-hour period

3. **Severe dehydration (greater than 10% fluid loss)**

   a. Patients will most likely require hospitalization for intravenous hydration.

   b. Normal saline solution 20 mL per kg of body weight infused until improved perfusion, heart rate, urine output, and mental status.

C. **Antimicrobial Therapy.** More useful in cases of diarrhea associated with invasive or inflammatory pathogens. Antimicrobial agents may also be beneficial for:

1. Patients less than 3 months or greater than 65 years of age.

2. Patients with malignancy, immunocompromised (e.g., HIV), inflammatory bowel disease (e.g., ulcerative colitis, Crohn disease), and/or corticosteroid use (especially in cases of salmonella infection).

3. Patients with cardiovascular disease, prosthetic device (e.g., heart valve, orthopedic device), hemolytic anemia, sickle cell disease, or on hemodialysis (also especially important in cases of salmonella infection).

4. Parasitic cases.

5. Patients with vascular grafts (e.g., abdominal aortic aneurysm repair); especially in cases of salmonella infection.

In general, the evidence does not support empiric antimicrobial therapy for routine acute diarrheal infection, except in cases of traveler's diarrhea where the likelihood of bacterial pathogens is high enough to justify the potential side effects of antibiotics. Furthermore, antibiotics should not be given for diarrhea due to Shiga toxin—E. coli, as there is an increased risk for the development of HUS. Finally, the use of antibiotics for community-acquired diarrhea should be discouraged as epidemiologic studies suggest that most community-acquired diarrhea is viral in origin (norovirus, rotavirus, and adenovirus) and is not shortened by the use of antibiotics.

Selected antimicrobial therapy for the more common causes of infectious diarrhea includes:

1. *Escherichia coli, Shigella* **spp,** *Aeromonas* **spp, or** *Plesiomonas* **spp.** Azithromycin 500 mg PO q24, levofloxacin 500 mg PO q24, ciprofloxacin 500 mg PO q12, or Bactrim (TMP 160 mg and SMZ 800 mg; pediatric dose is TMP 5 mg/kg and SMZ 25 mg/kg) PO q12 for *3 days. Single-dose therapy using azithromycin 1,000 mg, ciprofloxacin 750 mg, or levofloxacin 500 mg may be considered and has been shown to be as effective as 3-day therapies for traveler's diarrhea due to noninvasive pathogens. Shigella* spp–related infections, however, are the exception and are usually treated for *5 days* in immunocompetent patients and *7 to 10 days* in immunocompromised patients.

2. *Campylobacter* **spp.** Erythromycin 500 mg PO q12 for 5 days.

3. *Salmonella* **spp (nontyphi).** Treatment is usually indicated for severe diarrhea and/or patients with the following conditions: (a) age less than 6 months or greater than 50 years; (b) prosthetic vascular or orthopedic device; (c) atherosclerosis or valvular heart disease; (d) immunocompromised (e.g., HIV/AIDS); and (e) malignancy. Ciprofloxacin 500 mg PO q12 or Bactrim (TMP

160 mg and SMZ 800 mg; pediatric dose is TMP 5 mg/kg and SMZ 25 mg/kg) PO q12 for 7 to 14 days (longer duration for immunocompromised patient).

4. ***Yersinia* spp**. Treatment is usually indicated for severe diarrhea, bacteremia, or immunocompromised patients. Usually a combination of ciprofloxacin 500 mg PO q12 and Bactrim (TMP 160 mg and SMZ 800 mg; pediatric dose is TMP 5 mg/kg and SMZ 25 mg/kg) PO q12 for 7 to 14 days (longer duration for immunocompromised patient).

5. ***Vibrio cholera* O1 or O139**. Doxycycline 300 mg single oral dose, Bactrim (TMP 160 mg and SMZ 800 mg; pediatric dose is TMP 5 mg/kg and SMZ 25 mg/kg) PO q12 for 3 days, or ciprofloxacin 500 mg single oral dose.

6. ***Giardia*.** Metronidazole 250 to 750 mg PO q8 for 7 to 10 days.

7. ***Entamoeba histolytica*.** Metronidazole 750 mg PO q8 for 5 to 10 days followed by paromomycin 500 mg PO q8 for 7 days.

8. ***Cryptosporidium* spp,*Isospora* spp,*Cyclospora* spp, and *Microsporidium* spp.** Most patients have chronic diarrhea with immunocompromised conditions (e.g., HIV/AIDS), and treatment requires a combination of antimicrobial agents that should involve the assistance of an infectious diseases specialist.

VI. PREVENTION. Frequent and effective handwashing and alcohol-based hand sanitizers are of limited value in preventing most forms of traveler's diarrhea but may be useful where low-dose pathogens are responsible for a diarrheal illness (*e.g., cruise ship outbreak of norovirus infection, institutional outbreak, or in endemic diarrhea prevention*).

Probiotics, prebiotics, and synbiotics for prevention of traveler's diarrhea are not effective; however, individuals should undergo pretravel counseling regarding high-risk food/beverage avoidance to prevent traveler's diarrhea.

BIBLIOGRAPHY

Casburn-Jones AC, Farthing MJ. Management of infectious diarrhoea. *Gut.* 2004;53(2):296–305.

DuPont HL. Clinical practice. Bacterial diarrhea. *N Engl J Med.* 2009;361(16):1560–1569.

Guerrant RL, Van Gilder T, Steiner TS, et al. Practice guidelines for the management of infectious diarrhea. *Clin Infect Dis.* 2001;32(3):331–351.

Riddle MS, DuPont HL, Connor BA. ACG clinical guideline: diagnosis, treatment, and prevention of acute diarrheal infections in adults. *Am J Gastroenterol.* 2016;E111:602–622.

Thielman NM, Guerrant RL. Clinical practice. Acute infectious diarrhea. *N Engl J Med.* 2004; 350(1):38–47.

20

CLOSTRIDIUM DIFFICILE COLITIS

Ryan S. Arnold
William F. Wright

I. INTRODUCTION

A. Definition. An inflammatory condition of the colon due to toxins produced by the bacterium *Clostridium difficile*.

B. Epidemiology

1. *Colonization of the colon with* C. difficile *occurs in newborns and infants* and is estimated to occur in 60% to 70% of persons. (*Early colonization may be related to person-to-person spread during hospitalization for birth or through food sources.*)

2. *Complete loss or a significant reduction in colonization naturally occurs around the age of 12 to 18 months* and coincides with the development of the normal colonic flora.

3. Approximately 3% of healthy adolescents and adults are colonized with the bacteria and remain asymptomatic.

4. For unclear reasons (presumed increased person-to-person spread), *colonization increases to 20% to 30% in the hospital setting and to approximately 50% in nursing home or long-term care hospital settings.*

5. While there is no sexual predilection or seasonal variation for colonization with this bacterium, *increasing age and length of stay in the hospital, nursing home, or long-term care facility are associated with increased colonization rates.*

6. While this bacterium has a worldwide distribution, the incidence of *C. difficile* disease in colonized patients varies with time, certain locations, antibiotic exposure, and bacterial strain (e.g., B1/NAP1/027). The incidence of disease has been estimated to be from 30 to 90 cases per 100,000 persons.

II. RISK FACTORS. The following are risk factors for developing *C. difficile* disease.

A. Antibiotics. This is the *most important risk factor* with **all** antibiotic classes carrying a risk for the disease. Approximately 96% of symptomatic *Clostridium difficile* infected patients received antibiotics within 14 days of infection, and 100% of affected patients were exposed to antibiotics within 3 months. Although any antibiotic can result in disease, the most frequently associated antibiotic classes include:

1. Penicillin (most commonly ampicillin or amoxicillin)

2. Cephalosporin

3. Clindamycin

4. Fluoroquinolones

Any inciting antimicrobial agent(s) should be discontinued immediately upon confirmation of Clostridium difficile *infection (CDI), if possible.*

  B. **Proton-Pump Inhibitors and Histamine-2 Blockers.** Reduction of the gastric acid barrier may allow more viable bacteria and spores to reach the colon.

  C. **Hospitalization, Nursing Home Resident, or Admission to a Long-Term Care Facility**

  D. **Age Greater than 65 Years**

  E. **Immunosuppression, Neutropenia, or Advanced HIV/AIDS**

  F. **Gastrointestinal Tract Disease, Surgery, or Invasive Procedure**

  G. **Comorbid Illnesses.** For example, renal failure, diabetes, cirrhosis, and malnutrition.

  H. **Peripartum Period.** Due to increased risk of colonization for the mother.

  I. **Chemotherapeutic Agents.** These agents alter the intestinal flora to allow for increased colonization and development of disease.

III. **PATHOGENESIS OF INFECTION.** A stepwise progression leading to infection is as follows:

  A. **Increased Colonization** (based on risk factors as noted previously).

  B. **Indigenous Change in Normal Colonic Flora.** Protective microflora of the colon is most commonly changed due to the use of antibiotic therapy (especially antibiotics with anaerobic coverage).

  C. **Increased Proliferation of Viable Bacteria With Toxin Production.** Ingested *C. difficile* bacteria and/or spores (*most commonly*), from a presumed person-to-person spread, proliferate in the colon (*spores convert to vegetative bacteria in response to alkaline pH and low-oxygen tension*) to produce exotoxins:

    1. Toxin A primarily recruits inflammatory cells but can induce intestinal permeability and cytoskeleton changes.

    2. Toxin B is the primary virulence factor associated with infection.

    3. Binary toxin. Primary function is unknown but may be associated with increased production of both toxins A and B.

While infants have high colonization rates that may be associated with toxin production, they rarely develop colitis due to an underdeveloped immune system or lack of toxin binding receptors in the colon.

Most colonized adults remain asymptomatic until their normal protective colonic flora is disrupted. *Disease develops when a critical threshold of bacteria and/or toxin is reached.*

IV. **MICROBIOLOGY OF *C. DIFFICILE*.** The bacterium was initially called *Bacillus difficilis* because it was a rod-shaped bacterium that was *difficult* to isolate and grow.

  A. Gram-positive spore-forming rod on Gram stain.

  B. Cultured colonies have a horse manure odor and appear as flat, yellow, and ground-glass colonies with a surrounding yellow halo.

  C. Grows best in anaerobic conditions.

V. CLINICAL MANIFESTATIONS OF *C*. DIFFICILE INFECTION. The *clinical spectrum of infection can range from mild diarrhea to fulminant colitis* and most commonly occurs shortly following antibiotic exposure (but can occur as long as 60 days after antibiotic therapy). The most common manifestations include:

A. Diarrhea. This is the most common manifestation and is typically characterized as more than three loose or watery stools per day for a duration of greater than 24 to 48 hours. Diarrhea can vary depending on the severity of disease as follows:

1. **Mild-to-moderate illness**. Usually nonbloody diarrhea with 3 to 12 stools per day. Additionally defined as a white blood cell (WBC) count less than 15,000 cells/mcL and a serum creatinine less than 1.5 mg/dL.

2. **Severe illness**. Usually associated with *pseudomembranous colitis*. Characterized by greater than 12 bloody stools per day. Additionally defined as a WBC count greater than 15,000 cells/mcL and a serum creatinine greater than 1.5 mg/dL.

3. **Fulminant disease**. This form of illness is usually associated with ileus and/ or *toxic megacolon* with reduced or absent bowel movements and hypotension (i e., shock).

Pseudomembranous colitis is characterized by raised, yellow, mucosal plaques consisting of leukocytes, tissue debris, blood, and mucus, overlying a necrotic colonic surface epithelium. Additional causes of pseudomembranous colitis include *Staphylococcus aureus* colitis; infections due to *Campylobacter* spp, *Salmonella* spp, and *Shigella* spp; diarrhea associated with *Escherichia coli* 0157:H7; cytomegalovirus (CMV) colitis; Crohn colitis; ischemic colitis; and medications (such as nonsteroidal anti-inflammatory drugs (NSAIDs), cyclosporine, and methotrexate). However, *the most common cause of* pseudomembranous colitis *is* C. difficile–*associated colitis.*

B. Abdominal Pain. Typically consists of abdominal cramps and localized discomfort in mild disease. Diffuse abdominal pain and tenderness occur with more severe disease.

C. Fever. Patients with mild illness are usually afebrile or have a low-grade temperature; however, patients with severe or fulminant disease are usually febrile (greater than 38.9°C).

D. Nausea and Vomiting. While nausea with vomiting usually occurs with severe fulminant disease, nausea alone may occur with mild disease.

VI. COMPLICATIONS OF *CLOSTRIDIUM DIFFICILE* INFECTION

A. Ileus

B. Toxic Megacolon

C. Colonic Perforation

D. Peritonitis

E. **Systemic Inflammatory Response Syndrome (SIRS) and Sepsis With Multiorgan Failure.** For example, respiratory and renal failure.

VII. APPROACH TO THE PATIENT

A. **History.** An accurate and complete history should be obtained with the physician to focus on the presence of risk factors, such as recent receipt of antimicrobials and/or recent hospitalizations or extended-care facility stays should also be elucidated. Characterization of symptoms should include the presence or absence as well as volume of diarrhea, severity and location of associated abdominal pain or cramping, and the presence of subjective fevers, nausea, or anorexia. Infection will almost always be associated with a history of abdominal distention, abdominal pain, and diarrhea.

B. **Physical Examination.** A complete examination should be performed, but physicians should focus on assessing the severity of illness in order to determine the need for a higher level of care or surgical consultation. *Altered mental status and hypotension both suggest severe disease.* With severe protein-losing enteropathy, patients may exhibit signs of ascites, pleural effusions, and soft-tissue edema. **Abdominal examination should evaluate for the presence of distention and peritoneal signs. Findings of localized or generalized peritonitis are a critically important finding, mandating admission to a monitored unit and urgent surgical consultation.**

C. **Laboratory Studies.** The diagnosis of *C. difficile* colitis is based on the following clinical and laboratory criteria: (a) **diarrhea** (defined as *greater than three unformed stools in less than 24 hours*) and (b) a **positive stool test** for toxigenic *C. difficile* itself or its toxins. Alternatively, the diagnosis can be presumed in the setting of colonoscopy or histopathology evidence of pseudomembranous colitis.

1. **Complete blood count (CBC) with differential.** Always ordered with severe infection indicated by an elevated WBC count greater than 15,000 cells/mcL.

2. **Complete metabolic panel and serum lactate.** These should always be ordered as severe infection may be indicated by acute kidney failure with an elevated serum creatinine (greater than 1.5 mg/dL), hypoalbuminemia (less than 4.0 mg/dL), hypokalemia (defined as less than 3.5 mmol/L), metabolic acidosis, and elevated lactic acid level (defined as a venous sample greater than 2.2 mmol/L and usually indicates poor tissue oxygenation with increased mortality).

3. **Stool studies for *C. difficile*.** The proper sample that should be submitted to the laboratory for testing is a watery, loose, or unformed stool. Rectal swab testing in the setting of ileus is *not* reliable for *C. difficile* toxin testing. Additionally, routine testing of multiple stools is *not* recommended due to the increase in false-positive results (especially in the clinical setting of a low pretesting probability for the disease).

    a. **Culture.** This is the *gold standard diagnostic test* but is limited by the need for special culture media, difficult culture conditions, and specialized laboratories required for this method.

    b. **Enzyme immunoassay (EIA) for toxins A and B.** This is the most common method utilized due to an easy and low-cost method; however, the sensitivity is reported as 63% to 94% and specificity is reported as 75% to 100%. In the setting of a high pretesting probability for the disease, a negative EIA should be confirmed by another method.

    c. **Cell cytotoxicity assay.** This method requires a specialized laboratory with cell culture lines (e.g., human foreskin fibroblast cells) in order to diagnose *C. difficile* infection and usually can take as long as 1 to 3 days for results.

This method relies on the principle of cytotoxic cell changes in the presence of *C. difficile* toxins and has a reported sensitivity of 67% to 100%.

d. *C. difficile* **common antigen, otherwise known as glutamate dehydrogenase (GDH)**. A rapid (3 hours) and inexpensive latex agglutination test associated with a sensitivity of 58% to 68% and specificity of 94% to 98%; therefore, the high negative predictive can be useful as a screening test. Newer methods use EIA technology with a sensitivity of 85% to 95% and specificity of 89% to 99%.

e. **Polymerase chain reaction (PCR)**. This method is expensive and requires specialized equipment with reported sensitivities of 96% and specificities of 96% to 100%. In general, this method targets the toxin A (*tcdA*) and toxin B (*tcdB*) gene.

Only stools from patients with diarrhea should be tested for **Clostridium** difficile *and testing for cure should not be done.*

D. Radiologic Studies

1. **Plain films (kidneys, ureters, and bladder or acute abdominal series)**. May detect free air below the diaphragm in the setting of perforation. Toxic megacolon may be suggested by marked colonic dilation (greater than 6 cm), bowel wall edema, and loss of haustration.

2. **CT**. Although findings are *not* specific for *C. difficile* colitis, CT is useful for detecting complications of severe infection (see the aforementioned complications). There are no current data to suggest that patients have *characteristic CT findings*, although CT will commonly demonstrate colonic wall thickening, nodular haustral thickening, or an "accordion pattern." In addition to these findings, fulminant forms of infection will frequently show ascites, fat stranding, and a prominent intravenous contrast enhancement of the layers of the colonic wall. Mesenteric venous gas, pneumatosis, and pneumoperitoneum are less common and signify severe life-threatening disease.

Although CT scans, diagnostic colonoscopies, and sigmoidoscopies are often obtained when evaluating patients with CDI, they are most useful in evaluating patients with more severe forms of infection in an effort to provide as much clinically relevant data as possible to help decide on the choice of therapy (medical vs. surgical). Colonoscopy and sigmoidoscopy are often performed to determine the extent of luminal disease (proctitis vs. left-sided colitis or pancolitis). However, the length of luminal disease has not been evaluated as an indicator of either the likelihood of the success of medical therapy or as an indicator of the need for surgical intervention. The primary benefit of a diagnostic lower endoscopy for these patients is mainly to distinguish CDI from other types of colitides, such as CMV, graft-versus-host disease, inflammatory bowel disease (IBD), and ischemic colitis. Colonoscopy introduces the risk of endoscopic perforation, and therefore, these studies and procedures largely remain an adjunct, chosen at the discretion of the physician.

VIII. MANAGEMENT OF *C. DIFFICILE* COLITIS

A. Medical Management

1. **Initial infection**

   a. **Mild–moderate disease**. Metronidazole 500 mg PO q8 for 10 to 14 days. Failure to respond to metronidazole therapy within 5 to 7 days should prompt consideration of a change in therapy to vancomycin at standard dosing (see the following). For patients who are intolerant (nausea, vomiting, and taste disturbance)/allergic to metronidazole and for pregnant/breastfeeding women, vancomycin should be used at standard dosing (see the following).

b. **Severe disease** (*i.e., serum albumin LESS than 3 g/dL PLUS WBC count greater than 15,000 cells/mcL or creatinine greater than 1.5 mg/dL*). Vancomycin 125 mg PO q6 for 10 to 14 days.

c. **Severe, complicated disease** (*i.e., intensive care unit [ICU] admission for hypotension, fever greater than 38.5°C, ileus or abdominal distention, altered mental status, WBC count greater than 35,000 cells/mcL or less than 2,000 cells/mcL, serum lactate greater than 2.2 mmol/L or end-organ failure*). Vancomycin delivered orally (125 mg four times per day) plus intravenous metronidazole (500 mg three times a day) is the treatment of choice in patients with severe and complicated CDI who have no significant abdominal distention. Vancomycin delivered orally (500 mg four times per day) and per rectum (500 mg in a volume of 500 mL four times a day) plus intravenous metronidazole (500 mg three times a day) is the treatment of choice for patients with complicated CDI with ileus or toxic colon and/or significant abdominal distention. Finally, intravenous immunoglobulin therapy at a dose of 150 to 400 mg/kg has also been used for patients not responding to initial therapy (*particularly in patients with hypogammaglobulinemia*).

2. **Recurrent disease**

   a. **First recurrence**. The choice of antibiotic is based on clinical severity as recommended for initial episodes (as in the preceding).

   b. **Second and subsequent recurrence**. While resistance to metronidazole has been rare, *do not* use metronidazole beyond the first recurrence due to risk of neurotoxicity. Vancomycin *taper dosing* is the choice of antimicrobial therapy and is suggested as follows:

      i. Vancomycin dosed as previously for severity of disease; then

      ii. Vancomycin 125 mg PO q6 for 10 to 14 days; then

      iii. Vancomycin 125 mg PO q12 for 7 days; then

      iv. Vancomycin 125 mg PO q24 for 7 days; then

      v. Vancomycin 125 mg PO q48–72 for 2 to 8 weeks

Pulse dosing regimen(s) may include a standard 10-day course of vancomycin at a dose of 125 mg given four times daily, followed by 125 mg daily pulsed every 3 days for 10 total doses.

3. **Newer agents**. Fidaxomicin 200 mg PO q12 for 10 to 14 days has been demonstrated to be noninferior to vancomycin with respect to clinical cure in two double-blind, randomized, controlled trials for mild-to-moderate infection. Compared to vancomycin, it has been shown to decrease rates of recurrent disease within 4 weeks of initial cure and to have superior cure rates in patients receiving concomitant antibiotics for underlying infections.

4. Patients with refractory disease (usually greater than three recurrent episodes) may be considered for **fecal intestinal microbiota transplantation**

(FMT) if conventional medical measures have failed. Fecal transplantation is performed with fresh stool obtained from a healthy donor and homogenized with water. The most common method of transplantation presently is via direct infusion of the stool into the cecum via colonoscopy, although it may be administered by nasogastric or nasoduodenal tube or retention enema. The rates of eradication of disease have been reported as high as 83% to 92% after a single treatment.

B. **Surgical Management.** Surgical consultation for *C. difficile* colitis should typically be reserved for patients with severe colitis that fails to improve with medical therapy, for generalized peritonitis or for rare cases of colonic perforation. Surgical consultation should also be considered in patients with any one of the following: hypotension requiring vasopressor therapy; clinical signs of sepsis and organ dysfunction (see Chapter 47); mental status changes; WBC count ≥50,000 cells/mcL; lactate ≥5 mmol/L; or failure to improve on medical therapy after 5 days.

Subtotal colectomy with ileostomy is typically the operative procedure of choice for *C. difficile* colitis; however, diverting loop ileostomy with colonic lavage may be an alternative. *A serum lactic acid level greater than 5 mmol/L as well as a WBC count greater than 50,000 cells/mcL has been associated with a much more pronounced perioperative mortality.*

C. **Prevention.** Infection-control practices are paramount to the management of *C. difficile* infections and include the following measures:

1. **Hand hygiene.** This is considered to be the most important infection-control practice to prevention. Handwashing should be performed with ***warm water and soap*** (*4% chlorhexidine gluconate soap is more effective than plain soap*) as this mechanically removes *C. difficile* spores from the hands. (Contaminated hands with spores are the most common mechanism of spread.) *Alcohol-based hand hygiene products are ineffective for the prevention of* C. difficile.

2. **Contact precautions**. The additional practice of ***wearing both gowns and gloves*** has decreased the transmission of *C. difficile*.

BIBLIOGRAPHY

Cohen SH, Gerding DN, Johnson S, et al. Clinical practice guidelines for *Clostridium difficile* infection in adults: 2010 update by the Society for Healthcare Epidemiology of America (SHEA) and the Infectious Diseases Society of America (IDSA). *Infect Control Hosp Epidemiol.* 2010;31(5):431–455.

Salkind AR. *Clostridium difficile*: an update for the primary care clinician. *South Med J.* 2010;103(9):896–902.

Shannon-Lowe J, Matheson NJ, Cooke FJ, et al. Prevention and medical management of *Clostridium difficile* infection. *BMJ.* 2010;340:641–646.

Steele SR, McCormick J, Melton GB, et al. Practice parameters for the management of Clostridium difficile infection. *Dis Colon Rectum.* 2015;58(1):10–24.

Surawicz CM, Brandt LJ, Binion DG, et al. Guidelines for diagnosis, treatment, and prevention of Clostridium difficile infections. *Am J Gastroenterol.* 2013;108(4):478–498.

INFECTIOUS GASTRITIS— *HELICOBACTER PYLORI*

William F. Wright

I. INTRODUCTION

A. Definition. An *inflammatory* condition involving the lining of the stomach due to chronic colonization from the bacterium *Helicobacter pylori*.

B. Epidemiology and Risk Factors. The bacterium colonizes approximately 50% of the world population and, in general, is slightly more common in men when compared to women.

The prevalence of colonization is lower among non-Hispanic Caucasians than other racial/ethnic groups (e.g., Asian Americans, African Americans, Hispanic Americans, Native Americans, and Alaska natives). Racial/genetic factors may have some role in predisposition as African Americans with a higher proportion of African ancestry have been reported to have higher rates of colonization compared to African Americans with a lower proportion of African ancestry. Asian and Hispanic immigrants have a much higher prevalence of colonization than first- or second-generation Asians and Hispanics who were born in North America.

H. pylori has a narrow host range and is found almost exclusively in humans. Acquisition of the bacterium occurs during childhood and is thought to occur as a consequence of direct **human-to-human transmission**, via either an **oral–oral** or **fecal–oral** route or both.

Risk factors associated with increased colonization include:

1. **Lower socioeconomic status**

2. **An infected parent, especially an infected mother**

3. **Increased number of siblings**

4. **Contaminated food or water supplies**

5. **Pet animals**. Considered a very rare and unusual risk factor

C. Classification. Classification of gastritis is principally based on causative factors, in order to cover the three most important and best defined categories of gastritis—namely:

1. *H. pylori*-induced

2. **Drug-induced.** Commonly nonsteroidal agents (nonsteroidal anti-inflammatory drug [NSAIDs])

3. **Autoimmune**

II. PATHOGENESIS OF DISEASE

A. **Gastritis and Gastric Ulcer Theory.** A **gastric gland** is a simple tubular structure that is formed first by invaginations called **gastric pits** and contains sections known as an isthmus, neck, and base. The lining **epithelium** of the stomach, and gastric pits, is entirely made up of **mucous columnar cells**. These cells produce a thick coating of mucus, which protects the gastric mucosa from acid and enzymes in the lumen of the stomach. **Parietal** (oxyntic) cells are concentrated in the isthmus region, also found in the base and neck of the glands, and are responsible for **hydrochloric acid** (when stimulated by histamine, gastrin from antral G cells, and acetylcholine from the vagus nerve) and **intrinsic factor** production, which is needed for digestion and absorption of vitamin B_{12} in the terminal ileum. Antral acidification in turn stimulates the release of somatostatin from antral D cells to inhibit gastrin release and reduce acid production (negative-feedback regulation).

The most widely held theory concerning the cause of gastritis and ulcer formation first involves *H. pylori* colonization of the gastric antrum. The bacterium then is able to penetrate the mucus gel layer lining the gastric mucosa, using its flagella and urease enzyme, to lie within the gastric pit. Within the gastric pit it is able to bind gastric mucosal cells using blood group antigen binding adhesins (*see Section III*) and lipopolysaccharides (LPS). The bacterium then releases two main virulence factors, vacuolating cytotoxin (VacA) and cytotoxin-associated antigen (CagA), that results in disruption of intracellular tight junctions and cytoplasmic vacuolization of gastric epithelial cells (e.g., apoptosis) as well as production of gastric interleukin 8 (IL-8) inducing inflammation (e.g., gastritis). In the gastric antrum, it is thought that D cells are selectively destroyed resulting in the development of hypergastrinemia in the fasting and postprandial state (e.g., loss of the negative-feedback regulation of gastrin). The resulting acid hypersecretion in turn leads to gastric ulcer formation.

B. **Duodenal Ulcer Theory.** Apoptosis of antral D cells, hypergastrinemia, and increased basal hydrochloric acid production result in an increased acid load to the duodenal bulb leading to ulcer formation.

C. **Gastric Cancer Theory (gastric adenocarcinoma and mucosa-associated lymphoid tissue [MALT] lymphoma).** CagA is thought to act as an oncogene promoting cell proliferation and increase pro-inflammatory signals in long-lived progenitor stem cells. Chronic *H. pylori*-induced inflammation can eventually lead to loss of the normal gastric mucosal architecture, with destruction of gastric glands and replacement by fibrosis and intestinal-type epithelium (e.g., gastric atrophy). The continuous production of reactive oxygen species that results from the ongoing inflammation can also give rise to DNA damage, thus inducing the multiple mutations thought to be required for initiation of the cancer cascade. This process of atrophic gastritis, intestinal metaplasia, and multiple mutations eventually results in dysplasia and gastric cancers.

III. MICROBIOLOGY OF *HELICOBACTER PYLORI*

A. **General Microbiology.** The morphology involves a gram-negative bacterium, measuring 2 to 4 μm in length and 0.5 to 1 μm in width. Although usually spiral-shaped, the bacterium can appear as a rod or coccoid shape. Coccoid shapes appear after prolonged in vitro culture or antibiotic treatment. The bacterium has two to six unipolar, sheathed flagella of approximately 3 μm in length, which often carry a distinctive bulb at the end. The flagella confer motility and allow rapid movement in viscous solutions such as the mucus layer overlying gastric epithelial cells.

B. **Culture Requirements**. *H. pylori* is a fastidious microorganism that requires complex growth media *and* standard microaerobic conditions of 85% N_2, 10% CO_2, and 5% O_2. Growth occurs at 34°C to 40°C, with an optimum of 37°C. Commonly used solid media for routine isolation and culture consist of Columbia or *Brucella* agar supplemented with either (lysed) horse or sheep blood or, alternatively, newborn or fetal calf serum.

C. **Virulence Factors**. The bacterium produces a 550-kDa, multimeric, nickel-containing **urease** that catalyzes the hydrolysis of urea to yield ammonia and carbonic acid. The *ure* gene cluster, composed of seven genes, encodes the two structural subunits **UreA** (26.5 kDa) and **UreB** (60.3 kDa), and five accessory proteins. Accessory proteins are required for the nickel ion insertion into the apoenzyme. The native protein consists of six copies each of UreA and UreB; two nickel ions are coordinated into each UreB active site. Urease is found in the cytosol and aids in colonization of the host by neutralizing gastric acid and providing ammonia for bacterial protein synthesis.

Other important virulence factors include:

1. **VacA**, *a cytotoxin secreted as a large 140-kDa polypeptide, which causes disruption of intracellular tight junctions and cytoplasmic vacuolization in gastric epithelial cells.*

2. **CagA**, *an oncoprotein produced from a 40-kb region of chromosomal DNA encoding approximately 31 genes that forms a type IV secretion system. Injected into the cytosol of gastric cells, via a pilus, it appears to be involved in the induction of gastric IL-8 production, a potent neutrophil-activating chemokine, inducing inflammation.*

3. **Blood group antigen binding adhesin (BabA)**, *encoded by the* babA2 *gene, has been shown to mediate adherence of* H. pylori *to the Lewis b blood group antigen on human gastric cells.*

IV. **CLINICAL MANIFESTATIONS.** Colonization with *H. pylori* is not a disease in itself but a condition that affects the relative risk of developing various clinical disorders of the upper gastrointestinal tract. Although gastric colonization with *H. pylori* induces histologic gastritis in all individuals, only a minority develop any apparent clinical signs of this colonization (referred to then as *H. pylori* infection due to the result of clinical disease).

Dyspepsia is characterized by *epigastric pain, discomfort,* or *burning sensation.* An important cause of dyspepsia is peptic ulcer disease (PUD), which includes gastric and duodenal ulcers.

Gastric or duodenal ulcers (commonly referred to as peptic ulcers) are defined as mucosal defects with a diameter of at least 0.5 cm penetrating through the muscularis mucosa. Gastric ulcers most commonly occur along the lesser curvature of the stomach, in particular the transition from corpus to antrum mucosa. Duodenal ulcers usually occur in the duodenal bulb, which is the area most exposed to gastric acid.

Development of these disorders depends on a variety of bacterial, host, and environmental factors.

Three main clinical phenotypes (e.g., manifestations) have been described:

A. **Simple Gastritis Phenotype (85% of patients).** Patients are typically asymptomatic and have normal acid secretion.

B. **Gastric and Duodenal Ulcer Phenotype (10%–15% of patients).** Patients typically have dyspepsia and high acid secretion due to antral-predominant gastritis.

C. **Gastric Cancer Phenotype (approximately 1% of patients).** Patients typically are asymptomatic and have achlorhydria and multifocal atrophic gastritis.

V. APPROACH TO THE PATIENT

A. **History.** A complete and chronologically accurate history should be obtained in all suspected cases. The history should focus on the timing of events, risk factors, comorbid conditions, medication allergies, family history, and recent antimicrobial therapy. **H. pylori *should be included in the differential diagnosis of any patient who presents with dyspepsia, PUD, gastric perforation, melanotic stools from an upper intestinal bleed, long-term low-dose aspirin or NSAID treatment, unexplained iron-deficiency anemia, idiopathic thrombocytopenic purpura (ITP), and/or a family history of gastric cancer.***

The characteristic ulcer symptom is *burning* epigastric pain on an empty stomach that is relieved by eating, drinking milk, or taking antacid therapy. The pain may be exacerbated by NSAIDs or spicy foods.

B. **Physical Examination.** Typically the first sign of disease is the complication of either gastrointestinal perforation or bleeding. A complete physical examination should be performed, but areas of focus include:

1. **Vital signs.** Patients may or may not demonstrate tachycardia or tachypnea.

2. **Head, eyes, ears, nose, and throat (HEENT) examination**. Conjunctival pallor may be observed in the setting of bleeding.

3. **Abdominal examination.** Examination may be associated with epigastric tenderness on palpation or peritoneal signs if there is an associated perforation.

4. **Anorectal examination.** Digital rectal examination should be performed for hemoccult positive stool.

C. **Laboratory Studies**

1. **Complete blood count (CBC)**. Routinely ordered and may reveal iron-deficiency anemia, anemia of chronic disease, or thrombocytopenia.

2. **Complete metabolic profile (CMP)**. Routinely ordered for medication safety monitoring but nonspecific for *H. pylori* infection.

3. **Blood cultures**. Should not be ordered and are of low yield.

4. **Urea breath test**. A noninvasive test used for both initial diagnosis (sensitivity 97%, specificity 100%) and test of cure. Requires oral ingestion of carbon 13 or carbon 14 labeled urea and a 6-hour fasting state for testing.

5. **Stool antigen test**. A noninvasive test that utilizes monoclonal antibodies to *H. pylori* (sensitivity 92%, specificity 94%). Proton-pump inhibitors (PPI) seem to affect the accuracy of the stool antigen test and should be stopped 2 weeks prior to testing.

6. **Serologic antibodies, immunoglobulin G**. Cannot be used to distinguish active infection or test of cure.

7. **Endoscopy with biopsy, histology, and rapid urease testing**. Should be performed in patients 55 years or older to evaluate for cancer. The rapid urease test (sensitivity 95%, specificity 100%) can be performed if patients have not taken PPIs for 2 weeks or have not taken bismuth or antimicrobial agents within 4 weeks of endoscopy. Biopsy with histologic confirmation of *H. pylori* infection should be performed if patients are suspected of having cancer or have been taking PPIs, bismuth agents, or antimicrobials within 2 weeks of endoscopy.

8. **Culture and molecular tests**. Not routinely ordered or available.

D. **Radiologic Studies.** In general, diagnostic imaging is not required except in the case of patients suspected of gastric ulcer perforation where either an acute abdominal series (AAS) plain-film or CT image of the abdomen and pelvis may reveal intraperitoneal free air.

VI. MANAGEMENT

A. **Medical Management.** Appropriate combination antimicrobial therapy with acid suppression therapy (e.g., proton-pump antagonists [PPI]) is generally recommended. Key questions prior to selecting a therapy regimen should include *penicillin-allergy history* and *previous macrolide exposure* for any reason. General antimicrobial therapy recommendations for the treatment of *H. pylori* include (dosing assumes normal renal function):

1. *Recommended first-line regimens (listed in order of preferred combination therapy).*

   a. **Clarithromycin triple therapy (Food and Drug Administration [FDA] approved).** A PPI (standard or twice daily dosing), clarithromycin 500 mg daily, and amoxicillin 1 g daily (clarithromycin-based triple therapy) for a duration of 14 days. Metronidazole 500 mg every 8 hours may be used as an alternative to amoxicillin for patients with an allergy to penicillin.

   Clarithromycin triple therapy is particularly attractive in patients without any previous macrolide exposure or where clarithromycin resistance is known to be less than 15%.

   Eradication rates for clarithromycin triple therapy have been reported to be approximately 70% to 85%.

   b. **Bismuth quadruple therapy.** A PPI or histamine-2 receptor antagonist (standard or twice daily dosing), bismuth subcitrate 120 to 300 mg four times daily or bismuth subsalicylate 300 mg four times daily, metronidazole 250 mg four times daily or 500 mg three times daily, and tetracycline 500 mg four times daily for a duration of 10 to 14 days.

   Pylera is an FDA-approved combination product containing a PPI, bismuth subcitrate, tetracycline, and metronidazole taken for 10 days.

   Bismuth quadruple therapy is particularly attractive in patients with any previous macrolide exposure or who are allergic to penicillin.

   Eradication rates for quadruple therapy have been reported to be approximately 77% to 85%.

c. **Concomitant therapy.** A PPI (standard or twice daily dosing), amoxicillin 1 g daily, clarithromycin 500 mg daily, and metronidazole 250 mg four times daily or 500 mg three times daily given together for 3 to 10 days.

   Eradication rates for concomitant therapy have been reported to be approximately 88%.

d. **Sequential therapy.** A PPI (standard or twice daily dosing) plus amoxicillin 1 g twice daily for 5 days, followed by a PPI (standard or twice daily dosing), clarithromycin 500 mg twice daily, and metronidazole 500 mg twice daily for an additional 5 days. *Levofloxacin 500 mg daily may be used as an alternative to clarithromycin for a regimen known as levofloxacin sequential therapy.*

   Eradication rates for sequential therapy have been reported to be approximately 84% to 85%.

e. **Levofloxacin triple therapy.** A PPI (standard or twice daily dosing), levofloxacin 500 mg daily, and amoxicillin 1 g twice daily for a duration of 10 to 14 days.

   Eradication rates have been reported to be approximately 79% to 84%.

f. **LOAD (*levofloxacin, omeprazole, nitazoxanide agent and doxycycline*) therapy.** A PPI (double dose daily), levofloxacin 500 mg daily, metronidazole 500 mg twice daily, and doxycycline 100 mg daily.

   Eradication rates for LOAD therapy have been reported to be approximately 89% to 90%.

2. **Recommended salvage therapy strategies (e.g., *persistent* H. pylori *infection*).** Antimicrobial resistance rates for *H. pylori* have been estimated at 35% for metronidazole, 17.5% for clarithromycin, and 14% for levofloxacin. Resistance rates for amoxicillin, rifabutin, and tetracycline are estimated at less than 2%. Therefore, the strategy of salvage therapy is based upon whether the patient initially received clarithromycin triple therapy or bismuth quadruple therapy as well as previous quinolone therapy and penicillin-allergy history.

   a. Initially received clarithromycin triple therapy. Bismuth quadruple therapy or levofloxacin salvage regimens are the preferred treatment options. Rifabutin 150 to 300 mg daily for 10 days as a triple therapy with PPI and amoxicillin may be considered in patients without penicillin allergy.

   b. Initially received bismuth quadruple therapy. Clarithromycin- or levofloxacin-containing salvage regimens are the preferred treatment options. Rifabutin 150 to 300 mg daily for 10 days as a triple therapy with PPI and amoxicillin may be considered in patients without penicillin allergy.

B. **Surgical Management.** The primary treatment of *H. pylori* gastritis remains combination antimicrobial therapy. Accepted indications for surgery in the management of PUD include bleeding, perforation, obstruction, intractable disease, and suspected malignancy

   1. **Perforations.** Perforated peptic ulcers are mainly located in the first part of the duodenum, accounting for about 35% to 65% of cases. The pylorus harbors about 25% to 45% and the stomach about 5% to 25% of perforated peptic

ulcers. While it is estimated that about 50% of the perforations seal spontaneously, when surgical management is required simple closure with an omental patch (Graham patch) is sufficient to treat peptic ulcer perforations in up to 90% of cases. Ulcers occurring within the stomach should be excised to obtain tissue for histologic investigation as gastric cancer occasionally presents as perforated gastric ulcer.

2. **Bleeding.** Some features of bleeding ulcers may predict ongoing or high probability of rebleeding. According to the Forrest endoscopic classification, these features are (a) spurting arterial bleeding (highest rebleeding risk), (b) oozing venous bleeding, (c) visible nonbleeding vessel, (d) adherent blot clot, and (e) flat spot or clean base (lowest rebleeding risk).

Hemostasis in bleeding peptic ulcers can be achieved by endoscopic treatment in 90% to 95% of cases; however, approximately 5% to 10% of bleeding peptic ulcers need emergency operation. While the majority of bleeding peptic ulcers requiring surgery are mainly located in the first part of the duodenum, accounting for about 75% of cases, bleeding gastric and pyloric ulcers account for about 20% and 5%, respectively. Although stitch ligation of the ulcer is sufficient to control peptic ulcer bleeding in most cases, extra-duodenal ligation of the gastroduodenal artery may be necessary to stop bleeding of large duodenal ulcers. About 25% of patients require some form of pyloroplasty, and about 10% of patients undergo gastric resection, mainly Billroth II resection. The presence of an ulcer with a diameter of more than 2 cm increases the likelihood that a gastric resection must be performed.

VII. PROBIOTICS

A. Adjuvant probiotics containing *Lactobacillus* and *Bifidobacterium* species may increase *H. pylori* cure rates.

B. Probiotic supplementation may also reduce the incidence of antimicrobial side effects (e.g., antimicrobial-associated diarrhea).

BIBLIOGRAPHY

Chey WD, Leontiadis GI, Howden CW, et al. ACG Clinical Guideline: treatment of Helicobacter pylori infection. *Am J Gastroenterol.* 2017;112(2):212–239.

Fashner J, Gitu AC. Diagnosis and treatment of peptic ulcer disease and H. pylori infection. *Am Fam Physician.* 2015;91(4):236–242.

Gerrits MM, van Vliet AH, Kuipers EJ, et al. Helicobacter pylori and antimicrobial resistance: molecular mechanisms and clinical implications. *Lancet Infect Dis.* 2006;6(11):699–709.

Kavitt RT, Cifu AS. Management of Helicobacter pylori infection. *JAMA.* 2017;317(15):1572–1573.

Kusters JG, van Vliet AH, Kuipers EJ. Pathogenesis of Helicobacter pylori infection. *Clin Microbiol Rev.* 2006;19(3):449–490.

Malfertheiner P, Megraud F, O'Morain CA, et al. Management of Helicobacter pylori infection: the Maastricht V/Florence consensus report. *Gut.* 2017;66(1):6–30.

McColl KE. Clinical practice. Helicobacter pylori infection. *N Engl J Med.* 2010;362(17):1597–1604.

Sugano K, Tack J, Kuipers EJ, et al. Kyoto global consensus report on Helicobacter pylori gastritis. *Gut.* 2015;64(9):1353–1367.

22

ANORECTAL ABSCESS AND FISTULA-IN-ANO

William F. Wright

I. INTRODUCTION

A. Definition. An *anorectal abscess* is a collection of pus in the area of the anus and rectum. An anorectal fistula (**fistula-in-ano**) is an abnormal communication between the anus and the perianal skin.

B. Epidemiology. The disease is more common in men (66%) when compared to women (34%). The majority of patients are between the ages of 21 and 40 years (66%).

C. Classification. The anatomic classification of anorectal fistula involves its relationship to sphincter muscles.

1. **Intersphincteric fistula.** Most common.

2. **Transsphincteric.**

3. **Suprasphincteric.**

4. **Extrasphincteric.** Least common.

Anal fistulas may also be classified as "simple" or "complex." "Complex" anal fistulas include transsphincteric fistulas that involve greater than 30% of the external sphincter; suprasphincteric, extrasphincteric, and horseshoe fistulas; and anal fistulas associated with inflammatory bowel disease (IBD), radiation, malignancy, preexisting fecal incontinence, or chronic diarrhea. "Simple" anal fistulas have none of these complex features.

II. PATHOGENESIS

A. Cryptoglandular Theory. The most widely held theory concerning the cause of anorectal abscess and resultant fistula-in-ano disease is *obstruction* of anal glands and ducts. Anal glands and ducts discharge mucus in the area called the *zone of transition* (the transition of somatic skin extending halfway along the anal canal to the rectal portion of the colon) around the base of anal crypts. Enteric microorganisms entering the anal gland channel initiate acute inflammation and resultant gland obstruction with abscess formation. Once an abscess has formed, infected material will migrate through any channel (or sinus tract) to the exterior. Fistula-in-ano is virtually a sinus tract opening secondary to an infected anal gland, which opens through a minute ductal opening in an area of the anal crypt.

III. MICROBIOLOGY OF ANORECTAL ABSCESS

A. **Aerobic and Anaerobic Bacteria (*Cryptoglandular abscess*).** The microbiology is best illustrated as a polymicrobial environment. Most common isolated microorganisms include:

1. *Staphylococcus aureus* spp, *Streptococcus* spp, and *Enterococcus* spp

2. *Escherichia coli* and *Klebsiella pneumoniae*

3. *Finegoldia magna* (formerly *Peptostreptococcus* spp)

4. *Fusobacterium* spp

5. *Prevotella* spp

6. *Bacteroides fragilis* group spp

7. *Porphyromonas* spp

8. *Clostridium* spp

B. ***Actinomyces* spp,** particularly *Actinomyces israelii* and *Actinomyces meyeri*, most commonly are the result of foreign body penetration wound, trauma, or neoplastic disease. Risk factors include diabetes mellitus and HIV infection.

C. **Lymphogranuloma venereum (LGV)** is usually associated as a sexually transmitted infection that can manifest as either a unilateral inguinal syndrome (e.g., painful inguinal lymphadenopathy) or anorectal syndrome characterized best as hemorrhagic proctocolitis. Unlike other *Chlamydia trachomatis* related infections, LGV serovars L1, L2, and L3 are associated with inflammatory lesions of lymphatic tissue. Most cases of anorectal syndrome involve serovar L2b and occur in men who have sex with men (MSM), particularly unprotected anal receptive intercourse.

D. **Mycobacterial Infections** include predominantly *Mycobacterium tuberculosis* as a result of pulmonary tuberculosis, supporting the most common mechanism of anorectal abscess as gastrointestinal tract ingestion of a large number of microorganisms.

E. **Fungal Pathogens** include *rarely Candida* species.

IV. CLINICAL MANIFESTATIONS OF ANORECTAL ABSCESS

A. **Pain** (100% of patients), **perianal swelling** (96% of patients), and **fever** (19% of patients) are considered the hallmarks associated with anorectal abscess.

B. **Additional symptoms may include:** gluteal pain, rectal bleeding, dysuria, and urinary retention.

V. APPROACH TO THE PATIENT

A. **History.** A complete and chronologically accurate history should be obtained in all suspected cases of anorectal abscess. The history should focus on the timing of events, risk factors, comorbid conditions, medication allergies, recent infections, and recent antimicrobial therapy. *An anorectal abscess should be included in the differential diagnosis of any patient who presents with anorectal pain, swelling, and fever.*

Crohn disease, obstetric trauma, or local irradiation can increase the risk of developing anorectal fistulas. Other comorbid conditions associated with anorectal abscess and fistula-in-ano disease include ulcerative colitis, episiotomy, prostatectomy, anorectal carcinoma, hematologic malignancy, and penetrating foreign body injury.

B. **Physical Examination.** A complete physical examination should be performed, but areas of focus include:

1. **Vital signs.** Fever is common; however, patients may or may not demonstrate tachypnea.

2. **Anorectal examination.** On physical examination, there may be spontaneous or digitally expressed discharge, an open sinus, granulation tissue, or a palpable cord. If the patient cannot tolerate a digital examination, anesthesia is needed.

   Goodsall and Miles's so-called *rule* states that fistulas with an external opening lying above a horizontal line drawn through the center of the anal canal, with the patient in the lithotomy position, usually drain directly into the anal canal. Fistulas lying below this horizontal line usually drain into the midline posteriorly. The predictive accuracy of this rule is 40% to 90% for posterior fistulas and 50% to 70% for anterior fistulas.

3. **Genitourinary examination.** Anorectal abscesses can be associated with sexually transmitted diseases (STDs) such as LGV (see the preceding), syphilis, gonorrhea, and chlamydia infection.

4. **Pulmonary examination.** Anorectal abscesses can be associated with pulmonary tuberculosis.

C. **Laboratory Studies**

1. **Complete blood count (CBC).** Routinely ordered and may reveal leukocytosis, leukopenia, and anemia of chronic disease.

2. **Basic metabolic panel (BMP).** Routinely ordered but nonspecific for anorectal abscess infections.

3. **Blood cultures.** Commonly two sets are ordered but are of low yield.

4. **Serum rapid plasma reagin (RPR) and urine for gonorrhea and chlamydia infection.** Should be obtained in patients with immunosuppressed conditions (e.g., HIV) or epidemiologically associated risk factors.

5. **Deep tissue sample for Gram stain and routine cultures** are more likely to yield results beneficial to guide further antimicrobial therapy in complicated disease (e.g., peritoneal abscess, secondary peritonitis, necrotizing skin and soft-tissue infection, and/or inflammatory bowel disease); however, superficial swab cultures from ulcer or sinus tracts may not identify the true bacteriologic pathogen because of bacterial colonization of wound surfaces with microorganisms typically not considered pathogenic (e.g., *Enterococcus* and/ or coagulase-negative *Staphylococcus* spp).

D. **Radiologic Studies.** Superficial abscesses and simple fistulas, in general, do not require diagnostic imaging.

1. **Endoanal ultrasound (EUS) and transperineal ultrasound (TPUS).** EUS is an imaging study performed in two or three dimensions, with or without peroxide enhancement, and it typically identifies an abscess and fistula-in-ano in 73% to 100% of the cases. TPUS is a noninvasive alternative to EUS with an estimated sensitivity of 85%.

2. **Abdominal and pelvic CT or MRI.** More useful for identifying smaller abscesses, recurrent fistula-in-ano, and perianal Crohn disease. The sensitivity of CT was 77% and 70% in immunocompetent and immunocompromised patients. An advantage of MRI over CT is better identification of both anorectal abscess and associated fistula tracts. MRI has an overall sensitivity of 82% to 90% for the identification of abscesses and fistula-in-ano.

3. **Fistulography.** A contrast-based injection study of the fistula under fluoroscopy may also be an effective means of studying an anal fistula.

VI. MANAGEMENT OF ANORECTAL ABSCESS

A. **Medical Management.** Appropriate antimicrobial therapy with routine incision and drainage of an uncomplicated anorectal abscess in healthy patients does not improve healing or reduce recurrence; therefore, it is not generally recommended. Selective use of antibiotics for patients with anorectal abscess complicated by cellulitis, systemic inflammation, leukocytosis, leukopenia, or immunosuppression (e.g., HIV, use of immunosuppressive therapy, prolonged use of corticosteroids, or absolute neutrophil count [ANC] less than $1000/mm^3$) has been advocated. General antimicrobial therapy recommendations for the treatment of anorectal abscesses include (dosing assumes normal renal function):

1. *Cryptoglandular type abscess.*
   a. Immunocompetent patient. Metronidazole 15 to 20 mg/kg orally divided into 3 or 4 doses daily with or without ciprofloxacin 500 mg once or twice daily for a duration of 5 to 10 days.
   b. Immunocompromised patient. Metronidazole 15 to 20 mg/kg orally divided into 3 or 4 doses daily with or without ciprofloxacin 500 mg once or twice daily for a duration of 2 to 4 weeks.
   c. Patients with Crohn disease. Metronidazole 15 to 20 mg/kg orally divided into 3 or 4 doses daily with or without ciprofloxacin 500 mg once or twice daily for a duration of 8 to 10 weeks.

2. **Mycobacterium tuberculosis** *type abscess*. The standard therapy is the 6-month antimicrobial course that is the same as for active pulmonary tuberculosis, which includes oral isoniazid 5 mg/kg daily, rifampin 10 mg/kg daily, pyrazinamide 20 to 25 mg/kg daily, and ethambutol 15 to 20 mg/kg daily.

3. **Actinomyces** *type abscess*. Penicillin G 10 to 20 million units intravenously divided four times daily followed by oral penicillin V 2 to 4 g divided four times daily for a duration of 2 weeks to 6 months. Oral doxycycline 100 mg twice daily is an alternative for patients with documented penicillin allergy.

4. *LGV type abscess.* Oral doxycycline 100 mg twice daily for a duration of 21 days.

B. **Surgical Management.** The primary treatment of anorectal abscess remains surgical drainage. In general, the incision should be kept as close as possible to the anal verge to minimize the length of a potential fistula, while still providing adequate drainage. Packing the wound has demonstrated equivalent or superior abscess resolution, with less pain and faster healing when compared to patients whose wounds are left unpacked.

The primary goal of operative treatment of anal fistula-in-ano is to obliterate the internal fistulous opening and any associated epithelialized tracks and to preserve anal sphincter function. Simple fistula-in-ano in patients with normal anal sphincter function may be treated with *fistulotomy*. In a fistulotomy the surgeon first probes to find the fistula's internal opening. Then the tract is cut open and scraped followed by having its contents flushed out. Then its sides are stitched to the sides of the incision in order to lay open the fistula. A more complicated fistula, such as a horseshoe fistula (where the tract extends around both sides of the body and has external openings on both sides of the anus), is treated by usually laying open just the segment where the tracts join and the remainder of the tracts are removed.

Marsupialization of the wound edges after fistulotomy has been associated with less postoperative bleeding and accelerated wound healing and may also reduce the need for postoperative analgesics. It is a surgical technique of cutting a slit into an abscess or cyst and suturing the edges of the slit to form a continuous surface from the exterior surface to the interior surface of the cyst or abscess. Sutured in this fashion, the site remains open and can drain freely.

Endoanal advancement flap is a sphincter-sparing technique that consists of curettage of the fistula tract, suture closure of the internal opening, and mobilization of a segment of proximal healthy anorectal mucosa, submucosa, and muscle to cover the site.

With complex anal fistulas, initial *seton placement* (a silk string or rubber band) to control infection is typically followed by a secondary, definitive procedure to eradicate the fistula. A seton (silk string or rubber band) is used to either create scar tissue around part of the sphincter muscle before cutting it with a knife or allow the seton to slowly cut all the way through the muscle over the course of several weeks. The seton may also aid in the drainage of the fistula.

VII. PROGNOSIS

A. Inadequate drainage, loculations, horseshoe-type abscess, and failure to perform primary fistulotomy have been identified as risk factors for recurrent anorectal abscess.

B. Factors associated with failed surgical fistula repair include prior radiation, underlying Crohn disease, active proctitis, rectovaginal fistula, malignancy, obesity, and the number of previously attempted fistula-in-ano repairs.

BIBLIOGRAPHY

Vogel JD, Johnson EK, Morris AM, et al. Clinical practice guideline for the management of anorectal abscess, fistula-in-ano, and rectovaginal fistula. *Dis Colon Rectum*. 2016;59(12):1117–1133.
Wright WF. Infectious diseases perspective of anorectal abscess and fistula-in-ano disease. *Am J Med Sci*. 2016;351(4):427–434.

CHOLECYSTITIS

William F. Wright

I. INTRODUCTION

A. Definition. An inflammatory condition of the gallbladder with a resultant secondary infection.

B. Classification. There are two types of inflammatory conditions of the gallbladder that are most commonly acute in nature.

1. **Acute calculous (stone) cholecystitis (ACC).** The most common type is due to gallstone impaction of the cystic duct leading to obstruction with the subsequent onset of inflammation. Stone types include:

   a. **Cholesterol stones** are most common and due to supersaturation of cholesterol.

   b. **Black-pigment stones** are primarily composed of bilirubin and thought to be associated with chronic hemolysis and/or liver cirrhosis.

   c. **Brown-pigment stones** are primarily composed of bilirubin but are particularly *associated with infections* (i.e., ascending bacteria from the gastrointestinal tract).

   The most important factors for excess secretion of cholesterol from the liver are obesity, age, rapid weight loss, pregnancy, and drugs (oral contraceptives). Supersaturated cholesterol in the bile initially appears as biliary sludge, which is then considered a risk factor for the formation of gallstones.

2. **Acute acalculous (no stone) cholecystitis (AAC).** Most commonly thought to occur in a hospitalized or critically ill patient with systemic hypotension and gallbladder ischemia. Risk factors include:

   a. Trauma and resuscitation from hemorrhagic shock

   b. Burns

   c. Recent major surgery

   d. Sepsis

   e. Prolonged fasting or total parenteral nutrition (TPN; sludge formation at 4 to 6 weeks)

   f. Mechanical ventilation with positive end-expiratory pressure

   g. Diabetes mellitus (secondary to atherosclerosis)

   h. Vasculitis

   i. Heart failure and/or cardiac arrest

    j. End-stage renal failure (secondary to atherosclerosis)

    k. Acute myelogenous leukemia (especially with elevated white blood cell [WBC] count or blast crisis)

C. Pathophysiology. The precipitating event in the development of *ACC* is *occlusion of gallbladder neck*, or cystic duct, by a gallstone. This results in an increased gallbladder intraluminal pressure and dilatation with mural (wall) edema. Other factors that contribute to the pathogenesis include mucosal ischemia (as a result of cystic artery compression), production of inflammatory mediators (i.e., lysolecithin and prostaglandins known to be toxic to mucosa), and direct mucosal injury from an impacted stone and concentrated bile.

    The precipitating event in the development of *AAC* is thought to result from ischemia due to *altered cystic artery blood flow* (i.e., arterial occlusion or hypotension).

II. MICROBIAL CAUSES OF CHOLECYSTITIS.
Gallbladder inflammation and edema surrounding the gallbladder are initially sterile, but a secondary bacterial (or other pathogen) infection can occur because of direct invasion or a disseminated infection.

A. Acute Calculous Cholecystitis. The most common pathogens include:

    1. Gram-negative enteric bacilli (e.g., Enterobacteriaceae)

    2. Enterococci species

    3. Intestinal anaerobes (e.g., *Bacteroides* spp, *Clostridium* spp)

B. Acute Acalculous Cholecystitis. Microorganisms include:

    1. Gram-negative enteric bacilli (e.g., Enterobacteriaceae)

    2. Intestinal anaerobes

    3. Chronic carriers of typhoidal and nontyphoidal Salmonella

    4. Hepatobiliary candidiasis (usually in neutropenic patients with recovery of blood counts)

    5. Cholera or *Campylobacter* enteritis or active diarrheal disease

    6. Gastrointestinal tuberculosis

    7. Leptospirosis (disseminated illness)

    8. Viral pathogens: hepatitis A and B, dengue fever, Epstein–Barr virus (EBV), and cytomegalovirus (CMV; usually renal transplant patients)

    9. Parasitic pathogens (by obstruction): *Ascaris lumbricoides, Echinococcus,* and liver flukes *Clonorchis sinensis* and *Opisthorchis viverrini*

    10. *Cryptosporidium* or microsporidium protozoa in HIV/AIDS patients with chronic diarrhea

III. CLINICAL MANIFESTATIONS OF CHOLECYSTITIS

A. Acute Calculous Cholecystitis. This illness typically begins with persistent localized right upper quadrant or epigastric pain (*known as biliary colic*) in a patient with previous colic pain. The pain follows oral food consumption, may radiate to the back, and is usually accompanied by nausea and vomiting. Fever is almost always present.

Jaundice is *uncommon* with ACC but if present should raise concerns for processes that obstruct the biliary duct (e.g., common bile duct stone or pancreatic mass). However, jaundice is *common* with AAC and thought to be secondary to intrahepatic cholestasis from systemic inflammatory response syndrome (SIRS)/sepsis.

B. **Acute Acalculous Cholecystitis.** Most patients with this illness are in a critical condition (e.g., surgical or medical intensive care unit) and cannot communicate biliary colic symptoms. **Therefore, physicians must maintain a high clinical suspicion for this diagnosis in critically ill patients with a fever and/or jaundice with no identified etiology.**

IV. APPROACH TO THE PATIENT

A. **History.** Typically ACC has an acute onset and patients usually have a prior history of biliary colic. *ACC should be considered in the differential diagnosis in patients with right upper quadrant or epigastric pain and fever* with the following risks:

1. Hyperlipidemia

2. Diabetes

3. Obesity or rapid weight loss

4. *Helicobacter pylori* gastritis (increases gallstone formation)

5. Oral contraception

An accurate history is usually unable to be obtained in cases of AAC as patients are critically ill.

B. **Physical Examination.** The physical examination in *AAC* is generally unreliable, but a thorough physical exam should be performed looking for other causes of fever. Jaundice is common with AAC.

For patients with *ACC,* a complete physical examination should be performed. The physician should focus on the abdominal examination findings:

1. Right upper quadrant or epigastric tenderness on palpation

2. Voluntary guarding on abdominal examination

3. Bowel sounds typically present

4. **Murphy sign:** an examination test performed by palpation of the right subcostal area while the patient inspires deeply. When this bedside examination test elicits a painful response from the patient, it is considered a positive result. This maneuver may have an associated sudden cessation of inspiration while the physician palpates the gallbladder during deep breathing that is termed *inspiratory arrest*. The estimated sensitivity of this sign is reported at 97.2% with a 48.3% specificity, 70% positive predictive value (PPV), and 93.3% negative predictive value (NPV).

C. **Laboratory Studies**

1. **Complete blood count (CBC).** Elevation of the WBC count is observed in the majority of patients.

2. **Complete metabolic profile (CMP)**. Liver function testing typically reveals a *cholestasis* hepatic pattern.

3. **C-reactive protein (CRP) and erythrocyte sedimentation rate (ESR)**. Values are typically elevated but nonspecific. However, the diagnosis of acute cholecystitis by elevation of CRP, 3 mg/dL or more, with supporting ultrasound findings (see the following) is reported to have a sensitivity of 97%, specificity of 76%, and PPV of 95%.

4. **Amylase**. An elevated level may suggest perforation or gangrenous cholecystitis.

5. **Blood cultures**. Are routinely ordered but rarely reveal a causative pathogen.

6. **Cultures**. Aseptically obtained pericholecystic fluid or gallbladder contents are not included as diagnostic criteria but may be helpful to identify pathogens in particular cases.

7. **Histology (from a surgically removed gallbladder)**. The gold standard for diagnosis of cholecystitis is pathologic examination of the gallbladder.

D. **Radiologic Studies**

1. **Plain films (kidneys, ureters, and bladder or acute abdominal series)** have minimal usefulness in the diagnosis of cholelithiasis, choledocholithiasis, or cholecystitis, as only approximately 20% of stones appear (presumably due to calcium bilirubinate content of stones).

2. **Ultrasonography** is the initial test of choice when evaluating cholecystitis. Abnormal findings include:

   a. Thickening of the gallbladder wall (single most reliable criterion): 4 mm or greater for ACC, 3.5 mm or greater for AAC, as long as the patient *does not* have chronic liver disease, ascites, or right-sided heart failure.

   b. Enlarged gallbladder. Long axis diameter of 8 cm or greater; short axis diameter of 4 cm or greater.

   c. Incarcerated gallstone and/or echo debris.

   d. Pericholecystic fluid. The presence of "gas" is suggestive of emphysematous cholecystitis secondary to a gas-producing bacteria (e.g., *Clostridium* spp).

   e. Right upper quadrant tenderness with ultrasound probe pressure (sonographic Murphy sign). A sonographic Murphy sign with evidence of cholelithiasis has a PPV of 92%.

   The absence of cholelithiasis or abnormal findings has an NPV of 95% for cholelithiasis.

3. **Hepatobiliary scintigraphy (HIDA) or technetium-labeled iminodiacetic acid** that is excreted into bile is 95% accurate for the diagnosis of ACC but has low sensitivity for AAC (68%). *The absence of gallbladder filling within 1 hour of administration is an indication of cystic duct obstruction and ACC.*

4. **CT** is as accurate as ultrasonography with similar findings but unreliable for the detection of cystic duct obstruction with ACC. Typical findings might include thickened gallbladder wall, pericholecystic fluid, enlarged gallbladder, and/or linear high-density areas in the pericholecystic fat tissue.

V. DIAGNOSTIC CRITERIA FOR CHOLECYSTITIS

A. Tokyo Guidelines for Diagnosis

1. *Signs/symptoms:* Murphy sign, right upper quadrant tenderness, right upper quadrant mass

2. *Systemic findings:* fever, elevated WBC count, elevated CRP

3. *Radiology findings:* positive findings on ultrasonography or HIDA (see Section IV.D)

   *The presence of one finding in each category suggests **DEFINITE** acute cholecystitis. The diagnostic sensitivity and specificity of definite acute cholecystitis by this criteria are reported as 91.2% and 96.9%, respectively.*

   *The presence of one finding in the category of signs/symptoms and systemic findings BUT NO imaging findings suggests **SUSPECTED** acute cholecystitis.*

B. Tokyo Guidelines for Severity of Illness

1. *Mild:* Mild inflammation and no organ dysfunction. This category can also be defined as acute cholecystitis in a healthy patient with no organ dysfunction.

2. *Moderate:* Cholecystitis with one or more of the following:

   a. WBC count greater than or equal to 18,000/mm^3

   b. Illness period greater than or equal to 72 hours

   c. Right upper quadrant palpable tender mass

   d. Findings of biliary peritonitis, abscess, gangrenous or emphysematous cholecystitis

3. *Severe:* Cholecystitis with one or more of the following:

   a. Hypotension–shock

   b. Altered mental status

   c. Acute respiratory distress syndrome (ARDS) or hypoxic respiratory failure, PaO$_2$/FiO$_2$ ratio LESS than 300

   d. Renal failure (creatinine greater than or equal to 2.0 mg/dL)

   e. Hepatic failure (international normalized ratio [INR] greater than or equal to 1.5)

   f. Thrombocytopenia (platelets less than or equal to 100,000/mm^3)

VI. MANAGEMENT OF CHOLECYSTITIS

A. Medical Management

1. Supportive care, intravenous (IV) fluid resuscitation, and fasting.

2. **Antimicrobial therapy** is often empirically initiated at initial diagnosis and hospitalization. However, indications of infection that warrant antimicrobial therapy include right upper quadrant pain with one of the following:

   a. WBC count greater than or equal to 12.5 cells/mm^3

   b. Fever greater than or equal to 38.5°C

   c. Radiographic findings of gas or abscess

3. Suggested antibiotics

a. **Piperacillin/tazobactam 3.375 g IV q6,** *or*

b. **Meropenem 500 to 1,000 mg IV q8,** *or*

c. **Cipro 400 mg IV q24** *plus* **metronidazole 500 mg IV q6–8**

If cholecystectomy is performed, the **treatment duration is 4 to 7 days** postoperatively. If cholecystectomy is *not* performed, the **treatment duration is typically 2 weeks.**

B. **Surgical Management**

1. **Cholecystectomy**. Early (within 72 hours) laparoscopic cholecystectomy is the treatment of choice for most patients with mild-to-moderate ACC.

   However, patients with a WBC count greater than or equal to 18 cells/mm³, age greater than or equal to 60, and symptoms lasting 72 hours or longer may need an open cholecystectomy. *A delayed surgical procedure (2–3 months) may be needed for severe cholecystitis or selected cases of moderate illness.*

2. **Percutaneous cholecystostomy**. Performed by interventional radiology with drain placement and is typically reserved for critically ill patients with ACC or AAC, severe cholecystitis, older adults, and patients who are poor operative candidates.

BIBLIOGRAPHY

Barie PS, Eachempati SR. Acute acalculous cholecystitis. *Gastroenterol Clin North Am*. 2010;39(2): 343–357.

Hirota M, Takada T, Kawarada Y, et al. Diagnostic criteria and severity assessment of acute cholecystitis: Tokyo guidelines. *J Hepatobiliary Pancreat Surg*. 2007;14:78–82.

Julka K, Ko CW. Infectious diseases and the gallbladder. *Infect Dis Clin North Am*. 2010;24(4): 885–898.

Solomkin JS, Mazuski JE, Bradley JS, et al. Diagnosis and management of complicated intra-abdominal infection in adults and children: guidelines by the Surgical Infection Society and Infectious Diseases Society of America. *Clin Infect Dis*. 2010;50:133–64.

Strasberg SM. Acute calculous cholecystitis. *N Engl J Med*. 2008;358(26):2804–2811.

Trowbridge RL, Rutkowski NK, Shojania KG. Does this patient have acute cholecystitis? *JAMA*. 2003;289(1):80–86.

Yokoe M, Takada T, Strasberg SM, et al. New diagnostic criteria and severity assessment of acute cholecystitis in revised Tokyo guidelines. *J Hepatobiliary Pancreat Sci*. 2012;19:578–585.

Yoshida M, Takada T, Kawarada Y, et al. Antimicrobial therapy for acute cholangitis: Tokyo guidelines. *J Hepatobiliary Pancreat Sci*. 2007;14:83–90.

ACUTE CHOLANGITIS

William F. Wright

I. INTRODUCTION

A. Definition. A clinical condition characterized by *obstruction of the biliary tract* resulting in a secondary bacterial infection.

B. Pathogenesis. Bile is normally sterile because of forward bile flow into the small intestine, antibacterial properties of bile salts, and bile IgA. Bacteria can be introduced into the biliary tract with an incompetent sphincter of Oddi, sphincterotomy (surgical division of the sphincter of Oddi), biliary stone stasis or passage, and/or biliary stent placement (for symptomatic jaundice from malignant obstruction of biliary stone removal). Acute cholangitis develops because of an ***obstructive process*** with the following sequence of events:

1. Reduced bile flow and IgA production due to obstruction.

2. Increased intrabiliary ductal pressure (greater than or equal to 14 cm H_2O).

3. Impaired biliary tight junctions.

4. Translocation of bacteria into the portal and systemic circulation.

C. Risk Factors. The risk factors for biliary obstruction leading to acute cholangitis include:

1. Cholelithiasis (most commonly from cholesterol stones passing into the biliary tract).

2. Choledocholithiasis (can be either a cholesterol stone or brown-pigment stone).

3. Malignancy with obstruction relieved by biliary stenting.

4. Prior endoscopic retrograde cholangiopancreatography (ERCP) with biliary stenting.

5. Diabetes mellitus.

6. Age greater than or equal to 75 years.

7. Certain parasitic infections (see Section II.G).

II. MICROBIAL CAUSES OF ACUTE CHOLANGITIS

A. *Escherichia coli* (most common).

B. *Klebsiella* spp.

C. *Enterobacter* spp.

D. *Enterococcus* spp. While the pathogenicity of enterococci has not been demonstrated, it may be an important pathogen in selected immunosuppressed patients, particularly hepatic transplantation.

E. **Anaerobic bacteria.** Most commonly, *Clostridium* spp or *Bacteroides* spp.

F. **Other pathogens.** Patients with recent biliary surgery or procedures, or indwelling stents, are more likely to be polymicrobial and harbor multidrug-resistant pathogens, *Pseudomonas* spp, methicillin-resistant *Staphylococcus aureus* (MRSA), vancomycin-resistant enterococci (VRE), and/or fungi (most commonly *Candida* spp).

G. **Parasites (unusual causes):** *Ascaris lumbricoides, Clonorchis sinensis* (flukes), *Opisthorchis felineus* (flukes), and *Fasciola hepatica* (flukes).

H. Cholangitis in HIV/AIDS patients may **include** *Cryptosporidium, Microsporidium,* or *Cyclospora.* A rare cause may include cytomegalovirus (CMV).

III. **CLINICAL MANIFESTATIONS OF ACUTE CHOLANGITIS.** Traditionally, the clinical symptoms of **fever** (the most consistent presentation) and **right upper abdominal quadrant tenderness** (indicating biliary tract pain) along with the sign of **jaundice** have been associated with acute cholangitis, known as **Charçot triad.** Analysis of cases indicates an estimated 26.4% to 82.6% sensitivity and 79.8% to 95.9% specificity of Charcot triad for acute cholangitis. Approximately 12% to 15% of acute cholangitis cases will demonstrate this classical triad.

Charcot triad with **hypotension** and **altered mental status**, known as **Reynolds pentad**, most likely signifies bacteremia and sepsis but only occurs in about 20% of patients.

IV. **APPROACH TO THE PATIENT**

A. **History.** Differentiating cholangitis and other biliary tract disorders can be challenging. *Physicians must have a high clinical concern for cholangitis in patients with fever and abnormal liver chemistries with a history of hepatobiliary disease.* When taking the history, focus on searching for an underlying risk factor (see the aforementioned risk factors).

B. **Physical Examination.** A complete physical examination should be performed but no findings on examination are specific for cholangitis. Areas of the physical examination to focus on include:

   1. *Conjunctival examination.* Elevated bilirubin appears as icteric sclera; bilirubin greater than or equal to 2 mg/dL.

   2. *Oral–pharyngeal examination.* Elevated bilirubin appears a sublingual icteric; bilirubin greater than or equal to 5 mg/dL. This most commonly signifies hepatic or biliary disease.

   3. *Abdominal examination* (to localize the pain and rule out other processes such as peritonitis).

C. **Laboratory Studies**

   1. **Complete blood count (CBC) with differential.** Most patients have an elevated white blood cell (WBC) count with or without neutrophilia predominance. Eosinophilia may suggest a parasitic etiology.

   2. **Complete metabolic profile (CMP).** Routinely ordered as electrolyte abnormalities and a low serum HCO_3 may suggest metabolic acidosis and sepsis.

Aspartate aminotransferase (AST) and alanine aminotransferase (ALT) are commonly abnormal but nonspecific. Alkaline phosphatase and total bilirubin (greater than 2 mg/dL) are commonly elevated. It is considered appropriate and practical that the threshold for abnormality is set at 1.5 times the normal upper limit for the liver function tests.

3. **Prothrombin time (PT)/partial thromboplastin time (PTT).** Chronic liver disease and/or thrombocytopenia of sepsis may create an abnormal bleeding time that would need to be corrected prior to any invasive test or procedure.

4. **Pancreatic enzymes.** An elevated amylase and lipase may suggest an associated pancreatitis.

5. **Blood cultures.** Both aerobic and anaerobic bottles (most commonly two sets) are routinely ordered with half of cases revealing a bacteria pathogen.

6. **Bile cultures.** Have the best yield for the identification of a microbial pathogen (positive in 80%–100% of cases). Most commonly obtained with ERCP or percutaneous drainage (20–40 mL of bile is commonly recommended). *In the absence of bile cultures, any positive blood cultures should guide antimicrobial therapy.*

7. **Stool ova and parasite.** May be helpful in cases suspected of parasitic etiology.

D. **Radiography Studies.** Imaging establishes the diagnosis of acute cholangitis.

1. **Transabdominal ultrasound.** A noninvasive imaging study that may be helpful as an *initial imaging test* to evaluate the gallbladder for stones or common bile duct dilatation.

2. **CT.** Useful for the evaluation of a distal common bile duct obstruction from a malignancy or pancreatic disorder.

3. **Magnetic resonance cholangiopancreatography (MRCP).** A noninvasive study and has a reported sensitivity of greater than 90% for stones greater than or equal to 6 mm.

4. **Endoscopic ultrasonography.** The *preferred diagnostic test* as it is more sensitive than CT or MRCP of stones less than 1 cm. Further, fine-needle aspiration with endoscopic ultrasonography is an additional modality for the diagnosis of other etiologies.

5. **ERCP.** The diagnostic gold standard as it is both diagnostic and therapeutic for acute cholangitis.

V. DIAGNOSTIC CRITERIA FOR ACUTE CHOLANGITIS

A. Tokyo Guidelines for Diagnosis

1. *Cholestasis:* jaundice and/or abnormal liver function tests (usually an elevation of 1.5 times the upper limit of normal)

2. *Systemic findings:* fever, chills, elevated WBC, and/or elevated C-reactive protein (CRP)

3. *Radiology findings:* biliary dilatation, stricture, stone, stent, and/or sludge

*The presence of one finding in each category suggests **DEFINITE** acute cholangitis. The diagnostic sensitivity and specificity of definite acute cholangitis by this criteria are reported as 95.1% and 66.3%, respectively.*

*The presence of one finding in the category of systemic inflammation findings and one finding from either category of cholestasis or imaging findings suggests **SUSPECTED** acute cholangitis. These diagnostic criteria for "suspected" disease allow early biliary drainage or infection source control among patients with acute cholangitis without waiting for a definitive diagnosis due to mortality risk with this disease process.*

B. **Tokyo Guidelines for Severity of Illness**

1. *Mild:* Mild inflammation and no organ dysfunction. This category can also be defined as acute cholangitis in a healthy patient with no organ dysfunction.

2. *Moderate:* Cholangitis with any two of the following:

   a. WBC count greater than or equal to $12,000/mm^3$ or less than or equal to $4,000/mm^3$

   b. High fever, greater than or equal to 39°C

   c. Age greater than or equal to 75 years

   d. Hyperbilirubinemia; total bilirubin greater than or equal to 5 mg/dL

   e. Hypoalbuminemia

3. *Severe:* Cholangitis with one or more of the following:

   a. Hypotension–shock

   b. Altered mental status

   c. Acute respiratory distress syndrome (ARDS) or hypoxic respiratory failure, PaO_2/FiO_2 ratio LESS than 300

   d. Renal failure (creatinine greater than or equal to 2.0 mg/dL)

   e. Hepatic failure (prothrombin time greater than or equal to 1.5)

   f. Thrombocytopenia (platelets less than or equal to $100,000/mm^3$)

VI. **TREATMENT.** The therapy for acute cholangitis consists of antimicrobial therapy and biliary drainage along with rehydration by intravenous (IV) fluids and correction of electrolyte abnormalities or coagulopathy (goal international normalized ratio [INR] less than 1.4).

A. **Antimicrobial Therapy**

1. Ampicillin with gentamicin was traditionally the antibiotic choice, but selected antibiotic regimens include:

   a. **Piperacillin/tazobactam** 3.375 g IV q6 *or*

   b. **Ampicillin/sulbactam** 3 g IV q6 *or*

   c. **Tigecycline** 100 mg IV one dose, then 50 mg IV q12 (usually reserved for multidrug-resistant pathogens or penicillin-allergic patients) *or*

   d. **Doripenem** 500 mg IV q8 *or* **meropenem** 500 to 1,000 mg IV q8 (usually reserved for multidrug-resistant pathogens or penicillin-allergic patients)

   e. **Levofloxacin** 500 mg IV/PO q24 *or* **moxifloxacin** 400 mg IV/PO q24

2. The *recommended duration has traditionally been **7 to 10 days**.* However, mild cholangitis may be treated for **2 to 3 days** following drainage and mod-

erate–severe cholangitis should be treated for a minimum of **5 to 7 days**. Acute cholangitis associated bacteremia should be treated for **14 days**.

3. Parasitic flukes are treated with either praziquantel 25 mg/kg PO q8 for three doses or albendazole 400 mg PO q12 for 7 days.

Ascariasis is usually treated with either albendazole 400 mg PO for one dose or mebendazole 100 mg PO q12 for 3 days.

B. **Biliary Drainage.** Almost always required to relieve obstruction and the source of infection.

1. **Endoscopic biliary decompression with ERCP** is the procedure of choice (98% successful). Complications include *pancreatitis, bleeding,* and *perforation*.

   a. **Mild cholangitis.** ERCP with sphincterotomy or balloon dilatation of the sphincter with stone extraction can be performed within 24 to 48 hours.

   b. **Moderate-to-severe cholangitis.** ERCP with stent placement for decompression may be performed with return for later sphincterotomy and stone extraction may be performed.

2. **Percutaneous transhepatic cholangiography (PTC)** should be performed if ERCP is not possible owing to:

   a. Altered surgical anatomy (e.g., Whipple or Billroth operation)

   b. Duodenal obstruction

   Complications include: *localized pain, bile peritonitis,* or *hemobilia* as well as a biliary venous fistula.

3. **Surgical decompression** is *not* recommended except for extreme cases where both ERCP and PTC cannot be performed.

BIBLIOGRAPHY

Attasaranya S, Fogel EL, Lehman GA. Choledocholithiasis, ascending cholangitis, and gallstone pancreatitis. *Med Clin North Am.* 2008;92(4):925–960.

Kinney TP. Management of ascending cholangitis. *Gastointest Endoscopy Clin North Am.* 2007;17(2):289–309.

Kiriyama S, Takada T, Strasberg SM, et al. New diagnostic criteria and severity assessment of acute cholangitis in revised Tokyo guidelines. *J Hepatobiliary Pancreat Sci.* 2012;19:548–556.

Lee JG. Diagnosis and management of acute cholangitis. *Nat Rev Gastroenterol Hepatol.* 2009;6(9):533–541.

Solomkin JS, Mazuski JE, Bradley JS, et al. Diagnosis and management of complicated intra-abdominal infection in adults and children: guidelines by the Surgical Infection Society and Infectious Diseases Society of America. *Clin Infect Dis.* 2010;50:133–164.

Tanaka A, Takada T, Kawarada Y, et al. Antimicrobial therapy for acute cholangitis: Tokyo guidelines. *J Hepatobiliary Pancreat Sci.* 2007;14:59–67.

HEPATIC ABSCESS

William F. Wright

I. INTRODUCTION

A. Definition. A bacterial, fungal, or parasitic enclosed collection of pus that involves the liver parenchyma.

B. Epidemiology

1. Bacterial liver abscesses most commonly occur in the sixth decade of life with equal sex distribution.

2. Fungal liver abscesses tend to occur in the fifth decade of life with equal sex distribution.

3. Parasitic liver cysts tend to occur in young populations with equal sex distribution in association with travel to an endemic region (e.g., East Asia, South America, East Africa, and Mediterranean).

C. Risk Factors. Liver abscesses or cysts are most commonly the result of direct extension to the liver or hematogenous extension to the liver.

1. Ascending cholangitis (most common cause of bacterial abscess).

2. Pyelophlebitis (suppurative thrombosis of the portal vein) from diverticulitis, pancreatitis, or appendicitis.

3. Hematogenous dissemination from bacterial endocarditis, catheter-related bloodstream infection, or intravenous (IV) drug abuse.

4. Biliary obstruction (benign or malignant) with instrumentation or stenting.

5. Caroli disease (congenital malformation of segmental bile ducts with multifocal dilatation).

6. Inflammatory bowel disease (e.g., Crohn disease and ulcerative colitis). Usually due to hematogenous portal extension of bacteria to the liver.

7. Diabetes mellitus and chronic renal failure (association with *Mycobacterium tuberculosis*).

8. Chronic granulomatous disease.

9. Hemochromatosis (more common with *Yersinia enterocolitica*).

10. Dogs and sheep-grazing areas (association with *Echinococcus* hepatic cysts). Consumption of raw, freshwater fish (e.g., *Clonorchis sinensis*) or contaminated water (e.g., *Ascaris lumbricoides* and *Entamoeba histolytica*). *It should be noted that these parasites are very rare infections and do not represent true abscesses but rather form a hepatic cyst.*

11. Chemotherapy and neutropenia (e.g., *Candida* spp).

II. MICROBIOLOGY

A. Bacterial or Pyogenic Etiology

1. **Gram-negative pathogens.** *Escherichia coli* and *Klebsiella* spp are the most common. *Klebsiella* are most commonly associated with gas-forming abscesses. Other pathogens include:

    a. *Pseudomonas* spp

    b. *Proteus* spp

    c. *Enterobacter* spp

    d. *Citrobacter* spp

    e. *Morganella* spp

    f. *Serratia* spp

    g. *Burkholderia pseudomallei*

2. **Gram-positive etiology.** *Enterococcus* and *viridans streptococci* (e.g., *Streptococcus milleri*) are common and usually associated with polymicrobial abscesses. Others include:

    a. *Staphylococcus aureus* (usually from a contiguous source and/or associated with chronic granulomatous disease)

    b. Beta-hemolytic streptococci

3. **Anaerobic bacteria.** Anaerobes are seldom recovered in culture but most commonly include *Bacteroides* spp (gram-negative). Others include:

    a. *Fusobacterium* spp (gram-negative)

    b. *Clostridium* spp (gram-positive)

    c. *Peptostreptococcus* spp (gram-positive)

B. Fungal Etiology. (*Patients are usually immunocompromised.*) Most commonly include *Candida* spp (e.g., *C. albicans, C. tropicalis, C. krusei,* and *C. parapsilosis*) in association with recovery from chemotherapy-induced neutropenia. Other fungal pathogens include:

1. *Aspergillus* spp

2. *Cryptococcus neoformans*

3. *Histoplasma capsulatum*

4. *Coccidioides immitis*

5. *Trichosporon* spp

C. Parasitic Causes. (These are *not* true abscesses but rather form hepatic cysts or invade the biliary tract with the exception of *Entamoeba histolytica*, which causes a true liver abscess.) *Echinococcus granulosus, E. multilocularis, Entamoeba histolytica, Clonorchis sinensis, Ascaris lumbricoides, Schistosoma (S. japonicum* and *S. mansoni),* and *Fasciola hepatica.*

D. Tuberculosis. Most commonly associated with the *miliary form* of *Mycobacterium tuberculosis.*

III. CLINICAL MANIFESTATIONS OF LIVER ABSCESS

A. Bacterial Liver Abscess. Clinical manifestations from hematologic extension usually occurred within 3 days while direct extension occurred from 3 to 42 days (usually within 1 month).

1. **Classic triad.** Fever, jaundice, and right upper quadrant pain occur in only 10% of cases. Jaundice occurs variably.

2. **Fever and chills.** Most common manifestation.

3. **Right upper quadrant pain or generalized abdominal pain, anorexia or malaise, and nausea with or without emesis** are additional manifestations.

B. Fungal Liver Abscess. Clinical manifestations are variable due to immunosuppression but may mimic bacterial liver abscess. Hepatosplenic candidiasis most commonly manifests as a fever 1 to 2 weeks following recovery from chemotherapy-induced neutropenia.

C. Parasitic Liver Cysts. Clinical manifestations are similar to those for bacterial liver abscesses except patients usually have more pronounced fever and right upper quadrant abdominal pain (especially *Hydatid cysts* with *Echinococcus* where hydatid fluid pressure can reach high levels). Patients may also present with cough and/or dyspnea (e.g., alveolar echinococcosis or Loeffler syndrome in association with *Ascaris lumbricoides*).

D. Tuberculous Liver Abscess. Most symptoms are constitutional with fever, weight loss, anorexia, fatigue, and night sweats. Patients typically have right upper quadrant pain. Patients may also have cough and/or dyspnea in association with pulmonary tuberculosis.

IV. APPROACH TO THE PATIENT

A. History. Liver abscess usually has a *subacute* onset but should be included in the differential diagnosis in patients with fever and abdominal pain. This history should focus on risk factors and travel history or exposures.

B. Physical Examination. A complete physical examination should be performed, but areas of additional focus include:

1. **Ophthalmologic examination** (to detect jaundice).

2. **Cardiovascular examination** (to detect murmurs suggestive of endocarditis).

3. **Pulmonary examination** (detect wheezing associated with parasitic illness [e.g., Loeffler syndrome] or focal findings for pneumonia/empyema).

4. **Abdominal examination** (to detect hepatic tenderness, hepatomegaly and/or splenomegaly, or findings to suggest diverticulitis, cholecystitis, or appendicitis).

C. Laboratory Studies

1. **Complete blood count (CBC).** Routinely ordered, and the white blood cell (WBC) count is almost always elevated with bacterial abscesses. Eosinophilia may suggest a parasitic etiology (except in the case of *Entamoeba histolytica*). Patients recovering from neutropenia in association with liver abscesses may indicate hepatosplenic candidiasis.

2. **Basic metabolic panel (BMP).** Usually nonspecific in liver abscess but hyperglycemia may indicate infection in diabetic patients. Hyponatremia may occur with tuberculous liver abscess.

3. **Liver function tests (LFTs).** Almost always demonstrate elevated levels of alkaline phosphatase and alanine aminotransferase (ALT); however, levels of total bilirubin are varied.

4. **Prothrombin time (PT)/partial thromboplastin time (PTT).** Variable but may be prolonged in patients on anticoagulants.

5. **Blood cultures.** Should be ordered on all patients and more likely to be positive (positive 50%; at least two sets) with polymicrobial bacterial infections but may occasionally grow *Candida* spp.

6. **Cultures.** Aspiration of abscess contents for Gram stain and culture should be performed in patients with suspected bacterial liver abscesses. Aspiration can be performed with ultrasonography or CT guidance or by simple percutaneous needle aspiration for small simple abscesses. Aspirated abscess contents may also confirm *Candidiasis*. Aspirations of amoebic abscesses appear as "anchovy paste" due to both inflammation and necrosis with hemorrhage into the abscess cavity.

7. **Serology.** Serologic testing is most commonly performed for *Entamoeba histolytica, Clonorchis sinensis, Fasciola hepatica,* and *Echinococcus* spp (as aspirated antigenic *Echinococcus* cystic fluid released into the circulation can cause an acute intense allergic reaction).

8. **Stool ova and parasites (O&P).** May identify *Entamoeba histolytica* cysts and/or trophozoites

D. **Radiography Studies.** Radiographic imaging studies are essential in the diagnosis of liver abscesses and either **ultrasonography** or **CT** is used.

1. **Ultrasonography.** This is the most common imaging test performed in patients suspected of biliary tract disease. Ultrasonography demonstrates good sensitivity with parasitic abscesses but has poor sensitivity with hepatosplenic candidiasis.

   Bacterial or amoebic abscesses can be either **microabscesses** (less than 2 cm) or **macroabscesses** (greater than or equal to 2 cm) that can appear as **hypoechoic** (most common) or **hyperechoic** lesions. **Echinococcus** lesions typically show well-defined, round to oval, **multiloculated cysts** with **internal septations** and varying degrees of calcifications.

   Tuberculosis-related liver abscesses usually manifest as multiple small hypoechoic lesions.

2. **CT**. Contrast-enhanced CT has improved sensitivity over ultrasonography, is superior for guided needle aspirations, and should be the initial test in patients suspected of hepatosplenic candidiasis. Bacterial abscesses are generally well defined with hypoattenuation. Amoebic lesions are typically well defined with fluid attenuation (10–200 Hounsfield units) and a 3 to 15 mm thick rim enhancement with or without septations. *Echinococcus* can show a well-defined lesion with hypoattenuation of fluid and rim enhancement (*E. multilocularis* typically show multiple, ill-defined, and

hypoattenuation lesions). Schistosomiasis hepatic cysts have the characteristic presence of calcified septations and appear as a "tortoise shell" (*S. japonicum*). Candidiasis usually appears as multiple round, discrete areas of low attenuation (2–20 mm).

V. **TREATMENT.** Traditionally, treatment has consisted of: (a) **drainage of abscess contents** (pericystectomy or formal hepatic resection for *Echinococcus*), (b) **administration of parenteral antimicrobial agents,** and (c) **treatment of the underlying condition.**

A. **Bacterial Abscesses.** Antibiotics without drainage should only be reserved for small lesions, lesions not amenable to drainage, or patients with unacceptable risks (e.g., bleeding). Duration is typically 2 to 3 weeks of parenteral therapy followed by 4 to 6 weeks of oral therapy. Options for **parenteral therapy** include:

   1. Piperacillin/tazobactam 3.375 g IV q6
   2. Ampicillin/sulbactam 3 g IV q6
   3. Meropenem 500–1,000 mg IV q8
   4. Moxifloxacin 400 mg IV q24

   Options for **oral therapy** include:

   1. Moxifloxacin 400 mg PO q24
   2. Ciprofloxacin 500 mg PO q12 *plus* metronidazole 500 mg PO q12

B. **Fungal Abscesses.** The antimicrobial of choice for fungi other than *Candida* spp is amphotericin B liposomal 3 to 5 mg/kg. However, the majority of cases are related to hepatosplenic candidiasis, and the treatment options include:

   1. **Non–albicans** *Candida.* Micafungin 100 mg IV q24 *or* caspofungin 70 mg IV load, then 50 mg IV q24 for 2 to 4 weeks.
   2. *Candida albicans.* Fluconazole 800 mg IV/PO load, then 400 mg IV/PO q24 for 2 to 4 weeks.

C. **Parasitic Organisms**

   1. *Entamoeba histolytica* **hepatic abscess.** Metronidazole 750 mg PO q8 for 7 to 10 days followed by treatment of intraluminal disease with paromomycin 500 mg PO q8 for 7 days.
   2. *Echinococcosis* **hepatic cyst**

      a. **Operable.** Surgical removal with albendazole 400 mg PO q12 for 1 to 6 months. Surgical removal is best performed after injection of the cyst with hypertonic saline, alcohol, or iodophor to kill daughter cysts.

      b. **Nonoperable.** Albendazole 400 mg PO q12 for 1 to 6 months.

   3. *Clonorchis sinensis.* Albendazole 400 mg PO q12 for 1 to 2 weeks.
   4. *Schistosomiasis.* Praziquantel 20 mg/kg PO q12 for three doses.
   5. *Ascaris lumbricoides.* Albendazole 400 mg PO q12 for 1 to 6 months.

D. **Tuberculosis Abscess.** Treatment is the same as for pulmonary tuberculosis.

BIBLIOGRAPHY

Branum GD, Tyson GS, Branum MA, et al. Hepatic abscess: changes in etiology, diagnosis, and management. *Ann Surg.* 1990;212(6):655–662.

Mortele KJ, Segatto E, Ros PR. The infected liver: radiologic-pathologic correlation. *Radiographics.* 2004;24(4):937–955.

Reid-Lombardo KM, Khan S, Sclabas G. Hepatic cysts and liver abscess. *Surg Clin North Am.* 2010;90(4):679–697.

26

HEPATITIS A

William F. Wright

I. INTRODUCTION

A. Definition. Hepatitis A virus (HAV) infection is an acute, most often self-limiting viral illness characterized as hepatitis and jaundice. HAV infection can sometimes be a fulminant illness.

B. Epidemiology

1. Most common cause of acute viral hepatitis in the United States.
2. More likely to occur in patients aged 5 to 14 years.
3. More likely to occur with American Indians, Alaskan Indians, and Hispanics (lowest occurrence in Caucasians, Asians, and African Americans).
4. More likely to occur in Central and South America, Africa, India, the Middle East, and parts of Asia (lowest in the United States and Japan).

C. Risk Factors. Most commonly transmitted by oral–fecal route; however, no identified source occurs in approximately 50% of cases.

1. Household or sexual contact (especially men who have sex with men).
2. Foreign travelers (particularly those to developing nations).
3. Contaminated food or water (particularly associated with green onions and strawberries).
4. Consumption of shellfish from contaminated water (a significant cause outside the United States).
5. Daycare children and daycare workers.
6. Blood transfusion or blood products are *very rarely* associated with HAV.
7. Injection and noninjection drug use.

II. MICROBIOLOGY

A. RNA picornavirus; *Hepatovirus* genus.

B. Nonenveloped virus (a lack of a lipid envelope confers resistance to bile lysis in the small intestine and liver).

C. Four genotypes and one serotype.

D. The coding region of the genome codes for four structural proteins and seven nonstructural proteins.

E. The virus replicates through a RNA-dependent polymerase in hepatocytes and gastrointestinal epithelial cells.

F. **Life Cycle of HAV**

 1. *Oral inoculation of fecally excreted virus.*

 2. *Transportation across gastrointestinal epithelium to mesenteric veins of liver (viremia).*

 3. *Taken up by hepatocytes, replicates, and shed into the bile canaliculi.*

 4. *Transported to the intestine and excreted into the feces.*

III. CLINICAL MANIFESTATION OF HAV

 A. **Classic HAV.** Acute onset of illness following an incubation period of approximately 1 month. The illness is typically self-limited (approximately 8 weeks) and consists of two phases:

 1. **Preicteric phase.** Characterized by fever, malaise, and fatigue (influenza-like) and nausea, emesis, and diarrhea approximately 1 week prior to the appearance of dark urine.

 2. **Icteric phase.** Characterized by jaundice and pale-colored stool. This phase is associated with hepatocyte injury (elevated aminotransferases) and eventual HAV clearance through cell-mediated and antibody-mediated processes. Commonly associated with hepatomegaly and splenomegaly.

 B. **Fulminant HAV.** Characterized by worsening jaundice and development of encephalopathy. This form of HAV infection is rare but more common with older adults (age greater than 49) and patients with chronic hepatitis B virus (HBV) and hepatitis C virus (HCV).

 C. **Relapsing HAV.** Uncommon, but characterized by recurrent HAV infection with a symptom-free interval.

 D. **Cholestasis HAV.** Uncommon, but characterized as a prolonged course of HAV infection (over months) associated with fever, jaundice, and pruritus. *Patients may present clinically similar to acute acalculous cholecystitis.*

IV. APPROACH TO THE PATIENT

 A. **History.** While the majority of adults are symptomatic, historical findings may be nonspecific. A complete history should be performed to review risk factors for HAV as well as for consideration of other causes of jaundice and hepatitis:

 1. Autoimmune hepatitis/systemic lupus erythematosus (SLE).

 2. Alcohol hepatitis.

 3. *Medications*: acetaminophen, isoniazid, rifampin, sulfonamides, and oral contraceptives.

 4. *Bacterial infections*: syphilis, typhoid, Rocky Mountain spotted fever (RMSF), Q fever, and leptospirosis.

 5. *Parasite infections*: liver flukes.

 6. Cholecystitis/choledocholithiasis.

 7. Metastatic disease (e.g., colon cancer, pancreatic cancer).

 8. *Viral infections*: cytomegalovirus (CMV), Epstein–Barr virus (EBV), HBV, HCV, varicella-zoster virus (VZV), herpes simplex virus (HSV).

B. Physical Examination. A complete physical examination should be performed, but areas to focus attention include:

1. **Ophthalmic examination** (to detect jaundice).

2. **Neurologic examination** (to evaluate mental status for signs of encephalopathy and asterixis).

3. **Abdomen examination** (to detect tender hepatomegaly and splenomegaly common in icteric phase of HAV).

4. **Lymphatic examination** (postcervical lymphadenopathy is occasionally observed in the icteric phase of HAV).

5. **Dermatologic examination** (to detect vasculitis as rarely HAV can be associated with cryoglobulinemia).

C. Laboratory Studies

1. **Serum anti-HAV immunoglobulin M (IgM) and immunoglobulin G (IgG).** The preferred confirmatory test for HAV.

   a. **Anti-HAV IgM.** Detected 1 to 2 weeks after HAV exposure and remains elevated for 3 to 6 months.

   b. **Anti-HAV IgG.** Detected 5 to 6 weeks after HAV exposure, remains elevated lifelong, and confers protective immunity against HAV.

2. **Complete blood count (CBC).** Routinely ordered on hospitalized patients but nonspecific.

3. **Basic metabolic panel (BMP).** Usually nonspecific but chronic renal insufficiency may suggest chronic liver disease (usually associated with thrombocytopenia).

4. **Prothrombin time (PT)/partial thromboplastin time (PTT).** A prolonged PTT may reflect extensive liver necrosis and/or need for liver transplantations (especially if PTT is greater than or equal to 25 seconds)

5. **Liver function test (LFT).** Alanine aminotransferase (ALT) and aspartate aminotransferase (AST) may be as high as 3,100 upper limit of normal (ULN), alkaline phosphatase is only minimally elevated, and total bilirubin is rarely greater than 10 ng/dL. (Total bilirubin greater than or equal to10 ng/dL may suggest cholestasis HAV.) *Antinuclear antibody (ANA), antineutrophil cytoplasmic antibody (ANCA), rapid plasma reagin (RPR), and serum antibodies to typhoid, RMSF, Q fever, and leptospirosis may be helpful in cases mimicking HAV infection with abnormal LFTs.*

6. **Blood cultures** are *not* recommended routinely. *Cultures may be helpful in cases with a fever and a concern for cholecystitis or choledocholithiasis.*

D. Radiographic Studies. A transabdominal ultrasonography or CT scan may be helpful to demonstrate hepatomegaly and splenomegaly in association with HAV infection (common in icteric phase of HAV) but usually reserved to evaluate cases with concerns for cholelithiasis and choledocholithiasis.

V. TREATMENT. Virus-specific therapy is *not* available for HAV; therefore, treatment is mainly supportive measures, avoidance of hepatic toxins (less than 2 g/day acetaminophen) and alcohol, vaccination, and prevention. *Indication for evaluation for liver transplantation includes:*

1. Fulminant HAV.

2. Jaundice lasting more than 7 days before encephalopathy (indicating extensive liver necrosis).

3. Serum bilirubin greater than or equal to 17 mg/dL.

Prevention measures primarily include: improved sanitation, pretravel vaccination, vaccination of high-risk patients, and postexposure prophylaxis. **Hand hygiene is most important for preventing transmission** *(since the virus can survive as fomites and resist freezing, detergents, and acids). Environmental control of surfaces should include inactivation of HAV by formalin and/or chlorine.*

A. Passive Immunization: Immune Globulin

1. Provides short-term protection through passive antibody transfer. When used as preexposure prophylaxis (e.g., travelers):

    a. A single intramuscular (IM) dose of 0.02 mL/kg protects for less than 3 months.

    b. A single IM dose of 0.06 mL/kg protects for 3 to 5 months.

    When used as postexposure prophylaxis within 2 weeks of exposure, a single IM dose of 0.02 mL/kg is 80% to 90% effective in preventing HAV.

2. *Not* contraindicated during pregnancy or lactation.

3. Consists of pooled plasma with anti-HAV (plasma is negative for HIV and treated to inactivate other viruses).

4. *Do not* give within 2 to 3 weeks following administration of live, attenuated vaccines (decreases immunogenicity of vaccine).

5. Wait 3 months for measles–mumps–rubella (MMR) vaccine administration following immunoglobulin (IG) administration and 5 months for varicella vaccine administration following immunoglobulin (IG) administration.

6. Immunoglobulin (IG) is recommended for:

    a. Persons with a recent HAV exposure (less than 2 weeks) and no history of HAV vaccine; a single dose of immunoglobulin (IG) at 0.02 mL/kg. HAV vaccine can be administered at the same time but in a separate anatomic location.

    b. Unvaccinated persons with regular household or sexual contact of individuals with serologically confirmed HAV.

    c. Unvaccinated staff and attendees of child daycare centers or homes with greater than one case are identified in children or employees. During an outbreak (defined as cases involving three or more families) immunoglobulin (IG) should also be administered to unvaccinated household members of children in daycare who wear diapers.

    d. For individuals aged greater than 40 years, immunoglobulin (IG) is preferred because of the absence of information regarding vaccine performance in this age group and because of the more severe manifestations of HAV in older adults. Vaccine can be used if immunoglobulin (IG) cannot be obtained. The magnitude of the risk of HAV transmission from the exposure should be considered in decisions to use vaccine or immunoglobulin (IG) in this age group.

e. For children aged less than 12 months, immunocompromised persons, persons with chronic liver disease, and persons who are allergic to the vaccine or a vaccine component, immunoglobulin (IG) should be used.

B. Active Immunization: *Vaccination*

1. Two licensed vaccines, Havrix and Vaqta, are derived from formalin inactivated cell-culture-propagated HAV. *HAV vaccine also exists in combination with HBV vaccine (Twinrix).*

2. Usually provided as two IM injections given 6 months apart.

3. Vaccination is recommended for the following:

   a. Persons working or traveling to high-risk areas

   b. Men who have sex with men

   c. Drug use history (injection or noninjection)

   d. History of chronic HBV and HCV (increased risk of fulminant HAV)

   e. HAV research laboratory workers

   f. Children (all children aged 12–23 months as routine vaccination)

BIBLIOGRAPHY

Advisory Committee of Immunization Practices (ACIP), Fiore AE, Wasley A, et al. Prevention of hepatitis A through active or passive immunization: recommendations of the Advisory Committee on Immunization Practices (ACIP). *MMWR Recomm Rep.* 2006;55(RR-7):1–23.

Brundage SC, Fitzpatrick AN. Hepatitis A. *Am Fam Physician.* 2006;73(12):2162–2168.

Kemmer NM, Miskovsky EP. Hepatitis A. *Infect Dis Clin North Am.* 2000;14(3):605–615.

HEPATITIS B

Luciano Kapelusznik
Rohit Talwani
William F. Wright

I. INTRODUCTION

A. **Definition.** Infection with hepatitis B virus (HBV) is either an acute, self-limited or chronic infection that can be characterized by hepatitis and jaundice. It can also be a fulminant illness in less than 1% of cases.

B. **Epidemiology.** The prevalence of HBV is higher in Southeast Asia, Pacific Basin (i.e., Japan, Australia, and New Zealand), sub-Saharan Africa, the Amazon Basin, the Middle East, and Eastern Europe where infection is more commonly obtained by perinatal transmission (mother to child at birth or during infancy). The prevalence of HBV is low (estimated to be less than 2%) in the United States but is more commonly obtained during adolescence and adulthood in association with certain risks.

C. **Risk Factors.** Most commonly transmitted by sexual contact as well as percutaneous injuries or needle puncture, and perinatal (mother to child at birth or during infancy).

   1. Injection drug use.

   2. Healthcare workers.

   3. Sexual or household contact with HBV-positive person (HBsAg positive).

   4. Men who have sex with men.

   5. Blood or blood product transfusion.

   6. Infants born to HBV-positive mothers (HBsAg positive).

   7. HIV infection.

   8. Comorbid illnesses needing chemotherapy or immunosuppression treatment (these are more commonly associated with reactivation of HBV rather than as a risk to acquire the virus).

   9. Travel to high-risk areas.

   10. People born in Asia, Africa, and other regions with moderate or high rates of hepatitis B.

   11. Unvaccinated people whose parents are from regions with high rates of HBV.

   12. Hemodialysis.

II. MICROBIOLOGY

A. DNA virus; hepadnavirus.

B. Covalently closed circular DNA with four reading **frames:**

1. Presurface–surface. Codes three surface antigens.

   a. HBsAg—most commonly tested for infection

   b. M protein—unknown function

   c. L protein—important for host cell binding and virion assembly/release

2. Precore–core. Codes two main antigens.

   a. HBcAg—commonly used in serology

   b. HBeAg—a marker for viral replication but has no direct role for replication or assembly

3. P coding region. Codes for viral polymerase.

4. X coding region. Involved with host cell signal transduction and required for replication and spread of virus.

C. The cardinal feature of viral replication is by reverse transcription (similar to HIV).

D. Eight different genotypes (A–H).

E. Double-shelled virus with an outer lipoprotein envelope (susceptible to bile acid lysis).

F. HBV predominantly infects liver cells and lymphocytes.

III. VIRAL LIFE CYCLE AND PATHOGENESIS

A. Primary HBV Infection. More commonly is an *asymptomatic, self-limited illness that is not directly cytotoxic to cells.*

1. HBV is transmitted in blood and secretions to primarily infect liver cells.

2. HBsAg becomes detected in the blood following a 4- to 10-week incubation period. Viremia is established during this period of detection. Patients are infectious.

3. HBcAg and anti-HBc immunoglobulin M (IgM) then begin to appear in the blood.

4. HBeAg usually becomes detectable. Some patients may be HBeAg negative due to gene mutations that either reduce or eliminate production of the antigen.

5. HBV replication is not directly cytotoxic to liver cells, but liver injury and symptoms are related to both the antiviral cytotoxic T-cell response and cytokines (e.g., tumor necrosis factor [TNF]).

6. In most cases involving adults, inflammatory cytokines (e.g., interferon-gamma and TNF-alpha) and an immunologic response result in the disappearance of HBsAg, HBcAg, and HBeAg, and **the presence of anti-HBs (HBsAb) indicates recovery and immunity.** However, low levels of HBV DNA may remain detectable but are not considered infectious. In cases of acquisition during infancy, most cases (up to 95%) will not clear the virus and become a chronic infection.

B. Persistent (Chronic) HBV Infection. In some patients the primary infection does not resolve (5%).

1. Characterized by persistent circulating HBsAg greater than or equal to 6 months. Antibodies to HBsAg are still produced but are undetected due to excess HBsAg in persistent infection.

2. HBeAg is detectable in some cases (except HBeAg-negative patients) but may disappear with the development of anti-HBe antibodies. The detection of HBeAg in the blood usually indicates high viral replication and viremia (patients are highly infectious). While anti-HBe antibodies suggest lower infectivity and reduced viral replication, low levels of HBV DNA might remain detectable.

3. Persistent infection may be classified as:

   a. Asymptomatic chronic HBV carriers. Patients have normal liver function tests (LFTs) and liver biopsy.

      i. HBeAg-negative carriers have a good prognosis

      ii. HBeAg-positive carriers with or without anti-HBe antibodies have a high risk of hepatocellular carcinoma (*see Section V.C.8 for the subset of patients who should be screened for hepatocellular cancer [HCC]*).

   b. Symptomatic chronic HBV infection. Patients have abnormal LFTs and liver biopsy with the risk of progression to cirrhosis (estimated to be 20% in 5 years) and/or HCC.

IV. CLINICAL MANIFESTATIONS OF HBV INFECTION

A. Acute HBV Infection. Usually lasts 2 to 4 months.

1. *Symptoms.* Typically nonspecific and include fatigue, anorexia (poor appetite), nausea, emesis, generalized or right upper quadrant abdominal pain, fever, jaundice, and dark urine (due to elevated urobilirubin).

2. *Signs.* Most commonly involve right upper quadrant tenderness (liver tenderness), hepatomegaly, splenomegaly, scleral icterus.

B. Chronic HBV Infection. Most patients remain asymptomatic but might develop signs or symptoms related to hepatic cirrhosis. These include: fatigue, weakness, anorexia, gynecomastia, palmar erythema, renal insufficiency, thrombocytopenia, anemia, and coagulopathy.

C. Extrahepatic HBV Manifestations

1. *Polyarteritis nodosa.* Small-vessel vasculitis characterized by neuropathy, dermatologic ulcers, fevers, hypertension, and abdominal pain.

2. *Glomerulonephritis.* Most commonly membranous glomerulonephritis characterized by hematuria and proteinuria.

V. APPROACH TO THE PATIENT

A. History. Adults are symptomatic in 30% to 50% of cases (children are rarely symptomatic); therefore, HBV should be included in the differential diagnosis of patients being **evaluated for abdominal pain, fever, and jaundice** (immunosuppressed patients or older adults may be asymptomatic). The history should focus on HBV risk factors and consideration for other etiologies.

B. Physical Examination. A complete physical examination should be performed, but areas to focus attention include:

1. Ophthalmologic examination (to detect jaundice).

2. Neurologic examination (to detect asterixis and other signs of encephalopathy).

3. Abdomen examination (to detect hepatomegaly and splenomegaly).

C. Laboratory Studies

1. The diagnosis of HBV usually involves the evaluation of HBsAg, HBsAb, HBcAb, and HBeAg/HBeAb. Tests should be performed with acute infection and 6 months following acute infection. Interpretation includes:

HBsAg	HBcAb	HBsAb	Status
–	–	–	Susceptible
–	–	+	Vaccinated
–	+	+	Natural infection but patient immune
+	+	–	Acute (if ≤6 months) or chronic (if ≥6 months); HBcAb IgM is also considered an indicator of acute infection

IgM, immunoglobulin M.

2. *HBV DNA.* Values vary based on clinical status and are more useful in chronic HBV treatment plans.

3. *Liver biopsy.* Important for therapy with chronic HBV.

4. *Complete blood count (CBC).* Routinely ordered but nonspecific. Anemia and thrombocytopenia may indicate chronic liver disease.

5. *Basic Metabolic Panel.* Renal insufficiency may be associated with chronic liver disease.

6. *LFTs.* Aminotransferase levels might be elevated but vary with status; in general, alanine aminotransferase (ALT) greater than aspartate aminotransferase (AST) greater than alkaline phosphatase. Albumin level may be low with chronic liver disease.

7. *Prothrombin time/partial thromboplastin time.* Prolonged in chronic liver disease or cirrhosis.

8. *Serum alpha-fetoprotein.* Marker of HCC usually performed one to two times per year in those individuals at high risk for HCC. The following patients should be screened for HCC:

   a. *Asian males greater than 40 years; Asian females greater than 50 years*

   b. *All cirrhotic hepatitis B carriers*

   c. *Family history of HCC*

   d. *African Americans greater than age 20*

   For noncirrhotic hepatitis B carriers not listed previously, the risk of HCC varies depending on the severity of the underlying liver disease, and current and past hepatic inflammatory activity. Patients with high HBV DNA concentrations and those with ongoing hepatic inflammatory activity also remain at risk for HCC.

9. *Blood cultures.* Not recommended routinely.

D. Radiographic Studies. A transabdominal ultrasonography or CT scan may be helpful to demonstrate hepatomegaly and splenomegaly in acute infection as well as demonstrate cirrhosis or screen for hepatocellular carcinoma in chronic infection.

VI. TREATMENT

A. Goals of Therapy

1. Reduction of viremia. Despite either self-limited HBV infection or seroconversion with treatment of chronic HBV, circulating viral DNA persists at low levels.

2. Reduction of hepatic dysfunction. Normalization of aminotransferase levels (e.g., ALT) is most commonly used for evaluation.

3. Successful therapy is defined as reduction or normalization of ALT, loss of circulating HBeAg, seroconversion to anti-HBe, and reduction of circulating viral DNA (e.g., less than 10–100).

4. Cure of HBV is *rare* but defined as complete resolution of HBV circulating viral DNA, HBsAg clearance, and HBsAb seroconversion; however, HBV DNA persists in hepatocytes.

B. Predictors for the Response to HBV Therapy

1. Elevated ALT level.

2. Low HBV DNA level.

3. Mild-to-moderate histology grading on liver biopsy.

4. Serotype (genotypes B and C are more likely to be associated with spontaneous resolution; genotype A treated with pegylated interferon is more likely to result in seroconversion).

5. Certain oral therapies are more likely to be associated with resistance in the YMDD motif of DNA polymerase domain C (e.g., lamivudine, telbivudine, and adefovir). Adefovir resistance is associated with B and D domain mutations. Resistance to lamivudine is sufficiently high to limit clinical utility in some cases.

C. Indications for Therapy. The guidelines for therapy are based on HBeAg status, HBV DNA level, ALT, and liver biopsy results as well as cirrhosis status.

1. HBeAg positive, ALT greater than or equal to two times the upper limit of normal (ULN), and HBV DNA greater than or equal to 20,000 IU/mL should be treated with or without a pretreatment liver biopsy.

2. HBeAg positive, ALT less than or equal to two times ULN (but liver biopsy with mild-to-severe inflammation or fibrosis), and HBV DNA greater than or equal to 20,000 IU/mL should be treated. If liver biopsy does *not* show inflammation or fibrosis, then treatment is *not* indicated as therapy in this case has minimal clinical benefit.

3. HBeAg negative, ALT greater than or equal to two times ULN, and HBV DNA greater than or equal to 2,000 IU/mL should be treated with or without liver biopsy.

4. HBeAg negative, ALT less than or equal to two times ULN (but liver biopsy with mild-to-severe inflammation or fibrosis), and HBV DNA greater than or equal to 2,000 IU/mL should be treated.

5. Compensated HBV cirrhosis with HBV DNA greater than or equal to 2,000 IU/mL (with or without a positive HBeAg) should be treated.

6. Compensated HBV cirrhosis with ALT greater than or equal to two times ULN and HBV DNA less than or equal to 2,000 IU/mL should be treated.

7. *Decompensated HBV cirrhosis (e.g., hepatic encephalopathy) and detectable HBV DNA should be considered for liver transplantation.*

D. Agents for Therapy. Usually divided by compensated or decompensated disease.

1. **Pegylated interferon alfa-2a and -2b.** A subcutaneously injected immunomodulating agent that is considered *first-line treatment* for **compensated disease**. The usual dose is 180 mcg by subcutaneous injection weekly for 48 weeks. The benefit of this agent is: (a) no drug resistance, and (b) likelihood of seroconversion (HBV DNA suppression is less profound than oral therapies). *Patients with high ALT, genotype A, and low-level HBV DNA tend to respond best to interferon therapy.* Tenofovir and entecavir are oral therapies that are also options considered as first-line therapies for compensated HBV.

    Oral therapies are the only option for treating **decompensated HBV liver disease** but are in some cases as effective as injectable pegylated interferon in compensated disease and patients who previously have not responded to nonpegylated interferon. *Oral therapies are nucleotide or nucleoside analogues that inhibit the reverse transcription from HBV RNA to DNA during the virus replication life cycle.* In general, oral therapy requires a longer duration for seroconversion, and all agents need monitoring of serum creatinine and dose adjustment for renal disease. Available oral therapies include:

    a. **Lamivudine (Epivir)** 100 mg PO q24 for 48 to 52 weeks. Usually well tolerated but is no longer considered first-line therapy due to resistance (up to 70% after 5 years) in the YMDD motif of the HBV DNA polymerase and also may be a reason to change therapy. This agent can be used with HIV coinfection.

    b. **Adefovir (Hepsera)** 10 mg PO q24 for greater than or equal to 48 weeks. An effective alternative in lamivudine-resistant HBV but is the least potent and slowest to suppress viral DNA. This agent has HIV activity at higher doses but is limited due to nephrotoxicity.

    c. **Entecavir (Baraclude)** 0.5 mg PO q24 for greater than or equal to 48 weeks is generally well tolerated, and the development of resistance is usually not of clinical significance in treatment-naïve patients. This agent has some activity for HIV.

    d. **Tenofovir (Viread)** 300 mg PO q24 for greater than or equal to 48 weeks is generally well tolerated and considered a preferred first-line therapy. Resistance rates have currently not been documented in patients after 5 years of follow-up, and this agent can be used with HIV coinfection.

    e. **Telbivudine (Tyzeka)** 600 mg PO q24 for greater than or equal to 52 weeks is more commonly associated with elevated creatine kinase (CK) levels and peripheral neuropathy, but resistance is low.

        Currently, the combination of HBV therapies with the hope of reducing resistance and improving markers of HBV infection has *not* shown an increased efficacy in treatment.

BIBLIOGRAPHY

Dienstag JL. Hepatitis B virus infection. *N Engl J Med.* 2008;359(14):1486–1500.

Ganem D, Prince AM. Hepatitis B virus infection—natural history and clinical consequences. *N Engl J Med.* 2004;350(11):1118–1129.

Wilkins T, Zimmerman D, Schade RR. Hepatitis B: diagnosis and treatment. *Am Fam Physician.* 2010;81(8):965–972.

HEPATITIS C

Rohit Talwani
Luciano Kapelusznik
William F. Wright

I. INTRODUCTION

A. Definition and Epidemiology. Hepatitis C is a viral infection of the liver characterized by chronic inflammation, sometimes leading to serious liver damage such as cirrhosis and hepatocellular cancer. First discovered in 1989, it is a major, global health problem affecting over 170 million people worldwide. In the United States, an estimated 2.7 million individuals are chronically infected with the hepatitis C virus (HCV). The most common mode of transmission is through contaminated *blood*.

B. Risk Factors. Risk factors for HCV infection include:

1. *Intravenous drug use (IVDU).* This is the most important risk factor for HCV infection.

2. *Recipient of blood transfusion or organ transplant prior to 1992.* Since 1992 when universal screening was instituted for blood donors, blood transfusion has become a rare mode of transmission, with an estimated risk of one in 1 million units of blood transfused.

3. *Persons infected with HIV born to HCV-infected mothers.*

4. *Persons with hemophilia receiving clotting factors prior to 1987.*

5. *Multiple sexual partners, sex with a partner infected with HCV, and/or divorced or separated.*

6. *Body piercing, body tattooing, and commercial barbering.* Mainly occurs from an unregulated establishment.

7. *Poverty and/or education level less than 12 years.*

8. *Healthcare workers.* Following a needle-stick injury, the likelihood of acquiring a blood-borne infection from an infected host follows the rule of three: 30% hepatitis B virus (HBV), 3% HCV, and 0.3% HIV.

9. *Persons receiving hemodialysis.*

II. MICROBIOLOGY/VIROLOGY

A. Classification. RNA virus of the family of flaviviruses (similar to West Nile virus, yellow fever virus, and dengue virus).

B. Genotypes. A single-stranded RNA virus of 9.5 kb that can be divided into *seven genotypes* from polymerase chain reaction (PCR) sequence analysis of the

5' noncoding region; however, most research has focused on genotypes 1 to 6. *Determining the genotype is important for treatment and treatment duration.*

HCV genotype 1 is the most commonly found genotype in the United States and Europe. Genotypes 1, 2, 4, and 5 are found as endemic infections in Africa, while genotypes 3 and 6 have evolved in Asia.

The HCV genome encodes a single polyprotein that produces both structural proteins and regulatory proteins. A structural protein that encodes the virus envelope, E2 envelope protein, contains a binding site for CD81 on hepatocytes and B lymphocytes (the primary cells in which the HCV virus replicates). *In vivo replication rates of HCV are much greater than for HIV or HBV infection.*

Hepatitis C polyprotein structure

5' end   3' end

C	E1	E2	p7	NS2	NS3	NS4A	NS4B	NS5A	NS5B

NS, nonstructural.

The polyprotein contains three structural proteins (core, E1 and E2) and seven NS proteins (p7, NS2, NS3, NS4A, NS4B, NS5A, and NS5B). It is cleaved by cellular and viral proteases into the following proteins: C (the core); E1 and E2 (envelope glycoproteins); P7 (a membrane protein that serves as an ion channel); NS2, NS3–NS4A, NS4B, NS5A, and NS5B. The NS2/3 cysteine protease starts a cascade of enzymatic reactions leading to the release of all subsequent proteins: NS3 serine protease and RNA helicase, NS3–4A serine protease, NS4B and NS5A RNA-binding proteins, and NS5B RNA-dependent RNA polymerase.

III. CLINICAL MANIFESTATIONS OF HCV INFECTION

A. **Acute Infection.** Patients are generally *asymptomatic*, and the infection usually goes undiagnosed at this stage. However, a minority of patients (less than or equal to 20%) develop *symptomatic* hepatitis that usually consists of: **jaundice, malaise, and/or nausea.**

   Acute infection is defined as an infection of less than 6 months' duration. Of those acutely infected, approximately 20% to 50% may spontaneously clear the infection. Spontaneous clearance of HCV is higher in symptomatic acute infection (presumed secondary to a robust immune response). *Fulminant hepatitis/hepatic failure is very rare.*

B. **Chronic Infection.** In the majority of patients the infection becomes chronic with a slow interval development (20–30 years) of hepatic cirrhosis and/or hepatocellular carcinoma (HCC; estimated to be 20% of those with chronic infection). HCC rarely occurs without cirrhosis. *Chronic infection is defined as an infection of greater than 6 months' duration.* The most common manifestation is *fatigue* but it can also be associated with findings of cirrhosis. Other manifestations include:

   1. Anorexia

   2. Gastrointestinal bleeding

   3. Altered mental status (hepatic encephalopathy or asterixis)

   4. Jaundice

5. Palmar erythema and/or spider angiomas

6. Ascites and splenomegaly

7. Testicular atrophy or gynecomastia

8. Dupuytren's contractures

Patients with HCV infection can develop diabetes due to insulin resistance.

C. **Extrahepatic Manifestations.** Most conditions are associated with either an autoimmune or lymphoproliferative disorder in association with chronic hepatic HCV infection.

1. **Lymphoproliferative**

   a. *Non-Hodgkin's B-cell lymphoma.* Chronic B-cell activation by HCV is associated with transformation to the development of B-cell non-Hodgkin's lymphoma (NHL). Type II mixed cryoglobulinemia is characterized by a combination of monoclonal and polyclonal immunoglobulins, with the monoclonal component directed against immunoglobulin G (IgG). The production of IgG is sustained by the clonal expansion of B cells. Mixed cryoglobulinemia is a lymphoproliferative disorder that predisposes patients to B-cell NHL.

2. **Autoimmune**

   a. *Cryoglobulinemia and vasculitis.* Cryoglobulinemia is a disease characterized by circulating immune complexes that precipitate at lower temperatures. It is divided into three types: monoclonal (type I), mixed (type II), and polyclonal (type III). Mixed-type cryoglobulinemia is most closely associated with HCV and results from clonal expansion of rheumatoid factor (RF) producing B cells. The B-cell produced RF (IgM) binds with HCV core proteins and IgG to form immune complexes that attach to the endothelial lining of small blood vessels resulting in a systemic vasculitis. Clinically, the classic triad involves: waning palpable purpuric skin lesions, arthralgias, and weakness.

   b. *Membranoproliferative glomerulonephritis (MPGN).* Usually occurs in the setting of cryoglobulinemia where immune complexes deposit in the glomerulus to provoke glomerular infiltration by macrophages. This results in microscopic hematuria, proteinuria, and renal impairment. A kidney biopsy will demonstrate inflammatory cells within the glomerulus and double contours of the basement membrane.

   c. *Lichen planus.* An inflammatory immune-mediated condition that can affect the skin, hair, nails, and mucous membranes. On the skin, it usually appears as purplish, often itchy, flat-topped bumps, developing over several weeks.

   d. *Sicca syndrome* (Latin *siccus*, meaning "dry"). An autoimmune disease, also known as *Sjogren syndrome*, that classically combines dry eyes, dry mouth, and another disease of connective tissue such as rheumatoid arthritis (most common), lupus, scleroderma, or polymyositis. Occurs in approximately 50% of patients with mixed cryoglobulinemia.

e. ***Porphyria cutanea tarda.*** This is a dermatologic condition whereby HCV inhibits the activity of uroporphyrinogen decarboxylase (UROD). Patients most commonly present with fluid-filled vesicles on sun-exposed areas of skin (e.g., hands, arms, face, and legs).

f. Other extrahepatic manifestations that may involve immune complex deposition include: ***type 2 diabetes***, ***autoimmune thyroiditis,*** and ***immune thrombocytopenia***.

Identification of extrahepatic manifestations of HCV is also a primary indication for antiviral therapy.

IV. APPROACH TO THE PATIENT

A. **History.** Acute HCV infection is often missed, but infection should be suspected in patients with an elevated alanine aminotransferase (ALT) and exposure risk (see the aforementioned risk factors).

Chronic infection with HCV should always be included in the differential diagnosis of patients being evaluated for:

1. Abnormal liver chemistry (ALT greater than or equal to aspartate aminotransferase [AST]).

2. Anemia and thrombocytopenia.

3. Findings suggestive of cirrhosis (see Section III.B).

B. **Physical Examination.** A complete examination should be performed, but areas of specific focus include:

1. Conjunctival examination (to detect jaundice).

2. Vascular examination (to detect signs of vasculitis and lymph node enlargement).

3. Neurologic examination (to detect encephalopathy or asterixis).

4. Abdominal examination (to detect ascites, cirrhosis, or splenomegaly).

5. Dermatologic examination (to detect rash or vasculitis).

C. **Laboratory Studies**

1. **Complete blood count (CBC).** Patients with chronic HCV may have anemia. Thrombocytopenia usually occurs in patients with hepatic cirrhosis. Pancytopenia is also a complication of combined HCV treatment.

2. **Basic metabolic panel (BMP).** Routinely ordered. MPGN should be suspected if creatinine is elevated.

3. **Liver function tests**. An ALT:AST ratio greater than or equal to 2:1, elevated alkaline phosphatase and bilirubin level, as well as a low albumin may suggest HCV. Liver chemistries are unreliable for predicting the severity of hepatic HCV, and normal results cannot rule out HCV-related liver disease or cirrhosis. *However, an AST:platelet ratio greater than or equal to 1.5 has a high positive predictive value (88%) for liver fibrosis calculated as:*

$$AST \ level \times 100/platelet \ count$$

4. **Prothrombin time (PT)/partial thromboplastin time (PTT).** An elevated PT may suggest cirrhosis.

5. **Thyroid-stimulating hormone (TSH)**. HCV therapy can induce an autoimmune thyroiditis; therefore, a baseline TSH may be helpful.

6. **Urinalysis**. Findings of glomerulonephritis may suggest HCV.

7. **Uric acid level**. Hyperuricemia can be a complication of HCV treatment; therefore, a baseline uric acid level may be helpful.

8. **Erythrocyte sedimentation rate (ESR) and C-reactive protein (CRP)**. Values are nonspecific but may be elevated with HCV.

Patients with chronic HCV infection should also be assessed for serologic evidence of HBV and HIV infections (see Chapters 27 and 43), which may accelerate liver fibrosis.

D. **Radiographic Studies**

1. Transabdominal ultrasound is adequate to evaluate for cirrhosis and splenomegaly as well as ascites.

E. **HCV-Specific Diagnostic Testing.** Diagnostic testing is generally divided into serologic assays for antibodies or molecular assays for HCV RNA.

1. **Serologic assay**. Most commonly involve enzyme immunoassays (EIAs) with HCV core protein and/or NS proteins to detect anti-HCV (IgG; sensitivity of 95%, specificity of 99%, positive likelihood ratio of 95, and negative likelihood ratio of 0.05). Assays can detect antibodies within 4 to 10 weeks but may take as long as 6 months.

   Recombinant immunoblot assay (RIBA) has traditionally been utilized to confirm positive EIA results in settings without molecular assays. A "positive" assay is defined as antibodies to greater than or equal to two HCV antigens. An "indeterminate" assay is defined as antibodies to greater than or equal to one antigen.

   Serologic testing for HCV should be performed initially in patients suspected of acute or chronic HCV. The U.S. Preventive Services Task Force and the Centers for Disease Control and Prevention recommend periodic HCV screening for all adults at high risk of infection and one-time screening in adults born between 1945 and 1965. The American Association for the Study of Liver Diseases recommends annual screening for intravenous drug users and for men who are HIV seropositive and have unprotected sex with men. False-negative screening test results occur infrequently with HIV, transplant immunosuppression, hemodialysis, or hypogammaglobulinemia with agammaglobulinemia.

2. **Molecular assay**. Most commonly involves the PCR technique and helpful for the determination of:

   a. **HCV quantitative RNA viral load.** Quantification of the viral load is relevant to therapy as a pretreatment viral load less than 800,000 IU/mL is associated with a sustained response to treatment.

   b. **HCV viral genotype.** Genotyping can help predict the therapy outcome as genotypes 1 and 4 are more resistant to treatment (and require a longer duration) than genotypes 2 and 3.

   Thus, HCV-RNA testing should be performed with: (a) a positive anti-HCV, (b) patients considered for treatment, and (c) patients with unexplained liver disease or immunosuppression with a negative anti-HCV as PCR is usually positive within 1 to 2 weeks of acute HCV. If the anti-HCV antibody test result is negative in a patient who may have been exposed to HCV within the previous 6 months, HCV RNA should be measured every 4 to 8 weeks for at least 6 months or follow-up anti-HCV antibody testing should be performed in 12 weeks. **HCV genotype should be ordered in patients considered for therapy.**

F. **Liver Biopsy Testing.** The diagnostic gold standard is to assess the level of liver inflammation and fibrosis. The liver biopsy is a histologic assessment for the *grade* (defines the extent of necroinflammatory activity) and the *stage* (establishes the extent of fibrosis or the presence of cirrhosis) in hepatic disease and helps to determine the urgency of treatment because the degree of liver fibrosis predicts disease progression and clinical outcomes. *Thus, a liver biopsy should be considered in patients with chronic HCV for prognosis or treatment considerations.*

The Metavir scoring system (Table 28.1) grades fibrosis from 0 to 4, and treatment should be considered in patients with substantial fibrosis (score of 2 or greater).
The prevalence of biopsy proven cirrhosis after 20 years of infection has varied from 7% (in retrospective studies) to 18% (in clinical referred settings). The risk of cirrhosis is increased in individuals abusing alcohol, those who acquire the disease at an older age, men with concomitant obesity, immunosuppressed HIV-positive patients, or those with recurrent HCV following liver transplantation.

The most efficient approach to fibrosis is the combination of direct serum biomarkers and vibration-controlled transient liver elastography.

V. **TREATMENT OF HCV.** *The goal of treatment is to prevent complications and death from chronic HCV infection.* Decisions for treatment should be made jointly by patients and clinicians. Factors that need to be considered are current level of liver fibrosis and inflammation, likelihood of continuous fibrosis progression, and probability of treatment response, and side effects. Factors that negatively affect prognosis include: (a) advanced age, (b) obesity (BMI 25), (c) HIV infection, (d) immunosuppression (e.g., transplant, corticosteroids), (e) patients who consume 50 g alcohol/day, (f) bridging fibrosis on biopsy, and (g) symptomatic cryoglobulinemia.

The current recommended therapy (Table 28.2) and available evidence supports treatment for ALL HCV-infected persons, except those patients who have a limited life expectancy (less than 12 months) due to a nonliver related comorbid condition. *The most important treatment objective is the achievement of sustained virologic response (SVR) to treatment defined as a negative HCV-RNA PCR 12 or more weeks following the completion of therapy.* SVR is a marker for virologic

TABLE 28.1 ■ Metavir Scoring System

Level of hepatic fibrosis	Score
1. No fibrosis	0
2. Minimal scarring	1
3. Positive scarring with extension beyond areas containing blood vessels	2
4. Bridging fibrosis with connection to other areas of fibrosis	3
5. Cirrhosis or advanced liver scarring	4

TABLE 28.2 ■ Recommended Treatment Regimens for Patients With Chronic HCV Not Previously Treated (Naïve)

Genotype	Without Cirrhosis	With Cirrhosis
1a	1. Ledipasvir 90 mg/Sofosbuvir 400 mg for 12 weeks or 2. Elbasvir 50 mg/Grazoprevir 100 mg for 12 weeks or 3. Paritaprevir 150 mg/Ritonavir 100 mg/Ombitasvir 25 mg plus dasabuvir 250 mg twice daily and weight-based ribavirin for 12 weeks or 4. Sofosbuvir 400 mg plus simeprevir 150 mg with or without weight-based ribavirin for 12 weeks or 5. Sofosbuvir 400 mg/Velpatasvir 100 mg for 12 weeks or 6. Daclatasvir 60 mg plus sofosbuvir 400 mg for 12 weeks	1. Ledipasvir 90 mg/Sofosbuvir 400 mg for 12 weeks or 2. Elbasvir 50 mg/Grazoprevir 100 mg for 12 weeks or 3. Elbasvir 50 mg/Grazoprevir 100 mg with weight-based ribavirin for 16 weeks is an alternative regimen for patients with baseline NS5A polymorphisms at amino acid positions 28, 30, 31, or 93 that confer resistance or 4. Sofosbuvir 400 mg/Velpatasvir 100 mg for 12 weeks or 5. Paritaprevir 150 mg/Ritonavir 100 mg/Ombitasvir 25 mg plus dasabuvir 250 mg twice daily and weight-based ribavirin for 24 weeks or 6. Sofosbuvir 400 mg plus simeprevir 150 mg with or without weight-based ribavirin for 24 weeks or 7. Daclatasvir 60 mg plus sofosbuvir 400 mg with or without weight-based ribavirin for 24 weeks
1b	1. Ledipasvir 90 mg/Sofosbuvir 400 mg for 12 weeks or 2. Elbasvir 50 mg/Grazoprevir 100 mg for 12 weeks or 3. Paritaprevir 150 mg/Ritonavir 100 mg/Ombitasvir 25 mg plus dasabuvir 250 mg twice daily and weight-based ribavirin for 12 weeks or 4. Sofosbuvir 400 mg plus simeprevir 150 mg with or without weight-based ribavirin for 12 weeks or 5. Sofosbuvir 400 mg/Velpatasvir 100 mg for 12 weeks or 6. Daclatasvir 60 mg plus sofosbuvir 400 mg for 12 weeks	1. Ledipasvir 90 mg/Sofosbuvir 400 mg for 12 weeks or 2. Elbasvir 50 mg/Grazoprevir 100 mg for 12 weeks or 3. Sofosbuvir 400 mg/Velpatasvir 100 mg for 12 weeks or 4. Paritaprevir 150 mg/Ritonavir 100 mg/Ombitasvir 25 mg plus dasabuvir 250 mg twice daily for 12 weeks or 5. *Sofosbuvir 400 mg plus simeprevir 150 mg with or without weight-based ribavirin for 24 weeks or 6. Daclatasvir 60 mg plus sofosbuvir 400 mg with or without weight-based ribavirin for 24 weeks

(continued)

TABLE 28.2 ■ Recommended Treatment Regimens for Patients With Chronic HCV Not Previously Treated (Naïve) (continued)

Genotype	Without Cirrhosis	With Cirrhosis
2	1. Sofosbuvir 400 mg plus Velpatasvir 100 mg for 12 weeks or 2. Daclatasvir 60 mg plus sofosbuvir 400 mg for 12 weeks	1. Sofosbuvir 400 mg plus Velpatasvir 100 mg for 12 weeks or 2. Daclatasvir 60 mg plus sofosbuvir 400 mg for 16–24 weeks
3	1. Sofosbuvir 400 mg plus Velpatasvir 100 mg for 12 weeks or 2. Daclatasvir 60 mg plus sofosbuvir 400 mg for 12 weeks	1. Sofosbuvir 400 mg plus Velpatasvir 100 mg for 12 weeks or 2. Daclatasvir 60 mg plus sofosbuvir 400 mg with or without weight-based ribavirin for 24 weeks (testing for Y93H polymorphism is recommended for cirrhotic patients and ribavirin should be included in regimen if present)
4	1. Ledipasvir 90 mg/Sofosbuvir 400 mg for 12 weeks or 2. Elbasvir 50 mg/Grazoprevir 100 mg for 12 weeks or 3. Paritaprevir 150 mg/Ritonavir 100 mg/Ombitasvir 25 mg plus dasabuvir 250 mg twice daily and weight-based ribavirin for 12 weeks or 4. Sofosbuvir 400 mg /Velpatasvir 100 mg for 12 weeks	1. Ledipasvir 90 mg/Sofosbuvir 400 mg for 12 weeks or 2. Elbasvir 50 mg/Grazoprevir 100 mg for 12 weeks or 3. Paritaprevir 150 mg/Ritonavir 100 mg/Ombitasvir 25 mg plus dasabuvir 250 mg twice daily and weight-based ribavirin for 12 weeks or 4. Sofosbuvir 400 mg /Velpatasvir 100 mg for 12 weeks
5 and 6	1. Ledipasvir 90 mg/Sofosbuvir 400 mg for 12 weeks or 2. Sofosbuvir 400 mg/Velpatasvir 100 mg for 12 weeks	1. Ledipasvir 90 mg/Sofosbuvir 400 mg for 12 weeks or 2. Sofosbuvir 400 mg/Velpatasvir 100 mg for 12 weeks

*The combination regimen sofosbuvir plus simeprevir should NOT be used in patients harboring the nonstructural protein 3 (NS3) Q80K polymorphism due to lower SVR rates.

The standard weight-based dosing of ribavirin is 1,000 mg daily for individuals who weigh less than 75 kg and 1,200 mg daily for individuals who weigh more than 75 kg.

Serious symptomatic bradycardia may occur in patients taking amiodarone with any combination regimen that uses sofosbuvir.

HBV reactivation may occur in patients treated with DAA medicines for hepatitis C virus. In a few cases, HBV reactivation in patients treated with DAA medicines may result in serious liver problems or death. HBV reactivation usually occurs within 4–8 weeks.

DAA, direct-acting antiviral; HBV, hepatitis B virus; HVC, hepatitis C virus; SVR, sustained virologic response.

cure and is associated with an estimated 70% reduction in the risk of HCC, an estimated 75% complete or partial remission with NHL, an estimated 90% risk reduction in the requirement for liver transplant, and reduction in symptoms associated with severe extrahepatic manifestations (including cryoglobulinemic vasculitis).

Patients with the **HIGHEST** priority for treatment include the following: (a) advanced hepatic fibrosis (Metavir 3), (b) compensated cirrhosis (Metavir 4), (c) organ transplant recipients, (d) cryoglobulinemic vasculitis, and/or (e) nephrotic syndrome and/or MPGN.

Patients with a **HIGH** priority for treatment include the following: (a) hepatic fibrosis (Metavir 2), (b) HIV and/or HBV coinfection, (c) insulin-dependent diabetes mellitus, (d) nonalcoholic steatohepatitis, (e) porphyria cutanea tarda, and/or (f) debilitating fatigue.

Patients who **may benefit from treatment** as a means to reduce transmission include: (a) men who have sex with men (including high-risk sexual practices), (b) patients with active IVDU, (c) incarcerated patients, (d) patients requiring long-term hemodialysis, (e) women of childbearing age, and/or (f) infected healthcare workers. These patients should also be counseled on ways to decrease transmission and minimize the risk of reinfection.

Treatment *mechanisms of action* include the following: (a) direct-acting antiviral (DAA) agents (*NS3/4A inhibitors simeprevir and grazoprevir; NS5A inhibitors daclatasvir, elbasvir, ledipasvir, and velpatasvir; and NS5B nucleoside inhibitor sofosbuvir*), (b) pegylated interferon that inhibits viral replication by antiviral, antiproliferative, and immunomodulatory effects, and (c) ribavirin that inhibits viral RNA polymerase, thereby inhibiting protein synthesis.

Treatment *monitoring* includes the following: CBC and complete metabolic panel (CMP) should be measured at week 4 of treatment and as clinically indicated. Baseline and every 12-week TSH level if pegylated interferon is used. Quantitative HCV viral load is recommended at week 4 of treatment, and at 12 and 24 weeks after completion of therapy.

Therapy should be DISCONTINUED if: (a) 10-fold increase in ALT at week 4 or (b) any increase in ALT associated with symptoms (e.g., weakness, nausea, vomiting, and/or jaundice).

A. The most common side effects from treatment include:

1. **Pegylated interferon**

   a. Influenza-like illness (fatigue, headache, fever, and rigors)

   b. Neutropenia (absolute neutrophil count [ANC] less than or equal to 1.5 units), anemia (hemoglobin less than or equal to 10 g/dL), or thrombocytopenia

   c. Autoimmune thyroiditis

   d. Anxiety, insomnia, psychosis, suicidal ideation

   e. Depression (usually respond to selective serotonin reuptake inhibitor [SSRI] antidepressants)

2. **Ribavirin**

   a. Lymphopenia

   b. Hemolytic anemia

   c. Hyperuricemia

      d. Rash

  3. Direct-acting agents

      a. Anemia

      b. Headache

      c. Nausea

      d. Fatigue

    Contraindications to therapy include: (a) uncontrolled depression or other neuropsychiatric illness, (b) untreated thyroid disease, (c) pregnancy, (d) age less than or equal to 2, (e) active autoimmune disease, (f) decompensated liver disease, (g) severe anemia, (h) recent organ transplantation, and (i) active cardiac disease.

B. Other specific treatment plans include:

  1. Acute HCV Infection. Unless required to prevent transmission to others, patients considered to have acute HCV infection should be monitored for 6 months. If spontaneous clearance does not occur, treatment should follow the same recommendations as for chronic HCV infection (Table 28.2).

  2. Chronic HCV infection in unique patient populations

    a. Decompensated hepatic cirrhosis. Patients considered to have decompensated hepatic cirrhosis (defined best as moderate or severe hepatic impairment; Child–Turcotte–Pugh class B or C) should be referred to specialty care centers (e.g., hepatology or transplant service).

    b. Retreatment of patients who failed prior therapy. Patients considered to have failed prior therapy should be referred to specialty care centers (e.g., HCV specialty clinic or hepatology service).

    c. HIV coinfection. Initiation of highly active antiretroviral therapy (HAART) in coinfected patients is associated with a higher risk of hepatotoxicity. However, it is felt that this is outweighed by the potential benefits of immune restoration that might lessen disease progression, and thus, initiation of HAART is generally recommended early in these patients. HCV/HIV coinfection is also associated with a higher rate of HCV persistence, faster progression rate to hepatic cirrhosis, and end-stage liver disease as well as higher HCV-RNA serum levels. Historically, coinfected patients also have a lower response rate to treatment using peginterferon with ribavirin.

      Currently, the treatment recommendations for HCV/HIV coinfection are the same as for patients with only chronic HCV infection (see Table 28.2). However, antiretroviral and HCV treatment interactions should be reviewed prior to initiating therapy.

C. The following drug interactions should be AVOIDED:

  1. Ledipasvir increases tenofovir levels (especially with a creatinine clearance (CrCL) less than 60 mL/min) and should be avoided with tenofovir with or without ritonavir-boosted HIV protease inhibitors.

2. **Sofosbuvir and fixed-dose combination ledipasvir/sofosbuvir should be avoided with cobicistat, elvitegravir, or tipranavir.**

3. **Simeprevir should not be used with efavirenz, etravirine, nevirapine, cobicistat, or any HIV protease inhibitor.**

4. **Paritaprevir/Ritonavir/Ombitasvir plus dasabuvir should not be used with raltegravir, dolutegravir, enfuvirtide, tenofovir, emtricitabine, lamivudine, atazanavir, efavirenz, rilpivirine, darunavir, and/or ritonavir-boosted lopinavir.**

5. **Ribavirin should not be used with didanosine, stavudine, and/or zidovudine.**

BIBLIOGRAPHY

Chung RT, Davis GL, Jensen DM, et al. Hepatitis C Guidance: AASLD-IDSA recommendations for testing, managing, and treating adults infected with Hepatitis C virus. *Hepatology.* 2015;62(3):932–947.

Feeney ER, Chung RT. Antiviral treatment of Hepatitis C. *BMJ.* 2014;348:g3308.

Liang TJ, Ghany MG. Current and future therapies for hepatitis C virus infection. *N Engl J Med.* 2013;368(20):1907–1917.

Webster DP, Klenerman P, Dusheiko GM. Hepatitis C. *Lancet.* 2015;385(9973):1124–1135.

Wilkins T, Akhtar M, Gititu E, et al. Diagnosis and management of Hepatitis C. *Am Fam Physician.* 2015;91(12):835–842.

URINARY TRACT INFECTIONS

Janaki C. Kuruppu
William F. Wright

I. INTRODUCTION

A. Definition. A bacterial infection of one or more structures in the urinary system.

B. Classification. Urinary tract infections (UTIs) can be classified according to anatomic location and complexity of clinical presentation.

1. **Anatomic localization**

   a. Lower tract

      i. *Urethritis*

      ii. *Cystitis*

   b. Upper tract and systemic (see Chapter 30, Pyelonephritis and Renal Abscess)

      i. Pyelonephritis

      ii. Renal or perinephric abscess

   c. Male accessory gland involvement

      i. Prostatitis

      ii. Epididymitis

      iii. Orchitis

2. **Clinical presentation**

   a. **Uncomplicated**. Previously healthy women without known anatomic or functional abnormality of the urinary tract.

   b. **Complicated**. All men, women, or children with functional, metabolic, or anatomic conditions that may increase risk of treatment failure or recurrence. Additional conditions considered as complicated include: a functional or anatomic urinary tract abnormality (e.g., polycystic kidney disease, nephrolithiasis, neurogenic bladder, pregnancy, or urinary tract instrumentation/catheterization) as well as any patient with diabetes mellitus, or with an immunocompromised status, either from comorbid condition or immunosuppressive therapy.

C. Risk Factors

1. Sexual intercourse (homosexuality and anorectal intercourse is also a risk factor for men).

2. New sexual partner within the past year.

3. Use of spermicides in women.

4. Prior UTI.

5. Lack of circumcision in men.

6. Recent urinary tract instrumentation or surgical procedure.

7. Benign prostatic hyperplasia (BPH).

8. Spinal cord injury with neurogenic bladder.

II. MICROBIOLOGY OF UTI

A. **Gram-Negative Rods.** Consists mainly of Enterobacteriaceae bacteria with *Escherichia coli* as the most common infecting organism (75%–90% in uncomplicated UTI); others include *Klebsiella pneumoniae* and *Proteus mirabilis.* *Pseudomonas* spp can cause UTIs but are commonly associated with urinary tract instrumentation or surgical procedures.

B. **Gram-Positive Cocci.** Commonly include *Staphylococcus saprophyticus, Enterococcus faecalis,* and *Streptococcus agalactiae* (group B streptococci).

C. **Fungal.** *Candida* spp commonly colonizes the urinary tract (especially in association with recent antimicrobial use, diabetes mellitus, and indwelling Foley catheterization) and does not typically represent a true urinary pathogen.

III. CLINICAL MANIFESTATIONS OF UTI

A. **Urethritis.** Urethral discharge, dysuria, urinary frequency, and pain or itching may signify this condition. There may be discomfort with ejaculation in men and vaginal discharge or irritation in women.

B. **Cystitis.** *Dysuria* (burning or pain on urination), *frequency* (frequent voiding of small volumes), *urgency* (sudden urge to void), suprapubic pain, and hematuria are most common. Women who present with any one of these symptoms have a greater than 50% likelihood of having a lower tract UTI and greater than 90% in women with dysuria and frequency *without* vaginal discharge or irritation (with the latter symptoms consider urethritis).

C. **Prostatitis.** Urinary frequency and/or dysuria may present with lower urinary tract obstruction secondary to edema. Fever, lower abdominal or suprapubic discomfort may also be presenting manifestations. Exquisite tenderness of the prostate can be elicited on digital rectal examination (DRE). Additionally, this condition can lead to chronic pelvic pain in men. Finally, some men develop chronic bacterial prostatitis that is *characterized by recurrent bacterial UTI with the same organism isolated repeatedly,* asymptomatic between episodes and often with normal rectal examination.

D. **Epididymitis.** Painful swelling of the scrotum, acute or gradual in onset, with or without dysuria or frequency. Usually unilateral and associated with urethral discharge.

E. **Orchitis.** Less common than prostatitis or epididymitis and usually caused by a viral infection (e.g., mumps, Coxsackie B); however, when present it is usually unilateral with testicular pain and swelling. Symptoms can be severe with nausea, fever, and constitutional symptoms. Pyogenic orchitis is rare and usually due to contiguous spread from epididymitis.

F. Pyelonephritis. Fever (temperature greater than 38°C), chills, flank pain, costovertebral-angle tenderness, and nausea or vomiting, with or without symptoms of cystitis (see Chapter 30 for details).

IV. APPROACH TO THE PATIENT

A. History. A complete and chronologically accurate history should be obtained in all patients suspected of a UTI. *A UTI should be included in the differential diagnosis of any patient who has symptoms of dysuria, frequency, and urgency.* The history should focus on the timing of events, risk factors, comorbid conditions, medication allergies, and recent antimicrobial therapy. Women should also be questioned about vaginal discharge or irritation.

Urethritis may have indolent onset, occur intermittently, and may be most noticeable in the morning with first micturition; however, cystitis generally has a more acute onset. Pyelonephritis tends to also have an acute onset but patients may or may not recall preceding lower urinary tract symptoms.

B. Physical Examination. While a complete physical examination should always be performed, the physical examination should emphasize these areas:

1. **Abdominal examination.** Discomfort on palpation or percussion of the lower abdominal area (e.g., suprapubic region) may occur with cystitis. While cystitis typically has no specific physical findings, *costovertebral-angle tenderness* (also known as Murphy's punch sign) is the only physical finding that increases the probability of UTI (indicating pyelonephritis).

2. **Genital–rectal examination.** Urethritis may demonstrate as vaginal discharge in women and a visible penile urethral discharge in men. A pelvic examination should be performed in sexually active women experiencing UTI symptoms with vaginal discharge and irritation. A DRE should be performed in men to evaluate the prostate gland. An enlarged or slightly boggy prostate is nonspecific; however, a swollen, firm, and exquisitely tender prostate is associated with acute prostatitis. A swollen, firm, and nontender prostate may suggest BPH.

C. Laboratory Studies

1. **Urinalysis.** The presence of leukocyte esterase *or* nitrite on urine dipstick has a sensitivity of 75% and specificity of 82%; however, negative results do not rule out infection in a patient with a strongly suggestive history for UTI. Microscopic examination of urine showing at least 10 white blood cells per cubic millimeter is considered significant pyuria. Hematuria (the presence of blood in the urine) is also commonly associated with cystitis.

2. **Urine culture.** Positive culture result indicating significant bacteriuria is traditionally defined as 10^5 colony-forming units per milliliter. Women with cystitis frequently have lower colony counts (10^2–10^4 colony-forming units per milliliter); therefore, in this clinical setting, urine culture generally does not add diagnostic accuracy but is helpful for the correct identification of the pathogen and determination of antimicrobial susceptibility. Growth of 10^3 colony-forming units per milliliter or more in men with dysuria may be considered as significant for a UTI. *Steps to obtaining a midstream clean-catch urine sample for culture include:*

   a. *Patients should be instructed to wash their hands.*

   b. *The vulva and glans penis should be cleaned by using three swabs with soap and sterile water.*

    c. *The first 10 mL of urine should be collected in a separate container or discarded as this represents the urethral urine.*

    d. *The midstream sample should be collected in a sterile container and transported to the laboratory immediately.* **Storage of a urine sample at room temperature for more than 2 hours results in significant increases in bacterial counts resulting in an unreliable sample.**

  3. Sequential urine cultures. In the evaluation of prostatitis, quantitative cultures of urine samples obtained before and after prostate massage can be helpful in isolating a particular pathogen. *Steps to obtaining a prostatic sample for evaluation include:*

    a. *The glans penis should be cleaned by using three swabs with soap and sterile water.*

    b. *The first 10 to 20 mL of urine should be collected in a separate container or discarded as this represents the urethral urine.*

    c. *The midstream sample should be collected in a sterile container and transported to the laboratory immediately.*

    d. *Prostatic massage is then performed by DRE with expressed prostatic secretions (EPS) collected in a separate container.* **Prostatitis is suggested by more than 15 white blood cells per high-power field on microscopic examination.**

    e. *Finally, 10 mL of urine should be collected following prostatic massage.*

D. Radiologic Studies. Uncomplicated UTIs *do not* require any imaging studies; however, imaging should be conducted if there is suspicion for an upper UTI, anatomic abnormalities predisposing to UTI, and in a patient with recurrent infection or failure to respond to appropriate therapy.

  1. Plain films (kidneys, ureters, and bladder). Useful to detect urinary calculi, calcification, soft tissue masses, and abnormal gas patterns.

  2. Ultrasonography. Allows characterization of size and contour of kidneys and bladder, identification of renal mass or abscess, visualization of certain calculi, and discernment of hydronephrosis.

  3. CT. Imaging modality of choice for nonpregnant women and men. Offers fine anatomic detail and can evaluate focal nephritis, renal or perirenal abscesses, and masses as well as both radiopaque and radiolucent calculi; however, caution must be used because renal injury may be aggravated by intravenous contrast material.

  4. MRI. Generally, there is *no advantage* of MRI over CT imaging for diagnosis of renal infection but MRI may be considered in patients who have allergy or other contraindication to iodinated contrast dye.

V. MANAGEMENT OF UTI

A. Urethritis. See Chapter 42, Sexually Transmitted Diseases.

B. Cystitis. *In randomized, controlled trials, placebo groups have spontaneous resolution of symptoms in 25% to 42% of women; therefore, antibiotic therapy is not mandatory but is generally prescribed to limit morbidity and speedy resolution of symptoms.* **Asymptomatic bacteriuria in pregnant women should**

always be treated with oral antimicrobial agents that are safe during pregnancy. Appropriate empirical oral antimicrobial choices include:

1. **Nitrofurantoin** 100 mg twice daily for **5 days.**

2. **TMP-SMX** 160 g/800 mg twice daily for **3 days.**

3. **Fosfomycin trometamol** 3 g sachet **single dose.**

4. **Ciprofloxacin** 250 mg twice daily (or 500 mg extended release once daily) for **3 days** (only if other options cannot be used).

C. **Prostatitis.** Acute prostatitis can be treated with agents appropriate for cystitis, pending results from urine culture to guide therapy. Cases of chronic prostatis may require 4 to 6 weeks of oral fluoroquinolones therapy.

D. **Epididymitis.** Most cases are due to *N. gonorrhoeae* or *C. trachomatis*; therefore, appropriately directed therapy for these agents is indicated and includes:

1. **Ceftriaxone** 250 mg intramuscular (IM), single dose

2. **Azithromycin** 1 g PO, single dose

In older men, drug therapy directed at *Escherichia coli* or *Pseudomonas* spp should be selected, such as **ciprofloxacin** 500 mg twice daily for **7 days.** Symptomatic improvement should be seen in 3 days; however, if no response, reevaluation is indicated.

E. **Orchitis.** Viral orchitis resolves within 2 weeks in most cases; however, antimicrobial treatment of bacterial orchitis should be based on culture results with the duration dictated by resolution of symptoms.

F. **Pyelonephritis.** See Chapter 30, Pyelonephritis and Renal Abscess.

VI. TREATMENT FAILURE OR RECURRENCE

A. Failure of symptoms to resolve should raise concern for resistant organisms. In the case of empiric therapy failing in the setting of cystitis, midstream urine collection should be sent for culture and sensitivity testing to identify the appropriate organism. Negative routine cultures with recurrent or persistent cystitis symptoms should raise concern for mycobacterial infection, or noninfectious causes of cystitis, such as malignancy or interstitial cystitis.

B. Gross hematuria or persistent microscopic hematuria may indicate malignancy, and CT imaging or cystoscopy are indicated for further evaluation.

C. Pyuria without bacteriuria suggests malignancy or mycobacterial infection.

VII. PROPHYLAXIS FOR RECURRENT CYSTITIS. Women who have recurrent cystitis without evidence of the aforementioned complications (malignancy, mycobacterial infection, interstitial cystitis) may be candidates for prophylaxis, or self-treatment. *Fluoroquinolone (e.g., ciprofloxacin) antimicrobial agents are not recommended for prophylaxis measures.*

With the exception of topical estrogen therapy in postmenopausal women, cranberry juice and D-mannose (bacterial adhesion blocker) have *no* proven role in reducing recurrent cystitis. Additionally, behavioral modifications with liberal fluid intake, immediate postcoital urination, elimination of douching and form-fitting underwear, and postdefecation maneuvers (e.g., wipe from front to back) have shown no benefit in reducing recurrent infections.

A. **Self-Treatment.** Women who have previously been diagnosed with cystitis have 85% to 95% accuracy in self-diagnosis and can be given prescriptions of usual first-line oral therapy to initiate treatment at first sign of UTI symptoms.

B. **Postcoital Antimicrobial Prophylaxis.** Single dose of any of the following as soon as possible after intercourse:

   1. **Nitrofurantoin** 50 to 100 mg

   2. **TMP-SMX** 40 mg/200 mg *or* 80 mg/400 mg

   3. **Trimethoprim** 100 mg

   4. **Cephalexin** 250 mg

C. **Continuous Prophylaxis.** This approach has shown significant reductions in recurrent cystitis. This treatment should be reserved for women with greater than three UTIs/12 months or greater than two UTIs/6 months. In general, a 6-month trial is provided with daily bedtime dosing of the following agents:

   1. **Nitrofurantoin** 50 to 100 mg (long-term continuous exposure with this agent can be associated with pulmonary hypersensitivity, hepatitis, and peripheral neuropathy)

   2. **TMP-SMX** 40 mg/200 mg (three times weekly)

   3. **Trimethoprim** 100 mg

   4. **Cephalexin** 125 to 250 mg

   5. **Fosfomycin** 3 g sachet *every 10 days* (this agent is *not* provided as a daily bedtime dose)

BIBLIOGRAPHY

Bent S, Nallamothu BK, Simel DL, et al. Does this woman have an acute uncomplicated urinary tract infection? *JAMA.* 2002;287:2701–2710.

Dielubanza EJ, Schaeffer AJ. Urinary tract infections in women. *Med Clin North Am.* 2011;95:27–41.

Gupta K, Hooton TM, Naber KG, et al. International clinical practice guidelines for the treatment of acute uncomplicated cystitis and pyelonephritis in women: a 2010 update by the Infectious Diseases Society of America and the European Society for Microbiology and Infectious Diseases. *Clin Infect Dis.* 2011;52:e103–e120.

Hooton TM. Uncomplicated urinary tract infection. *N Engl J Med.* 2012;366:1028–1037.

PYELONEPHRITIS AND RENAL ABSCESS

Jason Bailey
Janaki C. Kuruppu
William F. Wright

I. PYELONEPHRITIS

A. Definition. An inflammatory process of the upper urinary tract system, specifically the renal parenchyma. Pyelonephritis can be classified according to the chronicity and/or complexity of clinical presentation. Classifications include:

1. **Acute pyelonephritis.** This is an acute inflammatory process of the renal parenchyma most commonly as the result of a bacterial infection. Acute pyelonephritis can also be further classified by the complexity of the clinical presentation:

   a. **Uncomplicated acute pyelonephritis.** This is typically defined as acute pyelonephritis involving a typical bacteria and a healthy immune-competent patient with normal renal function and urinary tract anatomy.

   b. **Complicated acute pyelonephritis.** This is typically defined as acute pyelonephritis involving a patient at the extremes of age (less than 5 years or greater than 65 years), an atypical bacterium (e.g., unusual pathogen or multidrug resistance), male sex, immunosuppression, significant medical or surgical comorbidities (e.g., diabetes mellitus, renal failure, hemodialysis, pregnancy, uronephrolithiasis, or chronic liver disease), and/or an abnormal renal function or urinary tract anatomy (e.g., urinary reflux, indwelling urinary catheter).

2. **Chronic pyelonephritis.** Also termed chronic interstitial nephritis (CIN) that either results from active recurrent upper urinary tract infections or renal changes due to a prior upper urinary tract infection. *This condition would be considered as a complicated pyelonephritis and can be associated with renal scarring and systemic hypertension, most commonly in children.*

B. Pathogenesis. Three mechanisms are considered for development of infection:

1. **Ascending mechanism.** This is the *most common mechanism* and results from the migration of bacteria from lower urinary tract upward to the kidneys.

2. **Hematogenous mechanism.** Infection of the kidney resulting from seeding of circulating bacteremia, from a distant site of infection.

3. **Lymphatic mechanism.** While considered unusual, lymphatic connections between the ureters and kidneys *may* contribute to the development of increased bladder pressures and increased lymphatic flow directed to the kidney, which may lead to the development of ascending infections.

C. **Risk Factors.** Similar to cystitis, or lower urinary tract infection, risk factors (see Chapter 29, Urinary Tract Infections) include:

1. Sexual intercourse (homosexuality and anorectal intercourse are also a risk factor for men)

2. New sexual partner within the past year (vaginal colonization with typical pathogens)

3. Use of spermicides in women

4. Prior urinary tract infection

5. Lack of circumcision in men

6. Recent urinary tract instrumentation (e.g., urinary catheter) or surgical procedure

7. Benign prostatic hyperplasia (BPH)

8. Spinal cord injury with neurogenic bladder

9. Renal transplantation (most commonly occurs within 60 days after transplant as a result of immunosuppression and surgical vesicular–ureteral reflux)

10. Comorbid medical conditions (e.g., diabetes and renal failure)

11. Pregnancy

D. **Microbiology of Pyelonephritis**

1. **Gram-negative rods.** Consists mainly of Enterobacteriaceae bacteria with *Escherichia coli* as the most common infecting organism (80%); others include *Klebsiella pneumoniae* and *Proteus mirabilis. Pseudomonas* spp can rarely cause pyelonephritis but are commonly associated with urinary tract instrumentation or surgical procedures.

2. **Gram-positive cocci.** May include *Staphylococcus saprophyticus, Enterococcus faecalis,* and *Streptococcus agalactiae* (group B streptococci).

3. *Mycobacterium tuberculosis.* Most commonly results from dissemination from a primary site of infection such as the lung or gastrointestinal tract (see Chapter 14, Tuberculosis).

E. **Clinical Manifestations of Pyelonephritis.** Symptoms and signs of pyelonephritis can vary based on patient age and comorbid conditions, and the clinical presentation can range from a silent illness (e.g., subclinical pyelonephritis) to severe sepsis. Patients may already have an established diagnosis of acute cystitis with *dysuria* (burning or pain on urination), *frequency* (frequent voiding of small volumes), *urgency* (sudden urge to void), suprapubic or lower abdominal pain, and hematuria; however, patients with pyelonephritis may also experience the additional following symptoms:

1. **Fever** (temperature greater than 38°C): may be the most reliable finding to differentiate an upper urinary tract infection

2. **Chills**: may be an indication of concurrent bacteremia

3. **Nausea**

4. **Vomiting**

5. **Flank or lower back discomfort**

6. **Delirium or confusion**: may be the sole presenting finding in elderly patients

Mycobacterium tuberculosis typically presents with dysuria, frequency, urgency, and flank or back pain, but fever, chills, nausea, and vomiting are commonly absent.

F. Approach to the Patient With Pyelonephritis

1. **History.** A complete and chronologically accurate history should be obtained in all patients suspected of an upper urinary tract infection. *Pyelonephritis should be included in the differential diagnosis of any patient who has a fever, especially when associated with symptoms of dysuria, frequency, urgency, and/or back or flank discomfort.* The history should focus on the timing of events, risk factors, comorbid conditions, medication allergies, and recent antimicrobial therapy.

2. **Physical examination.** While a complete physical examination should always be performed, the physical examination should emphasis these areas:

   a. **Abdominal examination.** Discomfort on palpation or percussion of the lower abdominal area (e.g., suprapubic region) may occur with cystitis. While cystitis typically has no specific physical findings, *costovertebral-angle tenderness* (also known as Murphy's punch sign) is the only physical finding that increases the probability of urinary tract infection (indicating pyelonephritis).

   b. **Genital–rectal examination.** A digital rectal examination (DRE) should be performed in men to evaluate the prostate gland. An enlarged or slightly boggy prostate is nonspecific; however, a swollen, firm, and exquisitely tender prostate is associated with acute prostatitis. A swollen, firm, and nontender prostate may suggest BPH.

3. **Laboratory studies**

   a. **Complete blood count (CBC).** Routinely ordered and has traditionally indicated both the severity of illness and response to therapy.

   b. **Basic metabolic panel (BMP).** Routinely ordered and nonspecific for pyelonephritis; however, it is most helpful for determining the renal function.

   c. **Erythrocyte sedimentation rate (ESR) and C-reactive protein (CRP).** The serum levels are usually elevated but nonspecific.

   d. **Blood cultures.** Routinely ordered but may only result in positive cultures in as many as 20% to 30% of cases.

   e. **Urinalysis. Pyuria is present in the majority of cases.** The presence of leukocyte esterase *or* nitrite on urine dipstick has a sensitivity of 75% and specificity of 82%; however, negative results do not rule out infection in a patient with a strongly suggestive history for urinary tract infection. Microscopic examination of urine showing at least 10 white blood cells (WBCs) per cubic millimeter is considered significant pyuria. The finding of urinary WBC casts in association with symptoms is strongly associated with pyelonephritis. Hematuria (the presence of blood in the urine) is also commonly associated with cystitis and pyelonephritis.

   f. **Urine culture. All patients should have a urine culture with antimicrobial sensitivity testing performed** (*steps to obtain a midstream clean-catch urine sample for culture can be found in Chapter 29*). A positive culture result (along with typical clinical findings) indicating acute uncomplicated pyelonephritis is traditionally defined as greater than 10^2 colony-forming units per milliliter; however, a positive culture result indicating significant bacteriuria (without symptoms this would be known as subclinical pyelonephritis) is traditionally defined as 10^5 colony-forming units per milliliter. *Routine urine cultures will not grow Mycobacterium tuberculosis; therefore, this condition is associated with the so-called sterile pyuria.*

4. **Radiology studies.** Requirements for imaging studies should be assessed depending on the severity of the patient presentation. A patient with symptoms of uncomplicated pyelonephritis most likely does not require initial imaging studies; however, imaging should be performed for *complicated pyelonephritis, men, recurrent urinary tract infections, comorbid medical or surgical conditions, an uncommon urinary pathogen, persistent symptoms or fever greater than 72 hours following the initiation of appropriate antimicrobial therapy.*

   Imaging modalities for pyelonephritis include:

   a. **Intravenous urography (IVU).** A very cost-effective imaging modality but not widely available and is associated with use of intravenous (IV) iodinated contrast.

   b. **Ultrasound.** A widely available and cost-effective imaging modality that is not associated with iodinated contrast or ionizing radiation. It is especially useful for evaluation in pregnant women but is limited due to patient body habitus and operator dependence.

   c. **CT.** This is the *preferred imaging modality* when used with IV contrast as it provides a global evaluation of the kidneys, detect renal calculi, and can detect complications of pyelonephritis such as abscesses. Classic findings include wedge-shaped areas of decreased attenuation or a "striated nephrogram" appearance of the renal cortex.

   d. **MRI.** A costly imaging modality that is least available but can provide detailed anatomy findings without the use of ionizing radiation or iodinated contrast.

G. **Treatment of Pyelonephritis.** The initial management for pyelonephritis is based on the requirements for hospitalization. While the majority of patients can be managed in an outpatient setting with oral antimicrobial therapy, indications for hospitalization include: *extremes of age, inadequate medical access or unreliable social support, complicated risk factors and/or infection, significant comorbid medical conditions, and persistent symptoms despite appropriate outpatient therapy.* **Pregnant women always require hospitalization for IV antimicrobial therapy and hydration due to the onset of contractions associated with the infection and treatment.** Although antimicrobial therapy should always be guided by available urine culture and sensitivity data, empirical therapy regimens, based on treatment setting, include:

1. **Hospitalized patient**

   a. **Initial therapy.** Ceftriaxone 1 g or gentamicin 5 to 7 mg/kg or ciprofloxacin 400 mg IV daily for 24 to 48 hours. Ciprofloxacin should be avoided in pregnant women.

   b. **Switch therapy.** When the patient has improved symptoms and/or laboratory parameters, the patient may be "switched" to *oral therapy* in preparation for hospital discharge. Antimicrobial regimens include (in order of preference):

    i. Ciprofloxacin 500 mg twice daily or 1,000 mg once daily for *7 days or*

    ii. Levofloxacin 750 mg daily for *5 days or*

    iii. Trimethoprim–sulfamethoxazole 160/800 mg twice daily for *14 days*

2. **Nonhospitalized patient**. Patients who do not require hospitalization can be successfully treated with the oral regimens listed previously under the switch therapy category. If symptoms have resolved upon completion of therapy, posttreatment urinalysis and culture are not recommended. Pregnant women with pyelonephritis *do require* posttreatment management with either monthly urine cultures or antimicrobial suppression therapy with **nitrofurantoin 100 mg daily** (long-term continuous exposure with this agent can be associated with pulmonary hypersensitivity, hepatitis, and peripheral neuropathy) until 4 to 6 weeks post partum because of increased risk of recurrence and adverse effects on the fetus.

II. RENAL ABSCESS

A. **Definition.** Renal abscesses are commonly classified into two major types based on anatomical location.

1. **Intrarenal abscess.** These abscesses are confined to the renal cortex or corticomedullary region. Most intrarenal abscesses are the result of either a metastatic spread of infection from a distant site (e.g., hematogenous source) or liquefaction necrosis and abscess formation due to pyelonephritis (most common). Risk factors include: diabetes mellitus, hemodialysis, IV drug use, urinary tract instrumentation, renal calculi, and recurrent urinary tract infections.

2. **Perinephric abscess.** This abscess commonly results from rupture of a cortical or corticomedullary abscess through the renal capsule (e.g., Gerota fascia) into the perirenal space.

B. **Microbiology of Renal Abscesses**

1. **Gram-positive bacteria.** Most commonly involves *Staphylococcus aureus*; however, occasionally may involve *Streptococcus* spp or *Enterococcus* spp.

2. **Gram-negative bacteria.** Most commonly involves *Escherichia coli* but may also include *Enterobacter* spp, *Klebsiella* spp, *Proteus* spp, *Citrobacter* spp, *Serratia* spp, and *Pseudomonas* spp.

3. **Anaerobic bacteria.** *Clostridium* spp, *Bacteroides* spp, and *Actinomyces* spp may occasionally be associated with renal abscesses.

4. **Fungi.** Most commonly involves *Candida* spp.

C. **Clinical Manifestations.** The clinical manifestations are similar to pyelonephritis; however, signs and symptoms may vary based on the patient age, comorbid medical conditions, and location of the abscess.

1. **Intrarenal abscesses.** Fever, chills, nausea, vomiting, and flank or back pain are common; however, urinary symptoms may be absent if the abscess does not communicate with the urinary excretory passages. Fatigue, malaise, and weight loss may be additional manifestations.

2. **Perinephric abscesses.** Fever, chills, and unilateral flank pain are common manifestations. Other symptoms may include fatigue, malaise, nausea, referred pain (e.g., hip, knee, thigh), and weight loss.

D. **Rare Variants of Intrarenal Abscesses**

1. **Emphysematous pyelonephritis** is an intrarenal abscess due to "gas-forming" bacteria that is almost exclusively seen in patients with diabetes mellitus and characterized clinically by severe illness with fever, chills, and flank pain.

2. **Xanthogranulomatous pyelonephritis.** Uncommon, severe form of chronic infection, most commonly as the result of obstruction due to a staghorn calculus, of the renal parenchyma in which destroyed tissue is replaced with lipid-laden macrophages (e.g., xanthoma cells).

E. **Approach to the Patient**

1. **History.** A complete and chronologically accurate history should be obtained in all patients suspected of a renal abscess. A renal abscess should be included in the differential diagnosis of all patients with a fever and prior urinary tract infection that has *not* responded to appropriate antimicrobial therapy within 72 hours.

2. **Physical examination.** A complete physical examination should always be performed with focus areas the same as for pyelonephritis. The most common findings include flank pain, flank mass, and costovertebral-angle tenderness; however, findings may also include nonspecific abdominal pain and/or rarely a draining sinus tract.

3. **Laboratory studies.** The laboratory evaluation is the same as for pyelonephritis; however, the urinalysis may be normal in as many as 30% of cases. In general, the WBC count is elevated in the majority of cases, and blood cultures may have positive results in as many as 40% of cases.

4. **Radiology studies.** While imaging modalities are similar to pyelonephritis, *CT is the preferred test.* The most common finding includes inflammatory stranding with a central low-attenuation mass (located either in an intrarenal or perirenal position) that may have a peripheral enhancing rim of varied thickness following the administration of contrast material. Emphysematous pyelonephritis will have "gas" visualized within the renal parenchyma and/ or collecting system. Xanthogranulomatous pyelonephritis is usually identified as an enlarged kidney with dilated calyces containing renal calculi that *does not enhance* following administration of contrast material (indicates a nonfunctioning kidney).

   Ultrasound findings are variable and may include either hyper- or hypoechoic areas that lack color Doppler flow.

5. **Treatment.** Treatment of renal abscesses depends on comorbid medical conditions, medical allergies, and the location and size of the abscess. Treatment may require a combined medical and surgical approach.

   a. **Intrarenal abscesses**. Most intrarenal abscesses respond to antimicrobial therapy alone and rarely require surgical measures.

      i. **Antimicrobial therapy.** Empirical antimicrobial therapy should be directed at the most likely pathogen but tailored to the renal function and antimicrobial susceptibilities obtained with culture data. **The** duration of antimicrobial therapy has traditionally been 4 to 6 weeks. Suggested regimens according to the likely pathogen include:

(a) *Staphylococcus aureus:*

- **Oxacillin or methicillin sensitive.** *Nafcillin 2 g IV q4–6*

- **Oxacillin or methicillin resistant.** *Vancomycin 15 mg/kg IV q12–24* **(the vancomycin dose may need adjustments to maintain a serum trough level between 15 and 20 mcg/mL)**

(b) **Streptococcus spp.** *Penicillin G 5 million units IV q6* (if the polymerase chain reaction [PCN] minimum inhibitory concentration [MIC] data indicate the bacteria is susceptible) or *ceftriaxone 2 g IV q24* .

(c) *Enterococcus* **spp:**

- **Penicillin-sensitive.** *Penicillin G 5 million units IV q6*

- **Ampicillin-sensitive.** *Ampicillin 2 g IV q4–6*

- **Ampicillin-resistant.** *Vancomycin 15 mg/kg IV q12–24* **(the vancomycin dose may need adjustments to maintain a serum trough level between 15 and 20 mcg/mL)**

The addition of **gentamicin** at 1 mg/kg IV q8 is also suggested (dosing 3 mg/kg IV q24 has been associated with less nephrotoxicity).

(d) **Enteric gram-negative rods.** *Ceftriaxone 2 g IV q24* , or *ciprofloxacin 400 mg IV q12* (or 500–750 mg PO q12), or *ertapenem 1,000 mg IV q24* (carbapenem antibiotics are reserved for multidrug-resistant organisms).

(e) *Pseudomonas aeruginosa. Ceftazidime* or *cefepime 2 g IV q8* in combination with an aminoglycoside antibiotic (see gentamicin in the preceding), or *piperacillin–tazobactam 3.375 g IV q6* , or *meropenem 1,000 mg IV q8* , or *doripenem 500 mg IV q8* , or *imipenem–cilastatin 500–1,000 mg IV q6.*

(f) **Anaerobes.** *Metronidazole 500 mg IV or PO q8.*

(g) **Fungal.** *Fluconazole* 200 mg *IV or PO q24* or *lipid complex amphotericin B 3 to 5 mg/kg IV q24.* (Do not use micafungin, caspofungin, or anidulafungin as these agents *do not* achieve adequate urinary concentrations.)

  ii. **Surgical therapy.** Abscesses *larger than 5 cm* may require percutaneous drainage with the assistance of ultrasound or CT guidance; however, smaller abscesses that have *not* responded to appropriate antimicrobial therapy may also require drainage.

b. **Perinephric abscesses.** These abscesses are associated with mortality rates as high as 50%; therefore, a *combined medical and surgical approach* should be considered in all cases. While antimicrobial therapy is the same as for intrarenal abscesses, surgical measures may require assisted percutaneous drainage, open surgical drainage, or nephrectomy. Diffuse or advanced-stage xanthogranulomatous pyelonephritis almost always requires nephrectomy.

BIBLIOGRAPHY

Craig WD, Wagner BJ, Travis MD. Pyelonephritis: radiologic-pathologic review. *Radiographics.* 2008;28(1):255–277.

Dembry LM, Andriole VT. Renal and perirenal abscesses. *Infect Dis Clin North Am.* 1997;11(3):663–680.

Gupta K, Hooton TM, Naber KG, et al. International clinical practice guidelines for the treatment of acute uncomplicated cystitis and pyelonephritis in women: A 2010 update by the Infectious Diseases Society of America and the European Society for Microbiology and Infectious Diseases. *Clin Infect Dis.* 2011;52:e103–e120.

Hooton TM. Uncomplicated urinary tract infection. *N Engl J Med.* 2012;366:1028–1037.

Lane DR, Takhar SS. Diagnosis and management of urinary tract infection and pyelonephritis. *Emerg Med Clin North Am.* 2011;29(3):539–552.

Nicolle LE. Uncomplicated urinary tract infection in adults including uncomplicated pyelonephritis. *Urol Clin North Am.* 2008;35(1):1–12.

Warren JW, Abrutyn E, Hebel JR, et al. Guidelines for antimicrobial treatment of uncomplicated acute bacterial cystitis and acute pyelonephritis in women. Infectious Diseases Society of America (IDSA). *Clin Infect Dis.* 1999;29(4):745–758.

31

CATHETER-RELATED URINARY TRACT INFECTIONS

Clare Rock
Kerri A. Thom
William F. Wright

I. INTRODUCTION

A. **Definition.** A urinary tract infection is an infection involving any part of the urinary system, including urethra, bladder, ureters, and kidney. When this infection occurs in a patient who has or has recently had (in the preceding 48 hours) a urinary catheter, it is termed a *catheter-associated urinary tract infection (CAUTI)*. **Additional definitions:**

1. **Short-term urinary catheter.** An indwelling urinary catheter placed for a duration of *less than 30 days*.

2. **Long-term urinary catheter.** An indwelling urinary catheter placed for a duration of *more than 30 days*.

3. **Catheter-associated asymptomatic bacteriuria (CA-ASB).** A short- or long-term urinary catheter with significant bladder bacterial levels (i.e., significant bacteriuria; see Section IV.C) **but** *no symptoms of urinary tract infection* (see Section III).

4. **CAUTI.** A short- or long-term urinary catheter with significant bladder bacterial levels (i.e., significant bacteriuria; see Section IV.C) **and** *symptoms of urinary tract infection* (see Section III).

B. **Epidemiology.** CAUTI is the most frequent healthcare-associated infection in the United States with an estimated 560,000 episodes occurring annually. Each episode costs approximately $589 leading to considerable expense to the U.S. healthcare system. Although, when compared with other hospital-acquired infections, morbidity and mortality rates from CAUTI are considered relatively low, the high prevalence of urinary catheter use leads to a large cumulative burden of infections. It is estimated that 13,000 deaths annually in the United States are attributed to CAUTI. Infections due to urinary catheters can have an effect beyond the urinary tract; indeed, approximately 20% of hospital-acquired bacteremia arises from the urinary tract.

C. **Pathogenesis.** Urinary catheters allow for easier entry of microbes into the bladder. The placement of a urinary catheter into the bladder disrupts the natural host defense mechanisms. The introduction of bacteria into the bladder may be done at the time of urinary catheter insertion or may ascend into the urogenital system after urinary catheter placement. Causative bacteria of CAUTI can be from the patient's own skin and urogenital flora or can be transmitted from healthcare workers or from inanimate objects in the health-care setting. Most bacteria are extraluminally acquired, meaning the bacteria ascend from the catheter–urethral interface up into the bladder; however, approximately 33% are intraluminally acquired, meaning that the bacteria ascend from the urinary catheter drainage bag. Once the urinary catheter is in place, formations of **biofilms,** microcolonies of bacteria that adhere to the inner and outer surfaces of the urinary catheter, occur that enhance the bacteria's reproduction and potential to cause infection. The biofilm also acts to protect the bacteria from the host immune system and from the effect of antimicrobial agents as well as may facilitate bacteria resistance to antibiotics. Finally, the urinary catheter also prevents the complete elimination of blad-der urine that may facilitate the growth of bacteria within a residual pool of stagnant urine.

D. **Risk Factors.** Identifiable risk factors are related to the development of signifi-cant bacteriuria or bacteremia and are due to either the catheter or host factors.

1. *Risk factors for developing bacteriuria:*

   a. *Prolonged catheterization greater than 6 days.* (This is the most impor-tant risk factor with nearly all catheters associated with bacteriuria by 30 days.)

   b. *Lack of appropriate catheter care and sterile techniques upon placement*

   c. *Diabetes mellitus* (increased perineal colonization and urine glucose that supports microbial growth)

   d. *Age greater than 50 years*

   e. *Bacterial colonization of the drainage bag*

   f. *Female sex* (due to shorter urethra and easier access of perineal bacteria to the urinary bladder)

   g. *Elevated serum creatinine* (greater than 2.0 mg/dL at the time of catheter placement)

   h. *Ureteral stent*

   i. *Malnutrition*

2. *Risk factors for developing a secondary bacteremia:*

   a. *Male sex*

   b. *Age greater than 70 years*

   c. *Infection with Serratia marcescens* (due to increased nosocomial transmission)

   d. *Benign prostatic hyperplasia (BPH) or nephrolithiasis*

II. **MICROBIAL CAUSES OF CAUTI.** CAUTIs are predominantly healthcare-associ-ated infections and are associated with increased resistance to antimicrobial agents. *Of note, while short-term catheters are more likely to become infected with a sin-gle pathogen (i.e., monomicrobial), those with long-term catheterization may be polymicrobial.* It is important to distinguish urinary colonization from true infec-tion, as long-term catheterization is associated with urinary tract colonization with potentially pathogenic bacteria, which should only be treated in the presence of symptoms (see Section III). Most infections are due to enteric gram-negative pathogens; common pathogens include:

A. Bacterial Pathogens

1. *Escherichia coli* (most common)
2. *Klebsiella pneumoniae*
3. *Serratia marcescens*
4. *Citrobacter* spp
5. *Enterobacter* spp
6. *Pseudomonas aeruginosa*
7. *Proteus mirabilis*
8. *Providencia stuartii*
9. *Morganella morganii*
10. *Enterococcus* spp

B. Fungal Pathogens

1. *Candida* spp; *C. albicans, C. glabrata, C. tropicalis,* or *C. krusei* (common cause of ASB but less common cause of CAUTI)

   The isolation of *Staphylococcus aureus*, *Pseudomonas aeruginosa*, *Salmonella* spp, and *Candida* spp in the urine of a catheterized patient should *always* prompt the search for a bloodstream infection from another source, as these organisms are not typically associated with an ascending catheter infection.

III. CLINICAL MANIFESTATIONS OF CAUTI

The majority of patients with short-term urinary catheters and significant bacteriuria are asymptomatic. Not all patients with significant bacteriuria progress to develop CAUTI. While *fever* is the most common manifestation of CAUTI, it is not always present. Additionally, patients may or may not have the following signs or symptoms:

A. Costovertebral-Angle (CVA) Tenderness (also known as Murphy's punch sign)
B. Suprapubic Tenderness
C. Delirium
D. Hematuria (presence of blood in the urine)
E. Urgency (urge to void immediately)
F. Dysuria (pain or burning on urination); very uncommon
G. Frequency (frequent voiding of small volumes); very uncommon
H. Rigors

Patients with **spinal cord injuries** and a CAUTI may also present with:

I. Spasticity of the Lower Extremities
J. Autonomic Dysreflexia. (usually spinal cord injuries above thoracic vertebrae 5 to 6 or central nervous system conditions such as stroke or multiple sclerosis); characterized by an increased sympathetic response with extremely elevated

blood pressures, profuse sweating, and an erythematous rash of the head and neck. This is a medical emergency that requires immediate therapy.

K. Urinary Incontinence

L. Delirium

M. Rigors

IV. APPROACH TO THE PATIENT

A. **History.** A complete and accurate history should be obtained; however, this can be challenging as most CAUTIs occur in the hospital setting with patients who may be noncommunicative owing to intubation in the intensive care, delirium, and/or dementia. Additionally, even if patients are communicative, the history is often nonspecific and may be unreliable. *Evaluation for CAUTI should be undertaken when patients with a urinary catheter develop fever or otherwise unexplained systemic manifestations compatible with infection (e.g., malaise, altered mental status, and hypotension).* The history should also focus on risk factors and the duration the urinary catheter has been in place, as longer duration increases the risk of CAUTI.

B. **Physical Examination.** While a complete physical examination should be performed, **fever** and/or **tachycardia** are often the only clinical signs of infection due to CAUTI. Although focal clinical signs of infection may be lacking, signs that may be of value include suprapubic tenderness and CVA tenderness on palpation; however, these findings are infrequently present. When ***Staphylococcus aureus, Pseudomonas aeruginosa, Salmonella* spp, and *Candida* spp are identified in the urine of a catheterized patient, this should prompt the clinician to search for another source of bacteremia.**

C. **Laboratory Studies**

1. **Complete blood count (CBC).** Elevation of the white blood cell count may be seen but has minimal predictive value for CAUTI.

2. **Basic metabolic panel (BMP).** Routinely ordered but nonspecific.

3. **Blood cultures.** Routinely ordered during evaluation and may reveal a catheter-associated bacteremia; however, **blood cultures should *always* be obtained with *Staphylococcus aureus, Pseudomonas aeruginosa, Salmonella* spp, and *Candida* spp in the urine of a catheterized patient.**

4. **Urinalysis.** May show leukocyte esterase, nitrates, and/or pyuria. Although the presence of leukocyte esterase, nitrates, and/or pyuria may signal inflammation, these findings are nonspecific and *not* diagnostic of CA-ASB or CAUTI. (*Pyuria is universal among catheterized patients with significant bacteriuria but does not distinguish between colonization and infection.*) The absence of pyuria is helpful to exclude significant bacteriuria. Finally, the odor (most commonly a foul smell of ammonia production) and appearance (i.e., cloudy) of the urine in a catheterized patient is *not* predictive of CA-ASB or CAUTI.

5. **Urine culture**

   a. *Urine collection.* Specimens should be collected by an aseptic method through the port (i.e., needle and syringe) in short-term catheters. For long-term catheters the sample should be collected in the same manner *only after* the catheter is replaced. A midstream urinary sample should be obtained if the urinary catheter has been completely removed.

   b. *Urine culture.* Urinary catheters in place for more than a few days can be coated with bacterial biofilm and give spurious culture results. *A CAUTI is defined as greater than or equal to 10^3 colony-forming units (cfu)/mL with greater than or equal to one bacterial species in the presence of symptoms or signs associated with infection* (see the preceding).

   Culture results should *always* be interpreted along with clinical signs and symptoms to differentiate between catheter colonization and true infection, as colonization may be present regardless of the duration of catheterization.

V. MANAGEMENT OF CAUTI. In patients with significant bacteriuria and a fever with no other cause, it is reasonable to initiate antibiotic therapy; however, a urine sample for urinalysis and urine culture (as well as blood cultures if appropriate) should *always* be obtained prior to therapy. *Antibiotic treatment for CA-ASB and asymptomatic candiduria is not recommended. All urinary catheters should be removed if there is not an appropriate indication for use* (see Table 31.1). Empiric antibiotic choices may depend on previous urine culture results, current hospital antibiograms of potential urinary pathogens, and/or immediate urine Gram stain results. Recommendations include (all antibiotics should be adjusted to the renal clearance):

A. *Ceftazidime 2 g intravenous (IV) q8* or *cefepime 2 g IV q8* or *piperacillin–tazobactam 4.5 g IV q6.* (These are the preferred first-line agents used by the authors.)

B. *Ciprofloxacin 400 mg IV q12 (500 mg PO q12)* or *levofloxacin 500 mg IV/PO q24.* (We would not recommend empirical quinolone use for CAUTI, as greater

---

TABLE 31.1 ■ Prevention Strategies to Reduce CAUTIs

- Reduction of inappropriate catheter use:
  - Only inserted when necessary (e.g., acute urinary retention, accurate measurement of urine output in critically ill patients); a urinary catheter should not be inserted as a substitute for nursing care in an incontinent patient.
  - Urinary catheters should be removed as soon as possible.
  - Use urinary catheters in operative patients only as necessary, rather than routinely.
  - Expedited removal done in postoperative period for those who required initial urinary catheterization.
  - Consider alternatives such as condom catheter or intermittent catheterization.
- Proper catheter insertion and care:
  - Only properly trained persons should insert or care for catheters.
  - Use aseptic technique and sterile equipment for catheter insertion.
  - Hand hygiene is vital before and after any manipulation of catheter.
  - Keep continuously closed sterile drainage system with unobstructed urine flow.
  - For urine sampling use sterile technique to aspirate from sampling port.
- Infection control:
  - Develop and implement written guidelines for use of catheters.
  - Implement a medical document for catheter use.
  - Ensure adequate personnel and other resources for catheter-use surveillance.
  - Maintain regular CAUTI surveillance for at-risk groups.

CAUTI, catheter-associated urinary tract infection.

than 20% of *E. coli* hospital isolates are resistant; however, these agents may be used if the isolate is susceptible to these agents.)

C. *Meropenem 1 g IV q8* or *ertapenem 1 g IV q24* or *doripenem 500 mg IV q8*. (For patients who are known to be previously infected or colonized with a multidrug-resistant organism [MDRO], the empiric antimicrobial should include coverage of that MDRO.)

No empirical antifungal therapy is recommended, as removal or replacement of the urinary catheter will assist in the clearing of candiduria; however, if patients are symptomatic (see the preceding), have neutropenia, have undergone renal transplantation, or are undergoing a urologic procedure with manipulation, the recommendation is to initiate **fluconazole 200 mg IV/PO q24 or lipid complex amphotericin B 3 to 5 mg/kg IV q24**. *(Do not use micafungin, caspofungin, or anidulafungin, as these agents do not achieve adequate urinary concentrations.)*

The final antibiotic choice should be adjusted based on the urine culture and sensitivity results. **Antibiotic duration is generally 7 to 14 days**, depending on severity of infection and response to treatment.

VI. PREVENTION OF CAUTI. CAUTI-prevention and monitoring strategies should be routine in acute care hospitals. A multidisciplinary approach using a CAUTI-prevention bundle yields the best results in reducing the incidence of infection. Table 31.1 shows some key interventions in preventing CAUTI that should be included in a prevention bundle.

BIBLIOGRAPHY

Hooton TM, Bradley SF, Cardenas DD, et al. Diagnosis, prevention, and treatment of catheter-associated urinary tract infection in adults: 2009 International Clinical Practice Guidelines from the Infectious Diseases Society of America. *Clin Infect Dis*. 2010;50(5):625–663.

Johnson JR. Microbial virulence determinants and the pathogenesis of urinary tract infection. *Infect Dis Clin North Am*. 2003;17(2):261–278.

Maki DG, Tambyah PA. Engineering out the risk for infection with urinary catheters. *Emerg Infect Dis*. 2001;7(2):342–347.

Nicolle LE. Urinary catheter-associated infections. *Infect Dis Clin North Am*. 2012;26(1):13–27.

Saint S, Kowalski CP, Kaufman SR, et al. Preventing hospital-acquired urinary tract infections in the United States: a national study. *Clin Infec Dis*. 2008;46(2):243–250.

MENINGITIS AND VENTRICULITIS

William F. Wright

I. INTRODUCTION

A. Definition. An inflammatory process usually involving the meninges and cerebrospinal fluid (CSF), without involvement of brain tissue, due to the presence of a bacterial or viral pathogen.

B. Pathophysiology. The brain is protected by the skull and the pia, arachnoid, and dural meninges as well as the blood–brain barrier. When any of these defenses are breached by a microbial pathogen an inflammatory response within the CSF occurs.

C. Classification and Risk Factors. Most commonly classified based on the infecting pathogen and location at the onset of illness.

    1. Community-acquired meningitis. Patients have not been recently hospitalized and/or undergone any recent procedures (e.g., CSF shunt). Predisposing factors include preexisting diabetes mellitus, otitis media, sinusitis, pneumonia, and alcohol abuse. Pathogens can include bacterial, viral, fungal, or parasitic agents.

    2. Nosocomial meningitis and ventriculitis. Most commonly related to infections associated with CSF shunts, CSF drains, intrathecal drug therapy, deep brain stimulation hardware, neurosurgery procedures, and head trauma. Also usually associated with a typical nosocomial bacterial pathogen (e.g., methicillin-resistant *Staphylococcus aureus* [MRSA] or vancomycin-resistant *Enterococcus* spp).

II. CAUSES OF MENINGITIS

A. Bacterial. Predisposing factors depend on age, comorbid status, immune state, and/or alcoholism.

    1. *Streptococcus pneumoniae*. Most common cause of both community and nosocomial infections despite the patient age or immune status. However, asplenia and agammaglobulinemia are also risk factors.

    2. *Haemophilus influenzae* type B. Also associated with asplenia and agammaglobulinemia as well as alcoholism in adults. Vaccination efforts have declined rates in children.

    3. *Neisseria meningitidis* (serogroups A, B, C, W135, and Y). Most common pathogen in healthy young adults, but patients with asplenia and terminal complement pathways are also at risk. Serogroup Y is predominant in the United States and the second most common in parts of Europe. Serogroup B is the most common strain across Europe. Serogroup A has been responsible for large outbreaks in the meningitis belt of Africa.

4. ***Listeria monocytogenes***. Most commonly occurs in infants and patients over the age of 50 years with cell-mediated immune deficits and/or alcoholism.

5. ***Streptococcus pyogenes* (group A beta-hemolytic streptococci)**. Usually secondary to otitis media.

6. ***Streptococcus agalactiae* (group B beta-hemolytic streptococci)**. Most often occurs in poorly controlled diabetic patients with an associated infection who are greater than 65 years of age.

7. ***Staphylococcus* (*S. aureus* or coagulase-negative staphylococcus)**. Most frequently occur in the setting of neurosurgical procedures or placement of CSF shunts.

8. **Gram-negative bacilli (*Pseudomonas* or enteric pathogens)**. Have been associated with nosocomial meningitis in patients over the age of 50.

9. ***Mycobacterium tuberculosis* (MTB)**. Usually occurs in the setting of extrapulmonary disseminated disease (see Chapter 14, Tuberculosis, for more information).

10. **Spirochetes**. *Treponema pallidum* (secondary syphilis) and *Borrelia burgdorferi* (Lyme disease); see Chapter 42, Sexually Transmitted Diseases, and Chapter 50, Lyme Disease, for more information on these conditions.

B. **Viral.** Most commonly affect children but can occur at any age.

1. **Enteroviruses (e.g., Coxsackie A and B, echovirus, poliovirus, and enterovirus 71)**. *Account for the majority of viral meningitis cases* with a fecal–oral transmission during late summer and autumn in temperate climates (occurs year-round in the tropics).

2. **Herpes simplex virus (HSV-1, HSV-2)**. HSV-2 accounts for the majority of cases in association with primary genital herpes. *In immunocompetent patients, pure HSV meningitis is a self-limiting condition, whereas HSV meningitis in immunocompromised hosts or HSV encephalitis is a life-threatening medical emergency requiring treatment.*

3. **Varicella-zoster virus (VZV)**. Almost always associated with reactivation (e.g., shingles) rather than primary infection (e.g., chickenpox).

4. **HIV**. Most often occurs in the setting of acute infection (e.g., acute retroviral syndrome—*lymphadenopathy, dermatitis, pharyngitis, and oral candidiasis*).

5. **Measles–mumps–rubella (MMR) viruses**. Rates have declined with vaccination efforts, but the most common cause in unvaccinated patients would involve *mumps* (more common in males with or without parotid gland swelling).

6. **Arthropod-borne viruses and West Nile virus**. Most commonly associated with meningoencephalitis (see Chapter 33, Infectious Encephalitis).

7. **Lymphocytic choriomeningitis virus and Hantavirus**. These are rare causes associated with contact by infected rodents.

C. **Fungal.** Pathogens most commonly occur in nosocomial infections or immunocompromised patients such as transplantation of stem cells or solid organs and with HIV/AIDS (i.e., CD4 cell count below 200 cells/mm³). While ***Candida*** and ***Aspergillus*** species are common, other pathogens include:

1. ***Cryptococcus neoformans***
2. ***Histoplasma capsulatum***
3. ***Coccidioides immitis***

D. Parasitic. Rare cause of community-acquired meningitis, but the freshwater amoeba *Naegleria fowleri* can cause **primary amebic meningoencephalitis**. Amoeba gain access to the meninges and brain through disruption of the cribriform plate and olfactory nerve and are nearly always fatal.

III. CLINICAL PRESENTATION OF MENINGITIS. While the clinical presentation of meningitis may vary in children and older adults, the **classic triad** is: *acute onset fever, neck stiffness, and altered mental status.*

A. Fever. Present in the majority of patients but may be absent in older adults or immunocompromised.

B. Neck Stiffness. Occurs in the majority of patients and most commonly associated with **headache.**

C. Altered Mental Status. Is typically defined as a *Glasgow coma score* of less than 12 or a change in the patient's baseline mental status (e.g., dementia).

1. **Glasgow Coma Scale (GCS).** A neurologic scale developed by the University of Glasgow in 1974 as an objective method to grade the conscious state of a patient. Patients are evaluated in three areas (eye, verbal, and motor responses) and assigned a score based on the level of response. A patient with minimal brain involvement (awake) has a GCS score greater than 13, moderate involvement (confused) has a GCS score 9 to 12, and severe involvement (comatose) has a GCS score less than 8. The scoring method is as follows (possible minimal score of 3 and maximum score of 15):

Area	Response	Score
Eye	Does not open to any stimuli	1
	Opens only to painful stimuli	2
	Opens to voice command	3
	Opens spontaneously	4
Verbal	No verbal response	1
	Unintelligible response	2
	Unsuitable response	3
	Confused response	4
	Normal verbal conversation	5
Motor	No movement	1
	Decerebrate (extension) posturing to stimuli	2

(continued)

Area	Response	Score
	Decorticate (flexion) posturing to stimuli	3
	Withdrawal to painful stimuli	4
	Localizes to painful stimuli	5
	Normal motor response	6

Patients may also present with signs and symptoms of:

D. Headache. Occurs in response to meningeal inflammation.

E. Photophobia. Reduced tolerance to bright light presumed to be due to meningeal inflammation of the trigeminal nerve (ophthalmic branch of cranial nerve 5). More commonly occurs with viral meningitis.

F. Nausea and Vomiting

IV. APPROACH TO THE PATIENT

A. History. Meningitis is a diagnosis that should always be included in the differential diagnosis when evaluating a patient with the classic triad of fever, neck pain, and/or confusion or headache. The majority of patients have at least two of the classic triad. Fever is the MOST sensitive of the classic triad signs followed by neck stiffness. Confusion or altered mental status is more commonly associated with bacterial meningitis. The absence of all three classic signs virtually eliminates the diagnostic consideration for meningitis. *The history should focus on the timing of events, recent surgical procedures, recent infections (particularly head and neck infections), comorbid illnesses, vaccination history, occupational exposures, and recent travels.*

Fever, new headache, nausea, lethargy, seizure, and/or change in mental status in a patient with a history of neurosurgical procedure or cranial trauma are suggestive of healthcare-associated ventriculitis and meningitis.

B. Physical Examination. In addition to a general complete examination, the examination should also emphasize:

1. **Funduscopic examination** (to detect papilledema).

2. **Head, eyes, ears, nose, and throat (HEENT) examination** (to detect a paranasal sinus, ear, or odontogenic infection). Oral thrush may indicate HIV.

3. **Neurologic examination.** Meningeal inflammation is detected by performing the **Kernig** and **Brudzinski signs**.

   The *Kernig test* is best performed with the patient lying supine and the hip flexed at 90 degrees. A positive test is present when extension of the knee in this position elicits resistance or pain in the lower back or posterior thigh.

   The *Brudzinski test* is best performed with the patient lying supine and a positive test is present when passive flexion of the cervical spine results also in flexion of the patient's knees and hips.

   An additional physical examination maneuver is the *jolt accentuation test*. This test is performed by asking the seated patient to rotate the head horizontally back and forth at a frequency of two to three rotations per second. A positive test is indicated by worsening headache.

However, increased intracranial pressure or extension of the infection may be indicated by: *focal neurologic deficits, worsening mental status,* or *papilledema.*

4. **Cardiovascular examination** (to detect murmur and/or evaluate for signs of endocarditis; see Chapter 7, Infective Endocarditis).

Austrian syndrome—*pneumonia, meningitis,* and *endocarditis*—is a very rare syndrome that can be caused by *Streptococcus pneumoniae.*

5. **Pulmonary examination** (to search for localized findings suggestive of pneumonia; see Chapter 11, Pneumonia).

6. **Dermatologic examination**. To search for peripheral manifestations of endocarditis (see Chapter 7). Petechiae or hemorrhagic bulla may indicate meningococcal infection; however, petechial, purpuric, and/or ecchymotic rashes can occur with *S. pneumoniae, H. influenzae,* or *L. monocytogenes.* A morbilliform rash on the chest or trunk may suggest HIV.

C. **Laboratory Studies.** The most important component of the laboratory studies is the analysis of CSF.

1. **Lumbar puncture (LP)**. Meningitis is a diagnosis that requires analysis of CSF. Cranial imaging should precede an LP in patients with the following:

   a. New-onset seizure

   b. Immunocompromised status

   c. Altered mental status (GCS score 8–11)

   d. Space-occupying lesion concern, increased intracranial pressure, or papilledema

   Therapy should be initiated prior to neuroimaging for patients with a delay in LP (*CSF values will not significantly change within 4 hours*).

   The LP is usually obtained from the L3–L4 or L4–L5 interspace with the patient in the lateral recumbent position with both knees flexed and slight neck flexion.

   Always be sure to document the opening pressure (normal; 60–180 cmH$_2$O or 6–14 mmHg).

   Typically, four tubes are obtained for analysis:

   i. **Tube 1**. Cell count/differential, glucose, and protein.

   ii. **Tube 2**. Polymerase chain reaction (PCR), serology, or other studies (e.g., acid-fast bacillus [AFB], cryptococcus antigen).

   iii. **Tube 3**. Gram stain and culture.

   iv. **Tube 4**. Cell count/differential, glucose, and protein. *Tube 4 is typically used for the cell count/differential, glucose, and protein with a traumatic LP for improved accuracy.*

2. **CSF analysis**. Normal CSF values are: glucose 45 to 80 mg/dL with a blood-to-CSF glucose ratio greater than or equal to 0.6; protein 15 to 45 mg/dL;

and white blood cell (WBC) count less than 5/mcL. CSF values should be obtained as soon as possible following LP, as delays can alter the cell count and glucose (falsely low values).

Typical CSF Findings for Meningitis

Pathogen	WBC Count	Differential	CSF/Serum Glucose	Protein
Viral	50–1,000	Lymphocytic*	≥0.6	Minimally elevated
Bacterial**	500–5,000	Neutrophilic	≤0.4	Elevated
Tuberculosis	50–300	Monocytic	≤0.3	Elevated
Cryptococcus	20–500	Monocytic	≤0.5	Elevated

*Can be neutrophilic with first 24 hours of infection.

**A CSF lactate value greater than or equal to 31 mg/dL (3.5 mmol/L) may be suggestive of bacterial meningitis. *In postneurosurgical patients, a CSF lactate value greater than 4.0 mmol/L performed better than the CSF/serum glucose ratio for bacterial meningitis with a sensitivity of 88% and specificity of 98%.*

CSF, cerebrospinal fluid; WBC, white blood cell.

3. **CSF Gram stain and culture.** Routine methods for CSF Gram stain have 60% to 90% sensitivity and 97% specificity for the diagnosis of bacterial meningitis.

Pathogen/Infection	Diagnostic Test for CSF
Enterovirus	PCR
HSV	PCR
VZV	PCR
HIV	IgM/IgG ELISA
Mumps	IgM/IgG ELISA
Lyme disease	IgM/IgG ELISA (serum EIA)
Syphilis	VDRL (serum RPR)
Tuberculosis	PCR (cutaneous PPD)
Cryptococcus	CSF latex agglutination

CSF, cerebrospinal fluid; EIA, enzyme immunoassay; ELISA, enzyme-linked immunosorbent assay; HSV, herpes simplex virus; IgG, immunoglobulin G; IgM, immunoglobulin M; PCR, polymerase chain reaction; PPD, purified protein derivative; RPR, rapid plasma regain; VDRL, Venereal Disease Research Laboratory; VZV, varicella-zoster virus.

4. **PCR and serology.** These methods are typically reserved for viral pathogens.

5. **Additional testing.** Always obtain serum glucose at the time of LP as well as basic metabolic panel (BMP). Liver function tests (LFTs) may be helpful for cytomegalovirus (CMV) or Epstein–Barr virus (EBV). Always obtain a complete blood count (CBC) and prothrombin time/international normalized ratio (PT/INR), as thrombocytopenia and coagulopathy may result in either a **subarachnoid hemorrhage** or **subdural** or **epidural hematoma**. Blood cultures are routinely ordered but rarely useful. Brain imaging with CT scan or MRI is routinely ordered to search for other etiologies and evaluate for evidence of intracranial pressure or space-occupying lesion.

An elevated CSF lactate (see the preceding tables) or CSF procalcitonin (cut-off value of 0.075 ng/mL was associated with a sensitivity of 96% and negative predictive value of 97.6%), or the combination of both, may be useful in the diagnosis of healthcare-associated bacterial ventriculitis and meningitis. Detection of beta-D-glucan and galactomannan in CSF may be useful in the diagnosis of fungal ventriculitis and meningitis.

V. **COMPLICATIONS OF MENINGITIS.** Most patients typically respond to therapy within 48 to 72 hours (*improvement of hypoglycorrhachia [low CSF glucose] and reduction of CSF lactate levels are usually the earliest indicators of improvement with therapy*); however, patients who do not respond should have **brain imaging** (e.g., CT or MRI) repeated and repeat **CSF analysis**. Possible complications include:

A. **Progression to Meningoencephalitis**

B. **Increased Intracranial Pressure**

C. **Subarachnoid Hemorrhage or Subdural/Epidural Hematoma**

D. **Seizures or Nonconvulsive Status Epilepticus**

E. **Subdural Empyema**

F. **Antimicrobial Treatment Failure** (microbial resistance, poor central nervous system [CNS] antibiotic dosing, or poor antibiotic penetration)

VI. **TREATMENT.** (*Antibiotics listed assume normal renal function.*) As it is difficult to differentiate bacterial from viral or fungal meningitis on clinical grounds alone, patients often are placed on empirical antimicrobial therapy based on the most likely pathogen that should be initiated as soon as the diagnosis is considered.

A. **Community-acquired bacterial meningitis.** With the increased rates of penicillin-resistant *Streptococcus pneumoniae*, the suggested treatments are:

   1. **Age less than 50 (*N. meningitidis, S. pneumoniae, H. influenzae*).** Vancomycin 15 mg/kg intravenous (IV) q12 *plus* ceftriaxone 2 g IV q12. Guidelines recommend fluoroquinolones (e.g., moxifloxacin 400 mg daily or levofloxacin 750 mg daily) as an alternative to third-generation cephalosporins plus vancomycin for meningitis caused by *S. pneumoniae* strains resistant to penicillin and third-generation cephalosporins. Guidelines also recommend cefepime (1–2 g q12–24) as a second-line agent in the treatment of *H. influenzae* meningitis.

   2. **Age greater than 50 (*S. pneumoniae, N. meningitidis, L. monocytogenes*).** Vancomycin 15 mg/kg IV q12 *plus* ceftriaxone 2 g IV q12 *plus* ampicillin 2 g IV q8.

   3. **Corticosteroids.** Dexamethasone 10 mg IV q6 should be given for 4 days and initiated at the start of antibiotic therapy due to a worsening inflammation associated with lysis of bacteria and antibiotic therapy.

   4. **Duration.** Trials investigating shorter (4–7 days) versus longer (7–14 days) antibiotic treatments for bacterial meningitis noted no difference in outcomes. Many authorities recommend at least 7 days of treatment for *Haemophilus*

spp and meningococcal meningitis, and 10 to 14 days of treatment for pneumococcal meningitis.

5. **Patients with *N. meningitidis* meningitis** require *respiratory isolation* for 24 hours following initiation of antibiotics, and close contacts must receive *chemoprophylaxis* with a single oral dose of ciprofloxacin 500 mg or a single intramuscular (IM) dose of ceftriaxone 250 mg (chemoprophylaxis is *not* required for other meningitis-related pathogens).

B. **Nosocomial Meningitis and Ventriculitis.** In patients with nosocomial healthcare-associated ventriculitis and meningitis, removal of an infected CSF shunt, drain, intrathecal infusion pump, and/or hardware is recommended.

Guidelines recommend vancomycin (see the aforementioned dosing) and either cefepime or ceftazidime (2 g every 8 hours) as empirical first-line treatment in patients with postneurosurgical meningitis. Meropenem (2 g every 8 hours as a standard or prolonged infusion [each dose administered over 3 hours]) is the carbapenem of choice in the treatment of bacterial meningitis when pathogens are resistant to cefepime or ceftazidime. Daptomycin (6–12 mg/kg once daily), usually combined with rifampin (300 mg every 8 hours or 450 mg every 12 hours), or standard doses of linezolid (600 mg every 12 hours) may be considered for meningitis caused by MRSA and vancomycin-resistant *Enterococcus* spp.

Patients should be treated for a duration of 10 to 14 days.

C. **Viral Meningitis**

1. **HSV**

   a. **Immunocompetent host.** Usually due to HSV-2 with primary genital herpes. Thus, the treatment is directed to genital herpes.

   b. **Immunocompromised host.** Usually treatment is with acyclovir 10 mg/kg IV q8 (adjusted for renal failure) for 14 to 21 days.

2. **VZV.** Usual treatment is the same as for shingles with acyclovir 10 mg/kg IV q8 for 7 to 10 days *or* valacyclovir 1 g PO q8 for 7 to 10 days.

BIBLIOGRAPHY

Attia J, Hatala R, Cook DJ, et al. The rational clinical examination. Does this adult patient have acute meningitis? *JAMA*. 1999;282(2):175–181.

Honda H, Warren DK. Central nervous system infections: meningitis and brain abscess. *Infect Dis Clin North Am*. 2009;23(3):609–623.

Logan SA, MacMahon E. Viral meningitis. *BMJ*. 2008;336(7634):36–40.

McGill F, Heyderman RS, Panagiotou S, et al. Acute bacterial meningitis in adults. *Lancet*. 2016;388(10063):3036–3047.

Straus SE, Thorpe KE, Holryd-Leduc J. How do I perform a lumbar puncture and analyze the results to diagnose bacterial meningitis? *JAMA*. 2006;296(16):2012–2022.

Tunkel AR, Hartman BJ, Kaplan SL, et al. Practice guidelines for the management of bacterial meningitis. *Clin Infect Dis*. 2004;39(9):1267–1284.

Tunkel AR, Hasbun R, Bhimraj A, et al. 2017 Infectious Diseases Society of America's clinical practice guidelines for healthcare-associated ventriculitis and meningitis. *Clin Infect Dis*. 2017 Feb 14. doi: 10.1093/cid/ciw861 [Epub ahead of print].

van de Beek D, de Gans J, Tunkel AR, et al. Community-acquired bacterial meningitis in adults. *N Engl J Med*. 2006;354(1):44–53.

van de Beek D, Drake JM, Tunkel AR. Nosocomial bacterial meningitis. *N Engl J Med*. 2010;362(2):146–154.

33

INFECTIOUS ENCEPHALITIS

William F. Wright

I. INTRODUCTION

A. Definition. An infectious process of the brain parenchyma, usually as the result of a viral pathogen, primarily associated with a degree of involvement of the leptomeningeal layers.

B. Pathogenesis. Pathogens typically gain access to the central nervous system (CNS) by one of two methods:

1. **Hematogenous spread.** Most common mechanism and usually initiated at the cutaneous site of an insect bite (e.g., mosquito or tick) with resultant viremia and subsequent CNS penetration (e.g., arthropod-borne viruses).

2. **Neuronal spread.** Usually initiated at a cutaneous site with neurologic involvement and subsequent CNS penetration (e.g., herpes simplex virus [HSV]).

II. IMPORTANT CAUSES OF INFECTIOUS ENCEPHALITIS. While viral pathogens are more likely associated with encephalitis, a list of important causes includes:

A. Viral Pathogens

1. **Herpes simplex virus (HSV-1 and HSV-2).** The most common cause of nonendemic, sporadic, and acute encephalitis. *HSV-1* is typically more common and observed mostly in *adults* but can occur in *children* greater than 6 months of age. *HSV-2* (which is the most common cause of genital herpes) causes infection in *neonates* (average age of 1–2 weeks but acquired by vertical transmission at birth).

2. **Cytomegalovirus (CMV).** *Occurs in patients with* HIV/AIDS (lower CD4 counts such as less than 50 cells/mm³) or immunosuppressed conditions (e.g., diabetes, chronic renal failure, or corticosteroid use).

3. **Other herpesviruses.** Examples such as *Epstein—Barr virus* (EBV), *varicella-zoster virus* (VZV), and *herpes B virus* can occur. (*Herpes B virus has been transmitted by the bite or scratch from a macaque monkey.*)

4. **Influenza A virus.** Associated with a late demyelination syndrome, known as *postinfectious encephalomyelitis*, following an upper respiratory infection.

5. **Measles, mumps, and rubella viruses.** Vaccination efforts have now made these viruses *rare* as causes of encephalitis except in countries or immigrants with poor vaccination rates.

6. **Enteroviruses.** *Poliovirus, coxsackievirus, echovirus,* and *enterovirus 71.* Infections are usually mild and self-limiting. Poliovirus infections have been

associated with postvaccination efforts (type 2 or 3 strain). Enterovirus 71 infection has been associated with *hand, foot, and mouth disease.*

7. **Rabies virus.** Transmitted by the bite of a rabid animal (e.g., foxes, bats, skunks, dogs, and cattle).

8. **Retroviruses.** *Human T-cell lymphotropic virus I (HTLV-I)* and *HIV.* HTLV-I is transmitted by blood products or sexual contact and associated with adult T-cell leukemia/lymphoma, myelopathy/tropical spastic paresis, or uveitis. The highest prevalence of HTLV-I occurs in Japan, Africa, the Caribbean Islands, and Central and South America.

9. **Arthropod-borne viruses.** Typically transmitted by either a tick or mosquito:

   a. **Mosquito-borne** (most commonly the *Culex* species)

      i. **Alphavirus. Eastern and Western equine**

      ii. **Flavivirus.** *St Louis encephalitis virus, Japanese B encephalitis virus, West Nile virus.* Japanese encephalitis is associated with travel to Asia during the rainy season. West Nile virus was once well described in Africa and the Middle East but now occurs in the United States (associated with avian crow deaths).

      iii. **Bunyavirus.** *California virus, La Crosse virus, Jamestown Canyon virus.*

   b. **Tick-borne** (most commonly transmitted by *Ixodes* or *Dermacentor* ticks)

      i. Colorado tick fever (Dermacentor)

      ii. Powassan virus (Ixodes)

10. **Hendra virus and Nipah virus.** Paramyxoviridae viruses transmitted to humans (via respiratory route) through infected pigs.

B. **Bacterial Pathogens (Rare Etiologies)**

   1. *Mycobacterium tuberculosis, Listeria monocytogenes,* and *Nocardia* **species.** Most commonly occur in patients with immunosuppression, cell-mediated immune deficits, or HIV/AIDS.

   2. *Leptospira.* Causes leptospirosis, a spirochete bacterial illness associated with water sports.

   3. *Borrelia burgdorferi* (late Lyme disease). Transmitted by an *Ixodes* tick.

   4. **Rickettsias.** *Rocky Mountain spotted fever (RMSF), Q fever (Coxiella), ehrlichiosis (Ehrlichia chaffeensis).* RMSF (caused by the bacterium *Rickettsia rickettsii*) is transmitted by the bite of a dog tick or wood tick (*Dermacentor* spp). *Ehrlichia chaffeensis* is transmitted by the bite of a Lone Star tick (*Amblyomma americanum*). Q fever is acquired by association with cattle birth exposure.

C. **Fungal Pathogens** (rare etiologies). These infections most commonly occur with immunosuppression or cell-mediated immune deficits or HIV/AIDS and include *Cryptococcus* and *Aspergillus* spp.

D. **Parasitic Pathogens** (rare etiologies). Can include both *malaria* (genus *Plasmodium*) and *Toxoplasma gondii* (most commonly in association with HIV/

AIDS and a CD4 count less than 100 cells/mm³). Primary amoebic meningoencephalitis (PAM) is a rare but extremely lethal cause associated with the amoeba *Naegleria fowleri* (typically during the summer and associated with freshwater swimming).

III. CLINICAL MANIFESTATIONS OF INFECTIVE ENCEPHALITIS

A. Classic Triad. *Fever* (acute onset), *headache*, and *altered mental status* (i.e., Glasgow Coma Scale score less than 12). Patients with meningitis usually have fever, headache, and neck pain but typically *not* altered mental status.

B. Neurologic Changes. Include speech or behavior changes, hemiparesis, seizures, ataxia, and cranial nerve deficits.

C. Parotid Gland Swelling. Can be associated with mumps.

D. Rash or Vesicular Lesions. May be seen with tick-borne or arthropod-borne diseases, and VZV (*shingles is characterized by pustule lesions on an erythematous base associated with radicular-type neurologic pain*).

E. Erythema Nodosum. Tender red nodules most commonly located on the anterior tibia but may also occur on the thigh, arm, trunk, neck, or face. May suggest tuberculosis, EBV, hepatitis C, or histoplasmosis infection.

F. Mucous Membrane Lesions and/or Ulcers. Primary HSV lesions can be associated with *herpetic gingivostomatitis* (ulcers on the gingiva) but usually occur in children. Recurrent HSV lesions in adults are most commonly known as *herpes simplex labialis* (i.e., cold sores or fever blisters) and typically occur on the lip or vermilion. Intraoral lesions in adults are rare but when present typically involve mucosa tightly adherent to *bone and associated with minimal pain*.

G. Cough, Pharyngitis, Myalgia, Arthralgia, and Dyspnea. May suggest influenza A or acute HIV (especially when associated with a rash).

Herpes simplex virus encephalitis is suggested by frontotemporal signs with aphasia, personality changes, and/or focal seizures.

IV. APPROACH TO THE PATIENT. *The initial evaluation should distinguish encephalitis from other causes such as encephalopathy or acute disseminated encephalomyelitis (ADEM).* Infectious encephalitis is usually characterized by **headache, fever, focal neurologic signs, focal seizures, cerebrospinal changes, and changes on neurologic imaging**. ADEM is more likely with *recent vaccination* in children or adults, visual impairment, and multifocal white matter changes on neuroimaging.

Some important causes of encephalopathy (noninfectious):

1. Renal failure (e.g., electrolyte abnormalities or elevated blood urea nitrogen [BUN])

2. Liver failure (e.g., elevated ammonia level; NH_4)

3. Diabetic ketoacidosis (DKA)

4. Stroke (ischemic or hemorrhagic)

5. Seizure (most commonly generalized but can occur with certain partial seizures)

6. Malignant hypertension (defined as severe hypertension with retinal bleeding)

7. Drug overdose (e.g., narcotics)

8. Nutritional deficiency (e.g., vitamin B_{12}/folate deficit) or metabolic abnormality (elevated calcium, sodium, or CO_2 level)

9. Dementia

10. Delirium secondary to a distant infection (e.g., urinary tract infection [UTI], pneumonia) or fever

A. **Patient History.** The diagnosis of encephalitis can be difficult and should be included in the differential diagnosis of a patient evaluated for **fever** and **altered mental status.** A complete history should be obtained and is usually provided by family members or relatives. It is important to obtain information about:

1. **Timing of events.** Encephalitis is usually acute in onset and occurs during late summer/autumn in temperate climates and year-round in the tropics.

2. **Recent travel and geographic location.** Can provide clues to risks of acquiring a particular pathogen endemic to a particular location (see the aforementioned pathogens).

3. **Exposures to animals or insects** (e.g., dogs, mosquitoes, or ticks).

4. **Comorbid illnesses.** May be helpful to identify conditions that mimic encephalitis and immunosuppressed patients who may be more susceptible to pathogens (e.g., CMV, *Listeria monocytogenes*, and *Cryptococcus neoformans*).

5. **Occupational history** (e.g., forestry worker may be more likely to have a tick-borne illness).

6. **Vaccination history.** May indicate ADEM.

7. **Recent history of infection(s).** May indicate delirium due to another infection.

B. **Physical Examination.** While the physical examination is unlikely to reveal the cause, both a complete examination and neurologic examination should be performed. Areas of the examination for the physician to focus include:

1. **Dermatologic examination** (to detect rashes or vesicular lesions).

2. **Neurologic examination** (to detect focal neurologic deficits and mental status changes).

C. **Laboratory Studies**

1. **Cerebrospinal fluid (CSF).** Evaluation is essential to differentiate encephalitis from bacterial/viral meningitis or encephalopathy (see Chapter 32, Meningitis and Ventriculitis). In general, CSF in viral encephalitis typically shows:

   a. Normal glucose

   b. Normal or mildly elevated protein

   c. Lymphocytic pleocytosis (uncommonly greater than 500 cells/mm³)

   A CSF-elevated red blood cell (RBC) count (greater than or equal to 500 cells/mm³) is typically associated with hemorrhagic and necrotizing encephalitis (e.g., HSV, listerial, or amoebic encephalitis).

*Tuberculosis meningoencephalitis is highly characterized by **lymphocytic pleocytosis** and **reduced glucose**.*

2. **Blood cultures and CSF cultures.** Routinely ordered but are of limited value. CSF serology and/or polymerase chain reaction (PCR; HSV, VZV, and CMV) are more useful for the identification of a particular pathogen.

3. **Complete blood count (CBC).** A relative lymphocytosis is common with encephalitis. Low white blood cell (WBC) and platelets may suggest a tick-borne etiology (e.g., rickettsia illness). Elevated monocytes may suggest ehrlichiosis.

4. **Complete metabolic profile (CMP).** Usually nonspecific but may reveal comorbid illnesses (e.g., renal failure, diabetes). Abnormal liver function tests (LFTs) may be suggestive of liver failure (most commonly identified by low albumin and elevated prothrombin time [PT]) or ehrlichiosis.

5. **Urinalysis and toxicology screen.**

6. **HIV** enzyme-linked immunosorbent assay **(ELISA; serum).**

7. **Lyme ELISA** (serum).

8. **Rabies.** Salivary real-time (RT) PCR or direct antigen testing on nuchal skin biopsy or corneal impressions.

D. **Radiologic Studies**

1. **Plain films.** A chest radiograph is suggested for patients to evaluate for the possibility of pulmonary infection due to *Mycoplasma*, *Legionella*, or tuberculosis.

2. **CT scan of brain.** Helpful to evaluate for space-occupying lesions, abscesses, or hemorrhage as well as evidence of elevated intracranial pressure (e.g., midline shift).

3. **MRI of brain.** The **image test of choice** for evaluation of a patient suspected of encephalitis. Characteristic changes from MRI include:

   a. **HSV.** Medial temporal lobe edema and edema of the orbital surface of frontal lobes, insular cortex, and cingulate gyrus.

   b. **CMV.** Periventricular changes.

   c. **Japanese encephalitis virus.** Hypodense lesions in the thalamus as well as basal ganglia and midbrain.

   d. **Eastern equine encephalitis.** Focal lesions of thalamus, basal ganglia, and midbrain.

   e. **Enteroviruses.** Hyperintense lesions in midbrain, pons, and medulla.

   f. **Hendra and Nipah viruses.** Small-vessel vasculitis (diffuse).

E. **EEG.** EEG is helpful to distinguish *encephalopathy* (e.g., diffuse, bihemispheric slow waves) from *encephalitis* (e.g., HSV, periodic lateralizing temporal lobe epileptiform discharges).

V. TREATMENT *(Antimicrobial agents listed assume normal renal function.)*

A. Specific treatment should target the suspected or identified pathogen.

B. Critical care support may be needed for patients with elevated intracranial pressure.

C. Treatment recommendations for selected pathogens include:

1. **HSV and VZV.** Acyclovir 10 mg/kg intravenous (IV) q8 for *14 days* involving VZV and immunocompetent patients with HSV infection; however, treatment is *21 days* for HSV and immunosuppressed patients. (Acyclovir must be adjusted for renal failure.) Valacyclovir (1 g orally q8) may be considered because higher serum concentrations can be achieved.

2. **CMV.** Ganciclovir 5 mg/kg IV q12 with or without foscarnet 90 mg/kg IV q12 (or 60 mg/kg IV q8) for 14 days. (Foscarnet is used in cases of ganciclovir-resistant CMV.) CMV immunoglobulin therapy 500 mg/kg IV q48 for 14 days is also used. Following IV ganciclovir the patient is given valganciclovir 900 mg PO q24 *plus* CMV immunoglobulin G (IgG) 100 mg/kg q48 for 3 months.

3. **Toxoplasma.** Pyrimethamine 200 mg PO once, then 50 mg (less than or equal to 60 kg body weight) or 75 mg (greater than or equal to 60 kg body weight) PO q24 *plus* sulfadiazine 1,000 mg (less than or equal to 60 kg) or 1,500 mg (greater than or equal to 60 kg) PO q6 *plus* leucovorin 10 mg PO q24. (Alternative is TMP–SMX [5 mg/kg TMP and 25 mg/kg SMX] PO or IV q12; or atovaquone 1.5 g PO q12 plus pyrimethamine or sulfadiazine 1.5 mg PO q6.

4. **Listeria.** Ceftriaxone 2 g IV q12 plus ampicillin 2 g IV q4 for 14 days. (Alternative is TMP–SMX 5 mg/kg IV q6 or chloramphenicol 500 mg IV q6.)

5. **Fungal pathogens.** Amphotericin B (liposomal) 3 to 5 mg/kg IV q24 (6 mg/kg/d with *Cryptococcus* and HIV) plus flucytosine 5-FC 25/kg PO q6.

BIBLIOGRAPHY

Chaudhuri A, Kennedy PG. Diagnosis and treatment of viral encephalitis. *Postgrad Med J.* 2002;78(924):575–583.

Kennedy PG. Viral encephalitis. *J Neurol.* 2005;252(3):268–272.

Steiner I, Budka H, Chaudhuri A, et al. Viral encephalitis: a review of diagnostic methods and guidelines for management. *Eur J Neurol.* 2005;12(5):331–343.

Tunkel AR, Glaser CA, Bloch KC, et al. The management of encephalitis: clinical practice guidelines by the Infectious Diseases Society of America. *Clin Infect Dis.* 2008;47(3):303–327.

Whitley RJ, Gnann JW. Viral encephalitis: familiar infections and emerging pathogens. *Lancet.* 2002;359(9305):507–513.

34

BRAIN ABSCESS

William F. Wright

I. INTRODUCTION

A. Definition. A focal collection of microorganisms and purulent material within the brain parenchyma surrounded by an infiltrate of white blood cells (WBCs) and well-vascularized capsule.

B. Epidemiology. The estimated incidence ranges from 0.4 to 0.9 cases per 100,000 population with a mean age of onset at 34 years and a male-to-female ratio of 2.4 to 1.0.

C. Risk Factors. Predisposing factors include:

1. Disruption of the protective brain barrier through trauma or neurosurgical procedure

2. Immunosuppressive medical conditions (e.g., HIV, diabetes mellitus [DM], chronic kidney disease)

3. Hematologic or solid-organ transplantation

4. Chronic long-term corticosteroid use

5. Systemic source of infection (e.g., endocarditis)

D. Pathophysiologic Stages. Characterized predominantly by cerebral inflammation.

1. **Early stage, days 1 to 3 (early cerebritis).** Characterized by inoculation of microorganisms with a perivascular inflammatory response surrounding an early necrotic center, with increased edema in the surrounding white matter.

2. **Late stage, days 4 to 9.** Expansion of cerebral inflammation and edema with initiation to the development of a capsule (resulting from the accumulation of fibroblasts and neovascularization) surrounding the necrotic center.

Following the cerebral inflammation stages a **ring-enhancing capsule** begins formation: (a) **early capsule stage (days 10–14)** has appearance of *fibrosis;* and (b) **late capsule stage (greater than day 14)** appears as a well-formed vascularized capsule.

II. PATHOPHYSIOLOGY AND MICROBIAL CAUSES OF BRAIN ABSCESSES

A. Risk Factors. Brain abscesses most commonly result from either:

1. **Contiguous** spread of infection from (most common mechanism):

   a. Oropharyngeal/odontogenic infection

   b. Otitis media/mastoiditis infection

    c. Paranasal sinus infection

    d. Cranial trauma/or surgical site infection

  2. Hematogenous spread of infection:

    a. Endocarditis

    b. Lung infection

    c. Intra-abdominal infection

    d. Urinary tract infection

B. Microbiology. While the most common causative microorganisms are *Streptococcus* and *Staphylococcus* species (comprising 52% of cultured bacteria), most abscesses are polymicrobial. Particular pathogens also depend on the initial site of infection.

General Microbiological Causes of Brain Abscesses

Source of Organism	Organism	Site of Abscess
Paranasal sinus/ odontogenic (teeth)	Aerobic/anaerobic streptococci *Bacteroides* spp (anaerobe) *Fusobacterium* spp (anaerobe) *Haemophilus* spp	Frontal lobe
Otogenic (ear)	*Streptococcus* spp Enteric gram-negative bacilli *Bacteroides* spp *Pseudomonas aeruginosa*	Temporal lobe or cerebellum
Trauma/postoperative	*Staphylococcus aureus* *Staphylococcus epidermidis* (most commonly postoperative) Enteric gram-negative bacilli *Clostridium* spp *Pseudomonas* spp	Wound site
Hematogenous	**Endocarditis**: *Staphylococcus aureus*, viridans streptococcus **UTI**: enteric gram-negative bacilli, *Pseudomonas* **Abdomen**: *Streptococcus* spp, enteric gram-negative bacilli, anaerobes **Lung**: *Streptococcus* spp, *Nocardia* spp, *Actinomyces* spp, and *Fusobacterium* spp	Commonly in MCA distribution with multiple abscesses

MCA, middle cerebral artery; UTI, urinary tract infection.

C. Special Clinical Causes of Brain Abscess

  1. Fungal abscess. Most commonly seen in transplant patients, patients with diabetes, or those receiving corticosteroids and are typically due to *Aspergillus* spp (most common), *Candida* spp, *Coccidioides immitis*, *Blastomyces dermatitidis*, *Histoplasma capsulatum*, or *Scedosporium apiospermum* (i.e., *Pseudallescheria boydii*). **Mucormycosis (*Mucor* spp, *Rhizopus* spp, or *Absidia* spp) typically occurs in patients with diabetic ketoacidosis, intravenous (IV) drug use history, prolonged corticosteroid use, or prolonged neutropenia.**

2. ***Mycobacterium tuberculosis.*** Rare but most commonly seen in patients with disseminated disease.

3. ***Nocardia* spp.** Most commonly seen in patients with cell-mediated immune defects (e.g., corticosteroids or transplant) and may occur with dissemination from a pulmonary or cutaneous infection.

4. ***Toxoplasma gondii.*** Most commonly involves HIV/AIDS patients.

5. **Neurocysticercosis (i.e., pork tapeworm; *Taenia solium*).** A central nervous system (CNS) parasitic infection due to the larval form of the tapeworm *Taenia solium*. This infection is *not* a true abscess; appears as a cystic or calcified lesion.

III. COMPLICATIONS OF BRAIN ABSCESS

A. **Intraventricular Rupture of a Brain Abscess** is associated with an extremely high mortality rate and usually results from a delay in diagnosis or failure to initiate timely medical and surgical therapy.

B. **Seizures** are frequent complications with the initial illness with a gradual decline following treatment. A new-onset seizure can be the presenting manifestation for some cases of brain abscess, especially abscesses secondary to neurocysticercosis.

C. Any delay in diagnosis, hospitalization, or treatment, findings of focal neurologic deficits, immune compromise status, poorly controlled diabetes, and altered mental status (Glasgow Coma Scale [GCS] less than or equal to 12) can be associated with **permanent neurologic deficits and/or death**.

IV. CLINICAL MANIFESTATIONS OF BRAIN ABSCESS. The clinical presentation varies but is influenced by the **size** of the lesion, **location** of the lesion, and underlying **source** of the lesion. **Classic hallmark symptoms are:** headache, fever, focal neurologic deficits, and altered mental status. *The classic triad of fever, headache, and focal neurologic deficits is present in approximately 20% of patients.*

A. **Headache.** Most common presenting symptom and often characterized as a poorly localized dull ache.

B. **Fever.** Found in only half of cases.

C. **Focal Neurologic Deficits** (e.g., hemiparesis, aphasia, ataxia). Occurs in about one third of patients. Patients with abscesses in the brainstem or cerebellum may present with a cranial-nerve palsy or gait disorder. Behavioral changes may occur in patients with abscesses in the frontal or right temporal lobes. Signs of nausea, vomiting, drowsiness, and delirium may indicate increased intracranial pressure (e.g., hydrocephalus).

An abrupt and severe headache most likely indicates acute bacterial meningitis or subarachnoid hemorrhage.

V. APPROACH TO THE PATIENT

A. **History.** Brain abscess is a diagnosis often missed; therefore, always include this in the differential diagnosis when evaluating a patient for *headache, fever, or stroke-like illness*. The history should focus on comorbid conditions or infections that could predispose the patient to a brain abscess.

B. **Physical Examination.** Evaluation of a brain abscess should include a complete examination. In addition to the general examination, emphasis should be placed on the following:

   1. **Funduscopic examination** (to detect papilledema); papilledema occurs in less than one fourth of cases but usually signifies increased intracranial pressure.

   2. **Head, eyes, ears, nose, and throat (HEENT) examination** (to detect a paranasal sinus, ear, or odontogenic infection).

   3. **Neurologic examination** (to *evaluate* mental status level and the presence of a neurologic deficit; see Chapter 32, Meningitis and Ventriculitis).

   4. **Cardiovascular examination** (to detect murmurs or evidence of endocarditis; see Chapter 7, Infective Endocarditis).

   5. **Dermatologic examination** (to search for signs of endocarditis; see Chapter 7).

   6. **Musculoskeletal examination** (to detect septic arthritis or osteomyelitis; see Chapter 37, Septic Arthritis and Chapter 35, Osteomyelitis).

C. **Laboratory Studies.** There are *no* pathognomonic findings for brain abscess from laboratory studies.

   1. **Complete blood count (CBC).** Patients can have a normal CBC, mildly increased WBC, and/or anemia (anemia of chronic disease). However, the CBC may reveal neutropenia and/or thrombocytosis.

   2. **Complete metabolic panel (CMP).** A CMP is rarely helpful but elevated aspartate aminotransferase (AST), alanine aminotransferase (ALT), or alkaline phosphatase may indicate a hepatobiliary source of the abscess.

   3. **Erythrocyte sedimentation rate (ESR) and C-reactive protein (CRP).** An elevated level is nonspecific but may indicate infection.

   4. **Urinalysis.** An abnormal urinalysis may indicate a urinary source of infection.

   5. **Lumbar puncture** is a potentially dangerous procedure that is ***rarely*** of clinical value. The risk of **brainstem herniation**, especially with intracranial hypertension signs (see the preceding) and papilledema is increased in this setting and should *not* be performed.

   6. **Blood cultures.** Two sets are routinely ordered but rarely helpful except in cases of hematogenous source infection (see the preceding).

   7. **Abscess cultures.** Most commonly obtained by diagnostic needle aspiration with CT guidance. A request for Gram stain, acid-fast stain, and mycology stain (i.e., calcofluor white, periodic acid–Schiff) and standard bacterial and mycology cultures should be performed.

   8. **Purified protein derivative (PPD) or interferon-gamma release assay (e.g., QuantiFERON-TB Gold).** May be helpful in cases suspected of *Mycobacterium tuberculosis* (see Chapter 14, Tuberculosis).

D. **Radiography Studies.** Cranial imaging should be performed in all patients.

   1. **CT scanning with IV iodinated contrast** provides good resolution for the identification of brain abscesses with abscesses typically having hypodense centers surrounded by a smooth, thin-walled capsule.

2. **MRI scanning with IV gadolinium** is superior to CT scan because of improved image resolution and detail. Findings include:

   a. **T1-weighted image.** *Hypointense lesion* with enhanced ring.

   b. **T2-weighted image.** *Hyperintense lesion* with a well-defined hypointense capsule.

   Serial CT scan or MRI performed either weekly (hospitalized patient) or biweekly (outpatient setting) can help demonstrate response to antibiotic therapy or need for modification to the management with an intervention or change in antibiotics.

   MRI combined with diffusion-weighted and apparent-diffusion-coefficient images has a sensitivity and specificity for the differentiation of brain abscesses from primary or metastatic cancers of 96% (positive predictive value, 98%; negative predictive value, 92%).

VI. TREATMENT

A. **Antimicrobial Therapy.** (*Antibiotics listed assume normal renal and hepatic function.*)

   1. Brain abscesses are typically polymicrobial and empiric therapy should be initiated after obtaining appropriate cultures.

      An appropriate empirical regimen for an *immunocompetent patient* might be:

      a. Ceftriaxone 2 g IV q12, ceftazidime 2 g IV q8, or cefepime 2 g IV q8 *plus*

      b. Vancomycin 15 mg/kg IV q12 (with *methicillin-resistant Staphylococcus aureus* [MRSA] concern) *plus*

      c. Metronidazole 500 mg IV/potassium oral (PO) q6–8

      An appropriate empirical regimen for an *immunocompromised patient* might be:

      a. Ceftriaxone 2 g IV q12, ceftazidime 2 g IV q8, or cefepime 2 g IV q8 *plus*

      b. Trimethoprim–sulfamethoxazole (TMP/SMX): 10 to 20 mg TMP plus 50 to 100 mg SMX per kilogram per day, administered in two to four divided doses (with MRSA and *Nocardia* spp concern) *plus*

      c. Metronidazole 500 mg IV/PO q6–8 *plus*

      d. Voriconazole 4 mg per kilogram q12 after a loading dose of 6 mg per kilogram q12 for two doses.

   2. Antimicrobial therapy for special pathogens may include:

      a. **Methicillin-susceptible *Staphylococcus aureus* (MSSA).** Nafcillin or oxacillin 2 g IV q4. Alternative therapy includes cefazolin 2 g IV q8.

      b. **MRSA.** Vancomycin 15 mg/kg IV q8–24 or linezolid 600 g IV q12 (linezolid is not considered bactericidal). *Daptomycin should **not** be used as it does **not** have adequate CNS penetration.*

      c. ***Pseudomonas* species.** Meropenem 2 g IV q8 or cefepime 2 g IV q8.

      d. **Extended-spectrum beta-lactamase (ESBL) pathogen.** Meropenem 2 g IV q8 or piperacillin–tazobactam 3.375 g IV q6 or cefepime 2 g IV q8.

e. ***Actinomyces* species.** Ceftriaxone 2 g IV q12 with metronidazole 500 mg IV q6–8.

f. *Mycobacterium tuberculosis.* Standard four-drug therapy (e.g., isoniazid, 300 mg q24 [oral]; rifampin, 600 mg q24 [oral]; pyrazinamide, 15 to 30 mg per kilogram q24 [oral]; ethambutol, 15 mg per kilogram q24 [oral]).

g. ***Toxoplasmosis gondii.*** Pyrimethamine 200 mg dose, then 50 mg (less than or equal to 60 kg) or 75 mg (greater than or equal to 60 kg) q24 plus sulfadiazine 1,000 mg (less than or equal to 60 kg) or 1,500 mg (greater than 60 kg) q6 plus leucovorin 10–25 mg q24.

h. **Fungal.** Amphotericin B (lipid) 3 to 5 mg/kg/day with or without flucytosine (5-FC) 25 mg/kg PO q6.

i. ***Nocardia* species.** Bactrim (TMP 5 mg/SMX 15 mg) IV q6 or sulfadiazine 6 to 12 g IV q6 initially, then switch to oral therapy when clinically stable for *6 months total therapy.* Alternative is doxycycline 100 mg IV q12 initially, then switch to oral therapy for *6 months total therapy.*

The typical duration of standard antimicrobial therapy is a 6- to 8-week course of parenteral therapy that is sometimes followed by a 2- to 3-month course of oral antibiotics.

B. **Surgical Therapy**

1. Prior to any surgical intervention, bleeding times (i.e., prothrombin time [PT], partial thromboplastin time [PTT]) and thrombocytopenia results should be normalized or corrected to an acceptable level.

2. *Small lesions* (less than 2.5 cm) that are located in well-vascularized areas may respond to antibiotics alone.

3. **Formal stereotactic needle biopsy** for the collection of samples for culture and drainage of abscesses greater than or equal to 2.5 cm or located within deeper critical regions is the preferred surgical therapy.

4. **Open craniotomy** for diagnostic and therapeutic aspiration or abscess excision should be reserved for:

   a. Multiloculated abscesses

   b. Unusual (e.g., neurocysticercosis) or more resistant pathogens (e.g., fungi, ESBL, *Nocardia*)

   c. Deep subcortical white matter lesions with poor blood supply

C. **Adjunctive Therapy.** The routine use of corticosteroids is controversial, as therapy may interfere with bacterial clearance, formation of granulation tissue, and delayed collagen deposition. However, patients with **life-threatening cerebral edema** or **impending cerebral herniation** may benefit from the addition of **dexamethasone** 10 mg IV or PO q6 for 3 days followed by a tapering dose over 3 to 7 days.

BIBLIOGRAPHY

Brouwer MC, Coutinho JM, van de Beek D. Clinical characteristics and outcome of brain abscess: systematic review and meta-analysis. *Neurology.* 2014;82(9):806–813.

Brouwer MC, Tunkel AR, McKhann GM, et al. Brain abscess. *N Engl J Med.* 2014;371(5):447–456.

Carpenter J, Stapleton S, Holliman R. Retrospective analysis of 49 cases of brain abscess and review of the literature. *Eur J Clin Microbiol Infect Dis.* 2007;26(1):1–11.

Honda H, Warren DK. Central nervous system infections: meningitis and brain abscess. *Infect Dis Clin North Am.* 2009;23(3):609–623.

Mathisen GE, Johnson JP. Brain abscess. *Clin Infect Dis.* 1997;25(4):763–779.

OSTEOMYELITIS

William F. Wright

I. INTRODUCTION

A. Definition. An inflammatory condition of bone (osteitis) and/or bone marrow (myelitis), usually caused by infection with either a bacteria or fungus, that eventually leads to bone destruction and necrosis.

B. Pathogenesis. Bone tissue and matrix are typically resistant to any infection; however, infection can result from either invasion of bone by a bloodstream infection from a distant site (hematogenous source), extension from an adjacent local infection (contiguous source), or direct inoculation following trauma. Certain bacteria (e.g., *Staphylococcus aureus*) can then produce binding molecules that allow attachment to bone matrix components (e.g., fibronectin, collagen, and laminin). As bacteria multiply, most species produce an extracellular polymer called ***biofilm*** that allows evasion from the immune response. While most bacteria produce biofilm, the more commonly associated organisms include:

1. *S. aureus* and *S. epidermidis*

2. Streptococci (particularly group A)

3. *Pseudomonas aeruginosa*

   Early bone infection (**acute osteomyelitis**) is associated with edema, vascular congestion, and small-vessel thrombosis that then compromise blood flow to the bone (ischemia). Local ischemia results in areas of dead bone (sequestra) and necrosis that is characteristic of late bone infection (**chronic osteomyelitis**).

C. Risk Factors. The risk factors leading to osteomyelitis include:

1. **Trauma.** Most commonly as the result of direct inoculation from an open fracture or corrective orthopedic surgery (e.g., open reduction internal fixation).

2. **Implantable prosthetic orthopedic device** (e.g., prosthetic knee or hip).

3. **Diabetes mellitus.** Most commonly results from a neuropathic ulcer with adjacent skin and soft-tissue infection.

4. **Intravenous (IV) drug abuse, intravascular catheter, and hemodialysis catheter.**

5. **Spinal cord injury.** Most commonly results in osteomyelitis as a result of the development of pressure ulcers.

6. **Tuberculosis** (especially extrapulmonary involvement).

7. **Alcoholism and immunosuppression** (e.g., chronic corticosteroid use).

8. **Peripheral vascular disease (PVD).**

9. **Male gender.**

II. CLASSIFICATION OF OSTEOMYELITIS

A. **Waldvogel Classification System.** A simple and practical system based on three factors:

1. **Duration. Acute osteomyelitis** occurs within 2 weeks of infection prior to bone destruction and necrosis. Osteomyelitis occurring from the time period from 2 to 6 weeks is referred to as **subacute osteomyelitis. Chronic osteomyelitis** is generally defined by the following:

   a. Infection duration greater than 6 weeks

   b. Persistent or relapsed infection

   c. Infection associated with prosthetic devices

   d. Histologic evidence of dead or necrotic cortical bone

2. **Mechanism.** Osteomyelitis can occur as a result of a *hematogenous* or a *contiguous* source. Acute hematogenous osteomyelitis results from bacteremic seeding of bone and is more common in children under 5 years of age as the metaphyseal (growing) regions of the long bones are highly vascular and susceptible to even minor trauma. Hematogenous osteomyelitis among adults typically involves the adjacent vertebral disc space from a distant focus, as the disc is avascular, but can occur in the long bones, pelvis, or clavicle. Patients with vertebral osteomyelitis often have underlying medical conditions (e.g., diabetes mellitus, cancer, chronic renal disease) or a history of intravenous drug use (IVDU). Chronic osteomyelitis is uncommon among children and generally occurs secondary to open fractures, bacteremia, or contiguous soft-tissue infection.

3. **Vascular status.** Osteomyelitis associated with or without local or generalized vascular disease.

B. **Cierny–Mader Staging System.** A more comprehensive system that considers other factors important to osteomyelitis treatment and prognosis. The system is based on two main factors:

1. **Anatomical osteomyelitis type**

   a. **Medullary osteomyelitis.** Usually is localized to the medullary component of bone as a result of early hematogenous infection or infection of an implanted intramedullary rod.

   b. **Superficial osteomyelitis.** Infection as a result of an adjacent wound or ulcer (e.g., diabetic foot ulcer).

   c. **Localized osteomyelitis.** Full thickness cortical bone infection that does not compromise the remaining bone (uninfected bone) stability.

   d. **Diffuse osteomyelitis.** A bilateral or circumferential full thickness cortical bone infection that does compromise the remaining bone (uninfected bone) stability.

2. **Physiologic host status type**

a. **Normal host** (A-type host)

b. **Non-normal host** (B-type host)

 i. **Systemic conditions.** Malnutrition, renal failure, hepatic disease, diabetes, chronic obstructive pulmonary disease (COPD)/chronic hypoxia, malignancy, immunodeficiency, central nervous system (CNS) disease or neuropathy, and extremes of age.

 ii. **Local conditions to the site of osteomyelitis.** Venous stasis, chronic lymphedema, vasculitis, thrombophlebitis, deep vein thrombosis (DVT), radiation fibrosis, PVD, and tobacco abuse.

c. **Osteomyelitis treatment worse than disease** (C-type host)

III. **BACTERIAL AND FUNGAL CAUSES OF OSTEOMYELITIS.** In general, hematogenous source of osteomyelitis is typically caused by a single bacterium (i.e., monomicrobial), whereas a contiguous source osteomyelitis is commonly caused by many bacteria (i.e., polymicrobial). Common organisms include:

A. *S. aureus* (most common overall)

B. *S. epidermidis* (foreign-body associated)

C. *Propionibacterium acnes* (foreign-body associated)

D. *Pseudomonas aeruginosa* (IVDU and nosocomial associated)

E. *Streptococcus pneumoniae* (sickle cell disease associated)

F. *Enterococcus* spp (urinary tract infection [UTI], hematogenous, and diabetic foot ulcer)

G. *Enterobacteriaceae* spp (UTI and nosocomial associated)

H. *Serratia marcescens* (IVDU associated)

I. *Salmonella* spp (sickle cell disease associated)

J. *Pasteurella multocida* (cat- or dog-bite associated)

K. *Eikenella corrodens* (human-bite associated)

L. *Streptococcus* spp (hematogenous source)

M. *Bartonella henselae* (HIV infection associated or occasionally associated with cat or dog bites)

N. *Brucella* spp (associated with direct contact with sheep, goats, swine, or dogs and/or ingestion of contaminated foods)

O. *Coxiella burnetii* (known as **Q fever** and most commonly associated with direct contact with infected cattle, sheep, goats, cats, and dogs)

P. *Aspergillus* and *Candida* spp (immunocompromised patient)

Q. *Mycobacterium tuberculosis* (hematogenous spread tends to localize to the cervical or thoracic spine)

R. **Anaerobic Bacteria** (most commonly associated with diabetic foot infections)

IV. **CLINICAL MANIFESTATIONS OF OSTEOMYELITIS.** *Localized pain and tenderness* of the involved bone segment is the most consistent presentation. However, pain may be significantly reduced or absent in diabetic patients with peripheral neuropathy. Pain and tenderness associated with hematogenous source osteomyelitis are usually indolent with occasional *fevers* (occurs half the time in association with vertebral osteomyelitis) and *constitutional symptoms.* Low-grade fevers in association with night sweats, weight loss, anorexia, and fatigue are more likely to occur with chronic osteomyelitis. Additionally, chronic pain with or without erythema over the affected bone, sinus tracts, and draining ulcers are more likely to occur with chronic osteomyelitis. A chronic draining sinus tract or abscess without erythema, warmth, tenderness, and edema, that is, "cold abscess," should prompt consideration for *M. tuberculosis.*

V. COMPLICATIONS OF OSTEOMYELITIS

A. **Brodie Abscess.** A chronic localized bone abscess from a hematogenous source that most commonly involves the distal tibia in patients less than 25 years of age.

B. **Vertebral Epidural or Subdural Abscess.** Results from *posterior extension* of vertebral osteomyelitis.

C. **Bacterial Meningitis.** An unusual complication of a *posterior extension* of vertebral osteomyelitis.

D. **Psoas, Paravertebral, Retropharyngeal, Mediastinal, Subphrenic and/or Retroperitoneal Abscess.** Usually results from an *anterior extension* of vertebral osteomyelitis.

E. **Squamous Cell Carcinoma.** Known as a *Marjolin ulcer,* which is usually associated with chronic osteomyelitis. These slow-growing ulcers most commonly occur on the extremities in association with well-defined edges and abundant granulation tissue. The most common symptoms and signs are a persistent ulcer with pain, bleeding, and drainage with foul odor.

F. **Amyloidosis (Most Commonly AA Amyloidosis).** Usually results from chronic osteomyelitis.

VI. APPROACH TO THE PATIENT WITH OSTEOMYELITIS

A. **History.** The diagnosis of osteomyelitis can be challenging in patients with or without the coexistence of diabetic-related neuropathy and/or vascular disease. *Physicians must have a high clinical concern for osteomyelitis in patients with pain and tenderness above a bone segment and/or an underlying risk factor* (see the preceding). *Physicians should also suspect the diagnosis of native vertebral osteomyelitis in patients with new or worsening back or neck pain and fever.* When taking the history, the clinician should focus on the duration of symptoms, duration of comorbid diseases, hospitalizations, prior infections, previous surgeries, implantable prosthetic devices, medications, and risk factors (see the preceding). Native vertebral osteomyelitis is typically associated with recalcitrant back pain unresponsive to conservative measures.

B. **Physical Examination.** A complete physical examination should be performed, but areas of the examination to focus on include:

1. **Musculoskeletal examination.** This is the most important aspect of the physical examination. A surgical scar overlying a bone segment or joint may indicate a prosthetic device. Synovial joint swelling and diminished joint range of motion may indicate septic arthritis and/or osteomyelitis. Tenderness palpated over a bone segment or joint space may indicate osteomyelitis.

2. **Vital signs.** Elevations in temperature, heart rate, respiratory rate, and pain score with changes in blood pressure are more likely associated with acute infection. Normal vital signs with a low-grade fever may suggest subacute or chronic infections.

3. **Dermatologic examination.** IVDU injection sites, prior vascular catheter site or existing catheter sites, nail-bed splinter hemorrhages, Janeway lesions, or Osler nodes may suggest a hematogenous source. Examination of surgical scars or ulcers (e.g., pressure or neuropathic ulcers) may suggest a contiguous source. (*Diabetic foot ulcers greater than 2 cm² in dimension are more likely associated with osteomyelitis; sensitivity 56% and specificity 92%.*)

   "Probe test." The physician probes the depth of any ulcer base (technically this should be performed with a sterile stainless steel eye probe). The test is positive if a *rock-hard and gritty* structure is observed. For osteomyelitis this test has a sensitivity of 66% and specificity of 85%.

   Cutaneous findings of *cellulitis* (e.g., erythema, warmth, edema, and tenderness) as well as *draining sinus tracts* (a draining sinus tract strongly suggests osteomyelitis) may also be associated with a contiguous source.

4. **Cardiovascular examination.** A new diastolic murmur or change with existing murmur may suggest a hematogenous source such as endocarditis. Examination of peripheral pulses, capillary refill, and signs of venous stasis changes may uncover vascular disease.

5. **Neurologic examination.** Evaluation of peripheral neuropathy is important in diabetic patients as any type of peripheral neuropathy predisposes to neuropathic ulcers and osteomyelitis (see Chapter 41, Diabetic Foot Infections). *In addition, with cases of vertebral osteomyelitis the findings of sensory deficits, decreased motor response, and vertebral bone pain (increased by neck flexion and Valsalva maneuvers) associated with constipation or incontinence may signify spinal cord compression and require prompt hospitalization and immediate referral to a surgeon, as paraplegia may occur within hours after the onset of symptoms.*

6. **Respiratory examination.** Focal findings to suggest a respiratory infection may indicate a hematogenous source osteomyelitis (most commonly vertebral osteomyelitis).

7. **Oropharyngeal examination.** Findings of poor oral anatomy (e.g., gingivitis), dental abscess, or foul breath may suggest a hematogenous source osteomyelitis.

C. **Laboratory Studies**

1. **Complete blood count (CBC).** Most patients have an elevated white blood cell (WBC) count with acute infection, while the count is usually mildly elevated or normal in chronic infection.

2. **Basic metabolic panel (BMP).** Routinely ordered but no findings suggest osteomyelitis. A low-serum HCO_3 may be associated with metabolic acidosis and infection.

3. **Liver function tests (LFTs).** This test is ordered to mainly determine the nutritional status of the host through measuring the albumin and prealbumin levels (see Section VII).

4. **Erythrocyte sedimentation rate (ESR)/C-reactive protein (CRP).** Levels are often elevated in acute and chronic infection. **An ESR value greater than 70 mm/hour is more often associated with osteomyelitis in patients with diabetic foot infections (sensitivity 90%; specificity 100%).** The greatest value of these tests is normalization of levels in response to therapy. **A rapid decline of the ESR (greater than 50%) within the first 4 weeks of therapy is less likely associated with treatment failure.**

5. **Blood cultures.** Routinely ordered but most often positive in cases of hematogenous source osteomyelitis. **In the setting of radiographic confirmation of osteomyelitis and positive blood cultures with a typical pathogen (e.g., _S. aureus_), the requirement for bone biopsy and culture may be eliminated.**

6. **Sinus tract or ulcer swab cultures.** In general, _not_ routinely recommended, as they do not predict the presence or absence of organisms that cause osteomyelitis (22% concordance rate). The concordance rate for _S. aureus_ (i.e., methicillin-susceptible _Staphylococcus aureus_ [MSSA] or methicillin-resistant _Staphylococcus aureus_ [MRSA]) may be as high as 50%.

7. **Bone biopsy and culture.** This is still the gold or criterion standard procedure for microbiological determination of the causative bacteria that can be obtained by open biopsy or CT guidance biopsy. Patients should be off antibiotics for a minimum of 48 hours and two samples obtained through uninfected skin. One sample is used for Gram stain, fungal stains (e.g., periodic acid-Schiff stain [PAS], calcofluor white), acid-fast bacillus (AFB) smear and culture. _The other sample is for histopathology confirmation._

   An image-guided aspiration biopsy in patients with suspected native vertebral osteomyelitis is helpful when a microbiological diagnosis for an associated organism has not been established. A second aspiration biopsy should be obtained with a nondiagnostic first image-guided aspiration biopsy or when the original image-guided aspiration biopsy specimen grew skin contaminant bacteria (e.g., coagulase-negative _Staphylococcus_ species except _S. lugdunensis_).

8. **Serology.** May be helpful in cases suspected to be due to brucellosis and Q fever.

D. **Radiography Studies.** Imaging establishes the diagnosis of osteomyelitis.

1. **Plain-film radiology.** Widely available and inexpensive but is most useful in chronic osteomyelitis, as 50% to 75% of bone matrix loss (manifested as osteopenia) must occur before characteristic changes such as **cortical erosions, lytic changes,** and/or **periosteal reactions** are visualized (typically evolves over 1 to 3 weeks). Two-view radiographs are typically the initial imaging test ordered, but a negative image cannot exclude the diagnosis (sensitivity 60%; specificity 70%).

2. **CT.** Widely available and provides improved resolution images when compared to plain-film radiology. CT scan is usually the second best option if an MRI cannot be obtained. A major limitation to CT scan is image degradation or scatter phenomenon in the presence of implanted prosthetic devices adjacent to infected bone. In chronic osteomyelitis, CT findings include thickened cortical bone with sclerotic changes and chronic draining sinus tracts (sensitivity 67%; specificity 50%).

3. Radionuclide studies. Generally more reliable in acute osteomyelitis but may not be readily available. Three of the most common studies include:

a. Technetium-99 polyphosphate scan. This isotope accumulates in areas of increased blood flow and new bone formation. While this study can be positive within 48 hours of infection onset, impaired blood flow (e.g., PVD or venous stasis) may limit the utility of this study (sensitivity 85%; specificity 45%).

b. Gallium citrate Ga-67 scan. This isotope attaches to **transferrin** and leaks into areas of inflammation, infection, and malignancy but does not distinguish well between bone and tissue inflammation.

c. Indium-111–labeled leukocyte scan ("tagged white blood cell scan"). More useful with acute osteomyelitis but only positive in 40% of cases.

If radionuclide studies are needed, the combined **indium-111–labeled leukocyte scan** and **technetium-99–labeled sulfur colloid scan** has the best performance for the diagnosis of osteomyelitis (sensitivity 80%; specificity 75%).

4. Nuclear MRI. This test is expensive but is the most useful imaging study to diagnose osteomyelitis (sensitivity 90%; specificity 80%). MRI is contraindicated in the presence of **ferromagnetic material** (iron-containing) but offers the best spatial resolution in differentiating bone and soft-tissue infection. MRI usually consists of two main sequences:

a. T1-weighted. Edema is **dark** on this image.

b. T2-weighted. Edema is **bright** on this image.

The addition of **gadolinium contrast** to MRI improves visualization of sinus tracts, fistulas, and abscesses.

MRI Characteristics		
Condition	T1-Weighted	T2-Weighted
Osteomyelitis	Decreased	Increased
Sinus tracts	Intermediate	Increased
Abscesses	Intermediate	Increased
Cellulitis	Intermediate	Increased

VII. TREATMENT. In general, antibiotic therapy alone is used to treat acute osteomyelitis, while antibiotic therapy in combination with surgical therapy is required for chronic osteomyelitis. Additional factors that involve successful treatment include:

1. Optimize nutrition for wound healing and bone healing.

2. Correct any vascular issues that may contribute to bone hypoxia or ischemia (e.g., arterial insufficiency, anemia).

3. Optimize any metabolic derangement or electrolyte abnormality.

4. Optimize diabetes control as elevated glucose (greater than or equal to 180 mg/dL) impairs neutrophil dysfunction and wound healing.

5. Offer smoking cessation, as smoking reduces blood flow to bones and contributes to ischemia as well as poor wound healing.

6. Minimize immunosuppression medications (e.g., corticosteroids, azathioprine) in an effort to improve neutrophil dysfunction with high doses and wound healing.

7. Optimize wound management.

A. **Antibiotic Therapy.** Antibiotics listed assume normal renal function. Traditionally, the duration of therapy is 4 to 6 weeks as based on animal models indicating that revascularization of bone following surgical debridement occurs in about 4 weeks. Selected antibiotic regimens include:

1. *Staphylococcus aureus*

   a. **Penicillin-sensitive.** Penicillin G 12 to 20 million units IV q24 or cefazolin 1 g IV q6–8. (Vancomycin 15 mg/kg IV q12–24 should be used for penicillin-allergic patients; however, *the vancomycin dose may need adjustments to maintain a serum trough level between 15 and 20 mcg/mL.*)

   b. **Penicillin-resistant but oxacillin-sensitive.** Nafcillin or oxacillin 1 to 2 g IV q4–6 or cefazolin 1 to 2 g IV q4–6. (Vancomycin should be used for penicillin-allergic patients.)

   c. **Oxacillin-resistant (e.g., MRSA).** Vancomycin 15 mg/kg IV q12–24. (*The vancomycin dose may need adjustments to maintain a serum trough level between 15 and 20 mcg/mL.*) Alternatives include daptomycin 6 to 12 mg/kg IV q24 (6 mg/kg dosing is recommended) or clindamycin 600 mg IV or PO q6 (should only be used if the organism is susceptible).

2. **Coagulase-negative staphylococci (e.g., *S. epidermidis*).** While the majority is oxacillin-resistant, treatment would be vancomycin 15 mg/kg IV q12–24. If oxacillin-sensitive, then use nafcillin or oxacillin 1 to 2 g IV q4–6.

3. **Streptococci.** Penicillin G 2 million units IV q4, or ampicillin 2 g IV q6, or ceftriaxone 1 to 2 g IV q24. (Clindamycin 600 mg IV q6 may be used in patients with a true anaphylactic reaction to penicillin.)

4. *Enterococcus.* Ampicillin 2 g IV q4 *plus or minus* gentamicin 1 mg/kg IV q8 or vancomycin 15 mg/kg IV q12–24. For isolates-resistant vancomycin, consider using daptomycin 6 to 12 mg/kg IV q24 (6 mg/kg dosing is most common) or linezolid 600 mg IV or PO q12.

5. **Enteric gram-negative rods (e.g., Enterobacteriaceae).** Ampicillin–sulbactam 1.5 to 3 g IV q6 (*use of this agent may be limited by high resistance rates*) or ceftriaxone 1 to 2 g IV q24 or ciprofloxacin 400 mg IV (or 500 mg PO) q8–12.

6. *Pseudomonas aeruginosa.* Cefepime or ceftazidime 2 g IV q8–12; ciprofloxacin 400 mg IV (500 mg PO) q8–12; meropenem 1 g IV q8.

7. *Propionibacterium acnes.* Penicillin G 20 million units IV q24 continuously or in six divided doses or ceftriaxone 2 g IV q24 or clindamycin 600 to 900 mg IV q8 or vancomycin IV 15–20 mg/kg q12.

8. *Salmonella species.* Ciprofloxacin PO 500 mg q12 (or 400 mg IV q12) or ceftriaxone 2 g IV q24.

9. **Anaerobes.** Clindamycin 600 mg IV or PO q6 or metronidazole 500 mg IV or PO q6–8.

B. **Surgical Therapy.** Generally accepted indications for surgery include antibiotic failure, infected surgical hardware, and chronic osteomyelitis with necrotic bone and soft tissue. Indications for surgery among patients with native vertebral osteomyelitis may include the development of neurologic deficits or symptoms of spinal cord compression and evidence of progression or recurrence despite proper antimicrobial therapy. The principles of operative treatment include:

1. Address vascular issues such as arterial insufficiency (e.g., vascular surgery consult, noninvasive vascular studies such as ankle–brachial index [ABI] measurement).

2. Adequate drainage of abscesses and extensive debridement of infected and necrotic tissue. Debridement should be performed until punctuate bleeding is noted and there is marginal resection of more than 5 mm.

3. Dead space management (i.e., bone grafts or antibiotic impregnated material) and appropriate soft-tissue coverage (i.e., muscle flaps).

4. Bone stabilization with plates, screws, rods, and fixation devices if needed.

C. **Prognosis and Recurrence.** Despite the use of appropriate long-term antimicrobial therapy in conjunction with surgical debridement, the recurrence rate of chronic osteomyelitis in adults is about 30% to 50% at 12 months.

BIBLIOGRAPHY

Berbari EF, Kanj SS, Kowalski TJ, et al. 2015 Infectious Diseases Society of America (IDSA) clinical practice guidelines for the diagnosis and treatment of native vertebral osteomyelitis in adults. *Clin Infect Dis.* 2015;61(6):e26–e46.

Calhoun JH, Manring MM. Adult osteomyelitis. *Infect Dis Clin North Am.* 2005;19(4):765–786.

Hatzenbuehler J, Pulling TJ. Diagnosis and management of osteomyelitis. *Am Fam Physician.* 2011;84(9):1027–1033.

Howell WR, Goulston C. Osteomyelitis· an update for hospitalists. *Hosp Pract (Minneap).* 2011;39(1):153–160.

Rao N, Ziran BH, Lipsky BA. Treating osteomyelitis: antibiotics and surgery. *Plast Reconstr Surg.* 2011;127(suppl 10):177S–187S.

Zimmerli W. Clinical practice. Vertebral osteomyelitis. *N Engl J Med.* 2010;362(11):1022–1029.

36

MANDIBULAR AND MAXILLARY OSTEOMYELITIS

William F. Wright

I. INTRODUCTION

A. **Definition and Normal Dental Anatomy.** Human teeth have an *outer layer of enamel* that is an extremely hard, highly mineralized, crystalline structure that covers and protects the tooth crown. The inner layer of the tooth contains *dentine* (the bulk of calcified tooth just beneath the enamel layer) and a *pulp chamber.* The pulp chamber contains blood vessels and nerves that connect to the jaw's vascular and nervous supply through the tooth apices. Finally, *tooth roots* attach to the surrounding *alveolar jawbone* of the tooth socket via the *periodontal ligament*. The alveolar jawbone has a lower component, mandible, and an upper component, maxilla.

Osteomyelitis is an inflammatory condition of the alveolar osseous medulla jawbone. *Osteitis* is a superficial inflammatory condition of the alveolar jawbone cortex.

B. **Pathogenesis.** Long bone infection (e.g., femur, tibia, fibula) can result from either invasion of bone by a bloodstream infection from a distant site (hematogenous source), extension from an adjacent local infection (contiguous source), or direct inoculation following trauma.

Osteomyelitis of the maxillofacial (e.g., jawbone) skeleton most commonly occurs as a result of extension from an adjacent local site (e.g., skin, oral cavity, or paranasal sinuses).

Certain bacteria (e.g., *Staphylococcus aureus*) can then produce binding molecules that allow attachment to bone matrix components (e.g., fibronectin, collagen, and laminin). As bacteria multiply, most species produce an extracellular polymer called *biofilm* that allows evasion from the immune response.

Early bone infection (**acute osteomyelitis [AO]**) is associated with edema, vascular congestion, and small-vessel thrombosis that then compromise blood flow to the bone (ischemia). Local ischemia results in areas of dead bone (sequestra) and necrosis that is characteristic of late bone infection (**chronic osteomyelitis**).

C. **Epidemiology and Risk Factors.** Mandibular osteomyelitis is more common than maxillary osteomyelitis. Men and women are affected equally. The risk factors that lead particularly to maxillofacial osteomyelitis include:

1. **Alcoholism.** This condition leads to malnutrition and impaired immune response.

2. **Bisphosphonates and chemotherapy.** Usually related to high doses and prolonged use of these medications that then leads to sterile bone necrosis.

3. **Chronic kidney and liver disease.** Due to impaired host immune response.

4. **Diabetes mellitus.** Usually associated with long-term uncontrolled diabetes leading to reduced neutrophil function (e.g., chemotaxis and oxidative burst), impaired vascular perfusion, and delayed wound healing.

5. **HIV infection and immunosuppression** (e.g., chronic corticosteroid use, malnutrition).

6. **Intravenous (IV) drug abuse.** Rarely related to metastatic spread from a distant infection source as a result of injection drug abuse.

7. **Implantable dental prosthetic device.**

8. **Peripheral vascular disease (PVD).** Results in reduced wound healing, reduced tissue oxygenation, and impaired host immune response.

9. **Radiation therapy.** Results in reduced wound healing and impaired host immune response.

10. **Smoking.** Associated with impaired vascular perfusion and delayed wound healing.

11. **Surgical procedure (e.g., dentoalveolar surgical wound) or trauma.** Most commonly as the result of direct inoculation from an open dental wound connected to the medullary bone space or corrective dental surgery.

II. CLASSIFICATION

A. **Zurich Classification System.** Developed at the University of Zurich, Switzerland Department of Cranio-Maxillofacial Surgery. A system based on the clinical appearance, course of disease, and radiologic features. This system results in three major groups:

1. **AO.** Occurs within 4 weeks of infection prior to bone destruction and necrosis.

2. **Secondary chronic osteomyelitis (SCO).** This stage is typically a suppurative condition that is considered an extension of AO. Occurs after 4 weeks of infection and is associated with bone destruction and necrosis.

3. **Primary chronic osteomyelitis (PCO).** A rare, nonsuppurative, chronic inflammation of an unknown cause.

III. BACTERIAL AND FUNGAL CAUSES

Common pathogenic microorganisms include:

A. *Staphylococcus aureus*

B. *Staphylococcus epidermidis (would be more commonly expected in the setting of implantable dental prosthetic devices)*

C. *Streptococcus* spp *(particularly v*iridans *streptococcus species and the* Streptococcus anginosus *group)*

D. *Actinomyces* spp *(particularly* A. israelii *and* A. dentalis*)*

E. *Nocardia* spp

F. *Eikenella corrodens*

G. *Prevotella, Porphyromonas,* and fusobacterium spp

H. *Rhodococcus equi*

I. *Candida albicans*

IV. CLINICAL MANIFESTATIONS

Clinical manifestations are varied and depend upon the stage of disease at presentation.

A. **Acute Maxillofacial Osteomyelitis.** Cases consistently present with jawbone intense pain, trismus, fevers, malaise, and purulent drainage. Additional symptoms with this stage include: regional adenopathy, bad breath (e.g., halitosis), and lower lip paresthesia/anesthesia due to involvement of the inferior alveolar nerve (e.g., Vincent's syndrome).

B. **Secondary Chronic Maxillofacial Osteomyelitis.** Symptoms of this stage typically reflect symptoms and signs of acute disease but are less extensive and intense. Jawbone pain is typically reduced to a dull ache and swelling is replaced by firm induration caused by the periosteal reaction. Sequestration and fistula formation are regarded as classic findings for this stage of illness.

C. **Primary Chronic Maxillofacial Osteomyelitis.** This form of infection has far fewer symptoms and signs of disease that typically characterize acute and chronic suppurative osteomyelitis.

V. CLINICAL CONDITIONS

A. **Alveolar Osteitis.** This condition is best known and referred to as "dry socket." The condition occurs in approximately 5% of patients undergoing dental extraction and is thought to be due to premature fibrinolysis of the postoperative platelet clot. The incidence is reported to be higher among patients with third molar extractions due to the higher vascularity at this location potentially leading to earlier fibrinolysis. The cardinal symptoms include jawbone pain that begins approximately 3 to 5 days after dental extraction that radiates along the trigeminal nerve distribution (e.g., radiates to either the ear or temporal region). This condition is not considered as a true infectious process of the bone. Treatment typically involves topical eugenol-based compounds on a nonresorbable carrier dressing.

B. **Dentoalveolar Abscess (Also Known as Periapical Abscess, Dental Abscess, or Abscessed Tooth).** This condition commonly occurs when dental caries destroy the tooth's protective enamel and dentin, allowing bacteria to reach the pulp. An abscess may develop when bacteria invade the nerves and blood vessels, filling the central cavity of the tooth (pulp) and causing the pulp to undergo necrosis. Symptoms include painful dental throbbing, swelling or reddening of the gums, extreme pain when biting or chewing, and sensitivity to heat and cold. Treatment typically involves incision and drainage followed by a short course of antimicrobial therapy (3–7 days).

1. **Ludwig's angina.** Originally described by Wilhelm Frederick von Ludwig in 1836, this is a rare but serious and potentially life-threatening complication of a dentoalveolar abscess. This condition originates most commonly from a dentoalveolar abscess of the second or third mandibular molars. These teeth have roots that lie at the level of the mylohyoid muscle, and abscesses here can spread to the submandibular space. Once infection is established in the submandibular space, the infection can then rapidly spread to adjacent structures such as the anterior neck, the pharyngomaxillary space, the retropharynx, and the superior mediastinum. Patients typically have a history of recent dental extraction and poor oral hygiene. Additional predisposing conditions include diabetes mellitus, neutropenia, alcoholism, aplastic anemia, glomerulonephritis, dermatomyositis, and systemic lupus erythematosus. Symptoms

include swelling and pain in the floor of the mouth and anterior neck, fever, dysphagia, odynophagia, drooling, trismus, toothache, fetid breath, hoarseness, stridor, respiratory distress, and decreased air movement. The presence of cyanosis and a "sniffing" neck position (i.e., the characteristic posture assumed by patients with impending upper airway compromise consisting of an upright posture with the neck thrust forward and the chin elevated) are all signs of impending airway catastrophe. Signs of this infection include elevation of the tongue, woody, brawny induration of the floor of the mouth and anterior neck, and nonfluctuant suprahyoid swelling. Bilateral submandibular edema, with marked tenderness on palpation and, occasionally, subcutaneous emphysema can be seen on the extraoral examination. Treatment typically involves airway control, prompt IV antimicrobial therapy directed at bacteria comprising the polymicrobial oral flora, and urgent surgical drainage.

C. **Osteonecrosis Associated With Radiation or Chemical Therapies**. Oncology-related radiation therapy and osteoporosis-related bisphosphonate therapy (typically high-dose therapy) cause a hypoxic, hypocellular, and hypovascular state leading to bone necrosis. While this condition is considered rare, it can lead to invasion of microorganisms and secondary infection (e.g., *Staphylococcus aureus* and *Actinomyces* species). Clinically, jawbone pain is the most common symptom. Radiographic findings include bone sclerosis, sclerotic lesions of the lamina dura surrounding dentition, and widening of periodontal ligaments. Treatment typically involves removal of the causative agent.

D. **Periostitis Ossificans (Garrés Sclerosing Osteomyelitis)**. This is a specific type of chronic nonsuppurative sclerosing osteomyelitis that primarily affects children and adolescents. It is merely a periosteal reaction in response to many nonspecific stimuli (such as dental decay, mild periodontitis, dental eruption, or previous dental extraction) that leads to the formation of new bone outside the normal cortical layer. The typical radiographic feature of Garre's osteomyelitis is known as the "onion skin" appearance due to the periosteal reaction. Clinically, this condition presents as a hard swelling of the jaw and subsequent facial asymmetry with which patients may present. The lesion is usually asymptomatic with no accompanying general and/or local signs of inflammation.

E. **SAPHO Syndrome.** This is a syndrome associated with synovitis, acne, pustulosis, hyperostosis, and osteitis. It is characterized by chronic nonsuppurative recurrent multifocal osteomyelitis. Low-grade bone pain and swelling are common. Bacterial cultures in this syndrome have in some case demonstrated growth of *Propionibacterium acnes*, *Actinomyces* species, and *Eikenella corrodens*. There is no consistent relationship among the radiographic findings of osteolysis, osteosclerosis, and periosteal reactions to be considered classic for this condition. The diagnostic criteria for this syndrome include: (a) chronic nonsuppurative multifocal osteomyelitis; (b) acute, subacute, or chronic arthritis with palmoplantar pustulosis, pustular psoriasis, or severe acne; or (c) severe osteitis with palmoplantar pustulosis, pustular psoriasis, or severe acne.

VI. APPROACH TO THE PATIENT

A. **History.** The diagnosis of maxillofacial osteomyelitis can be challenging in patients with or without the coexistence of diabetic-related neuropathy and/or vascular disease. *Physicians must have a high clinical concern for* *maxillofacial osteomyelitis in patients with pain and tenderness above a jawbone segment and/or an underlying risk factor* (see the preceding). When taking the history, the clinician should focus on the duration of symptoms, duration of comorbid diseases, hospitalizations, prior infections, previous surgeries, implantable prosthetic devices, medications, and risk factors (see the preceding).

B. Physical Examination. A complete physical examination should be performed, but areas of the examination to focus on include:

1. **Vital signs.** Elevations in temperature, heart rate, respiratory rate, and pain score with changes in blood pressure are more likely associated with acute infection. Normal vital signs with a low-grade fever may suggest subacute or chronic infections.

2. **Oropharyngeal examination.** This is the most important aspect of the physical examination and includes evaluation of the oral hard and soft tissues, pharynx, tongue, gingiva, and dentition. Specific examination areas include:

    a. Lips and labial mucosa. Normal findings are indicated by a wet, shiny, and salmon pink appearance.

    b. Buccal and vestibular mucosa. Normal findings are indicated by a wet, shiny, and salmon pink appearance. The clinician should evaluate the salivary gland openings of **Stensen's** (on the buccal mucosa adjacent to the second molar) and **Wharton's ducts** (at the base of the frenum) for purulence.

    c. Hard and soft palate. Infections may have the appearance of ulcers, erythema, leukoplakia, and focal areas of swelling.

    d. Tongue. Infections may have the appearance of ulcers, erythema, leukoplakia, and focal areas of swelling. A yellow-golden hue consistent with nicotine stomatitis may indicate a smoking history. The tongue is also the most common site for oral malignancies.

    e. Gingiva. Normal findings are indicated by a wet, shiny, and salmon pink appearance. Infections may have the appearance of ulcers, erythema, bleeding, and focal areas of swelling.

    A dentoalveolar abscess (e.g., periapical abscess) may be suggested by the presence of a pus-filled sac in the tissue around the root of a tooth, a draining sinus tract from the root of the tooth, and/or elevated loose tooth from the socket.

    f. Periodontium. Dental caries is a bacterial disease of teeth characterized by demineralization of tooth enamel and dentine by acid produced during the fermentation of dietary carbohydrates by oral bacteria, predominately *Streptococcus mutans.* Dental decay presents visually as opaque white areas of enamel with gray undertones. Where there is visual breakdown of a tooth surface, it is classified as a cavitated carious lesion. Advanced active root caries are suggested by well-defined areas of yellowish to light brown discoloration with the presence of a softening/leathery consistency on direct dental probing. Arrested caries can be observed as intact but discolored spots (usually darker brown to black).

    Alveolar osteitis (e.g., dry socket) is suggested by an area of extracted dentition with an inflamed gingival margin, exposed jawbone, and tenderness on direct palpation. Acute jawbone osteomyelitis is suggested by an area of extracted dentition with an inflamed gingival margin, purulence, exposed jawbone, and tenderness on direct palpation.

3. **Head and neck (extraoral) examination.** The extraoral head and neck examination should focus on the evaluation of facial or jawline asymmetries, lymph node enlargement, and cutaneous changes (such as previous surgical scars). The lymph node examination should include the anterior and posterior cervical chain, supraclavicular region, and preauricular lymph nodes. An abnormally large and tender node may be an indication of infection.

4. **Musculoskeletal examination.** Tenderness palpated over a bone segment or joint space may indicate osteomyelitis. Synovial joint swelling and diminished joint range of motion with the additional findings of palmoplantar pustulosis, pustular psoriasis, or severe acne may suggest the SAPHO syndrome.

5. **Dermatologic examination.** The presence of palmoplantar pustulosis, pustular psoriasis, or severe acne may suggest the SAPHO syndrome.

   Cutaneous findings of *facial cellulitis* (e.g., erythema, warmth, edema, and tenderness) as well as *draining sinus tracts* (a draining sinus tract strongly suggests osteomyelitis) may also be associated with a dental source infection.

6. **Cardiovascular examination.** A new diastolic murmur or change with existing murmur may suggest a hematogenous source such as endocarditis. Examination of peripheral pulses, capillary refill, and signs of venous stasis changes may uncover vascular disease.

7. **Respiratory examination.** Focal findings to suggest a respiratory infection may indicate a hematogenous source osteomyelitis.

8. **Neurologic examination.** Evaluation of peripheral neuropathy is important in diabetic patients.

C. **Laboratory Studies**

1. **Complete blood count (CBC).** Most patients have an elevated white blood cell (WBC) count with acute infection, while the count is usually mildly elevated or normal in chronic infections.

2. **Basic metabolic panel (BMP) and hemoglobin A_{1c}.** Routinely ordered but *no* findings suggest osteomyelitis. A low-serum HCO_3 may be associated with metabolic acidosis and infection. This test is ordered to mainly determine the creatinine clearance and diabetes status of the host to assist with medical management.

3. **Liver function tests (LFTs).** This test is ordered to mainly determine the nutritional status of the host through measuring the albumin and prealbumin levels.

4. **Erythrocyte sedimentation rate (ESR)/C-reactive protein (CRP).** Levels are often elevated in acute and chronic infection. The greatest value of these tests is normalization of levels in response to therapy.

5. **Blood cultures.** Routinely ordered but are *not* often positive except in rare cases of hematogenous source osteomyelitis. However, in the setting of radiographic confirmation of osteomyelitis and positive blood cultures with

a typical pathogen (e.g., *S. aureus*), the requirement for bone biopsy and culture may be eliminated.

6. **Sinus tract or ulcer swab cultures.** In general, *not* routinely recommended, as they *do not* always accurately predict the presence or absence of organisms that cause osteomyelitis.

7. **Bone biopsy and culture.** This is still the gold or criterion standard procedure for microbiological determination of the causative bacteria that can be obtained by open biopsy or CT guidance biopsy. Patients should be off antibiotics and two samples obtained through uninfected skin. One sample is used for Gram stain, fungal stains (e.g., periodic acid-Schiff stain [PAS], calcofluor white), acid-fast bacillus (AFB) smear and culture. The other sample is for histopathology confirmation.

8. **Serology.** May be helpful in cases suspected to be related to HIV infections (see Chapter 43, HIV and AIDS).

D. **Radiography Studies.** Imaging establishes the diagnosis of osteomyelitis.

1. **Conventional plain-film radiology.** Widely available and inexpensive but is most useful in chronic osteomyelitis, as 50% to 75% of bone matrix loss (manifested as osteopenia) must occur before characteristic changes such as **cortical erosions**, **lytic changes**, and/or **periosteal reactions** are visualized (typically evolves over 1 to 3 weeks). Panoramic projection radiographs are typically the initial imaging test ordered for maxillofacial cases, but a negative image cannot exclude the diagnosis.

2. **CT.** Widely available and provides improved resolution images when compared to plain-film radiology. Cone beam CT scan is usually the second best option if an MRI cannot be obtained. A major limitation to CT scan is image degradation or scatter phenomenon in the presence of implanted prosthetic devices adjacent to infected bone. In chronic osteomyelitis, CT findings include thickened cortical bone with sclerotic changes and chronic draining sinus tracts.

3. **Radionuclide studies.** Generally more reliable in acute maxillofacial osteomyelitis or SAPHO syndrome but may not be readily available. Three of the most common radioactive substances used to identify alterations of bone physiology include:

   a. **Technetium-99–labeled methylene polyphosphate scan.** This isotope accumulates in areas of increased blood flow and new bone formation. While this study can be positive within 48 hours of infection onset, impaired blood flow (e.g., PVD or venous stasis) may limit the utility of this study.

   b. **Gallium citrate Ga-67 scan.** This isotope attaches to **transferrin** and leaks into areas of inflammation, infection, and malignancy but does not distinguish well between bone and tissue inflammation.

   c. **Indium-111–labeled leukocyte scan ("tagged white blood cell scan").** More useful with AO.

   If radionuclide studies are needed, the combined **indium-111–labeled leukocyte scan** and **technetium-99–labeled sulfur colloid scan** has the best performance for the diagnosis of osteomyelitis.

4. **Nuclear MRI.** This test is expensive but is the most useful imaging study to diagnose osteomyelitis. MRI is contraindicated in the presence of **ferromagnetic material** (iron-containing) but offers the best spatial resolution in differentiating bone and soft-tissue infection when gadolinium is used as a contrast agent. MRI usually consists of two main sequences:

a. **T1-weighted.** Edema is **dark** on this image.

b. **T2-weighted.** Edema is **bright** on this image.

The addition of **gadolinium contrast** to MRI also improves visualization of sinus tracts, fistulas, and abscesses.

MRI Characteristics		
Condition	T1-Weighted	T2-Weighted
Osteomyelitis	Decreased	Increased
Sinus tracts	Intermediate	Increased
Abscesses	Intermediate	Increased
Cellulitis	Intermediate	Increased

VII. TREATMENT. In general, antibiotic therapy in combination with surgical therapy is required for successful management of maxillofacial osteomyelitis. Additional factors that involve successful treatment include:

1. Optimize nutrition for wound healing and bone healing.

2. Correct any vascular issues that may contribute to bone hypoxia or ischemia (e.g., arterial insufficiency, anemia).

3. Optimize any metabolic derangement or electrolyte abnormality.

4. Optimize diabetes control as elevated glucose (greater than or equal to 180 mg/dL) impairs neutrophil dysfunction and wound healing.

5. Offer smoking cessation, as smoking reduces blood flow to bones and contributes to ischemia as well as poor wound healing.

6. Minimize immunosuppression medications (e.g., corticosteroids, azathioprine) in an effort to improve neutrophil dysfunction and wound healing.

7. Optimize wound management.

A. **Antibiotic Therapy.** Antibiotics listed assume normal renal function. Traditionally, the duration of therapy for maxillofacial osteomyelitis is 4 to 6 weeks as based on animal models indicating that revascularization of bone following surgical debridement occurs in about 4 weeks.

Selected antibiotic regimens include:

1. *Staphylococcus aureus*

a. **Penicillin-sensitive.** Penicillin G 12 to 20 million units IV q24 or cefazolin 1 g IV q6–8. (Vancomycin 15 mg/kg IV q12–24 should be used for penicillin-allergic patients; however, *the vancomycin dose may need adjustments to maintain a serum trough level between 15 and 20 mcg/mL.*)

b. **Penicillin-resistant but oxacillin-sensitive.** Nafcillin or oxacillin 1 to 2 g IV q4–6 or cefazolin 1 to 2 g IV q4–6. (Vancomycin should be used for penicillin-allergic patients.)

   c. **Oxacillin-resistant (e.g., methicillin-resistant *S. aureus*).** Vancomycin 15 mg/kg IV q12–24. (*The vancomycin dose may need adjustments to maintain a serum trough level between 15 and 20 mcg/mL.*) Alternatives include daptomycin 6 to 12 mg/kg IV q24 (6 mg/kg dosing is recommended) or clindamycin 600 mg IV or PO q6 (should only be used if the organism is susceptible).

  2. **Coagulase-negative staphylococci (e.g., *S. epidermidis*).** While the majority is oxacillin-resistant, treatment would be vancomycin 15 mg/kg IV q12–24. If oxacillin-sensitive, then use nafcillin or oxacillin 1 to 2 g IV q4–6.

  3. ***Streptococcus* species.** Penicillin G 2 million units IV q4, or ampicillin 2 g IV q6, or ceftriaxone 1 to 2 g IV q24. (Clindamycin 600 mg IV q6 may be used in patients with a true anaphylactic reaction to penicillin.)

  4. ***Enterococcus* species.** Ampicillin 2 g IV q4 *plus or minus* gentamicin 1 mg/kg IV q8 or vancomycin 15 mg/kg IV q12–24. For isolates-resistant vancomycin, consider using daptomycin 6–12 mg/kg IV q24 (6 mg/kg dosing is most common) or linezolid 600 mg IV or PO q12.

  5. **Enteric gram-negative rods (e.g., Enterobacteriaceae).** Ampicillin-sulbactam 1.5 to 3 g IV q6 (*use of this agent may be limited by high resistance rates*) or ceftriaxone 1 to 2 g IV q24 or ciprofloxacin 400 mg IV (or 500 mg PO) q8–12.

  6. ***Pseudomonas aeruginosa.*** Cefepime or ceftazidime 2 g IV q8–12; ciprofloxacin 400 mg IV (500 mg PO) q8–12; meropenem 1 g IV q8 hours.

  7. ***Propionibacterium acnes.*** Penicillin G 20 million units IV q24 continuously or in six divided doses or ceftriaxone 2 g IV q24 or Clindamycin 600 to 900 mg IV q8 or vancomycin IV 15–20 mg/kg q12.

  8. **Anaerobes.** Clindamycin 600 mg IV or PO q6 or metronidazole 500 mg IV or PO q6–8.

B. **Surgical Therapy.** It is generally accepted that a combination of antimicrobial and surgical therapy is required for a successful outcome. Maxillofacial surgical corrective measures include sequestrectomy, saucerization, and decortication. The principles of operative treatment include:

  1. Early diagnosis that reduces morbidity and extent of disease.

  2. Adequate drainage of abscesses and extensive debridement of infected and necrotic tissue. Debridement should be performed until punctuate bleeding is noted and there is marginal resection of more than 5 mm.

  3. Dead space management (i.e., bone grafts or antibiotic impregnated material) and appropriate soft-tissue coverage (i.e., muscle flaps).

  4. Bone stabilization with plates, screws, rods, and fixation devices if needed.

BIBLIOGRAPHY

Bernier S, Clermont S, Maranda G, et al. Osteomyelitis of the jaws. *J Can Dent Assoc.* 1995;61(5):441–442, 445–448.

Douglass AB, Douglass JM. Common dental emergencies. *Am Fam Physician.* 2003;67(3):511–516.

Krakowiak PA. Alveolar osteitis and osteomyelitis of the jaws. *Oral Maxillofac Surg Clin North Am.* 2011;23(3):401–413.

Morrison A, Khan A, Tetradis S, et al. Osteonecrosis of the jaw: an update for dentists. *J Can Dent Assoc.* 2015;81:f19.

Robertson D, Smith AJ. The microbiology of the acute dental abscess. *J Med Microbiol.* 2009; 58(2):155–162.

Schuknecht B, Valavanis A. Osteomyelitis of the mandible. *Neuroimaging Clin North Am.* 2003;13(3): 605–618.

Suei Y, Taquchi A, Tanimoto K. Diagnosis and classification of mandibular osteomyelitis. *Oral Surg Oral Med Oral Pathol Oral Radiol Endod.* 2005;100(2):207–214.

37

SEPTIC ARTHRITIS

William F. Wright

I. INTRODUCTION

A. Definition. An inflammatory disorder of a joint, or multiple joints (arthritis), caused by infection with a microorganism (septic) that can lead to joint destruction.

B. Epidemiology. The incidence of septic arthritis ranges widely, between 4 and 40 cases per 100,000 person-years.

C. Pathogenesis. Normally, the **synovium** (similar to egg white) consists of two layers that are sterile:

1. **Outer; subintimal layer.** A fibrous layer containing small blood vessels.

2. **Inner; intimal layer.** The layer that contains a **membrane** with **fibroblasts** and **macrophages**. Fibroblasts produce a lubricating polysaccharide called **hyaluronan**. This layer lacks a protective basement membrane.

   Most commonly, septic arthritis is the result of bacteria that deposit within the synovial membrane as a result of a bloodstream infection (e.g., bacteremia). Less commonly, bacteria can be introduced by **direct inoculation** such as trauma, surgical procedures, or iatrogenic needle stick as with corticosteroid injection.

   Following deposition of bacteria within the joint, an inflammatory response is initiated with inflammatory cells (e.g., neutrophils), cytokines, reactive oxygen species, and proteinases that lead to joint destruction. Additionally, the inflammatory response induces a **joint effusion** that adds to joint destruction through increasing joint-space pressure, mechanically reducing blood flow (ischemia), and reducing joint-space nutrients.

D. Risk Factors. The risk factors for septic arthritis are associated with conditions that **increase the risk of bacteremia** or **predispose the joint to infection** (joint inflammation or damage) and include:

1. **Joint predisposition.** Inflammatory or noninflammatory joint injury. Abnormal joint architecture is one of the most important risk factors for septic arthritis as seen in patients with rheumatoid arthritis (RA), crystal-induced arthritis, and Charcot's arthropathy. Although underlying joint disease is a primary risk factor for septic arthritis, disease-modifying antirheumatic drugs (DMARDs) that may limit joint destruction due to rheumatologic disease appear to paradoxically increase the risk of joint infection.

   Risk factors include:

   a. RA or systemic lupus erythematosus (SLE)

   b. Osteoarthritis

    c. Trauma or prior surgery (e.g., prosthetic joint placement)

    d. Gout or pseudogout

    e. Joint-space injection with corticosteroids

  2. Predisposition to bacteremia

    a. Intravenous (IV) catheters, hemodialysis catheter, and intravenous drug use (IVDU)

    b. Diabetes mellitus

    c. Cirrhosis

    d. Chronic kidney disease

    e. Hypogammaglobulinemia or complement deficiency

    f. Hematologic or solid organ malignancy and chemotherapy

    g. Alcoholism, low socioeconomic and education status

    h. Extremes of age

    i. Psoriasis, eczema, and cutaneous ulcers or infection

    j. Anti-inflammatory or immunosuppressive therapy

    k. Urinary tract or gastrointestinal-related infections

    l. Promiscuity and/or male homosexuality (e.g., gonorrhea infection)

    m. Menstruation or pregnancy (i.e., concurrent disseminated gonorrhea infection)

E. Differential Diagnosis. Other conditions that can occur either alone or simultaneously with septic arthritis that should be considered include:

  1. Crystal-induced arthritis. Monosodium urate gout or calcium pyrophosphates dehydrate gout.

  2. Reactive arthritis (e.g., psoriasis, inflammatory bowel disease).

  3. Chronic inflammatory arthritis (e.g., RA, systemic lupus, psoriatic arthritis).

II. MICROBIOLOGY OF SEPTIC ARTHRITIS. Traditionally, the microorganisms causing septic arthritis have been classified as:

A. Gonococcal-Related Septic Arthritis. Most commonly caused by *Neisseria gonorrhoeae* organisms that belong to the protein 1-A serotype (i.e., more invasive serotype). Associated with high-risk sexual activity and/or terminal complement deficiencies.

B. Nongonococcal-Related Septic Arthritis

  1. Bacteria. Most common group of microorganisms.

    a. *Staphylococcus aureus* (accounts for approximately 60%–75 % of joint infections). Most common and more likely associated with RA, diabetes mellitus, or IVDU.

    b. *Streptococcus* **spp.** Second most common group with *S. pyogenes* often associated with autoimmune diseases, chronic skin conditions, or trauma. Groups B, C, F, and G are more often associated with immunodeficiency, *diabetes mellitus*, malignancy, or genitourinary or gastrointestinal infections.

   c. **Coagulase-negative staphylococci.** Usually in association with prosthetic devices.

   d. **Enteric gram-negative rods.** *Escherichia coli* is the most common in association with IVDU and genitourinary or gastrointestinal infections. *Shigella* spp, *Yersinia* spp, *Salmonella* spp (especially in association with sickle cell disease and iron overload states), or *Campylobacter* spp may cause septic arthritis in association with infectious diarrhea.

   e. *Pseudomonas aeruginosa.* Most commonly associated with IVDU, nosocomial infections, or puncture wounds of the foot through a shoe.

   f. **Anaerobes.** Unusual and commonly associated with diabetes mellitus or bite wounds.

   g. *Kingella kingae.* A leading cause of septic arthritis in children.

   h. *Eikenella corrodens.* Associated with a human bite.

   i. *Pasteurella multocida.* Associated with a dog or cat bite.

   j. *Streptobacillus moniliformis.* Associated with a rat bite or scratch.

   k. *Borrelia burgdorferi.* Lyme tick exposure.

   l. *Brucella* spp. Associated with ingestion of unpasteurized dairy products.

   m. *Mycoplasma hominis* and *Ureaplasma urealyticum.* Associated with hypogammaglobulinemia.

   n. *Mycobacterium tuberculosis* and *M. marinum.* *M. tuberculosis* is associated with immunocompromised patients and either pulmonary or extrapulmonary disease. *M. marinum* usually involves small joints and associated with exposure to fish water (e.g., domestic fish tanks).

   o. *Tropheryma whippelii* **(Whipple disease).** Migratory arthritis in association with diarrhea, weight loss, and malabsorption.

   p. *Neisseria meningitidis.*

2. **Fungi.** Usually a chronic arthritis involving one or more joints in association with immunosuppression and/or a particular geographic location.

   a. *Sporothrix schenckii.* Associated with soil exposure and/or gardening.

   b. *Coccidioides immitis.* Most commonly involves the knee and residence, or recent travel, in the Southwestern United States.

   c. *Blastomyces dermatitidis.* Associated with soil or dust exposure containing decomposed wood (north-central and southern United States).

   d. *Paracoccidioides brasiliensis*

   e. *Candida albicans* (yeast)

   f. *Pseudallescheria (Scedosporium) boydii*

   g. *Histoplasma capsulatum*

3. **Viral.** Most viral-related cases are thought to *be an immune-mediated process* rather than *direct viral invasion.*

   a. **Rubella and mumps viruses**

   b. **Parvovirus B19**

    c. **Hepatitis B and C viruses**

    d. **Lymphocytic choriomeningitis virus**

    e. **Human T-cell lymphotropic virus I (HTLV-1) and HIV**

III. CLINICAL MANIFESTATIONS OF SEPTIC ARTHRITIS

  A. **Nongonococcal Septic Arthritis.** Classically, the clinical symptom of fever and an acutely swollen and painful joint with limited range of motion has been associated with bacterial septic arthritis.

    1. **Fever.** A fever greater than 37.5°C occurs 60% of the time.

    2. **Rigors.** Occurs with 6% of cases.

    3. **Sweats.** Occurs with 15% of cases.

    4. **Pain.** Occurs with 85% of cases.

    5. **Swelling with limited range of motion.** Occurs with 80% of cases.

    While any joint may be involved, the most common joint involved is the knee (45%), followed by the hip (15%), ankle (9%), elbow (8%), wrist (6%), and shoulder (5%). **Septic arthritis that is associated with cartilaginous joints (e.g., sternoclavicular, costochondral, sacroiliac, and pubic symphysis) is most commonly associated with IVDU.** Polyarticular arthritis is unusual with nongonococcal septic arthritis; however, it is more likely to occur in association with *S. pneumoniae*, Group B streptococci, and enteric gram-negative rods as well as be asymmetric and with at least four involved joints (10%–20% of cases).

  B. **Gonococcal Septic Arthritis.** Traditionally, gonococcal septic arthritis symptoms occur in young, sexually active individuals in association with disseminated gonococcal infection. Characteristics of gonococcal septic arthritis include:

    1. **Sex.** Gonococcal septic arthritis occurs with homosexual males, but 75% of cases are associated with menstruating or pregnant **women** (increased risk of disseminated gonococcal infection).

    2. **Arthritis.** Commonly involves multiple joints (75% of cases), is asymmetric, and migrates from one joint to the next. This is otherwise known as ***migratory arthritis*** and involves the distal joints (e.g., hands, wrists, ankles, and knees).

    3. **Dermatitis.** The characteristic rash *(erythematous papules that progress to vesicle or pustular lesions)* only occurs in 40% to 50% of cases.

    4. **Tenosynovitis.** Characterized as pain, swelling, and periarticular erythema and occurs in 21% of cases (most commonly the wrist).

    5. **Urethritis or vaginal discharge.** Occurs in 30% of cases.

IV. APPROACH TO THE PATIENT

  A. **History.** Differentiating septic arthritis and other causes of an acutely swollen, painful joint (e.g., gout, pseudogout) can be challenging. **Physicians must have a high clinical concern for septic arthritis in a patient presenting with acute onset of joint(s) pain, swelling, and restricted motion, as this is a common medical emergency.**

Constitutional symptoms such as fever, chills, or rigors may be present in patients with septic arthritis, although their sensitivities are very low.

When taking the history, focus on:

1. Identification of an underlying risk factor (see the preceding).

2. Comorbid illnesses, medications (especially medications that predispose to immunosuppression or gout such as corticosteroids, chemotherapy, and diuretics), and exposures (e.g., ticks).

3. A detailed sexual history should be obtained to determine the risk of a sexually transmitted infection, especially gonococcal disease.

B. **Physical Examination.** A complete history and physical examination should be performed, but no finding on examination is specific for septic arthritis. Areas of focus on the physical examination include:

1. **Vital signs.** Elevated fever and pulse rate in association with a decreased blood pressure may suggest bacteremia and sepsis.

2. **Conjunctiva.** Subconjunctival hemorrhages may suggest staphylococcal bacteremia and endocarditis.

3. **Cardiovascular examination.** A new diastolic murmur (indicating valvular regurgitation) or change with existing murmur may suggest endocarditis. Tachycardia with associated hypotension may also suggest bacteremia and sepsis. It is also important to identify any vascular catheters that may lead to a bloodstream infection (e.g., peripherally inserted central catheter [PICC], hemodialysis catheter).

4. **Abdominal examination.** Localized pain such as right upper quadrant (RUQ; biliary tract infection), right lower quadrant (RLQ; appendicitis), left lower quadrant (LLQ; diverticulitis), suprapubic discomfort (cystitis), and costovertebral angle (CVA) tenderness (pyelonephritis) may suggest a gastrointestinal or genitourinary cause for bacteremia and septic arthritis. Splenomegaly in association with adenopathy may suggest immunosuppression due to a hematologic malignancy.

5. **Dermatologic examination.** The findings of nail-bed splinter hemorrhages, Janeway lesions, and Osler nodes may suggest endocarditis. Subcutaneous nodules may suggest rheumatoid arthritis or gout (gouty tophi). Erythematous papules may suggest gonococcal disease. Surgical scars overlying joints may suggest implanted prosthetic devices. Additional skin lesions to identify that may be helpful in cases of polyarthritis as well as with determining immune status include: **psoriatic plaques** (this may suggest psoriatic arthritis and is characterized by well-demarcated areas of hyperkeratosis on extensor surfaces), **eczema lesions,** and **acanthosis nigricans** (hyperpigment of skin folds associated with diabetes).

6. **Musculoskeletal examination.** This is the most important aspect of the physical examination and should always be performed to detect joint swelling (i.e., joint effusion), changes with range of motion, and joint deformities (i.e., subluxation). *An infected joint is usually indicated by a single joint in association with rapid fluctuant swelling and joint pain and tenderness with diminished range of **passive** motion. Severe limitation of **active** range of motion may be involved but tends to suggest involvement of muscles and/or ligaments and tendons.*

C. Laboratory Studies

1. **Complete blood count (CBC).** A peripheral white blood cell (WBC) count is often elevated in nongonococcal septic arthritis and elevated in half the cases of gonococcal septic arthritis.

2. **Erythrocyte sedimentation rate (ESR) and C-reactive protein (CRP).** Elevated levels are common but nonspecific. Additionally, evaluation of serial levels may be helpful in monitoring the response to therapy.

3. **Complete metabolic profile (CMP).** Electrolyte, renal, and liver tests are routinely ordered but nonspecific to the diagnosis of septic arthritis. Abnormalities (such as a reduced serum HCO_3 or elevated serum creatinine) are poor prognostic indicators and may alter the choice and dosing of antibiotic therapy.

4. **Prothrombin time (PT)/partial thromboplastin time (PTT).** Anticoagulation studies should be evaluated prior to any invasive test or procedure.

5. **Blood cultures.** At least two sets (a set is equal to one aerobic and one anaerobic bottle) should be ordered prior to initiating antibiotics. Positive cultures are found in half the cases of nongonococcal septic arthritis and rarely with gonococcal disease.

6. **Gonococcal and *Chlamydia trachomatis* DNA testing.** Nucleic acid detection methods are generally associated with very high sensitivities (97%–98%) and specificities (99%) but can be associated with a 5% false-negative rate.

   First-void urine samples are commonly used, but swab samples of the urethra, endocervix, vagina (obtained exclusively in prepubertal females), pharynx, and rectum may also be collected for testing.

7. **Uterine endocervix culture.** Approximately 80% to 90% of women with gonococcal septic arthritis show positive cultures (grown on chocolate or Thayer–Martin media).

8. **Pharyngeal and/or urethral cultures.** Approximately 50% to 75% of men with gonococcal septic arthritis demonstrate positive cultures.

9. **Urinalysis.** Gonococcal nucleic acid amplification testing may be helpful if cultures are not obtained (see the preceding).

10. **Synovial fluid analysis.** Traditionally, a synovial fluid WBC count greater than 50,000 cells/mm³ was an indication for antibiotics in native joints (the cutoff for WBC count is much lower in prosthetic joint septic arthritis). However, 33% of patients with native joint septic arthritis have counts less than 50,000 cells/mm³. The most important indicator of septic arthritis is a rising synovial WBC count and greater than 90% neutrophils on differential. Evaluation of synovial fluid glucose and protein may be performed, but abnormalities are nonspecific for septic arthritis. Synovial fluid lactate dehydrogenase (LDH) is 100% sensitive for septic arthritis, but the specificity is poor. *Synovial fluid should also be examined by polarizing microscopy for crystals of gout and pseudogout; however, crystal-induced arthropathy and infection can occur simultaneously.*

11. **Synovial fluid culture.** The Gram stain and culture of synovial fluid is the best diagnostic tool for septic arthritis.

  a. **Nongonococcal septic arthritis**

    i. **Gram stain.** Effective in 50% of cases.

    ii. **Culture.** Positive in 90% of cases (especially when inoculated into blood culture bottles rather than solid media).

  b. **Gonococcal septic arthritis**

    i. **Gram stain.** Often negative.

    ii. **Culture.** Positive in less than 50% of cases.

    iii. **Polymerase chain reaction (PCR).** Some assays demonstrate 78% sensitivity and 96% specificity.

  12. **Serology.** May be helpful in cases suspected to be due to Lyme disease, brucellosis, and Q fever.

D. **Radiography Studies.** In general, imaging tests are not helpful in the discrimination between septic arthritis and nonseptic inflammatory arthritis.

  1. **Plain-film radiography.** This imaging method is commonly ordered and most helpful as the infectious process develops with the most common findings to include soft-tissue changes of **fat-pad displacement** (joint capsule distention) and **joint-space widening** (due to localized edema). Late changes noted on plain films may include findings of **joint-space narrowing** (due to cartilage destruction) and/or **osteomyelitis**.

  2. **Ultrasonography.** The best method of detecting early intra- and extra-articular effusions as well as guide aspiration and/or drainage procedures, which is also noninvasive and devoid of ionizing radiation.

  3. **CT.** Of limited utility with early septic arthritis but is more sensitive in visualizing soft-tissue changes (e.g., joint capsule distention, joint-space widening, and bone erosions or osteitis).

  4. **MRI.** Most helpful for early detection of infections (e.g., effusions, abscesses, sinus tracts, and osteomyelitis) and soft-tissue edema (seen as high signal on T2-weighted images).

Proposed Case Definition for Bacterial Septic Arthritis

The case definition of septic arthritis requires one of four points to be met:
(1) Isolation of an organism from an affected joint
(2) Isolation of an organism from another source with a concomitant swollen, warm joint
(3) Clinical features and turbid joint fluid in the presence of previous antibiotic therapy, and/or
(4) Histologic or radiologic evidence consistent with septic arthritis

Source: From Newman JH. Review of septic arthritis throughout the antibiotic era. *Ann Rheum Dis.* 1976;35:198–205; Mathews CJ, Weston VC, Jones A, et al. Bacterial septic arthritis in adults. *Lancet.* 2010;375:846–855.

V. **TREATMENT.** Septic arthritis is considered a **true medical emergency** owing to rapid joint destruction and increased mortality rate (ranging from 7%–15%); therefore, the therapy for nongonococcal septic arthritis consists of **antimicrobial therapy** and **early joint-space drainage (less than 72 hours)** because of the potential for significant joint-space destruction. Surgical drainage of gonococcal septic arthritis is rarely indicated, and treatment usually consists of antimicrobial therapy alone.

A. Gonococcal Septic Arthritis

1. **Antibiotic treatment.** Traditionally, the duration of therapy has been **10 to 14 days**. Suggested therapy includes ceftriaxone 1 g intramuscular (IM) or IV q24 or ciprofloxacin 500 mg IV or PO q12. *Ciprofloxacin is usually not considered first-line therapy owing to the emergence of fluoroquinolone-resistant strains.*

   Patients should also receive 1 g azithromycin orally or doxycycline 100 mg orally twice daily for 7 days for dual coverage of gonococcal infection and potential Chlamydia trachomatis *coinfection.*

2. **Surgical treatment.** Usually only required for the initial synovial fluid aspirate needed for analysis.

B. Nongonococcal Septic Arthritis

1. **Antibiotic treatment.** The duration of therapy is usually **21 to 28 days,** but if osteomyelitis is present then a duration of **4 to 6 weeks** is recommended. Selected antibiotic regimens may include:

   a. *Staphylococcus aureus*

   i. **Penicillin-sensitive.** Penicillin G 2 million units IV q4 or cefazolin 1 g IV q6–8. (Vancomycin 15 mg/kg IV q12–24 should be used for penicillin-allergic patients, but *the vancomycin dose may need adjustment to maintain a serum trough level between 15 and 20 mcg/mL.)*

   ii. **Penicillin-resistant but oxacillin-sensitive.** Nafcillin or oxacillin 1 to 2 g IV q4–6 or cefazolin 1 to 2 g IV q4–6. (Vancomycin should be used for penicillin-allergic patients.)

   iii. **Oxacillin-resistant (e.g., methicillin-resistant** *S. aureus*). Vancomycin 15 mg/kg IV q12–24. (*The vancomycin dose may need adjustment to maintain a serum trough level between 15 and 20 mcg/ mL.)* Alternatives include daptomycin 6–12 mg/kg IV q24 (6 mg/kg dosing is most common) or clindamycin 600 mg IV or PO q6 (should only be used if the organism is susceptible).

   b. **Coagulase-negative staphylococci (e.g.,** *S. epidermidis*). Owing to the majority of isolates being oxacillin-resistant, treatment would be with vancomycin 15 mg/kg IV q12–24. (*The vancomycin dose may need adjustments to maintain a serum trough level between 15 and 20 mcg/mL.)* If oxacillin-sensitive, then use nafcillin or oxacillin 1 to 2 g IV q4–6.

   c. **Streptococci.** Penicillin G 2 million units IV q4 or ampicillin 2 g IV q6 or ceftriaxone 1 to 2 g IV q24. (*Clindamycin 600 mg IV q6 should be used in patients with a true anaphylactic reaction to penicillin.)*

   d. **Enterococcus.** Ampicillin 2 g IV q4 *plus or minus* gentamicin 1 mg/kg IV q8 or vancomycin 15 mg/kg IV q12–24. For isolates resistant to vancomycin, consider using daptomycin 6 to 12 mg/kg IV q24 (6 mg/kg dosing is most common) or linezolid 600 mg IV or PO q12.

   e. **Enteric gram-negative rods (e.g., Enterobacteriaceae).** Ampicillin–sulbactam 1.5 to 3 g IV q6 (*use of this agent is limited by high resistance rates*) or ceftriaxone 1 to 2 g IV q24 or ciprofloxacin 400 mg IV (or 500 mg PO) q8–12.

       f. _Pseudomonas aeruginosa._ Cefepime or ceftazidime 2 g IV q8–12; ciprofloxacin 400 mg IV (500 mg PO) q8–12; meropenem 1 g IV q8.

       g. Anaerobes. Clindamycin 600 mg IV or PO q6; metronidazole 500 mg IV or PO q6–8.

  2. Surgical treatment. Joint drainage through a single or daily arthrocentesis typically drains infected material, resolves effusions, and improves pain. Arthrocentesis improves blood flow for delivery of nutrients and antibiotics as well as removes bacteria, toxins, and enzymes that can lead to joint destruction. Persistent effusion despite 7 days of arthrocentesis, soft-tissue extension of infection (e.g., abscess), or osteomyelitis is an indication for arthroscopy or open surgical drainage.

  3. Adjuvant corticosteroid treatment. Joint destruction in infectious arthritis is driven primarily by the inflammatory response to the invading organism. With this in mind, systemic corticosteroid administration may be considered as adjunctive therapy. IV dexamethasone 0.15 mg/kg per dose q6 for a duration of 4 days beginning before or within 2 hours of antibiotic treatment may be considered as adjuvant therapy.

BIBLIOGRAPHY

Horowitz DL, Katzap E, Horowitz S, et al. Approach to septic arthritis. *Am Fam Physician.* 2011;84(6):653–660.

Margaretten ME, Kohlwes J, Moore D, et al. Does this adult patient have septic arthritis? *JAMA.* 2007;297(13):1478–1488.

Mathews CJ, Weston VC, Jones A, et al. Bacterial septic arthritis in adults. *Lancet.* 2010;375(9717): 846–855.

Newman JH. Review of septic arthritis throughout the antibiotic era. *Ann Rheum Dis.* 1976;35: 198–205.

Ross JJ. Septic arthritis. *Infect Dis Clin North Am.* 2005;19(4):799–817.

Sharff KA, Richards EP, Townes JM. Clinical management of septic arthritis. *Curr Rheumatol Rep.* 2013;15(6):332 (9-pages).

Shirtliff ME, Mader JT. Acute septic arthritis. *Clin Microbiol Rev.* 2002;15(4):527–544.

PERIPROSTHETIC JOINT INFECTIONS

William F. Wright

I. INTRODUCTION

A. Definition. An inflammatory condition that involves an implanted prosthetic orthopedic device (i.e., joint arthroplasty), most commonly the knee or hip joint, which is caused by infection with either bacteria or fungi.

B. Classification. There are three traditional classifications for periprosthetic joint infections based on the onset of infection following implantation.

1. **Early prosthetic infection.** Usually occurs within 1 to 3 months after prosthetic implantation.

2. **Delayed prosthetic infection.** An infection occurring within 3 to 24 months.

3. **Late prosthetic infection.** An infection occurring after 24 months.

An alternative classification system divided prosthetic joint infections by the duration of symptoms and may be more relevant to treatment and outcomes:

4. **Symptoms less than 4 weeks**. Implant can likely be preserved.

5. **Symptoms greater than 4 weeks**. Implant likely needs to be removed.

C. Pathogenesis. In general, both early and delayed infections are most often associated with skin bacteria (e.g., *Staphylococcus* or *Streptococcus*) introduced (or inoculated) during the immediate perioperative period. Additionally, early postoperative infections (i.e., secondarily infected hematoma or surgical incision site) can also provide a contiguous source infection. Late infections are more commonly associated with a bloodstream infection caused by a distant infection (e.g., urinary tract infection [UTI], gastrointestinal or biliary tract infection, dental infection, or endocarditis).

While prosthetic devices are sterile on implantation, they lack a microcirculation needed for immune defense (i.e., a periprosthetic immune-incompetent inflammatory area). Additionally, neutrophils that come into direct contact with prosthetic devices are activated with the release of granule contents important for immune defense. Release of these contents deactivates neutrophils for subsequent interactions with microorganisms. Prosthetic joint infections develop because of the following sequence of events:

1. Microorganisms gain access by direct inoculation or by a bloodstream infection (e.g., bacteremia, sepsis).

2. Microorganisms have a greater affinity to prosthetic material.

3. Microorganisms attach to the prosthesis and multiply as a result of a reduced local host defense.

4. Microorganisms produce a glycocalyx film or polysaccharide matrix called *biofilm* that protects the microbes from immune defenses.

D. **Epidemiology.** In general, the incidence of infection following implantation of a prosthetic orthopedic joint is less than 2%. Specific rates include:

1. **Knee prosthetic infections.** 0.8% to 1.9% incidence.

2. **Hip prosthetic infections.** 0.3% to 1.7% incidence.

E. **Risk Factors.** The risk of developing a prosthetic joint infection is based on two main factors:

1. **Patient-related risks.** These factors are derived from the patient, and this group is further divided into:

   a. **Systemic factors.** These factors increase infection risk because of increased risk of bloodstream infection or poor wound healing and include:

      i. **Advanced age** (age greater than or equal to 65)

      ii. **Obesity** (body mass index [BMI] greater than or equal to 30)

      iii. **Diabetes mellitus** (more commonly associated with chronic, uncontrolled disease)

      iv. **Rheumatoid arthritis** (especially patients receiving immune modulating medications)

      v. **Malignancy** (especially patients receiving chemotherapy)

      vi. **Corticosteroid administration** (most commonly long-term administration)

      vii. **Immunosuppression** (e.g., HIV, transplant patients)

      viii. **Tobacco abuse**

      ix. **Alcohol abuse**

      x. **Intravenous drug use (IVDU)**

      xi. **UTI**

   b. **Local factors.** These are local factors that increase the risk of infection and include:

      i. **Revision of a prosthetic joint** involving the same joint

      ii. **Emergent or urgent implantation** of a prosthetic joint to treat a fracture

      iii. **Anatomical location** (the risk of infection is greater for the knee as compared to the hip)

      iv. **Perioperative wound complication** (e.g., cellulitis, seroma, or hematoma). The persistent drainage of a wound for greater than 5 days following implantation and/or wound site hematoma may be more likely to result in infection

      v. **Postoperative complications** such as UTI, uncontrolled atrial fibrillation, acute coronary event, or requirement for blood transfusion

2. **Nonpatient-related risks.** These factors include surgeon experience and centers with low-volume surgical procedures and high rates of nosocomial infections.

II. MICROBIOLOGICAL CAUSES OF PERIPROSTHETIC JOINT INFECTIONS.
Although no microorganism may be identified (most commonly related to prior antibiotic administration) in as many as 11% of cases, the most commonly identified microorganisms include:

A. **Coagulase-Negative Staphylococci** *(e.g., S. epidermidis).* Most common and account for 30% to 40% of cases.

B. ***Staphylococcus aureus.*** Second most common organism accounting for 10% to 20% of cases.

C. **Streptococci (e.g., Group A or B streptococci).** May account for 10% of cases.

D. **Enterococci.** May account for 5% to 10% of cases.

E. **Enteric Gram-Negative Rods (e.g.,** *Escherichia coli***) and** *Pseudomonas aeruginosa.* Account for 1% to 5% of cases.

F. **Anaerobic Bacteria.** Unusual to cause prosthetic joint infections but may account for 1% to 5% of cases. Microbes include *Bacteroides* spp, *Clostridium* spp, *Prevotella* spp, and *Veillonella* spp.

G. **Polymicrobial.** May account for as many as 20% of cases (most commonly *S. aureus* and anaerobes).

Microorganisms that are **uncommonly** associated with prosthetic joint infections include:

H. **Bacteria**

   1. ***Propionibacterium acnes.*** Commonly associated with shoulder prosthetic joints

   2. ***Corynebacterium jeikeium***

   3. ***Listeria monocytogenes.*** Associated with the consumption of unpasteurized dairy products, extremes of age, and immunocompromised patients

   4. ***Actinomyces* spp and *Nocardia* spp.** Associated with immunocompromised patients

   5. ***Salmonella* spp.** Associated with infection in patients with sickle cell disease, collagen vascular disease, and HIV

   6. ***Haemophilus influenzae.*** Associated with infection in patients with systemic lupus erythematosus (SLE), hypogammaglobulinemia, EtOH abuse, and multiple myeloma

   7. ***Moraxella catarrhalis.*** Associated with collagen vascular diseases or chronic lung diseases (e.g., interstitial lung diseases)

   8. ***Brucella melitensis.*** Transmitted from animals through unpasteurized infected milk

   9. ***Pasteurella multocida.*** Associated with skin infections following the bite of a dog or cat

  10. ***Mycobacterium tuberculosis* and nontuberculous mycobacteria.** Associated with infection in immunocompromised patients

  11. ***Tropheryma whipplei***

I. **Fungi.** Rare causes but more common in immunocompromised patients.

 1. *Candida* **spp** (yeast pathogen)

 2. *Aspergillus* **spp**

 3. *Histoplasma capsulatum*

 4. *Sporothrix schenckii*

III. **CLINICAL MANIFESTATIONS OF PERIPROSTHETIC JOINT INFECTIONS.** The clinical manifestations of prosthetic joint infections are variable, but the most common symptom is *pain*. This symptom occurs with or *without adequate joint motion* and may be the result of joint swelling and inflammation and/or implant loosening or instability. Although there are no classic manifestations, additional symptoms and signs include:

A. **Fever.** This occurs in the majority of patients; however, elderly or immunocompromised patients may not be able to manifest a fever response. Late infections due to a bloodstream infection may present with tachycardia and hypotension (e.g., sepsis).

B. **Joint Swelling (Effusion), Redness (Erythema), and Warmth.** This is a more common finding in early infections. The formation of draining sinus tracts is more common with delayed or late infections.

C. **Other** systemic symptoms of **chills/rigors**, **night sweats**, **malaise**, **anorexia**, and **arthralgias** may present with infection. Weight loss is more common with low-grade chronic infections.

D. **Abdominal Discomfort, Flank Pain, Dysuria or Urinary Frequency, Tooth or Jaw Pain, and Shortness of Breath or Cough** are nonspecific but in association with prosthetic joint pain may manifest with late infections.

IV. **APPROACH TO THE PATIENT**

A. **History.** A complete and accurate history should be obtained as prosthetic joint infection can be difficult to differentiate from other complications of total joint arthroplasty (i.e., dislocation or noninfectious [aseptic] loosening and fracture of the prosthesis or bone). Therefore, *always include prosthetic joint infection in the differential diagnosis for complications or failure of a prosthetic joint.* When taking a history, be sure to focus on: when and where the implant was placed, complications or prior implant infection, comorbid illnesses, medications, unusual exposures, and risk factors (Section I.E).

B. **Physical Examination.** A complete physical examination should be performed, but findings for a prosthetic joint infection are variable. There are few classic findings on examination; therefore, **physicians must have a high clinical concern for a prosthetic joint infection in patients with a prosthetic joint and new (or changing) joint pain.** Areas of the physical examination to focus on include:

 1. **Funduscopic and conjunctival examination** to detect Roth spots or hemorrhages to suggest bacteremia or endocarditis.

 2. **Cardiovascular examination** to detect a new diastolic or regurgitate murmur to suggest endocarditis.

3. **Abdominal examination** to detect localized abnormalities or pain to suggest an underlying infective process (such as UTI, biliary or gastrointestinal infection).

4. **Dermatologic examination** to detect areas of cellulitis, *sinus tracts* (sinus tracts are considered pathognomonic for prosthetic joint infections), abscesses, wound dehiscence or drainage, and old surgical scars, as well as to search for Osler nodes, Janeway lesions, and splinter hemorrhages that may suggest bacteremia and endocarditis. **Subcutaneous nodules** may suggest underlying rheumatoid arthritis (especially over joint prominences and tendon sheaths). **Acanthosis nigricans** along skin folds may suggest underlying diabetes mellitus. Additionally, "track marks" may indicate IVDU.

   Early periprosthetic infections often present with local signs of erythema, swelling, wound drainage, and/or delayed wound healing.

5. **Musculoskeletal examination.** This is the most important aspect of the physical examination and should always be performed to detect joint swelling (i.e., joint effusion), changes with range of motion, and joint deformities (i.e., subluxation that may indicate prosthetic loosening). *An infected prosthetic joint is usually indicated by a single joint in association with rapid fluctuant swelling and joint pain and tenderness with diminished range of passive motion.*

   Late periprosthetic infections often present characterized as an acute septic arthritis syndrome (see Chapter 37, Septic Arthritis).

C. **Laboratory Studies.** Patients with a new joint pain, fever, and a prosthetic joint with multiple medical comorbidities as well as examination findings concerning for infection should be admitted to the hospital for further evaluation with an orthopedic surgeon.

1. **Complete blood count (CBC).** An elevated white blood cell (WBC) count is more likely to be found with early infections and may or may not be elevated in delayed or late infections.

2. **Complete metabolic profile (CMP).** Routinely ordered, as an elevated creatinine would require dosing adjustments for certain antibiotics. Correcting abnormal electrolytes, improving nutritional parameters (e.g., albumin and prealbumin), and normalizing glucose values (especially in patients with diabetes) are helpful to the overall care of the patient. Abnormal liver enzymes may suggest an underlying biliary tract infection.

3. **Prothrombin time (PT)/partial thromboplastin time (PTT).** Abnormal values should be corrected prior to any invasive test or procedure.

4. **C-reactive protein (CRP)/erythrocyte sedimentation rate (ESR).** Markers of inflammation are routinely ordered by serial measurements (e.g., every week or every other week) and are more helpful in determining response to therapy. Preoperative values are routinely ordered but have limited value for the diagnosis of infection (especially in patients with an underlying inflammatory condition such as rheumatoid arthritis).

5. **Blood cultures.** Routinely ordered but often negative (most helpful with late infections associated with bloodstream infections). Two sets (one set is equal to one aerobic bottle and one anaerobic bottle) should be ordered prior to starting antibiotics.

6. **Sinus tract or wound swab cultures.** The correlation of these cultures to deeper periprosthetic cultures is poor (approximately 20%–50%) and most often reflect colonizing skin organisms; therefore, these cultures should be avoided.

7. **Procalcitonin level.** Elevated levels may suggest infection, but this finding is nonspecific.

D. **Synovial Fluid and Joint-Space Studies.** The most useful preoperative evaluation in a patient suspected of a prosthetic joint infection is a diagnostic aspiration of synovial fluid for analysis that should be performed over normal skin.

1. **Synovial fluid analysis.** These are studies performed prior to surgery.

   a. **Cell count and differential.** A WBC count greater than 1,700 cells/mm^3 with greater than 65% neutrophils may be suggestive of a prosthetic joint infection (most commonly with the knee; sensitivity 94%–97%; specificity 88%–98%).

   b. **Gram stain.** Routinely recommended for guidance of empirical antibiotic therapy; however, staining is often negative (sensitivity 26%; specificity 97%).

   c. **Culture.** The most reliable method for detection of a microorganism and samples should be inoculated in blood culture bottles for the best results (sensitivity 56%–75%; specificity 95%–100%).

   d. **Synovial fluid biomarkers, alpha-defensin and CRP.** The alpha-defensin and CRP assays are optimized to a cutoff value of 5.2 mg/L and 3.0 mg/L, respectively (sensitivity of 97.3% and specificity of 100%).

2. **Joint-space analysis (i.e., periprosthetic tissue analysis).** These studies are done with sample obtained at the time of surgery.

   a. **Periprosthetic tissue analysis.** At least three samples, optimally five or six, should be taken from areas of inflammation for:

      i. **Histopathologic examination.** Greater than 5 to 10 neutrophils per high-power microscopic field suggests infection (sensitivity 50%–93%; specificity 77%–100%); however, some consider as low as 1 neutrophil per high-power field may suggest infection.

      ii. **Gram stain.** Gram stain has low yield due to low bacteria count with or without prior antibiotics.

      iii. **Prosthetic culture.** Culture of various samples from a prosthetic joint that has been removed may aid in the identification of a causative microbe. Culture is also the most reliable method for detecting a microorganism and should be plated to the appropriate solid media (sensitivity 65%–94%; specificity 98%).

      Sonication culture is a method used to culture bacteria that form biofilms on the surface of prosthetic devices. This method requires removal of the prosthetic device that is then sonicated for 5 minutes after the addition of sterile lactated Ringer's solution. The resultant fluid is then cultured with appropriate bacteriologic media.

E. **Radiography Studies.** Imaging studies are rarely utilized because of their expense, limited availability, and/or image distortion due to the prosthesis.

1. **Plain-film radiography.** Limited in value for the diagnosis of infection, but periprosthetic lucency, subperiosteal reaction, prosthetic migration, and osteolysis may suggest infection.

2. **CT.** Provides improved resolution between normal and abnormal tissue but is limited due to image artifacts caused by prosthetic joint implants.

3. **MRI.** Contraindicated in patients with ferromagnetic material and can still be associated with image distortion due to nonferromagnetic implants (e.g., titanium or tantalum) but provides excellent resolution to soft-tissue changes associated with prosthetic joint infections.

4. **Nuclear scintigraphy.** Is considered the test of choice when imaging is required for the diagnosis of a prosthetic joint infection. The best method is an indium-111–labeled WBC combined technetium-99–labeled colloid imaging for the most accurate diagnosis. Technetium-99 imaging is sensitive for detecting failed implants, while an indium-111–labeled WBC image improves the detection of infection.

MSIS and IDSA Criteria for Periprosthetic Joint Infection

A. Major Criteria
1. A sinus tract that communicates with the prosthesis
2. Isolation of a virulent pathogen (e.g., *Staphylococcus aureus*) on two separate tissue or fluid culture samples obtained (perioperative aspirate and/or intraoperative) from the affected prosthesis

B. Minor Criteria
1. Purulence within the affected joint
2. Erythrocyte sedimentation rate >30 mm/hour and C-reactive protein level >10 mg/L
3. Synovial fluid leukocyte count >3,000 cells/mcL
4. Synovial fluid neutrophil percentage >65%
5. Isolation of a virulent pathogen on one separate tissue or fluid culture sample obtained (perioperative aspirate and/or intraoperative) from the affected prosthesis
6. Greater than five neutrophils per high-powered field in five high-powered fields observed on histologic analysis of periprosthetic tissue at 400× magnification

Definite PJI
1. One major criterion *or* two. Four of six minor criteria

Possible PJI
1. The presence of PJI is possible even if the aforementioned criteria are not met; the clinician should use his or her clinical judgment to determine whether this is the case after reviewing all the available preoperative and intraoperative information

---

IDSA, Infectious Diseases Society of America; MSIS, Musculoskeletal Infection Society; PJI, periprosthetic joint infection.

V. TREATMENT. The optimal goals of treatment include: remove the infection, prevent the recurrence of infection, resolve pain and clinical symptoms, and restore joint stability and function through a combined medical and surgical approach. *Alternatively, the goal for some patients may involve achieving a stable and pain-free joint with retention of a functional infected device followed by suppressive antibiotic therapy* (see the following). Unstable or acutely ill patients should be admitted to the hospital and immediately placed on empirical antimicrobial therapy.

A. Medical Therapy. *(Listed antibiotic dosing presumes normal renal function and dosing would need to be adjusted with the level of renal function.)* Although the optimal medical care for prosthetic joint infections has not been established, most agree on appropriate selection and dosing of antimicrobial agents, correction of electrolyte and metabolic abnormalities, and optimal management of comorbid illnesses (e.g., diabetes, peripheral arterial occlusive disease).

In general, the duration of antibiotic therapy is intravenous (IV) administration for **2 to 6 weeks** followed by PO administration to complete **3 months** total of therapy for **prosthetic hip infections** and **6 months** total of therapy for **prosthetic knee infections** *with implant retention or a one-stage surgical exchange procedure* (see Section V.B). The duration of therapy for patients undergoing *permanent or transient resection arthroplasty*, with or without planned reimplantation, is **4 to 6 weeks** of antimicrobial therapy for either prosthetic hip or knee infections. Total elbow, total shoulder, and total ankle periprosthetic infections can be managed the same as total hip arthroplasty (THA) related infection protocols discussed earlier. Finally, the duration of medical therapy following amputation, or joint disarticulation, of a limb involving a periprosthetic infection is either 4 to 6 weeks if there is residual infected bone and soft tissue or 24 to 48 hours if all infected bone and soft tissue have been removed.

Suggested microorganism-specific therapy includes:

1. *Staphylococcus aureus* **or coagulase-negative staphylococci.**
   a. **Oxacillin- or methicillin-sensitive.** *Nafcillin 2 g IV q4–6, cefazolin 1 to 2 g IV q8, or ceftriaxone 1 to 2 g IV q24.*
   b. **Oxacillin- or methicillin-resistant.** *Vancomycin 15 mg/kg IV q12–24 or daptomycin 6 mg/kg IV q24.* (The vancomycin dose may need adjustment to maintain a serum trough level between 15 and 20 mcg/mL.)

   The addition of *rifampin 300 mg PO q8 or 450 mg PO q12 or 900 mg PO q24* has also been suggested for rifampin-susceptible isolates in patients treated with debridement and retention or one-stage exchange surgical procedures, as this antibiotic is effective against biofilm-producing microorganisms but is associated with significant side effects.

2. *Streptococcus* **spp.** *Penicillin G 5 million units IV q6* (if the penicillin minimum inhibitory concentration [MIC] data indicate the isolate is susceptible) or *ceftriaxone 2 g IV q24.*

3. *Enterococcus* **spp**
   a. **Penicillin-sensitive.** *Penicillin G 20 to 24 million units IV q24 as a continuous infusion or q4–6 as an intermittent dosing schedule.*
   b. **Ampicillin-sensitive.** *Ampicillin 2 g IV q24 as a continuous infusion or q4–6 as an intermittent dosing schedule.*
   c. **Ampicillin-resistant.** *Vancomycin 15 mg/kg IV q12–24 or daptomycin 6 mg/kg IV q24.* (The vancomycin dose may need adjustments to maintain a serum trough level between 15 and 20 mcg/mL.)

   The addition of ***ceftriaxone*** 1 to 2 g IV q12 or ***gentamicin*** at 1 mg/kg IV q8 has also been suggested for their synergy effects and should be used for a duration of 2 to 4 weeks (gentamicin dosing 3 mg/kg IV q24 has been associated with less nephrotoxicity).

4. **Enteric gram-negative rods.** Ceftriaxone 2 g IV q24, or ciprofloxacin 400 mg IV q12 or 500 to 750 mg PO q12, or imipenem 500 to 1,000 mg IV q6 (or equivalent carbapenem antibiotic) for multidrug-resistant organisms.

5. *Pseudomonas aeruginosa. Ceftazidime* or *cefepime 2 g IV q8* in combination with an aminoglycoside antibiotic. The aminoglycoside is administered for a duration of 2 weeks.

6. **Anaerobes.** *Clindamycin 600 mg IV q6–8* or *metronidazole 500 mg IV or PO q8.*

7. *Propionibacterium acnes. Penicillin G 20 million units IV q24 as a continuous infusion or q6 as an intermittent dosing schedule. An alternative therapy is ceftriaxone 2 g IV q24.*

B. **Surgical Therapy.** The most important factors that will determine the surgical option are both device stability and patient preference. An unstable device should *always* be removed. In general, the options for surgical therapy include:

1. **Debridement with retention of the original prosthetic joint.** This option is best for patients with early infections (less than or equal to 3 months), short duration of symptoms (less than or equal to 3 weeks), intact soft tissue (i.e., no sinus tracts or tissue necrosis), or stable prosthetic joint; patients unable to tolerate a more intensive surgical procedure (i.e., full explanation of the prosthetic device); and/or those with low virulent microorganisms (*this option is not recommended for* S. aureus–*related infections*) and consists of removing infected bone or tissue and evacuating hematomas or abscesses. Exchangeable prosthetic components (e.g., polyethylene liners) that do not require complete removal are also exchanged. (*Removal of these components alone is associated with a very low cure rate.*)

2. **Revision of prosthetic joint with debridement and removal of the prosthetic device.** This option is best performed in patients with delayed or late infection (implantation greater than or equal to 3 months), long duration of symptoms (greater than or equal to 3 weeks), unstable prosthetic implant or compromised periprosthetic soft-tissue, and multidrug-resistant bacteria or a fungus. Debridement is performed as in the preceding but prosthetic removal and subsequent replacement includes:

   a. **One-stage revision.** The prosthetic device is removed followed by debridement with immediate reimplantation of a new prosthetic joint.

   b. **Two-stage revision.** The prosthetic device is removed followed by debridement with immediate implantation of a spacer that in most cases involves joint-space cement material mixed with antibiotics (e.g., vancomycin). IV antibiotics are administered with reimplantation of new prosthetic joint. This seems to be the preferred method with most success and is associated with a cure rate of 85% to 90%.

3. **Resection arthroplasty.** This is the ***permanent removal*** of a prosthetic joint when an unacceptable joint function is expected following surgery; when the surgery will not provide benefit; when refractory infections occur following multiple surgical attempts; in nonambulatory patients; or in patients with limited bone stock, poor soft-tissue coverage, or infections involving highly resistant pathogens to which there are very limited medical therapy options.

This option may also be used in immunocompromised patients or patients with active intravenous drug abuse. This option may then involve limb amputation or arthrodesis (known as "joint fusion" and is the artificial induction of joint ossification between two bones).

BIBLIOGRAPHY

Del Pozo JL, Patel R. Clinical practice. Infection associated with prosthetic joints. *N Engl J Med.* 2009;361(8):787–794.

Marculescu CE, Berbari EF, Cockerill FR, et al. Unusual aerobic and anaerobic bacteria associated with prosthetic joint infections. *Clin Orthop Relat Res.* 2006;451:55–63.

Marculescu CE, Berbari EF, Cockerill FR, et al. Fungi, mycobacteria, zoonotic and other organisms in prosthetic joint infection. *Clin Orthop Relat Res.* 2006;451:64–72.

Osmon DR, Berbari EF, Berendt AR, et al. Infectious Diseases Society of America. Diagnosis and management of prosthetic joint infection: clinical practice guidelines by the Infectious Diseases Society of America. *Clin Infect Dis.* 2013;56(1):e1–e25.

Zimmerli W, Trampuz A, Ochsner PE. Prosthetic-joint infections. *N Engl J Med.* 2004;351(16): 1645–1654.

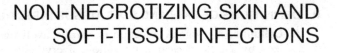

NON-NECROTIZING SKIN AND SOFT-TISSUE INFECTIONS

William F. Wright

I. **INTRODUCTION.** Skin and soft-tissue infections are the result of an acute, spreading pyogenic infection that typically involves both the epidermis and dermis that manifests as a localized area of erythema. Additionally, these infections can be classified as **uncomplicated** or **complicated**.

    A. **Uncomplicated Infections.** Defined as infections that respond to either standard antibiotics alone or a minor incision and drainage alone in a fairly healthy host.

    B. **Complicated Infections.** Defined as infections that do not respond to standard therapy, involve unusual or multidrug-resistant pathogens, are more invasive, require extensive debridement, involve systemic signs of infection, and/or a host with significant underlying comorbid illnesses.

    Furthermore, skin and soft-tissue infections can be classified as **nonpurulent** or **purulent** with classification of **mild, moderate, or severe** infection.

    C. **Nonpurulent Infections.** Cutaneous nonsuppurative inflammation devoid of pus. *Mild infection*: patients with nonpurulent infection and without systemic signs of infection. *Moderate infection*: patients with nonpurulent infection with systemic signs of infection. *Severe infection*: patients who have failed oral antibiotics or those with systemic signs of infection such as temperature greater than 38°C, tachycardia (heart rate greater than 90 beats per minute), tachypnea (respiratory rate greater than 24 breaths per minute), or abnormal white blood cell (WBC) count (greater than 12,000 or less than 400 cells/mcL) or immunocompromised patient.

    D. **Purulent Infections.** Cutaneous inflammation resulting in large amount of pus, which consists of neutrophils, dead cells, and fluid. *Mild infection*: patients with purulent infection without systemic signs of infection. *Moderate infection*: patients with purulent infection with systemic signs of infection. *Severe infection*: patients who have failed incision and drainage plus oral antibiotics or those with systemic signs of infection such as temperature greater than 38°C, tachycardia (heart rate greater than 90 beats per minute), tachypnea (respiratory rate greater than 24 breaths per minute), or abnormal WBC count (greater than 12,000 or less than 400 cells/mcL) or immunocompromised patient.

    Finally, skin and soft-tissue infections can be classified as **non-necrotizing** or **necrotizing**.

    E. **Non-Necrotizing Infections.** Usually not invasive and are devoid of devitalized or necrotic tissue.

F. **Necrotizing Infections.** Usually invasive to deeper tissues and demonstrate devitalized or necrotic areas on surgical debridement (see Chapter 40, Necrotizing Skin and Soft-Tissue Infections).

II. DEFINITIONS OF SKIN AND SOFT-TISSUE INFECTIONS

A. **Cellulitis.** A pyogenic infection primarily involving the **dermis**. It is characterized by a lack of clear demarcation of erythema, and the skin is usually not indurated.

B. **Erysipelas.** An infection involving **lymphatic tissue** and more superficial skin layers. It is typically indurated with a raised border that is clearly demarcated from normal skin.

C. **Folliculitis.** An infection involving hair follicles that typically manifests as a **pustule**.

D. **Impetigo.** A superficial skin infection that is associated with pustules or blisters (bullae) but is most commonly encountered as "honey-colored" crusts.

E. **Tinea.** Typically confined to the superficial epidermis and caused by fungi. These forms of infection usually manifest with scaling patches, plaques, or papules.

F. **Herpes.** Typically involves formation of **intraepidermal** blisters.

G. **Furuncles and Carbuncles.** Defined as **nodular** lesions within the **dermis** containing purulent material; commonly referred to as an **abscess**.

III. RISK FACTORS OF SKIN AND SOFT-TISSUE INFECTIONS

A. Any alteration of normal intact skin such as a wound, ulcer, or dermatologic **condition**

B. Trauma such as burns, crush injuries, or open **fractures**

C. Following surgical **incisions**

D. Irradiation of skin during cancer **therapy**

E. Injection drug **use**

F. Human or animal **bites**

G. Skin maceration and breakdown from exposure to saltwater or **freshwater**

H. Comorbid illnesses (e.g., diabetes, chronic renal failure, liver failure, or neutropenia) and lymphedema or arterial **insufficiency**

I. Occupational exposures (e.g., butchers, fishermen, and **veterinarians)**

IV. MICROBIAL CAUSES OF SKIN AND SOFT-TISSUE INFECTIONS. The microorganisms that are most frequently involved in **pyogenic** (bacterial) infections include: *Staphylococcus aureus* (methicillin-susceptible *Staphylococcus aureus* [MSSA] and methicillin-resistant *Staphylococcus aureus* [MRSA]) and **beta-hemolytic streptococci** (groups A, B, C, and G). However, certain conditions or exposure may provide acquisition of other specific pathogens:

A. **Diabetes.** *Staphylococcus aureus* (MSSA or MRSA), *Pseudomonas* spp, and/or *Bacteroides* spp (anaerobes).

B. **Cirrhosis.** Vibrio vulnificus (usually presents as sepsis and associated with saltwater exposure).

C. **Butcher or Veterinarian.** *Erysipelothrix* spp.

D. **Fisherman.** *Erysipelothrix* spp.

E. **Fish-Tank Exposure (for Pet Fish).** *Mycobacterium marinum.*

F. **Hot Tub Exposure.** *Pseudomonas* spp.

G. **Dog Bite.** *Pasteurella multocida* and *Capnocytophaga canimorsus.*

H. **Cat Bite.** *Pasteurella multocida.*

I. **Rat Bite.** *Streptobacillus moniliformis.*

J. **Intravenous Drug Use (IVDU).** MRSA and *Pseudomonas* spp.

K. **Tick Bite.** *Borrelia burgdorferi.*

L. **Hemochromatosis or Thalassemia.** *Vibrio vulnificus* (usually associated with ingestion of raw oysters).

M. **Systemic Lupus Erythematosus (SLE) and Nephritic Syndrome.** *Streptococcus pneumoniae.*

N. **Freshwater Exposure.** *Aeromonas* spp.

O. **Saltwater Exposure.** *Vibrio vulnificus.*

P. **Tinea Infections** are most commonly caused by three genera of fungi, also known as dermatophytes: ***Trichophyton*** (most common), ***Microsporum,*** and ***Epidermophyton***.

Q. **Candidiasis (most commonly *Candida albicans*)** often is represented as an intense erythema (beefy red) with pustules.

R. ***Malassezia furfur* Causes a Superficial Fungal Infection (Known as Tinea Versicolor) That Results in Alteration of Pigmentation (i.e., Hypo- or Hyperpigmentation).**

S. **Herpes Infections** are most commonly related to herpes simplex virus (HSV) or varicella-zoster virus (VZV).

V. **CLINICAL MANIFESTATIONS OF SKIN AND SOFT-TISSUE INFECTIONS.** The clinical manifestations of skin and soft-tissue infections are variable and depend on the anatomical site, host comorbid illnesses, immune response, and pathogen. Some manifestations have been presented (Section II).

A. **Classic Findings.** Usually include signs of inflammation: ***redness*** (rubor; due to increased blood flow to the affected area), ***warmth*** (calor; due to increased blood flow to the affected area), ***swelling*** (tumor; due to exudation of fluid), and ***tenderness or pain*** (dolor; due to mechanical and/or chemical mediators of inflammation). Often not all of the cardinal findings are found because of early treatment or the comorbid status of the host.

B. **Fever.** Usually occurs with skin and soft-tissue infections but may be absent owing to early treatment or immunodeficiency.

C. **Other Symptoms.** Fatigue, malaise, arthralgias, and myalgias (typically in association with Lyme disease) may be present. Chills may indicate associated bacteremia.

D. **Pain.** Mild tenderness and pain are part of the classic findings, but **significant pain may indicate a necrotizing skin infection**. HSV and VZV infections are

TABLE 39.1 ■ Criteria for Streptococcal Toxic Shock Syndrome

A. Isolation of group A Streptococcus by culture (from a sterile or nonsterile site)
B. Hypotension (systolic blood pressure less than 90 mmHg) and two or more of the following:
   1. Renal impairment (serum creatinine greater than 2 mg/dL)
   2. Thrombocytopenia (platelet count less than 100,000 cells/mcL or DIC
   3. Hepatic impairment (AST, ALT, or total bilirubin greater than twice the upper limit of normal)
   4. Lung injury related to inflammatory response (PaO_2/FiO_2 ratio less than 250)
   5. Generalized erythematous macular rash with a tendency to desquamate and/or involve soft-tissue necrosis

Definite case is defined as isolation of group A Streptococcus from a sterile site, hypotension, and two or more of the clinical and laboratory abnormalities.
Probable case is defined as isolation of group A Streptococcus from a nonsterile site, hypotension, and two or more of the clinical and laboratory abnormalities.

ALT, alanine aminotransferase; AST, aspartate aminotransferase; DIC, disseminated intravascular coagulopathy.

Source: Adapted from Defining the group A streptococcal toxic shock syndrome. Rationale and consensus definition. The Working Group on Severe Streptococcal Infections. *JAMA.* 1993;269:390–391.

typically associated with neuropathic pain. Diabetic patients may have decreased pain due to neuropathy.

   E. Purulent Drainage. Typically associated with abscesses caused by MRSA. While **foul-odor** drainage may indicate **anaerobic** infection, a **sweet (or fruity) odor** may indicate a ***Pseudomonas*** infection.

Toxic shock syndrome (TSS) is a rare, life-threatening clinical manifestation with certain types of skin and soft-tissue infections (Tables 39.1 and 39.2). Often TSS results from toxins produced by *Staphylococcus aureus* bacteria, but the condition may also be caused by toxins produced by group A *Streptococcus* bacteria. *Staphylococcus* TTS has been associated primarily with the use of superabsorbent tampons.

VI. APPROACH TO THE PATIENT

TABLE 39.2 ■ CDC Case Definition for Staphylococcus Toxic Shock Syndrome

A. Fever, temperature greater than 38.9°C
B. Rash, diffuse macular erythroderma with or without desquamation
C. Hypotension, systolic blood pressure less than 90 mmHg
D. Systems involvement, three or more of the following:
   1. Gastrointestinal: nausea, vomiting, or diarrhea at illness onset
   2. Musculoskeletal: myalgia or elevated serum CPK
   3. Mucous membrane hyperemia
   4. Renal: sterile pyuria and elevated BUN and serum creatinine
   5. Hematologic and hepatic abnormalities: AST, ALT, or total bilirubin greater than twice the upper limit of normal and platelet count less than 100,000 cells/mcL
   6. Central nervous system: disorientation or alterations in consciousness without focal neurologic signs

Proven case is defined as meeting ALL four criteria.
Probable case is defined as having three of the four criteria.

ALT, alanine aminotransferase; AST, aspartate aminotransferase; BUN, blood urea nitrogen; CDC, Centers for Disease Control and Prevention; CPK, creatine phosphokinase.

A. History. A complete and careful history is important in determining the potential exposure and cause of the infection. Additionally, obtain a history of IVDU, pets, recent procedure or surgery, particular hobbies/employment, and diet (e.g., raw oysters).

B. Physical Examination. A complete physical examination should be performed, as it is important to differentiate skin and soft-tissue infection from other conditions such as the following:

1. Deep vein thrombosis (DVT).

2. Acute gout (uric acid level may be elevated).

3. Drug-hypersensitivity reaction.

4. Contact dermatitis.

5. Pyoderma gangrenosa (inflammatory bowel disease).

6. Sweet disease (neutrophilic dermatosis).

7. Toxic epidermal necrolysis (TEN; usually a drug-associated exposure).

8. Carcinoma erysipeloides (most often associated with breast cancer with lymphatic involvement).

C. Laboratory Studies. These studies are important for identification of the pathogen and severity of illness.

1. **Complete blood count (CBC).** A marked elevated WBC count may indicate an invasive infection. A dramatic rise in the WBC count (greater than 50 cells/mcL) and hematocrit (HCT; greater than 60%) may suggest an infection due to **Clostridium spp.** Anemia and intravascular hemolysis may also suggest an infection due to **Clostridium perfringens**.

2. **Basic metabolic panel (BMP).** Serum chemistries may identify comorbid diseases such as diabetes or renal failure. Additionally, a low serum HCO_3 may indicate metabolic acidosis with bacteremia and/or sepsis.

3. **Uric acid.** May help differentiate a skin infection from gout.

4. **Blood cultures.** Are rarely helpful in uncomplicated skin and soft-tissue infections (less than 5%). However, blood *cultures may be helpful* in the following:

   a. Cellulitis with lymphedema

   b. Orbital cellulitis

   c. Patients with saltwater or freshwater exposure

   d. Patients hospitalized for complicated infections

   e. Patients with fever and chills (suggestive of bacteremia)

5. **Wound cultures.** *Superficial swab cultures from nonpurulent infections are **not** recommended; however, Gram stain and culture of the pus or exudates in association with purulent infections are recommended.* Cultures of skin needle aspirates or punch biopsies from nonpurulent infections are helpful in about 50% of cases involving *S. aureus* but are not practical in routine, uncomplicated cases. Needle-aspirated contents from intact bullae or vesicles may also yield positive cultures. Finally, deep cultures from abscesses or surgically obtained sources are most helpful to identify a causative pathogen.

If an unusual pathogen is suspected, the clinical microbiology laboratory should be notified for the correct culture methods.

6. **Radiography**

a. **Plain films** may be useful in identifying *gas in tissues* from an anaerobic infection such as from *Clostridium* spp.

b. **Ultrasonography** may be helpful in detecting a subcutaneous abscess. Venous duplex can also evaluate for DVT that may mimic infection.

c. **CT scan** may be helpful to identify deeper fluid collections, necrotizing fasciitis, or adjacent osteomyelitis.

d. **MRI** is helpful to identify necrotizing fasciitis (see Chapter 40).

VII. INDICATIONS FOR HOSPITALIZATION

A. Rapidly spreading area of infection.

B. Systemic signs of infection (e.g., chills and fever greater than or equal to 37.8°C).

C. Clinically significant comorbid diseases (e.g., diabetes and renal failure).

D. Immunocompromised host.

E. Need for surgical incision and drainage (e.g., abscesses or necrotizing fasciitis).

F. Limb-threatening infection (e.g., necrotizing fasciitis).

G. Complex or complicated skin infection.

H. Unusual exposure or pathogen (e.g., multidrug resistance).

I. Inadequate home situation or risk for nonadherence to medical therapy.

VIII. TREATMENT OF SKIN AND SOFT-TISSUE INFECTIONS. *(Antibiotic dosing is based on normal renal function.)*

Early surgical *incision and drainage* with systemic antimicrobial therapy is the recommended treatment for inflamed epidermoid cysts, carbuncles, abscesses, and large furuncles.

A. **Uncomplicated Infections**

1. Most cases of infections are mild to moderate in severity with a fairly normal host and due most commonly to *beta-hemolytic streptococci* or *S. aureus.*

2. *Uncomplicated abscesses less than 5 cm in diameter (most commonly due to S. aureus) can be treated effectively with incision and drainage alone.*

3. **Oral therapy** can be effectively provided in most cases, and recommended agents are:

a. **MSSA**. Dicloxacillin 500 mg q6 or cephalexin 500 mg q6.

b. **MRSA**. Doxycycline 100 mg twice daily or trimethoprim–sulfamethoxazole (TMP–SMX) DS twice daily. **Clindamycin** 300 mg three times daily may be an alternative (depending on antibiotic susceptibilities) for penicillin-allergic patients. **Linezolid** 600 mg twice daily is also an alternative for MRSA-related infections.

c. **Beta-hemolytic streptococci.** Penicillin V 250 mg three times daily, amoxicillin 250 to 500 mg three times daily, or clindamycin 300 mg three times daily.

The typical duration of treatment has *not* been well characterized but is usually *5 days* (*treatment should be extended to 10 days if the infection has improved within this time period*).

B. **Complicated Infections**

1. Patients are typically hospitalized and started on **intravenous (IV)** antibiotics.

2. Patients can usually be changed to **oral** therapy (see the preceding) when the vital signs and laboratory values are improving (or normalized) and skin findings are improving.

3. Recommendations for suggested IV antibiotics are:

   a. **MSSA.** Nafcillin 2 g q4 or cefazolin 2 g q8.

   b. **MRSA.** *Vancomycin 15 mg/kg q12, daptomycin 4 mg/kg daily, linezolid 600 mg twice daily, or tigecycline 100 mg IV load, then 50 mg intravenously twice daily.

   c. **Beta-hemolytic streptococci.** Penicillin G 2 million units q4–6, cefazolin 2 g q8, or clindamycin 600 mg q8 or ceftriaxone 2 g daily.

The duration of antimicrobial therapy has *not* been well defined but is usually a total of 5 days AFTER incision and drainage of purulent infection and resolution of systemic signs of infection for both purulent and nonpurulent infections (*treatment should be extended to 10 days if the infection has improved within this time period*). The recommended duration of therapy for pyomyositis is 2 to 3 weeks (14–21 days). A treatment of 21 to 28 days or longer may be needed for certain multidrug-resistant pathogens and/or complex infections (see the following).

C. **Recommended Antibiotics for Particular Pathogens or Conditions**

1. Diabetes. Piperacillin/tazobactam 3.375 g IV q6, *or* clindamycin 300 mg IV/PO q8 *plus* ciprofloxacin 400 mg IV q12 (500 mg PO q12) *or* meropenem 500 mg IV q8.

2. Human **or animal bite.** Ampicillin–sulbactam 3 g IV q6 *or* tigecycline 100 mg IV load, *then* 50 mg IV q12. Oral therapy can be Augmentin 250 to 500 mg q12 *or* doxycycline 100 g q12.

3. Freshwater **exposure.** Moxifloxacin 400 mg IV or PO q24, levofloxacin 500 mg IV or PO q24, *or* TMP–SMX 2.5 mg/kg IV q6 or PO q12.

4. Saltwater **exposure.** Doxycycline 200 mg IV q12 for *3 days*, then 100 mg IV q12 for a duration of *11 days*; *or* moxifloxacin 400 mg IV or PO q24 *or* levofloxacin 500 mg IV or PO q24 for a duration of *14 days*.

5. Burns. Piperacillin/tazobactam 3.375 g IV q6, doripenem 1 g IV q8, *or* meropenem 1 g IV q8.

6. Butcher, **fisher, or veterinarian.** Amoxicillin 500 mg PO q8 *or* PCN-G 12–20 MU IV q24.

7. Fish-tank **exposure (e.g.,** Mycobacterium **spp).** TMP–SMX DS PO q12 *plus* ethambutol 15 mg/kg PO q24 for 3 months *or* doxycycline 100 mg PO q12 for *3 months*.

Vancomycin is still the empirical drug of choice.

8. **Rat bite.** PCNG IV q4, *or* amoxicillin 1 g PO q8 *or* doxycycline 200 mg IV/PO q12 for *3 days*, *then* 100 mg IV/PO q12 for a duration of *11 days*.

9. **Herpes infection**

   a. **HSV.** Acyclovir 400 mg PO q8 for a duration of *10 days* or valacyclovir 1 g PO q12 for a duration of *7 to 10 days*.

   b. **VZV.** Acyclovir 800 mg PO q6 for a duration of *5 days* or valacyclovir 1 g PO q8 for a duration of *5 days*.

10. **Tinea/candidiasis.** Topical clotrimazole 1% cream q12 *or* fluconazole 200 to 400 mg PO daily for a duration of *14 days*.

D. **Recommended Adjunct Anti-Inflammatory Agents Used for Skin and Soft-Tissue Infections.**

Systemic corticosteroids (e.g., prednisone 40 mg daily for a duration of *7 days*) could be considered in nondiabetic adult patients.

BIBLIOGRAPHY

Daum RS. Clinical practice. Skin and soft-tissue infections caused by methicillin-resistant *Staphylococcus aureus*. *N Engl J Med*. 2007;357(4):380–390.

Defining the group A streptococcal toxic shock syndrome. Rationale and consensus definition. The Working Group on Severe Streptococcal Infections. *JAMA*. 1993;269:390–391.

May AK. Skin and soft-tissue infections. *Surg Clin North Am*. 2009;89(2):403–420.

Ramakrishnan K, Salinas RC, Aqudelo Hiquita NI. Skin and soft tissue infections. *Am Fam Physician*. 2015;92(6):474–483.

Stevens DL, Bisno AL, Chambers HF, et al. Infectious Diseases Society of America. Practice guidelines for the diagnosis and management of skin and soft tissue infections: 2014 update by the Infectious Diseases Society of America. *Clin Infect Dis*. 2014;59(2):e10–e52. Erratum in Stevens DL et al. *Clin Infect Dis*, 2014;59:147–159.

Stevens DL, Eron LL. Cellulitis and soft-tissue infections. *Ann Intern Med*. 2009;150(1):ITC11.

Swartz MN. Clinical practice. Cellulitis. *N Engl J Med*. 2004;350(9):904–912.

NECROTIZING SKIN AND SOFT-TISSUE INFECTIONS

William F. Wright

I. **INTRODUCTION.** Necrotizing fasciitis (NF) and necrotizing skin and soft-tissue infections are pyogenic infections of subcutaneous tissue and fascia characterized by devitalized tissue and necrosis with or without involvement of underlying muscle.

   A. **Epidemiology.** NF is a rare disease that occurs in both men and women. NF more frequently occurs during the winter months and with increasing age. The condition is associated with significant morbidity and mortality.

   B. **Pathophysiology.** Microbial invasion of tissues may occur from a breach in skin (most common) or extension from a perforated bowel. Endotoxins and exotoxins are produced leading to extensive cytokine release (systemic inflammatory response syndrome [SIRS]) with shock and multisystem organ failure.

   Fournier gangrene, named after French physician Jean Alfred Fournier, is NF of the perineum, penis, scrotum, and/or vulva. The average age at onset is 50 to 60 years. Eighty percent of patients have significant underlying diseases, particularly diabetes mellitus.

II. **MICROBIOLOGICAL CLASSIFICATIONS AND CAUSES OF NECROTIZING FASCIITIS/NECROTIZING SKIN AND SOFT TISSUES.** Three basic microbiological types have been proposed; however, classically this condition has been caused by group A beta-hemolytic streptococci (*S. pyogenes*).

   A. **Type 1 Infections (most common).** Polymicrobial.

      1. *Staphylococcus aureus.*

      2. *Streptococcus* spp (e.g., *S. pyogenes*).

      3. *Klebsiella* spp.

      4. *Escherichia coli.*

      5. **Anaerobes**: *Bacteroides* spp (e.g., *B. fragilis* group) or *Clostridium* spp (e.g., *C. welchii* and *C. septicum*). **C. septicum–related infections require gastrointestinal evaluation with its association to carcinoma of the colon.**

   B. **Type 2 Infections.** Monomicrobial.

      1. *Streptococcus pyogenes* (group A *Streptococcus*).

      2. *Staphylococcus aureus.*

C. **Type 3 Infections.** Typically involve infections due to *Vibrio vulnificus* with most patients having chronic cirrhosis or hepatitis B infection and exposure to warm saltwater.

III. RISK FACTORS FOR NECROTIZING FASCIITIS/NECROTIZING SKIN INFECTIONS

A. **Type 1 (Polymicrobial) Infections.** Typically occur in patients with the following risk factors:

1. Immunocompromised condition (e.g., cancer, renal failure, HIV infection, chronic corticosteroid use, and solid-organ or stem cell transplantation)

2. Diabetes mellitus

3. Peripheral vascular disease

4. Obesity (defined as a body mass index greater than 30)

5. Chronic alcohol abuse

6. Intravenous drug use (IVDU)

7. Surgical incisions

8. Blunt trauma

9. Insect bites

10. Indwelling catheters

B. **Type 2 (Monomicrobial) Infections.** Typically occur in healthy immunocompetent patients with the following risks:

1. Trauma

2. Surgical incisions

3. IVDU

C. **Type 3 Infections.** Associated with risks of infections from *Vibrio vulnificus* (section II.C).

IV. APPROACH TO THE PATIENT

A. **History.** A complete and careful history is important in determining the potential exposure and/or cause of the infection. Physicians must have a **high index of suspicion** with all skin and soft-tissue infections. The **classic symptoms** associated with NF/necrotizing skin infections are:

1. **Pain**. Pain is usually significant and out of proportion to the exam. **However, as tissue necrosis progresses, the involved area may become insensate.** Diabetic neuropathy may also limit a pain response.

2. **Anxiety**

3. **Diaphoresis**

B. **Physical Examination.** A complete physical examination should be performed. Common findings include: localized erythema or pallor; swelling; warmth; and pain and tenderness. Not all of the cardinal features of infection may be present as the infection and necrosis evolve. A staging system has been proposed:

1. **Early stage.** Involves erythema, tenderness, swelling, and pain out of proportion to exam.

2. **Late stage.** Manifests as insensate skin, subcutaneous emphysema, and skin necrosis with discoloration (typically violaceous, black, or gray).

Additional clinical findings include:

1. Fever and tachycardia

2. Hemorrhagic bulla

3. **Drainage of "dishwater" fluid.** This can be determined by a bedside **finger test** that involves gentle probing of the index finger through a small incision (greater than 2 cm). Lack of resistance to blunt dissection also may signify NF.

4. **Low tissue oxygen saturation.** Oxygen saturation less than 70% has 100% sensitivity and 97% specificity for NF.

C. Laboratory Evaluation

1. *The **gold standard** for the diagnosis of NF/necrotizing skin infections is surgical exploration and intraoperative biopsy for histology, Gram stain, and culture.* Findings suggestive of the diagnosis include:

   a. **Histology.** Superficial epidermal necrosis, dermal edema, and infiltration of polymorphonuclear leukocytes (PMNs).

   b. **Gram stain and culture** (see Section II). Samples obtained at the edge of living and necrotic tissue usually give the best results. Culture of skin surface samples and bulla (blister) fluid is rarely helpful.

   c. **Surgical exploration.** Typically reveals "dishwater" or foul-smelling fluid, necrosis, lack of bleeding, and loss of normal resistance to blunt probing along tissue planes.

2. **Laboratory studies** that may be helpful include:

   a. **Complete blood count (CBC).** The majority of patients will have an elevated white blood cell (WBC) count. Additionally, anemia may be present.

   b. **Basic metabolic panel (BMP).** In addition to identifying renal failure, hyponatremia, and hyperglycemia, low serum bicarbonate (HCO_3) may indicate metabolic acidosis and SIRS/sepsis.

   c. **Erythrocyte sedimentation rate (ESR), C-reactive protein (CRP), and procalcitonin.** Elevated levels are nonspecific but may suggest NF/ necrotizing skin infection.

A group of laboratory parameters, known as the **Laboratory Risk Indicator for Necrotizing Fasciitis (LRINEC) score,** has been introduced as a diagnostic tool for NF (Table 40.1). The developmental study by Wong et al. reported that a LRINEC score ≥6 had a sensitivity of 89.9%, specificity of 96.9%, positive predictive value of 92.0%, and negative predictive value of 96.0%.

3. **Radiologic studies**

   a. **Plain films** are helpful to identify edema and gas in tissues. However, these findings are not always present, and their absence does not exclude the diagnosis.

   b. **US** is generally not useful for the diagnosis of NF/necrotizing skin infections.

   c. **CT** is helpful for the identification of tissue inflammation, fascia edema and thickening, and gas (sensitivity 80%).

TABLE 40.1 ■ The LRINEC Score

Laboratory Parameter	Score
A. CRP: greater than 150 mg/dL	A. 4 points
B. Leukocytosis (WBC × 10^6/mm^3): 1. Less than 15 2. 15–25 3. Greater than 25	B. Points as follows: 1. 0 points 2. 1 point 3. 2 points
C. Hemoglobin (g/dL): 1. Greater than 13.5 2. 11–13.5 3. Less than 11	C. Points as follows: 1. 0 points 2. 1 point 3. 2 points
D. Sodium (mmol/L): less than 135	D. 2 points
E. Creatinine (mg/dL): greater than 1.6	E. 2 points
F. Glucose (mg/dL): greater than 180	F. 1 point

A score greater than 6 indicates possible necrotizing fasciitis and a score greater than 8 should strongly suggest necrotizing fasciitis.

CRP, C-reactive protein; LRINEC, Laboratory Risk Indicator for Necrotizing Fasciitis; WBC, white blood cell.

Source: From Wong CH, Khin LW, Heng KS, et al. The LRINEC (Laboratory Risk Indicator for Necrotizing Fasciitis) score: a tool for distinguishing necrotizing fasciitis from other soft tissue infections. *Crit Care Med.* 2004;32:1535–1541.

       d. MRI is the image test of choice (sensitivity 90%–100%) and has good resolution to identify soft-tissue and fascia changes (typically on T2-weighted image).

V. TREATMENT. The most important treatment modality for NF/necrotizing skin infections is *surgical debridement*; therefore, **prompt surgical consultation is recommended!** Additional management involves immediate institution of critical care support (i.e., hemodynamic support), fluid resuscitation, and intravenous (IV) broad-spectrum antibiotics. *The most important factor determining mortality is the timing of initial surgical debridement.*

A. Surgical Therapy

    1. The initial surgical debridement should occur as soon as possible, as antibiotic therapy cannot penetrate necrotic tissue adequately.

    2. Surgical excision of devitalized, necrotic, and infected tissue should be to the level of **healthy, bleeding tissue.**

    3. Serial surgical debridement is often required.

    4. Fournier gangrene may need a **temporary diverting colostomy** to facilitate wound healing and plastic reconstructive repair.

    5. Wounds are usually left open with **wet-to-dry dressings** during the initial hospitalization and then changed to **vacuum-assisted closure dressings**.

B. Antimicrobial Therapy. *(Antibiotic dosing listed assumes normal renal function.)* Since the majority of infections are polymicrobial, initiation of broad-spectrum antibiotics is recommended.

1. **Type 1 infection**. Piperacillin/tazobactam 3.375 g IV q6, meropenem 500 mg IV q8, or moxifloxacin 400 mg VI q24 can be used for infections without concern for methicillin-resistant *Staphylococcus aureus* (MRSA).

   If MRSA is of concern, then add either vancomycin 15 mg/kg IV q12, daptomycin 6 mg/kg IV q24, or linezolid 600 mg IV q12. Additionally, if MRSA is of concern, then monotherapy with tigecycline 100 mg IV load, then 50 mg IV q12 can also be used in selected patients.

2. **Type 2 infection**. Clindamycin 600 mg IV q8 is a useful agent for *Streptococcus pyogenes* (group A) as it also inhibits production of M proteins and exotoxins. Coverage for *Staphylococcus aureus* would be the same as type 1 infections.

3. **Type 3 infection**. Broad-spectrum antibiotics are used empirically, but with isolation of *Vibrio* spp the antibiotics can be changed to doxycycline 200 mg IV q12 × 3 days, then 100 mg IV q12 × 11 days *or* moxifloxacin 400 mg IV/ potassium oral (PO) q24 *or* levofloxacin 500 mg IV/PO q24.

4. *Clostridium*-**related infections**. PCN-G 10 MU IV q4 *and/or* clindamycin 600 mg IV q8.

In the absence of definitive clinical trials, the ***duration of antimicrobial therapy*** should be administered until further debridement is no longer necessary, the patient has improved clinically, and fever has been absent for 48 to 72 hours. A practical approach to this recommendation might be for a duration of 5 days AFTER the last major surgical debridement if the patient remains afebrile.

   C. **Intravenous Immunoglobulin (IVIG) Therapy**. Considered as an additional modality with surgical and medical therapy due to the theoretical mechanism of binding either streptococcal or staphylococcal exotoxins and decreasing SIRS/ sepsis. However, its efficacy remains to be proved; moreover, it is costly and not Food and Drug Administration (FDA) approved for treatment of NF/necrotizing skin infections.

   D. **Hyperbaric Oxygen Therapy**. Considered an additional modality of therapy that may or may not be of benefit for the treatment of NF/necrotizing skin infections.

BIBLIOGRAPHY

Hasham S, Matteucci P, Stanley PR, et al. Necrotizing fasciitis. *BMJ*. 2005;330(7495):830–833.

Ramakrishnan K, Salinas RC, Aqudelo Hiquita NI. Skin and soft tissue infections. *Am Fam Physician*. 2015;92(6):474–483.

Sarani B, Strong M, Pascual J, et al. Necrotizing fasciitis: current concepts and review of the literature. *J Am Coll Surg*. 2009;2008(2):279–288.

Shimizu T, Tokuda Y. Necrotizing fasciitis. *Intern Med*. 2010;49(12):1051–1057.

Stevens DL, Bisno AL, Chambers HF, et al. Infectious Diseases Society of America. Practice guidelines for the diagnosis and management of skin and soft tissue infections: 2014 update by the Infectious Diseases Society of America. *Clin Infect Dis*. 2014;59(2):e10–e52. Erratum in Stevens DL et al. *Clin Infect Dis*, 2014;59:147–159.

Wong CH, Khin LW, Heng KS, et al. The LRINEC (Laboratory Risk Indicator for Necrotizing Fasciitis) score: a tool for distinguishing necrotizing fasciitis from other soft tissue infections. *Crit Care Med*. 2004;32:1535–1541.

41

DIABETIC FOOT INFECTIONS

William F. Wright

I. INTRODUCTION

A. Definition. Diabetic foot infections are defined as any infectious process below the ankle in a patient diagnosed with diabetes.

B. The most common and classic lesion is the *mal perforans* foot ulcer (i.e., neuropathic ulcer).

C. Risk Factors. Those associated with diabetic foot infections include:

1. Peripheral **motor neuropathy** (e.g., claw toes, subluxed metatarsophalangeal joints, or callus formation).

2. Peripheral **sensory neuropathy.**

3. Peripheral **autonomic neuropathy** (e.g., dry, cracking skin).

4. Neuro-osteoarthropathy (e.g., Charçot disease).

5. Peripheral vascular disease (PVD).

6. Hyperglycemia or chronic kidney disease (CKD).

7. Inappropriate footwear or hygiene.

II. MICROBIOLOGICAL CAUSES OF DIABETIC FOOT INFECTIONS. In general, **acute infections** are often due to a **single microbial pathogen**, and **chronic infections** are often due to **multiple microbial pathogens.** Most infections are due to either a bacterial or fungal pathogen and include:

A. Bacterial Pathogens. Most infections are considered polymicrobial.

1. **Beta-hemolytic streptococcus** (groups A, B, and C) usually occur with acute infections such as an infected ulcer or cellulitis.

2. *Staphylococcus aureus* (methicillin-susceptible *Staphylococcus aureus* [MSSA] or methicillin-resistant *Staphylococcus aureus* [MRSA]) usually occur with both acute and chronic infections.

3. Gram-negative bacilli, **Enterobacteriaceae** (e.g., *Escherichia coli, Klebsiella* spp, *Proteus* spp), occur most often in patients with a previously treated infected ulcer, chronic and long-standing ulcer or wound, and in necrotic ulcers or wounds.

4. *Pseudomonas aeruginosa* most commonly occurs with ulcers or wounds of long duration or with **macerated** ulcers or wounds.

5. **Enterococci** (vancomycin-resistant *Enterococcus* [VRE] or non-VRE) most commonly occur with ulcers or wounds of long duration, with or without necrosis.

6. **Multidrug-resistant pathogens** (e.g., MRSA, VRE, or extended-spectrum beta-lactamase [ESBL]) can occur in patients exposed to prolonged, broad-spectrum antibiotic therapy.

7. **Obligate anaerobes** (e.g., *Bacteroides* spp) most commonly occur with necrotic or gangrene-associated infections.

B. **Fungal Pathogens.** Most commonly involve *Candida* spp and usually occur in association with ulcers or wounds of long duration and/or exposure to prolonged broad-spectrum antibiotic therapy.

III. CLASSIFICATION OF DIABETIC FOOT INFECTIONS. The concept for the classification of these infections includes these factors:

A. Because all skin wounds or ulcers contain microorganisms (i.e., colonization), *infection of the diabetic foot must be determined clinically.* Infection is typically suggested by one or more of the following:

1. **Systemic signs** (e.g., fever, chills, elevated white blood cell [WBC] count prior to surgery).

2. **Purulent drainage or foul odor.**

3. **More than two classic signs of infections** (e.g., warmth, swelling, redness, or tenderness).

4. **Delayed wound healing** in chronic wounds.

B. Based on the preceding, a validated clinical classification system has been developed (Table 41.1). It is presumed this classification system is used to describe a diabetic patient with a foot ulcer in order to determine whether there is an infection or not and the degree of infection (if present):

1. **Noninfected diabetic foot.** An ulceration that lacks either drainage and/ or classic manifestations of infection (see the preceding) in the surrounding tissues.

TABLE 41.1 ■ The International Working Group Classification of Diabetic Foot Infection*

Clinical Manifestation	Grade
The presence of at least two or more of the following: localized swelling, erythema, tenderness/pain, warmth, and/or purulence (e.g., localized infection)	1
Localized infection of skin and soft tissue only with erythema less than 2 cm and no systemic signs of infection (see the following)	2
Localized infection with erythema greater than 2 cm, involvement of deeper tissues (e.g., abscess, septic arthritis, osteomyelitis) but no systemic signs of infection (see the following)	3
Localized infection with erythema greater than 2 cm, involvement of deeper tissues (e.g., abscess, septic arthritis, osteomyelitis), and the presence of systemic signs of infection (e.g., temperature greater than 38°C or less than 36°C, heart rate greater than 90 beats per minute, respiratory rate greater than 20 breaths per minute or $PaCO_2$ less than 32 mmHg, and/or white blood cell count greater than 12,000 cells/microliter or less than 4,000 cells/microliter)	4

*A validated classification system known as PEDIS (P, perfusion; E, extent of infection; D, depth of infection; I, infection characteristics; and S, sensation). This classification system is endorsed by the Infectious Diseases Society of America (IDSA).

2. **Mild diabetic foot infection.** Demonstrated by an ulcer with purulent drainage and/or greater than two classic manifestations of infection. Also, cellulitis and/or erythema that does *not* extend more than 2 cm beyond the ulcer or wound edge.

3. **Moderate diabetic foot infection.** The same as mild infection *except* the patient has one of the following: (a) cellulitis greater than 2 cm beyond a wound or ulcer edge, (b) lymphangitic spread, (c) localized abscess, or (d) a deep space infection (e.g., osteomyelitis).

4. **Severe diabetic foot infection.** The same as moderate infection *except* the patient has **systemic toxicity** and/or **metabolic abnormalities.**

IV. **COMPLICATIONS OF DIABETIC FOOT INFECTIONS.** Osteomyelitis is the most common and serious complication of diabetic foot infections. This complication most commonly occurs in long-standing (greater than 1 month) ulcers, recurrent ulcers, or wounds that are either:

A. Large (more than 2 cm in diameter) and deep (more than 3 mm in depth), *or*

B. Exposed bone in a wound or ulcer bed

V. **APPROACH TO THE PATIENT**

A. **History.** A complete and accurate history should be performed to obtain information about risk factors (see the preceding), comorbid illnesses (e.g., PVD, CKD), duration and therapy of diabetes, and prior or recent infections and antibiotic therapy.

B. **Physical Examination.** In addition to a complete history, evaluation and examination should involve the entire patient as well as the infected wound or ulcer as to the extent and depth of infection. Additional suggestions are:

1. **Funduscopic examination** (to determine retinopathy).

2. **Dermatologic examination** (to detect signs of infection or exposed bone). *A diabetic foot ulcer greater than 2 cm in diameter is more likely associated with osteomyelitis; sensitivity 56% and specificity 92%.*

   a. **Probe test.** The physician probes the depth of any ulcer base (technically this should be performed with a sterile stainless steel eye probe). The test is positive if a *rock-hard and gritty* structure is observed. *For osteomyelitis this test has a sensitivity of 66% and specificity of 85%.*

3. **Neurologic examination** (to detect neuropathy). Usually performed at the bedside with a 10 g nylon monofilament.

4. **Cardiovascular examination** (to detect PVD). Absent dorsalis pedis and posterior tibial pulses with a reduced ankle–brachial index (ABI) can suggest PVD. An ABI is measured by using the resting systolic blood pressure in the ankle and arm.

   a. ABI 0.91 to 1.30 is normal.

   b. ABI 0.41 to 0.90 indicates mild-to-moderate PVD.

   c. ABI less than 0.41 indicates advanced ischemia.

5. **Musculoskeletal examination** (to detect joint involvement or Charçot changes).

C. Laboratory Studies

1. **Complete blood count (CBC).** A WBC count greater than 12,000 cells/mm^3 may be suggestive of a deep space infection (i.e., abscess) and/or osteomyelitis.

2. **Basic metabolic panel (BMP).** Most cases of diabetic foot infections will be associated with hyperglycemia; however, low serum bicarbonate (HCO$_3$) may indicate metabolic acidosis and/or severe infection.

3. **Erythrocyte sedimentation rate (ESR) and C-reactive protein (CRP).** Elevated levels are nonspecific and typically associated with infection and inflammation; however, an elevated *ESR value of greater than 70 mm/hour* may suggest osteomyelitis **(sensitivity 90%; specificity 100%)**. Additionally, levels are helpful in monitoring the response to therapy.

4. **Blood cultures.** Routinely ordered but are *rarely* useful in patients with mild-to-moderate infections.

5. **Wound cultures.** *Swab cultures from superficial ulcers, wounds, or sinus tracts are unreliable and should **not** be performed* (correlation of swab culture to deep space cultures ranges from 20% to 50%). Scraping the base of the ulcer with a scalpel or curette and surgically obtained samples are most reliable for culture of a pathogen. Needle aspiration of an abscess or tissue fluid by aseptic methods is an acceptable alternative.

   An appropriate Gram-stained smear of a wound sample has an overall sensitivity of 70% for identifying the growth of a bacterial pathogen.

6. **Deep tissue or bone culture (Table 41.2).** This is still the gold or criterion standard procedure for microbiological determination of the causative bacteria that can be obtained by open biopsy or CT guidance biopsy.

   Patients should be off antibiotics for a minimum of 2 weeks for any bone biopsy to AVOID false-negative cultures.

   Two to three bone samples should be obtained through uninfected skin. One sample is used for Gram stain, fungal stains (e.g., periodic acid-Schiff stain **[PAS], calcofluor white), AFB smear and culture.** *The other sample is for histopathology confirmation.* **Osteonecrosis and infiltration with leukocytes or chronic inflammatory cells, such as lymphocytes or plasma cells, are the criteria most commonly used for osteomyelitis on histopathologic examination.**

   The International Working Group on the Diabetic Foot developed a classification system to help physicians standardize the characteristics, severity, and

---

TABLE 41.2 ■ Recommended Indications for Bone Biopsy*

1. Diagnostic uncertainty regarding osteomyelitis (bone biopsy provides definitive diagnosis)
2. Absence of bacterial growth on soft-tissue cultures
3. Failure of empirical antimicrobial therapy as evidenced by persistently elevated inflammatory markers or bone deterioration on imaging
4. Soft-tissue and/or blood cultures with demonstrated growth of antimicrobial resistant bacteria (bone biopsy provides more accurate culture directed osteomyelitis therapy)

---

*A bone specimen should be submitted for bone culture and histology.

outcomes of infections (Table 41.1). The classification system uses both the clinical and laboratory data to generate a clinical severity score. In general, the majority of infections classified as grade 3 or higher typically require hospitalization. Furthermore, the majority of infections classified as grade 4 may ultimately require amputation to control infection.

D. Radiographic Studies. Imaging establishes the diagnosis of osteomyelitis.

1. **Plain-film radiology.** Widely available and inexpensive but is most useful in chronic osteomyelitis, as 50% to 75% of bone matrix loss (manifested as osteopenia) must occur before characteristic changes such as **cortical erosions**, **lytic changes**, and/or **periosteal reactions** are visualized (typically evolves over 1–3 weeks). Two-view radiographs are typically the initial imaging test ordered, but a negative image cannot exclude the diagnosis (sensitivity 60%; specificity 70%).

2. **CT.** Widely available and provides improved resolution images when compared to plain-film radiology. CT scan is usually the second best option if an MRI cannot be obtained. A major limitation to CT scan is image degradation or scatter phenomenon in the presence of implanted prosthetic devices adjacent to infected bone. In chronic osteomyelitis, CT findings include thickened cortical bone with sclerotic changes and chronic draining sinus tracts (sensitivity 67%; specificity 50%).

3. **Radionuclide studies.** Generally more reliable in acute osteomyelitis but may not be readily available. Three of the most common studies include:

   a. **Technetium-99 polyphosphate scan.** This isotope accumulates in areas of increased blood flow and new bone formation. While this study can be positive within 48 hours of infection onset, impaired blood flow (e.g., PVD or venous stasis) may limit the utility of this study (sensitivity 85%; specificity 45%).

   b. **Gallium citrate (Ga-67) scan.** This isotope attaches to **transferrin** and leaks into areas of inflammation, infection, and malignancy but does not distinguish well between bone and tissue inflammation.

   c. **Indium-111–labeled leukocyte scan ("tagged WBC scan").** More useful with acute osteomyelitis but only positive in 40% of cases (sensitivity 75%; specificity 70%).

   If radionuclide studies are needed, the combined **indium-111–labeled leukocyte scan** and **technetium-99–labeled sulfur colloid scan** has the best performance for the diagnosis of osteomyelitis (sensitivity 80%; specificity 75%).

4. **MRI.** This test is expensive but is the most useful imaging study to diagnose osteomyelitis (sensitivity 90%; specificity 80%). MRI is contraindicated in the presence of **ferromagnetic material** (iron containing) but offers the best spatial resolution in differentiating bone and soft-tissue infection. MRI usually consists of two main sequences:

   a. **T1-weighted.** Edema is **dark** on this image.

   b. **T2-weighted.** Edema is **bright** on this image.

   The addition of **gadolinium contrast** to MRI improves visualization of sinus tracts, fistulas, and abscesses.

Characteristic Findings on MRI		
Condition	T1-Weighted	T2-Weighted
Osteomyelitis	Decreased	Increased
Sinus tracts	Intermediate	Increased
Abscesses	Intermediate	Increased
Cellulitis	Intermediate	Increased

Overall Diagnostic Accuracy of Selected Imaging Studies		
Diagnostic Imaging	Sensitivity	Specificity
Plain films	43%–75%	65%–83%
Radionuclide scan	69%–100%	38%–83%
CT scan	24%–67%	50%
MRI	82%–100%	75%–96%

VI. TREATMENT *(Antibiotic dosing listed assumes normal renal function.)*

A. For diabetic foot infections, the most important initial treatment plan is to determine the need for hospitalization with restoration of fluid and electrolyte balances and treatment of hyperglycemia, acidosis, and azotemia.

Characteristics that may suggest need for hospitalization:

1. Acute or rapidly progressive infection.

2. Deep space infection or abscess.

3. Severe inflammation/cellulitis, crepitus, bulla, necrosis, or gangrene.

4. Systemic signs of infection (e.g., fever, chills).

5. Metabolic abnormalities (e.g., hyperglycemia, metabolic acidosis).

6. Hemodynamic instability.

7. Renal failure.

8. Patients unable or unwilling to comply with antibiotic therapy.

B. The majority of infections require a combination of medical and surgical therapy. Further, a multidisciplinary team approach is important for optimizing glucose control (goal glucose values of less than 140 mg/dL), nutritional status, and wound healing.

1. Antibiotic therapy. *Suggested antibiotic regimens for diabetic foot infections are based on the severity of infection and include:*

  a. Mild/moderate infections involving soft tissue only. Most infections can be treated as an outpatient with oral therapy for a duration of 1 to 3 weeks depending on clinical response to therapy. Options include:

   i. Cephalexin 500 mg PO q6 or dicloxacillin 500 mg PO q6

   ii. Amoxicillin/clavulanate 875/125 mg PO q12

   iii. Clindamycin 300 mg PO q8

   iv. Doxycycline 100 mg PO q12

   v. Trimethoprim–sulfamethoxazole DS (two tablets) PO q12

b. **Moderate/severe infections involving soft tissue only.** Most infections *without osteomyelitis* require intravenous (IV) therapy until clinically stable, which then can be changed to an oral regimen as previously. The duration of therapy is from 1 to 4 weeks depending on clinical response to therapy. Initial IV options include:

i. **Ampicillin–sulbactam 3 g IV q6 or piperacillin–tazobactam 3.375 to 4.5 g IV q6**

ii. **Clindamycin 450 mg IV q6** *with* **ciprofloxacin or levofloxacin 750 mg IV q12**

iii. **Clindamycin 600 mg IV q8** *with* **ceftazidime or cefepime 2 g IV q8**

iv. **Imipenem–cilastatin 500 mg IV q6** *or* **meropenem 1 g IV q8** *(usually used for multidrug-resistant pathogens such as ESBL)*

v. **Vancomycin 15 mg/kg IV q12–24** *with* **aztreonam 2 g IV q8 or cefepime 2 g IV q8 or ceftazidime 2 g IV q8** *with* **metronidazole 7.5 mg/kg IV q6**. The vancomycin dose may need adjustments to maintain a serum trough level between 15 and 20 mcg/mL. Additionally, for *Enterococcus* spp–resistant vancomycin, consider using daptomycin 6 to 12 mg/kg IV q24 (6 mg/kg dosing is most common) or linezolid 600 mg IV or PO q12.

Infections with osteomyelitis require IV therapy until clinically stable, which then can be changed to an oral regimen as previously. The duration of therapy is typically from 4 to 6 weeks depending on clinical response to therapy; however, guidelines suggest some patients (e.g., patients who cannot undergo surgical intervention) may be treated for as long as 3 months.

2. **Surgery.** The main goal of surgery is to control deep space infections and salvage the limb. In the majority of infections this involves drainage of purulent material, removal of all necrotic or infected tissue, and creation of a healthy wound bed. *In some cases, revascularization may be indicated by a low ABI (less than 0.90) or toe pressure (greater than 45 mmHg).* Requirements for amputation include:

a. **Digit or ray amputation.** Usually utilized with minor involvement of a digit, good blood flow, and only one metatarsal associated with osteomyelitis.

b. **Transmetatarsal amputation.** Usually utilized when multiple digits are associated with osteomyelitis.

c. **Above-ankle amputation.** Usually utilized with a gangrenous forefoot, multiple involved digits, heel necrosis, patients not medically able to have multiple salvage operations, and/or foot instability.

The duration of antimicrobial therapy after surgical intervention depends upon the presence of residual infected tissue and/or bone. The duration of therapy is 2 to 5 days if there is no residual infected bone or soft tissue (e.g., definitive amputation with clean margins). If there is only residual infected soft tissue the duration is typically between 1 and 3 weeks after surgical intervention. Infections with residual osteomyelitis require IV therapy until clinically stable, which then can be changed to an oral regimen as previously for a duration of therapy that is typically from 4 to 6 weeks after surgical intervention.

BIBLIOGRAPHY

Andersen CA, Roukis TS. The diabetic foot. *Surg Clin North Am*. 2007;87(5):1149–1177.

Bader MS, Brooks A. Medical management of diabetic foot infections. *Postgrad Med*. 2012;124(2): 102–113.

Butalia S, Palda VA, Sargeant RJ, et al. Does this patient with diabetes have osteomyelitis of the lower extremity? *JAMA*. 2008;299(7):806–813.

Dinh MT, Abad CL, Safdar N. Diagnostic accuracy of the physical examination and imaging tests for osteomyelitis underlying diabetic foot ulcers: meta-analysis. *Clin Infect Dis*. 2008;47(4): 519–527.

Lipsky BA, Berendt AR, Cornia PB, et al. 2012 Infectious Diseases Society of America clinical practice guideline for the diagnosis and treatment of diabetic foot infections. *Clin Infect Dis*. 2012;54(12):e132–e173.

van Baal JG. Surgical treatment of the infected diabetic foot. *Clin Infect Dis*. 2004;39(suppl 2): S123–128.

42

SEXUALLY TRANSMITTED DISEASES

Eric Cox
Leonard A. Sowah

I. INTRODUCTION

A. Definition. Sexually transmitted diseases (STDs) are diseases that are propagated among humans through intimate sexual contact.

B. Pathogenesis. Upon inoculation, an acute inflammatory response to the infectious agents usually leads to symptoms at the entry site. Most STDs thus present with urethral or vaginal discharge and/or anogenital ulcers.

C. Risk Factors. The risk factors for most STDs include, but are not limited to, the following:

1. Sexually active adolescents older than 15 years and young adults aged 18 to 24 years.

2. Multiple sexual partners or new partners.

3. Exchanging sex for drugs or money.

4. Low socioeconomic status.

5. Lack of circumcision in men.

6. Previous history of STD.

7. Prior or current illicit drug use.

8. History of domestic violence.

9. Homosexual or bisexual male.

10. Use of erectile dysfunction medications, especially among elderly males.

II. MICROBIAL CAUSES OF STDs.
The organisms responsible for most of the common STDs are shown under the appropriate categories in Table 42.1.

III. CLINICAL MANIFESTATIONS OF STDs.
There are four major syndromes of STDs: **genital ulcer disease, urethral discharge, vaginal discharge,** and **lower abdominal pain.** Urethritis in men generally presents as discharge with dysuria, whereas women may have only dysuria. Urinary frequency with dysuria usually suggests bacterial cystitis (see Chapter 29, Urinary Tract Infections).

IV. APPROACH TO THE PATIENT

A. History. A complete and chronologically accurate history should be obtained in all patients suspected of a sexually transmitted infection. ***An STD should be included in the differential diagnosis of any sexually active patient who***

TABLE 42.1 ■ Common Microbial Agents Causing STDs by Type of Clinical Syndrome

Genital Ulcer Disease	Urethritis/Vaginal Discharge	Others
Chancroid (*Haemophilus ducreyi*)	Gonorrhea (*Neisseria gonorrhoeae*)	Human papillomavirus
Syphilis (*Treponema pallidum*)	Chlamydia (*C. trachomatis*)	Hepatitis B
Genital herpes (HSV-2)	Trichomoniasis (*Trichomonas vaginalis*)	HIV
Donovanosis (*Klebsiella granulomatis*)	*Giardia lamblia*	
LGV (*Chlamydia trachomatis*)	*Mycoplasma genitalium*	
	Ureaplasma urealyticum	
	Bacterial vaginosis	

HSV, herpes simplex virus; LGV, lymphogranuloma venereum; STD, sexually transmitted disease.

has symptoms of urinary dysuria, frequency, and urgency with vaginal/urethral discharge or genital ulceration. The history should focus on the timing of events, risk factors, comorbid conditions, accurate social and sexual history, and travel history (some diseases may be associated with geographic clustering). In resource-limited settings, a syndromic approach is often applied for urethral discharge, vaginal discharge, or anogenital ulcer diseases.

The patient should be asked the following questions as part of the standard complete history:

1. Do you have any new sexual partners?

2. What are your engaged sexual practices and genders?

3. What are your numbers of partners within the last year? Monogamous patients should be asked about concerns of extra sexual activity by their partner outside the relationship.

4. With what frequency and usual settings do you use condoms?

B. **Physical Examination.** While a complete physical examination should always be performed, the physical examination should emphasize:

1. **Genital examination.** A pelvic examination should be performed in all sexually active women suspected of a sexually transmitted infection. Urethritis may demonstrate as vaginal discharge in women (a mucopurulent discharge from an inflamed cervical os) and a visible penile urethral discharge in men with or without an erythematous, edematous, and everted meatus. External genital ulcerative lesions may present as a syphilis ulcer (hard chancre; an ulcerative lesion with a smooth but indurated ulcer that is painless and not associated with necrosis or suppuration), donovanosis ulcer (soft chancre; an ulcerative lesion with an irregular border that is beefy red with central necrosis and profuse suppuration), or herpes ulcer (a superficial painful ulcer). Vulvovaginal candidiasis (VVC) and trichomoniasis are associated with vaginal wall erythema.

2. **Anorectal examination.** Anal and genital warts (condyloma) may be detected on careful examination. Condyloma acuminatum warts appear as villous projections and are due to human papillomavirus (HPV). Condyloma latum warts appear as flat lesions and are due to syphilis.

V. URETHRITIS/CERVICITIS SYNDROME

Urethritis and cervicitis are characterized by inflammation. Symptoms, if present, typically include dysuria; urethral pruritus; and mucoid, mucopurulent, or purulent discharge. Although *N. gonorrhoeae* and *C. trachomatis* are well established as clinically important infectious causes, *Mycoplasma genitalium* has also been associated with this syndrome.

In the setting of symptoms, urethritis can be documented by any of the following: (a) mucoid, mucopurulent, or purulent discharge on examination, (b) Gram stain of urethral secretions demonstrating ≥2 WBCs (white blood cells) per oil immersion field, or (c) positive leukocyte esterase test on first-void urine or microscopic examination of sediment from a spun first-void urine demonstrating ≥10 WBCs per high-power field.

Two major diagnostic signs characterize cervicitis: (a) a purulent or mucopurulent endocervical exudate visible in the endocervical canal or on an endocervical swab specimen (commonly referred to as mucopurulent cervicitis) and (b) sustained endocervical bleeding easily induced by gentle passage of a cotton swab through the cervical os.

A. **Chlamydia/Gonorrhea.** The discharge associated with gonorrhea is more purulent and copious than with chlamydia infection. In general, differences between men and women include:

1. **Men** usually present with a mucopurulent urethral discharge, urinary dysuria, epididymitis, or prostatitis (usually manifests as pelvic pain).

2. **Women** are usually asymptomatic (especially for chlamydia infections) but can present with a mucopurulent discharge at the cervical os, urinary dysuria, or abdominal/pelvic pain (this may be an indication of pelvic inflammatory disease [PID]). Asymptomatic chlamydia infections must be treated on account of long-term effects including infertility and risk of ectopic pregnancy.

B. **Nongonococcal Urethritis (NGU).** NGU is confirmed in symptomatic men when staining of urethral secretions indicates inflammation without gram-negative diplococci. *M. genitalium*, which can be sexually transmitted, is associated with symptoms of urethritis as well as urethral inflammation and accounts for 15% to 25% of NGU cases. *T. vaginalis* can cause NGU in heterosexual men.

To minimize transmission and reinfection, men and women treated for urethritis and cervicitis should be instructed to abstain from sexual intercourse until they, and all their sex partner(s) within the past 60 days, have been adequately treated for 7 days after single-dose therapy or until completion of a 7-day regimen (see Section XI) and symptoms resolved. Patients with a specific diagnosis of chlamydia infection, gonorrhea, or trichomoniasis should be instructed to return in 3 months after treatment for repeat testing because of high rates of reinfection. Patients should also specifically be tested for both HIV and syphilis.

VI. VAGINAL DISCHARGE SYNDROMES

These syndromes are characterized by vaginal discharge, itching, or odor. The three diseases most frequently associated with vaginal discharge are bacterial vaginosis (BV), *T. vaginalis* infection, and candidiasis. BV is the replacement of normal vaginal flora by an overgrowth of anaerobic bacteria including *Prevotella* spp, *Mobiluncus* spp, *Gardnerella Vaginalis*, *Ureaplasma* spp, *Mycoplasma* spp, and numerous fastidious or uncultivated anaerobes. VVC is usually not transmitted sexually. Vaginal irritation is common in all three conditions; however, VVC is associated with an intense vaginal pruritus.

A. BV, Trichomoniasis, and VVC. Characteristics of each infection include:

1. **VVC.** *Candida albicans* is the yeast responsible for the majority of cases. Typical symptoms include pruritus, vaginal soreness, dyspareunia, external dysuria, and/or abnormal vaginal discharge. The discharge of vaginal candidiasis is usually odorless with a thick light creamy color. The diagnosis is suggested by the presence of signs and symptoms of vaginitis when either (a) a wet preparation (saline, 10% potassium hydroxide [KOH]) or Gram stain of vaginal discharge demonstrates budding yeasts, hyphae, or pseudohyphae; or (b) a culture or another test yields a positive result for a yeast species. *Candida vaginitis* is associated with a normal vaginal pH (<4.5).

2. **Trichomonas.** *Trichomonas vaginalis* is an anaerobic, flagellated, motile protozoan. The incubation period ranges from 5 to 28 days prior to the development of a diffuse malodorous yellow-green vaginal discharge with vulvar irritation. The discharge associated with *T. vaginalis* is usually grayish, has a thin consistency, and tends to have a foul fishy odor. The classic yellow-green frothy discharge occurs in only 25% of cases. Microscopic evaluation of vaginal secretions is time dependent and associated with a low sensitivity (60%–70%). Food and Drug Administration (FDA) approved additional testing includes the OSOM Trichomonas Rapid Test, an immunochromatographic test, and a nucleic acid probe test, all of which are associated with a high sensitivity and specificity (83% and 97%).

   T. vaginalis infection is associated with two- to threefold increased risk for HIV acquisition, preterm birth, and other adverse pregnancy outcomes among pregnant women. Among women with HIV infection, *T. vaginalis* infection is associated with increased risk for PID.

3. **BV.** It is associated with having multiple male or female partners, a new sex partner, douching, lack of condom use, and lack of vaginal lactobacilli. Women with BV are at increased risk for the acquisition of other STDs such as HIV, *N. gonorrhoeae*, *C. trachomatis*, and/or herpes simplex virus 2 (HSV-2) infection. The discharge of BV is gray-white and typically covers the majority of the vaginal wall.

   BV can be diagnosed by the use of ***Amsel's Diagnostic Criteria***, which require three of the following symptoms or signs: (a) homogeneous, thin, white discharge that smoothly coats the vaginal walls, (b) clue cells (e.g., vaginal epithelial cells studded with adherent coccobacilli) on microscopic examination, (c) pH of vaginal fluid >4.5; or (d) a fishy odor of vaginal discharge before or after addition of 10% KOH (the whiff test).

VII. GENITAL ULCER SYNDROMES

A. **Syphilis, Chancroid (H. ducreyi), Lymphogranuloma Venereum (LGV), Donovanosis, and Genital Herpes.** Skin and mucous membrane ulcers occur as a primary symptom of these conditions. Characteristics of each infection include:

1. The chancre of syphilis is *painless* with a well-defined, punched-out edge; it is usually single but may be multiple.

2. The ulcers of chancroid are *painful* and have a well-defined undermined edge. The base usually has yellowish gray exudates.

3. Donovanosis usually presents with relatively *painless* beefy-red ulcers associated with a smooth, rolled-up edge. These ulcers can spread with further damage to local tissue if not treated in a timely manner.

4. Genital herpes usually presents on the external genitalia as clusters of *painful* papules and vesicles that eventually erode to ulcers.

5. LGV usually presents as inguinal lymphadenopathy with an indurated genital ulcer; however, an anogenital syndrome with ulceration and proctocolitis with fistula formation may occur in homosexual men.

VIII. OTHER CLINICAL MANIFESTATIONS OF STDs

A. **Pelvic Inflammatory Disease.** This condition commonly comprises a spectrum of inflammatory disorders of the upper female genital tract, including any combination of endometritis, salpingitis, tubo-ovarian abscess, and pelvic peritonitis, which is associated with sudden fever, urinary dysuria, vaginal discharge, and suprapubic pain and tenderness in a sexually active woman (most commonly following cessation of menses). Women with PID (symptomatic or asymptomatic) have the potential for significant damage to reproductive health and increased risk of infertility.

1. The minimal Centers for Disease Control and Prevention (CDC) criteria for the ***presumptive diagnosis of PID*** include uterine or adnexal tenderness or cervical motion tenderness on pelvic examination. One or more of the following additional criteria can be used as ***supportive criteria***: (a) elevated WBC count on saline microscopy of vaginal fluid, (b) elevated values of C-reactive protein (CRP) and erythrocyte sedimentation rate (ESR), (c) a fever greater than 38.3°C, (d) an ultrasound ruling out tubo-ovarian abscess or ectopic pregnancy, and (e) abnormal cervical mucopurulent discharge or cervical friability with or without laboratory documentation of cervical infection with *N. gonorrhoeae* or *C. trachomatis*.

   The criteria for a ***definitive diagnosis of PID*** include: (a) endometrial biopsy with histopathologic evidence of endometritis; (b) transvaginal sonography or MRI techniques showing thickened, fluid-filled tubes with or without free pelvic fluid or tubo-ovarian complex, or Doppler studies suggesting pelvic infection (e.g., tubal hyperemia); or (c) laparoscopic findings consistent with PID.

2. PID is usually treated on an outpatient basis; however, suggested ***indications for hospitalization*** include: (a) severe systemic symptoms (e.g., nausea, vomiting, fever), (b) pregnant women, (c) presence of tubo-ovarian abscess (or other surgical emergency), and/or (d) unable to tolerate and/or evidence of failure with outpatient therapy.

3. The risk for PID associated with intrauterine contraceptive device (IUD), copper-containing and levonorgestrel-releasing, use is primarily confined to the first 3 weeks after insertion.

B. **Acute Perihepatitis or Fitz-Hugh and Curtis Syndrome.** This syndrome is classically associated with fever and right upper quadrant abdominal pain in a female with a genital tract gonococcal or chlamydia infection. It is associated with fibrinous inflammation of the liver capsule and adjacent parietal peritoneum. It often occurs in the setting of acute salpingitis; however, symptoms of salpingitis may be mild or even absent in some cases. Treatment is with antibiotics directed against gonorrhea and chlamydia as in PID. Adhesions between diaphragm and liver can occur as sequelae and may require laparoscopic adhesiolysis.

C. **Gonococcal Septic Arthritis.** This condition is the result of gonococcal dissemination manifesting as septic arthritis of large joints (usually monoarticular or pauciarticular). Classically, it manifests as a triad of migratory polyarthralgia, dermatologic lesions (macules and papules with central necrosis), and tenosynovitis, which tends to affect the knees, wrists, ankles, and elbows in decreasing order. This more often occurs in sexually active women with a male-to-female ratio of 1:3, as opposed to Reiter syndrome.

D. **Proctitis, Proctocolitis, and Enteritis.** Sexually transmitted gastrointestinal syndromes (predominantly among persons who participate in receptive anal intercourse) include proctitis (rectal inflammation of the distal 10–12 cm), proctocolitis (inflammation of the colonic mucosa extending to 12 cm above the anus), and enteritis that can be associated with anorectal pain, tenesmus, or rectal discharge. The most common pathogens include *N. gonorrhoeae*, *C. trachomatis* (including LGV serovars), *T. pallidum*, and HSV. Proctocolitis can be acquired through receptive anal intercourse or by oral–anal contact and is associated with symptoms of diarrhea or abdominal cramps. Enteritis is usually acquired by oral–anal contact and is also associated with symptoms of diarrhea or abdominal cramps. Evaluation for these syndromes includes diagnostic procedures such as anoscopy or sigmoidoscopy for stool examination and culture of any anorectal exudate for polymorphonuclear leukocytes.

E. **Reiter Syndrome.** Commonly associated with the triad of: conjunctivitis, urethritis, and arthritis. This condition is more common in young adult men with HLA-B27.

F. **Epididymitis.** Usually an acute clinical syndrome consisting of unilateral testicular pain, swelling, and inflammation of the epididymis that lasts less than 6 weeks. It is most frequently caused by *C. trachomatis* or *N. gonorrhoeae*. Acute epididymitis caused by sexually transmitted enteric organisms (e.g., *Escherichia coli*) also occurs among men who are the insertive partner during anal intercourse. Chronic infectious epididymitis is characterized by a greater than 6-week history of symptoms and is most frequently seen in the setting of *Mycobacterium tuberculosis* (TB) infection.

The criteria for a ***diagnosis of acute epididymitis*** include any of the following: (a) Gram stain of urethral secretions demonstrating ≥2 WBCs per oil immersion field containing intracellular gram-negative diplococci; (b) positive leukocyte esterase test on first-void urine; (c) microscopic examination of sediment from a spun first-void urine demonstrating ≥10 WBCs per high-power field; and/or (d) positive urine testing for *C. trachomatis* and/or *N. gonorrhoeae* by nucleic acid amplification test (NAAT).

IX. LABORATORY STUDIES. Clinical evaluation and local epidemiologic situation must guide appropriate testing. Testing for HIV and hepatitis B and C must be offered to all patients.

A. Nucleic Acid Amplification Test. Highly sensitive in combination or as individual tests for chlamydia or gonorrhea. Samples are collected from urethral swabs, cervical samples, or urine.

B. Serologic Tests for LGV. Serology for the L strains of *Chlamydia trachomatis* must be done in cases of suspected LGV. Consider this serologic test in all cases of positive chlamydia tests with an anorectal specimen.

C. Dark Field Microscopy. Samples from ulcer edges would reveal typical spiral organisms suggestive of syphilis. In regions with endemic *Treponema pallidum pertenue* (causative organism for yaws), this may reveal misleading results.

D. Rapid Plasma Reagin (RPR). RPR and the Venereal Disease Research Laboratory (VDRL) nontreponemal tests are used to screen for syphilis, but are nonspecific and must be confirmed with a treponemal tests such as fluorescent treponemal antibody absorption (FTA-ABS) or microhemagglutination assay for antibodies to *Treponema pallidum* (MHA-TP).

E. Cerebrospinal fluid (CSF) Examination. CSF fluid positive for VDRL with an elevated CSF leukocyte count and high CSF protein may suggest neurosyphilis.

F. Viral Culture for HSV. Fluid from vesicles has a high yield for viral cultures and can differentiate HSV-1 and HSV-2.

G. Tzanck Smear. In herpetic lesions, ulcer base smears show multinucleated giant cells. This test does not differentiate between HSV-1 and HSV-2.

H. Herpes Simplex Type 2 Serology. Specific HSV-2 serology may be done in cases of suspected genital herpes. Asymptomatic screening is not recommended.

I. Wet Mount. Wet saline microscopy of vaginal fluid may show the motile *Trichomonas* spp or clue cells (which are bacterial-covered squamous epithelial cells) suggesting BV.

J. KOH Test. 10% KOH added to a sample of vaginal discharge that produces a fishy odor is suggestive of the diagnosis of BV.

K. Urethral/Cervical/Anal/Pharyngeal Swab. Different organisms require specific culture media, and samples must list suspected organisms to aid laboratory personnel. This is a testing modality that is very useful for STD specimens from extragenital sites in which NAAT are not FDA approved (e.g., oral or anorectal specimens).

L. Gram Stain. This can be valuable in cases of urethritis. A urethral sample from a male with gram-negative intracellular diplococci highly suggests gonorrhea infection (high specificity [>99%] and sensitivity [>95%]). Chancroid has a classic railroad-track or school-of-fish appearance of the gram-negative rods of *Haemophilus ducreyi*.

M. HIV Rapid Testing. Should be offered to all patients being evaluated for an STD (see Chapter 43, HIV and AIDS).

X. SPECIFIC PATHOGEN CHARACTERISTICS

A. Chancroid. *Haemophilus ducreyi* is a gram-negative rod associated with this infection. The incubation period ranges from 5 to 14 days prior to the onset of a soft painful ulcer with undermined edges and unilateral lymphadenopathy. This bacterium is difficult to culture and requires special media.

B. **HSV Infection.** Historically HSV-2 caused the majority of genital herpes outbreaks, but HSV-1 is increasing in genital herpes outbreaks. The incubation period ranges from 2 to 7 days prior to the onset of multiple vesicular lesions or ulcers, which are painful. Tzanck smear and viral cell culture are insensitive; therefore, polymerase chain reaction (PCR) is recommended.

C. **Lymphogranuloma Venereum.** *Chlamydia trachomatis* (serovar L1, L2, and L3) is associated with this infection. The incubation ranges from 3 to 30 days before the onset of unilateral inguinal or femoral lymphadenopathy. Rectal exposure can result in proctocolitis. Untreated infection may develop colorectal fistula. Aspirations from buboes or genital lesions can be sent for culture, direct immunofluorescence, or nucleic acid detection.

D. **Syphilis.** *Treponema pallidum* is a spirochete bacteria associated with this infection. The incubation period ranges from 10 to 90 days prior to the development of a chancre. Primary infection is characterized by a painless ulcer or chancre. Secondary infection can include a copper-colored symmetric maculopapular skin rash (commonly involving the palms and soles), mucocutaneous ulcers, and lymphadenopathy as well as neurologic signs. *Condylomata lata (flat warts located around the anus or in moist regions) are highly contagious*. Tertiary infection can be associated with cardiovascular disorders (aortic valve insufficiency or aortic inflammation), gummas, dementia, or lymphocytic meningitis. In primary infection, dark field microscopy of lesions is most helpful to establish the diagnosis. Serology most commonly involves screening with nontreponemal tests (e.g., VDRL and RPR). Treponema-specific tests include fluorescent treponemal antibody absorbed tests (FTA-ABS), the *T. pallidum* passive particle agglutination assays, enzyme immunoassays, and chemiluminescence immunoassays. Nontreponemal test antibody titers may correlate with disease activity and response to treatment (defined as a fourfold drop in antibody titers). Treponema-specific tests often remain positive lifelong. For neurosyphilis, CSF-VDRL analysis is most helpful to establish the diagnosis.

E. **Pediculosis Pubis (Pubic Lice).** Usually transmitted by sexual contact and associated with pruritus. Usually managed the same as other lice syndromes (permethrin 1% cream rinse applied to affected areas and washed off after 10 minutes or ivermectin 250 mcg/kg once orally).

F. **Scabies (*Sarcoptes scabiei*).** The predominant symptom is pruritus. Usually managed with permethrin 5% cream applied to all areas of the body from the neck down and washed off after 8 to 14 hours or ivermectin 200 mcg/kg orally.

G. **HPV Infections.** Most infections are self-limited and are asymptomatic. HPVs are double-stranded DNA viruses that cause genital warts (e.g., condylomata acuminata) and nearly 90% of cases are associated with types 6 and 11; however, types 16, 18, 31, 33, and 35 are associated with cervical cancer as well as other anogenital cancers. The incubation period is approximately 3 to 4 months prior to the development of soft papules with an irregular, verrucous surface. Persistent oncogenic HPV infection (types 16 and 18) is the strongest risk factor for development of HPV-associated cervical and anorectal precancers and cancers.

XI. TREATMENT

A. Antimicrobial Therapy

1. **PID.** *In general, patients should demonstrate clinical improvement within 3 days after initiation of therapy. Diagnostic laparoscopy for alternative diagnoses should be considered in patients who do not have clinical improvement within 3 days. Also, IUDs do not need to be removed unless patients do not demonstrate clinical improvement within 3 days after initiation of therapy.*

   Recommended inpatient empirical regimens include cefotetan 2 g intravenous (IV) every 12 hours *plus* doxycycline 100 mg orally or IV every 12 hours or cefoxitin 2 g IV every 6 hours *plus* doxycycline 100 mg orally or IV every 12 hours or clindamycin 900 mg IV every 8 hours *plus* gentamicin loading dose IV or intramuscular (IM) 2 mg/kg, followed by a maintenance dose 1.5 mg/kg every 8 hours (single daily gentamicin dosing [3–5 mg/kg] can be utilized as well).

   Alternative empirical inpatient regimen(s) include: ampicillin/sulbactam 3 g IV every 6 hours *plus* doxycycline 100 mg orally or IV every 12 hours.

   Oral therapy can be used 24 to 48 hours after clinical improvement to complete a total 14 days of therapy.

   Recommended outpatient IM and oral regimens include: ceftriaxone 250 mg IM in a single dose *plus* doxycycline 100 mg orally twice a day for 14 days with or without metronidazole 500 mg orally twice a day for 14 days or cefoxitin 2 g IM in a single dose and probenecid 1 g orally administered concurrently in a single dose *plus* doxycycline 100 mg orally twice a day for 14 days with or without metronidazole 500 mg orally twice a day for 14 days or other parenteral third-generation cephalosporin (e.g., ceftizoxime or cefotaxime) *plus* doxycycline 100 mg orally twice a day for 14 days with or without metronidazole 500 mg orally twice a day for 14 days. *While cefoxitin, a second-generation cephalosporin, has better anaerobic coverage than ceftriaxone, ceftriaxone has better coverage against* N. gonorrhoeae.

   The use of fluoroquinolones (levofloxacin 500 mg orally once daily or moxifloxacin 400 mg orally once daily) with metronidazole for 14 days (500 mg orally twice daily) can be considered in patients with a history of cephalosporin allergy.

   Patients should abstain from sex until they and their sex partners have completed treatment. Among all sexually active women with chlamydial or gonococcal PID repeat testing within 3 months after completing therapy is recommended.

2. **Urethritis or vaginal discharge (without ulcers) treatment suggestions include:**

   a. **Gonorrhea.** Ceftriaxone 250 mg single IM dose *plus* either azithromycin 1 g single oral dose *or* doxycycline 100 mg twice daily for 7 days. Ceftriaxone is the preferred cephalosporin because it provides high, and sustained, bactericidal blood levels. Alternative regimen(s) include: cefixime 400 mg single oral dose *plus* azithromycin 1 g single oral dose or dual treatment with single doses of IM gentamicin 240 mg *plus* oral azithromycin 2 g (*for patients with a history of penicillin allergy or allergic reaction to first-generation cephalosporins or for patients who failed standard cephalosporin therapy*).

Quinolones are *not* recommended owing to increasing quinolone-resistant *N. gonorrhoeae*.

Test of cure to detect therapeutic failure (e.g., repeat testing 2 weeks after completing therapy) is recommended only when therapeutic adherence is in question, after treatment with an alternative regimen, if symptoms persist, or when reinfection is suspected.

b. *Chlamydia* **infection.** Suggested treatment regimens include: azithromycin 1 g single oral dose or doxycycline 100 mg twice daily for 7 days. Azithromycin versus doxycycline for the treatment of urogenital chlamydial infection is equally efficacious, with microbial cure rates of 97% and 98%, respectively. However, doxycycline is contraindicated in the second and third trimesters of pregnancy.

Alternative regimens include: erythromycin base 500 mg or erythromycin ethylsuccinate 800 mg four times daily for 7 days, or levofloxacin 500 mg daily for 7 days. Mycoplasma and ureaplasma urethritis will respond to the same therapy for chlamydia infection. Azithromycin or erythromycin is recommended for pregnant women.

Test of cure to detect therapeutic failure (e.g., repeat testing 3–4 weeks after completing therapy) is not recommended unless therapeutic adherence is in question, symptoms persist, or reinfection is suspected. The use of chlamydial NAATs at less than 3 weeks after completion of therapy can lead to false-positive testing because of the presence of nonviable organisms.

c. **Mycoplasma infection (*M. genitalium*).** Suggested treatment regimens include: azithromycin 1 g single oral dose or doxycycline 100 mg twice daily for 7 days. Currently responds better to azithromycin than doxycycline, although azithromycin efficacy might be declining. The most common cause of persistent or recurrent NGU is *M. genitalium*, especially following doxycycline therapy. Azithromycin 1 g orally in a single dose should be administered to men initially treated with doxycycline. Men who fail a regimen of azithromycin should be retreated with moxifloxacin 400 mg orally once daily for 7 days.

d. **Trichomoniasis (*T. vaginalis*).** Metronidazole 2 g, metronidazole 500 mg orally twice a day for 7 days, or tinidazole 2 g as a single oral dose. *Alcohol consumption should be avoided during, and 72 hours after, treatment with nitroimidazoles to reduce the possibility of a disulfiram-like reaction.* While treatment of asymptomatic male partners may prevent reinfection, treating asymptomatic pregnant women does not reduce preterm labor.

Patients should abstain from sex until they and their sex partners have completed treatment.

Test of cure among all sexually active women (e.g., repeat testing within 2 weeks to 3 months after completing therapy) is recommended owing to high reinfection rates. In the setting of persistent or recurrent infection when reinfection is excluded, the patient (and partner[s]) can be treated with metronidazole 500 mg orally twice daily for 7 days.

e. **BV.** Oral treatment options include metronidazole 500 mg twice daily for 7 days, tinidazole 2 g daily oral dose for 2 days, or clindamycin 300 mg twice daily for 7 days. Topical intravaginal (5 g applications) treatment options include metronidazole 0.75% gel at bedtime for 5 days or clindamycin 2% cream at bedtime for 7 days. In pregnancy, this is associated with preterm labor, premature rupture of membranes, and postpartum endometritis. Treatment before 20 weeks may reduce preterm delivery.

Alcohol consumption should be avoided during, and 72 hours after, treatment with nitroimidazoles to reduce the possibility of a disulfiram-like reaction.

Test of cure or follow-up visits are unnecessary if symptoms resolve.

3. **Acute epididymitis.** *In general, patients should demonstrate clinical improvement within 3 days after initiation of therapy.*

   For acute epididymitis most likely caused by sexually transmitted chlamydia and gonorrhea: ceftriaxone 250 mg IM in a single dose *plus* doxycycline 100 mg orally twice a day for 10 days.

   For acute epididymitis most likely caused by sexually transmitted enteric organisms (men who practice insertive anal sex): ceftriaxone 250 mg IM in a single dose *plus* levofloxacin 500 mg orally once a day for 10 days or levofloxacin 500 mg orally once daily for 10 days.

   Patients should abstain from sex until they and any of their sex partners from the past 60 days have completed treatment.

4. **HPV-associated external anogenital warts (e.g., penis, groin, scrotum, vulva, perineum, external anus, and perianus).** While most respond within 3 months of therapy, treatment does not cure the virus itself and it is common for genital warts to recur. Treatment regimens are classified as either patient-applied or provider-administered modalities and clinicians usually employ combination therapy.

   Recommended patient-applied regimens include: Imiquimod 3.75% cream or 5% cream applied once at bedtime, three times a week for up to 16 weeks or podofilox 0.5% solution or gel is applied twice a day for 3 days, followed by 4 days of no therapy (this cycle can be performed up to four cycles) and/ or sinecatechins 15% ointment (a green-tea extract) applied three times daily for up to 16 weeks (catechins are not recommended for persons with HIV infection, pregnancy, or other immunocompromised conditions). Podofilox is contraindicated in pregnancy.

   Recommended provider-administered therapies include: Cryotherapy with liquid nitrogen or cryoprobe or surgical removal either by tangential scissor excision, tangential shave excision, curettage, laser or electrosurgery, or trichloroacetic acid (TCA) or bichloroacetic acid (BCA) 80% to 90% solution.

   Prevention can be accomplished with two available vaccines (FDA approved): Cervarix and Gardasil. Gardasil is approved for men and women from 9 to 26 years of age.

5. **Proctitis, proctocolitis, and enteritis.** Ceftriaxone 250 mg single IM dose *plus* doxycycline 100 mg twice daily for 7 days. Presumptive treatment for LGV includes doxycycline 100 mg twice daily orally for a total of 3 weeks.

   Test of cure to detect therapeutic failure (e.g., repeat testing 3 months after completing therapy) is recommended for infection associated with gonorrhea or chlamydia.

6. **Genital ulcer disease.** tTreatment suggestions include:

   a. **Syphilis**. Treatment is based on stage of illness;

      i. **Primary and secondary syphilis**. Benzathine penicillin G 2.4 million units IM single dose (infants and children are treated with 50,000 units/kg IM; maximum dose 2.4 million units).

      ii. **Latent syphilis**. Early latent infection is infection of less than 2 years. Late latent infection is more than 2 years from initial infection. Early latent syphilis treatment includes benzathine penicillin G 2.4 million units IM single dose. Late latent syphilis or syphilis of unknown duration treatment includes benzathine penicillin G 7.2 million units in three divided doses weekly. In HIV-positive individuals with neurologic symptoms, lumbar puncture with CSF examination for pleocytosis is recommended. In the presence of CSF pleocytosis, HIV-infected patients with late latent syphilis should be treated as for neurosyphilis.

      iii. **Neurosyphilis**. Syphilis with any neurologic symptom is defined as neurosyphilis. The recommended treatment includes IV penicillin G 18 to 24 million units daily (3–4 million units IV q4 or by continuous infusion). Response to treatment is regarded as a fourfold decline in nontreponemal serum antibody titers (these values should be checked at 6, 12, and 24 months).

      iv. **Alternate therapy.** Doxycycline 100 mg twice daily for 14 days can be used in primary and secondary syphilis in nonpregnant patients who have a penicillin allergy.

      v. **Pregnancy.** All pregnant women should be screened and treated with parenteral penicillin G; however, if the patient has a penicillin allergy, the woman should undergo desensitization prior to treatment.

   b. **Genital herpes**. Initial infections can be treated with oral acyclovir 200 mg five times daily for 10 days, or oral famciclovir 500 mg twice daily for 7 to 10 days, or oral valacyclovir 1g twice daily for 3 days. Recurrent infections should be managed with the assistance of an infectious-disease specialist; however, recommended suppressive therapy for recurrent genital herpes includes: acyclovir 400 mg orally twice a day or valacyclovir 500 mg orally once a day or valacyclovir 1 g orally once a day or famciclovir 250 mg orally twice a day. All pregnant women should be screened for herpes and asked about prodromal symptoms before labor. A cesarean section should be performed if there are active lesions at the time of delivery.

   c. **Chancroid**. Treatment regimens include: azithromycin 1 g single oral dose, or ceftriaxone 250 mg single IM dose, or ciprofloxacin 500 mg twice daily for 2 days, or erythromycin 500 mg three times daily for 7 days. Ciprofloxacin should not be used in pregnant or nursing women.

   d. **Donovanosis.** This is otherwise known as granuloma inguinale and caused by an intracellular gram-negative bacterium called *Klebsiella granulomatis*. It commonly manifests as a painless genital ulcer with the definitive diagnosis by skin biopsy. Treatment regimens include: doxycycline 100 mg twice daily, azithromycin 1 g weekly, erythromycin 500 mg four times daily, *or* trimethoprim–sulfamethoxazole one double-strength

(160 mg/800 mg) tablet twice daily for at least 21 days. HIV-seropositive patients may require longer therapy to ensure complete healing of all ulcers.

  e. **Lymphogranuloma venereum.** Doxycycline 100 mg twice a day for 21 days is considered the treatment of choice; however, an alternate regimen of erythromycin 500 mg four times daily for 21 days can be used (especially during pregnancy).

  f. **VVC.** Over-the-counter topical intravaginal applications (5 g applications) are available and most commonly include: clotrimazole 1% cream for 7 to 14 days, clotrimazole 2% cream for 3 days, miconazole 2% cream for 7 days, or miconazole 4% cream for 3 days. A single oral dose of fluconazole 150 mg can also be used for treatment. Only topical azole therapies, applied for 7 days, are recommended for use among pregnant women.

XII. PREVENTION. The public health and economic costs involved with an STD are very high; therefore, partner notification and treatment are recommended for all patients being evaluated for an STD (including HIV) in order to prevent reinfection and to reduce community spread. **Expedited partner therapy** is a CDC recommendation that allows a healthcare professional treating a patient for an STD to deliver treatment and/or a prescription to a partner without a full clinical evaluation of the partner. This is permissible in certain states and localities.

BIBLIOGRAPHY

Biggs WS, Williams RM. Common gynecologic infections. *Prim Care.* 2009;36(1):33–51.

Brill JR. Sexually transmitted infections in men. *Prim Care.* 2010;37(3):509–525.

Kaliaperumal K. Recent advances in management of genital ulcer disease and anogenital warts. *Dermatol Ther.* 2008;21(3):196–204.

Lee KC, Ngo-Metzger Q, Wolff T, et al. Sexually transmitted infections: recommendations from the U.S. Preventive Services Task Force. *Am Fam Physician.* 2016;94(11):907–915.

Workowski KA, Berman S; Centers for Disease Control and Prevention (CDC). Sexually transmitted diseases treatment guidelines, 2010. *MMWR Recomm Rep.* 2010;59(RR-12):1–110. Erratum in *MMWR Recomm Rep.* 2011;60(1):18.

Workowski KA, Bolan GA, Centers for Disease Control and Prevention (CDC). Sexually transmitted diseases treatment guidelines, 2015. *MMWR Recomm Rep.* 2015;64(RR-03):1–137. Erratum in *MMWR Recomm Rep.* 2015;64(33):924.

HIV AND AIDS

Shivakumar Narayanan
Guesly Delva
Robert R. Redfield
Bruce L. Gilliam

I. INTRODUCTION

A. Definitions

1. HIV is a **retrovirus** that infects humans.

   a. The clinically asymptomatic phase can last 3 to 12 years.

   b. It eventually leads to symptoms of disease such as opportunistic infections (OIs) and other noninfectious diseases that constitute the syndrome known as AIDS.

2. AIDS is defined by the Centers for Disease Control and Prevention (CDC) as any person with HIV infection and a CD4 lymphocyte count below 200 cells/mcL (or a CD4 count below 14%) or having an AIDS-indicator condition (see Table 43.1).

B. Pathogenesis.
The *primary route of transmission of the HIV virus is by entering the mucosal surface (predominantly sexual contact)*. Following mucosal entry, the virus binds to peripheral circulating T cells and macrophages (e.g., dendritic cells) that express the CD4 and CCR5 receptors. As the disease progresses to later stages after years of infection, the virus uses the CD4 and CXCR4 receptor to primarily enter T cells. Hosts with a congenitally deleted CCR5 receptor generally fail to establish a productive infection. Once the virus enters the intended target cell, it replicates by converting RNA to DNA by an *RNA-dependent DNA polymerase* (**reverse transcriptase**). This DNA is integrated in the host genome and leads to the production of new viruses that result in a burst of HIV viremia and widespread dissemination. HIV establishes a chronic infection and elicits a robust humoral and cell-mediated immune response. The infection results in the reduction of CD4 T cells as the result of HIV-induced cytolysis and T-cell-induced cytolysis. *The course of HIV infection to AIDS parallels the reduction of CD4 T cells and the amount of circulating virus in the blood.*

C. Risk Factors.
Risk factors for the transmission of HIV include:

1. Sexual contact, *which is the most common mode of transmission.* This includes both heterosexual (most common worldwide) and men who have sex with men (MSM).

TABLE 43.1 ■ AIDS-Indicator Conditions

Candidiasis of bronchi, trachea, lungs, or esophagus	Bacterial pneumonia, recurrent
PCP	*Mycobacterium tuberculosis*, any site (pulmonary or extrapulmonary)
Salmonella spp bacteremia or sepsis, recurrent	*Mycobacterium* spp disease, other species, or unidentified species (disseminated or extrapulmonary)
Cryptosporidiosis, chronic intestinal (greater than 1 month's duration)	Toxoplasmosis of the brain
Cytomegalovirus retinitis or disease (other than liver, spleen, or nodes)	Kaposi's sarcoma
Herpes simplex virus infection; chronic ulcer(s) (greater than 1 month's duration); or bronchitis, pneumonitis, esophagitis	Cervical cancer, invasive
Histoplasmosis (disseminated or extrapulmonary)	Encephalopathy, HIV-related
Isosporiasis, chronic intestinal (greater than 1 month's duration)	Lymphoma, primary of the brain
Mycobacterium avium complex or *Mycobacterium kansasii* (disseminated or extrapulmonary)	Lymphoma (Burkitt, immunoblastic, or equivalent term)
Coccidioidomycosis (disseminated or extrapulmonary)	PML
Cryptococcosis, extrapulmonary	Wasting syndrome due to HIV

PCP, *Pneumocystis jirovecii* pneumonia; PML, progressive multifocal leukoencephalopathy.

    a. Risk per coital (sexual) act:

        i. Unprotected receptive anal intercourse (1.4%)

        ii. Insertive anal intercourse (0.11%)

        iii. Receptive vaginal intercourse (0.08%)

        iv. Insertive vaginal intercourse (0.04%)

    b. Risk factors associated with increased transmission:

        i. *In the host transmitting the virus* (i.e., HIV-infected person)

            (a) High viral load

            (b) Genital ulcers/sexually transmitted disease

            (c) Acute HIV infection

            (d) Advanced disease stage

            (e) Substance abuse

        ii. *In the exposed individual* (generally non-HIV-infected person)

            (a) Lack of circumcision in men

(b) Genital ulcers/sexually transmitted disease

iii. *Infected blood and blood products*—8% of overall infections, risk varies.

(a) Injection drug use (IDU)/needle sharing (0.67%)

(b) Occupational needle-stick exposure (0.3%)

(c) Blood and component transfusion including platelets, plasma, leukocytes (90%)

iv. *Infected mothers to infants* (intrapartum, peripartal, or postpartum via breast milk).

(a) Risk factors for increased vertical transmission:

(1) High maternal HIV viral load

(2) Low maternal CD4 count

(3) Prolonged interval between membrane rupture and delivery

(4) Sexually transmitted diseases

(5) Hard drug use

(6) Cigarette smoking during pregnancy

(7) Preterm delivery

(8) Invasive obstetric procedures except for planned or nonemergent

D. Epidemiology

1. **HIV-1.** Majority of worldwide cases

   a. Group M represents approximately 90% of human infections

   i. *Subtypes*: A, B, C, D, F, G, H, J, and K

   (a) A—Eastern Europe, Central Asia, East and Central Africa

   (b) B—North America, Western Europe, Australia, Central and South America, East Asia, Oceania

   (c) C—Southern/Eastern Africa, India

   (d) D—Eastern Africa

   (e) F—South America, Eastern Europe, Central Africa

   (f) G, H, J, K—Central/West Africa

   ii. *Circulating recombinant forms (CRFs)*—combinations of two subtypes

   (a) AE(CRF01)—Southeast Asia

   (b) AG(CRF02)—West Africa

   b. Groups N, O, P—Rare. West/Central Africa/Cameroon

2. **HIV-2.** Predominantly in West Africa

   a. Lower transmission rates than HIV-1, slower disease progression. (This may be accounted for by lower viral load.)

   b. Certain HIV drugs are not active against HIV-2 (e.g., nonnucleoside reverse transcriptase inhibitors [NNRTIs] and enfuvirtide).

II. CLINICAL MANIFESTATIONS OF HIV AND AIDS

A. Acute HIV Infection

1. Characterized by high viral loads with dissemination and widespread dissemination to lymphoid organs.

   a. CD4 counts may be depressed in this period and recover once the host immune response controls viremia.

   b. Viral loads drop to their set point following this initial infection with high viral loads.

2. **Acute retroviral syndrome** occurs in 50% to 70% of infected individuals 3 to 6 weeks after infection.

   a. Patients are **highly infectious** during this period and often may not recognize that they are infected.

   b. Symptoms are those of a viral-like illness and may occur at frequencies as noted: *fever (96%), lymphadenopathy (74%), pharyngitis (70%), rash (70%), myalgia or arthralgia (54%), diarrhea (32%), headache (32%), nausea/vomiting (27%), hepatosplenomegaly (14%), weight loss (13%), thrush (12%), neurologic symptoms (12%).*

   c. OIs may also occur during this time.

   d. *Differential diagnosis of acute retroviral syndrome includes*: Epstein–Barr virus or *cytomegalovirus* (CMV) mononucleosis, primary herpes simplex virus (HSV) infection, influenza, viral hepatitis, rubella, drug reaction, secondary syphilis, and measles (as these conditions can mimic acute retroviral syndrome).

B. Asymptomatic Stage

1. Lack of clinically evident symptoms despite persistent viremia. Median duration of this stage in untreated patients is 10 years in the United States and Europe. *Untreated patients follow a course of inexorable viral replication and immunologic decline with the average rate of CD4 decline of approximately 50 cells/mL per year.*

2. A small subset of untreated patients is able to maintain relatively high CD4 counts and suppress HIV viremia to low levels without antiretroviral therapy (ART). These hosts are called **long-term nonprogressors**, and subsets of these who have no detectable virus are called **elite controllers** or **natural viral suppressors**.

C. Symptomatic Disease (AIDS)

1. Characterized by clinical symptoms of immune dysfunction or dysregulation.

   a. OIs are the most common reason for the clinical symptoms (see Table 43.2) encountered. Following the introduction of combination ART and widespread use of guidelines for the prevention of OIs, the incidence of these secondary infections has decreased dramatically.

2. Non-AIDS defining illnesses. These conditions, such as cancers and cardiovascular, kidney, and liver disease, tend to dominate the disease burden in patients whose disease is controlled on ART.

(*Text continues on page 350*)

TABLE 43.2 ■ Selected HIV-Related Diseases and Opportunistic Infections and Their Treatment or Prophylaxis

Disease/Clinical Syndrome	Signs and Symptoms	Etiologic Agent	Typical CD4 Count (copies/mL)	Diagnosis, Lab Results, or Other Studies	Initial Treatments or Comments	Prophylaxis/Prevention
Dermatologic						
Bacillary angiomatosis	Red, pedunculated, often friable skin nodules/lesions, can resemble KS. Can also have peliosis hepatis, osteomyelitis, endocarditis, CNS disease	*Bartonella* spp	<50	Biopsy of tissue (H&E, silver stains) PCR of tissue Blood culture	Doxycycline 100 mg PO BID x at least 3–4 months Alternatives: Erythromycin 500 mg PO q6 or azithromycin 500 mg PO daily or clarithromycin 500 mg PO BID Consider IV therapy with rifampin in peliosis hepatis, osteomyelitis, endocarditis, CNS disease	HAART; *Mycobacterium avium complex* prophylaxis with clarithromycin or azithromycin
Cryptococcosis	Can resemble molluscum; can also be pustules, plaques, etc.	*Cryptococcus neoformans*	<50	Skin biopsy Serum cryptococcal antigen	Fluconazole 200–400 mg PO daily if no CNS or disseminated disease	HAART; continue fluconazole treatment until CD4 >200 × 6 months
Herpes simplex	Vesicular lesions or ulcers in orolabial or genital regions; chronic MC disease in late-stage patients	HSV	Any (chronic MC disease usually <100)	Viral culture from swab HSV DNA PCR or antigen	Acyclovir 400 mg PO TID or famciclovir 500 mg PO BID or valacyclovir 1 g PO BID x 14 days; severe disease: acyclovir 5 mg/kg IV q8 until improved, then PO	Consider prophylaxis with one of the three drugs for recurrent or chronic MC disease; HAART
Herpes zoster (shingles)	Painful/pruritic rash in dermatomal distribution	VZV	Any	Clinical: vesicular rash in dermatomal distribution	Famciclovir 500 mg PO TID or valacyclovir 1 g PO TID × 7–14 days Alternative: acyclovir 800 mg PO 5 ×/day	Varicella immune globulin with exposure; consider varicella vaccine in those with CD4 >200

(continued)

TABLE 43.2 ■ Selected HIV-Related Diseases and Opportunistic Infections and Their Treatment or Prophylaxis   *(continued)*

Disease/Clinical Syndrome	Signs and Symptoms	Etiologic Agent	Typical CD4 Count (copies/mL)	Diagnosis, Lab Results, or Other Studies	Initial Treatments or Comments	Prophylaxis/Prevention
KS	Skin: violaceous or red skin or oral lesions, may be raised or flat Systemic disease: see the following	HHV-8	<200 but can occur at higher if not on HAART	Skin: clinical appearance, biopsy Biopsy: spindle cells and endothelial proliferation seen	Single lesion: HAART Limited lesions: cryotherapy or laser ablation, vinblastine lesions	HAART
Molluscum contagiosum	Dome-shaped papules with central umbilication	Pox virus	Usually <100	Biopsy: intraepidermal molluscum bodies	Liquid nitrogen; curettage or electrosurgery; imiquimod cream	HAART
Gastrointestinal						
Oral lesions: aphthous ulcers/candidiasis/oral hairy leukoplakia/histoplasmosis	Pain in mouth or with swallowing, may interfere with eating (oral hairy leukoplakia is usually without symptoms)	Aphthous ulcers: unknown *Candida* spp Oral hairy leukoplakia: EBV	<50 for aphthous ulcers Others: varies	Aphthous ulcers: yellow-gray pseudomembrane with erythematous "halo" Diagnosis of exclusion Candidiasis: curdy, white plaques. May cause erythematous lesions Hairy leukoplakia presents as white frond-like plaques on lateral surface of tongue	Aphthous ulcers: HAART Topical: clobetasol 0.05% or fluocinonide 0.05% ointment in Orabase Systemic: prednisone 40–60 mg/day × 1–2 weeks then taper *or* thalidomide 200 mg PO daily × 4–6 weeks Candidiasis: topical-clotrimazole 10 mg troche 5× per day for 7–14 days Alternative: nystatin 100,000 U/mL: 4–6 mL 4× per day for 7–14 days Systemic: fluconazole 100–200 mg per day PO for 7–14 days	HAART

(continued)

TABLE 43.2 ■ Selected HIV-Related Diseases and Opportunistic Infections and Their Treatment or Prophylaxis (continued)

Disease/Clinical Syndrome	Signs and Symptoms	Etiologic Agent	Typical CD4 Count (copies/mL)	Diagnosis, Lab Results, or Other Studies	Initial Treatments or Comments	Prophylaxis/Prevention
Candida esophagitis	Dysphagia, odynophagia, retrosternal pain, usually have thrush as well	Candida spp	100	Clinical presentation leads to empiric treatment with endoscopy if no response Endoscopy reveals white plaques in esophagus	Fluconazole 400 mg PO daily × 14–21 days	HAART; fluconazole 200 mg PO daily for recurrent disease only
CMV esophagitis or colitis	Esophagitis: odynophagia, retrosternal pain Colitis: diarrhea, fever, abdominal pain, weight loss	CMV	<50	Endoscopy revealing ulcers Biopsy pathology: intranuclear and intracytoplasmic inclusions	Valganciclovir 900 mg PO BID × 4 weeks or ganciclovir 5 mg/kg IV q12 × 4 weeks HAART	HAART
HSV esophagitis	Esophagitis: odynophagia, retrosternal pain	HSV	<50	Endoscopy revealing ulcers Biopsy pathology: multinucleated giant cells PCR positive	Acyclovir 5 mg/kg IV q8 × 14 days Until improvement then acyclovir 400 mg TID or valacyclovir 500 mg PO q12	HAART; acyclovir or valacyclovir for recurrent disease
Diarrhea—Bacterial	Watery stool, abdominal pain, nausea, vomiting	Salmonella, Shigella, Campylobacter, Vibrio, Yersinia, Escherichia coli Clostridium difficile	Depends on pathogen	Fecal WBC, Stool culture Stool C. difficile. toxin/ PCR Blood cultures Endoscopy with biopsy and culture	Ciprofloxacin 500–750 mg PO BID (for 14 days with CD4 >200, for 4–6 weeks for CD4 <200, for up to 6 months and start HAART with recurrent Salmonella) C. difficile: metronidazole 500 mg PO QID × 10–14 days	HAART

(continued)

Disease/Clinical Syndrome	Signs and Symptoms	Etiologic Agent	Typical CD4 Count (copies/mL)	Diagnosis, Lab Results, or Other Studies	Initial Treatments or Comments	Prophylaxis/Prevention
Diarrhea—Parasitic	Watery stool, abdominal pain, nausea, vomiting	*Entamoeba, Giardia, Cryptosporidium, Cyclospora, Microsporidia, Isospora*	Any	Fecal WBC Stool O&P stool antigen (*Giardia*), stool modified acid fast (*Cryptosporidium, Isospora, Cyclospora*) stain and trichrome stain (*Microsporidia*) Endoscopy with biopsy and culture	*Entamoeba, Giardia:* tinidazole 2 g PO × 1–5 days or metronidazole 500–750 mg PO QID × 7–14 days or nitazoxanide 500 mg BID × 3 days *Cyclospora, Isospora:* TMP/SMX DS PO QID × 10 days (continue three times/week in AIDS patients) *Cryptosporidium:* nitazoxanide 0.5–1 g PO BID × 14–30 days (and HAART) *Microsporidia:* HAART and albendazole 400 mg PO BID × 3 weeks	
Perianal lesions: HPV-associated warts Others: mucocutaneous HSV, KS	Mild pruritus, discomfort. Lesions can be intra-anal in MSM. Cauliflower-like on moist partly keratinized skin. Can be popular, flat, or keratinized	Human papillomavirus 6, 11 (low risk), 16, 18, 31, 33, 35 (high-risk oncogenic types)	Varies	Visual inspection; can confirm with biopsy. Serologic test for syphilis recommended HSV: viral culture from swab, PCR, or antigen KS: biopsy	Podofilox gel (0.55) BID × 3 days of a week × 4 weeks Imiquimod 5% cream OD at bedtime three times a week for 16 weeks Cryotherapy with liquid nitrogen/cryoprobe Trichloroacetic acid chemical cautery Surgical removal of recalcitrant lesions HSV: see the preceding	HPV4 vaccine (*Gardasil*) between ages 9 to 26. Protects against HPV types 6, 11, 16, 18

(continued)

TABLE 43.2 ■ Selected HIV-Related Diseases and Opportunistic Infections and Their Treatment or Prophylaxis (*continued*)

Disease/Clinical Syndrome	Signs and Symptoms	Etiologic Agent	Typical CD4 Count (copies/ mL)	Diagnosis, Lab Results, or Other Studies	Initial Treatments or Comments	Prophylaxis/Prevention
Neurologic						
Cerebral toxoplasmosis	Headache, altered mental status, focal deficits, seizures, can have fever but is less common	*Toxoplasma gondii*	<100 (most cases occur at <50)	Compatible clinical syndrome + IgG-positive serology + CT or MRI imaging with multiple corticomedullary lesions	Sulfadiazine: 1–1.5 g PO QID + pyrimethamine 200 mg PO × 1 then 50 mg PO daily + folinic acid 10–25 mg PO daily *or* TMP/SMX 5 mg/kg IV/PO QID	Primary:TMP/SMX800/160 mg 1 tablet PO daily
	Risk factors include consumption of uncooked meat, handling of cat litter			With edema and contrast enhancement; PCR-positive CSF (96% specificity; 50% sensitivity) Definitive diagnosis with brain biopsy	Alternative: clindamycin 600 mg PO QID + pyrimethamine + folinic acid	Alternative: dapsone 50 mg PO daily + pyrimethamine + leucovorin Secondary: continue treatment until asymptomatic and CD4 >200 × 6 months
PML- orJC-virus-associated encephalopathy	Cognitive dysfunction, progressive limb weakness (focal deficit) and/or sensory loss, ataxia, speech and/or visual disturbances, seizure, CN deficits	JC virus	<100	MRI usually shows hyperintense lesions on T2-weighted and fluid attenuated inversion recovery sequences, hypointense on T1-weighted sequences, typically in parietal and occipital lobes CSF positive for JC virus; DNA PCR (sensitivity 76%; specificity 100%)	HAART in treatment-naïve patients. HAART intensification in treatment experienced	Prevention of progressive HIV-related immunosuppressionwith HAART

(*continued*)

TABLE 43.2 ■ Selected HIV-Related Diseases and Opportunistic Infections and Their Treatment or Prophylaxis *(continued)*

Disease/Clinical Syndrome	Signs and Symptoms	Etiologic Agent	Typical CD4 Count (copies/ mL)	Diagnosis, Lab Results, or Other Studies	Initial Treatments or Comments	Prophylaxis/Prevention
Cryptococcal meningitis	Headache, fever +/− meningeal signs, cranial nerve palsies, altered mental status, motor or sensory deficits, seizures Immune reconstitution phenomena are common with worsening infection and elevation of intracranial pressures when ART is begun early in meningitis	*Cryptococcus neoformans*	<100	Positive CSF +/− blood (75%) cryptococcal antigen Abnormal CSF +/− elevated opening pressure on lumbar puncture Positive CSF India ink Basilar contrast enhancement, ventricle enlargement on CT	Amphotericin B 0.7 mg/kg IV daily (or lipid amphotericin 6 mg/kg) + flucytosine 100 mg/kg daily in four divided doses for ~2 weeks, then fluconazole 400 mg PO daily for 8 weeks for maintenance Alternatives: amphotericin B + fluconazole IV/PO 400 mg daily or fluconazole (400–800 mg daily) + flucytosine	Primary prophylaxis not recommended Secondary: fluconazole 200 mg PO daily until CD4 >200 × 6 months
CMV encephalitis or polyradiculomyelopathy	Encephalitis: confusion, lethargy, cranial nerve palsies, ataxia Polyradiculitis: leg paresis, bowel/ bladder dysfunction	CMV	<50	Positive CSF PCR CSF: increased protein, PMNs or mononuclear pleocytosis; periventricular contrast enhancement	Ganciclovir 5 mg/kg IV BID until symptoms improve then valganciclovir 900 mg PO daily	Valganciclovir 900 mg PO daily until CD4 count >100 × 6 months and no active disease

(continued)

TABLE 43.2 ■ Selected HIV-Related Diseases and Opportunistic Infections and Their Treatment or Prophylaxis *(continued)*

Disease/Clinical Syndrome	Signs and Symptoms	Etiologic Agent	Typical CD4 Count (copies/mL)	Diagnosis, Lab Results, or Other Studies	Initial Treatments or Comments	Prophylaxis/Prevention
Tuberculous meningitis	Fever, headache, meningismus, decreased level of consciousness, focal deficits	*Mycobacterium tuberculosis*	<350	CT/MRI: may have intracerebral lesions CSF: WBC 5–2,000 Protein nl-500 Glucose low AFB smear positive in 20% PCR positive; culture positive CXR: active TB up to 50%	Isoniazid, rifampin, pyrazinamide, ethambutol until cultures return (~8 weeks) then, if sensitive, isoniazid and rifampin for a total of 12 months therapy (see Chapter 14, Tuberculosis, for dosing) May substitute rifabutin 150 mg every other day for rifampin if on boosted PIs	See section on pulmonary tuberculosis later
Result of HIV Infection						
HIV encephalopathy, or dementia	Evolves to involve both cognitive and motor abnormalities Early: memory, concentration and attention decreased Later: ataxia, coordination decreased to paraplegia, dementia	HIV	<200	CSF: increased cells and protein MRI: atrophy, increased T2 signal/white matter hyperintensities Neuropsychologic testing: dementia Must rule out other OIs	HAART treatment/ intensification	

(continued)

TABLE 43.2 ▪ Selected HIV-Related Diseases and Opportunistic Infections and Their Treatment or Prophylaxis   *(continued)*

Disease/Clinical Syndrome	Signs and Symptoms	Etiologic Agent	Typical CD4 Count (copies/mL)	Diagnosis, Lab Results, or Other Studies	Initial Treatments or Comments	Prophylaxis/Prevention
Noninfectious/Neoplastic						
Primary CNS lymphoma	Headache, focal deficits or nonfocal signs, altered mental status with slow onset, seizures, no fever	EBV	≤50	MRI ring-enhancing lesions; less prominent contrast enhancement as compared to toxoplasmosis. Carcinomatous meningitis in CSF in up to 20% Positive CSF EBV PCR. Positive cytology rare	Radiotherapy +/− chemotherapy with rituximab-based regimens Patients should be treated with HAART	
Ophthalmologic						
CMV retinitis	Asymptomatic or can have decreased acuity, field deficits, floaters, scotomata	CMV	<50	Funduscopic exam by ophthalmologist: yellow-white perivascular infiltrates ± hemorrhages	Valganciclovir 900 mg PO BID × 14–21 days *or* ganciclovir 5 mg/kg IV q12 × 14-21 days *or* foscarnet 60 mg/kg IV q8 × 14–21 days	Secondary: 900 mg PO daily until disease inactive and CD4 >100 × 6 months Alternative: ganciclovir 5 mg/kg IV daily *or* foscarnet 90 mg IV once daily
ARN or PORN	ARN: ocular or periorbital pain, floaters, blurred vision PORN: floaters, decreased vision, decreased visual fields	VZV	PORN: <50 ARN: Any	Often have history of cutaneous herpes zoster; may occur bilaterally in 2/3 Funduscopic exam by ophthalmologist ARN: vasculitis	ARN: acyclovir 10 mg/kg IV q8 × 10–14 days followed by oral therapy for up to 14 weeks PORN: acyclovir 10 mg/kg IV q8 *or* ganciclovir 5 mg/kg IV q12 *or* foscarnet 60 mg/kg IV q8. May need lifelong maintenance with IV	HAART

(continued)

Disease/Clinical Syndrome	Signs and Symptoms	Etiologic Agent	Typical CD4 Count (copies/mL)	Diagnosis, Lab Results, or Other Studies	Initial Treatments or Comments	Prophylaxis/Prevention
Pulmonary						
Bacterial pneumonia	Acute fevers, chills, rigors, chest pain, cough productive of purulent sputum, and dyspnea as in non-HIV-infected individuals	Mainly *Streptococcus pneumoniae*, *Hemophilus* spp	Any	Positive sputum and/or blood culture, chest radiography; lobar infiltrate	Depends on organisms (see Chapter 11)	Pneumococcal and influenza vaccine recommended for HIV patients
PCP	Subacute, progressive dyspnea; fever, nonproductive cough	*Pneumocystis jirovecii*	<200	Hypoxemia, elevated LDH, demonstration of organisms in tissue, bronchoalveolarlavage fluid, or induced sputum CXR: normal to diffuse ground glass opacities CT chest: ground glass opacities and cysts	Trimethoprim–sulfamethoxazole 800/160 mg PO/IV q8 for 21 days Add steroids if severe illness (pO$_2$ < 70) Alternatives: dapsone 100 mg PO daily + trimethoprim 5 mg/kg/day q8 *or* primaquine 15–30 mg PO daily 1 clindamycin 600–900 mg IV q6–8 or 300–450 mg PO q6–8 *or* atovaquone 750 mg PO BID	Trimethoprim–sulfamethoxazole 800/160 mg one tablet PO daily or 400/80 mg one tablet daily until CD4 count >200 × 6 months Alternatives: dapsone 100 mg PO daily *or* dapsone 50 mg PO daily + pyrimethamine 50 mg PO weekly leucovorin 25 mg PO weekly *or* aerosolized pentamidine 300 mg monthly *or* atovaquone 1,500 mg PO daily

(*continued*)

TABLE 43.2 ■ Selected HIV-Related Diseases and Opportunistic Infections and Their Treatment or Prophylaxis *(continued)*

Disease/Clinical Syndrome	Signs and Symptoms	Etiologic Agent	Typical CD4 Count (copies/mL)	Diagnosis, Lab Results, or Other Studies	Initial Treatments or Comments	Prophylaxis/Prevention
Pulmonary tuberculosis	Fever—subacute to acute, productive cough, night sweats, weight loss, lymphadenopathy	*Mycobacterium tuberculosis*	Any (higher risk as CD4 declines)	LTBI: diagnosed with tuberculin skin test or IGRA. Active disease: sputum smear AFB positive or sputum culture Positive or nucleic acid amplification test of sputum positive CXR: infiltrate, cavity, effusion in higher CD4; may have infiltrate/effusion only in low CD4	DOT is recommended for all patients with HIV-related TB Rifampin 600 mg PO daily + isoniazid 300 mg PO daily + ethambutol 15–25 mg/kg/day and pyrazinamide 15–25 mg/kg/day (maximum dose 2,000 mg) PO daily May substitute rifabutin 150 mg every other day for rifampin when the patient is given with boosted PIs	Primary: LTBI treatment is isoniazid 300 mg PO daily + pyridoxine 50 mg PO daily for 9 months
Disseminated Disease						
Mycobacterium avium complex disease	Fever, diarrhea, weight loss, night sweats, abdominal pain.	*Mycobacterium avium* complex	<50	Blood or bone marrow culture (>85% positive with disseminated disease) Anemia, elevated alkaline phosphatase, low albumin Endoscopy with biopsy Lymphadenopathy on CT abdomen in disseminated disease	Clarithromycin 500 mg PO BID or azithromycin 600 mg PO daily + ethambutol 15 mg/kg daily ± third agent (rifabutin 300 mg PO daily [adjust dose with PIs] or quinolones)	HAART Primary (CD4 < 50): azithromycin 1,200 mg PO once weekly or clarithromycin 500 mg PO BID Secondary: continue treatment × 12 months and until CD4 >100 × 6 months

(continued)

TABLE 43.2 ■ Selected HIV-Related Diseases and Opportunistic Infections and Their Treatment or Prophylaxis *(continued)*

Disease/Clinical Syndrome	Signs and Symptoms	Etiologic Agent	Typical CD4 Count (copies/mL)	Diagnosis, Lab Results, or Other Studies	Initial Treatments or Comments	Prophylaxis/Prevention
Disseminated cryptococcosis	Cough, fever, malaise, dyspnea, pleuritic pain	*Cryptococcus neoformans*	<100	Positive blood or respiratory culture; positive serum cryptococcal antigen	Amphotericin B 0.7 mg/kg IV daily (or lipid amphotericin 6 mg/kg) + flucytosine 100 mg/kg daily in four divided doses for ~2 weeks, then fluconazole 400 mg daily for 8 weeks for maintenance	Primary prophylaxis not recommended Secondary:fluconazole200 mg PO
				CXR: nodules or focal infiltrate	Alternatives: amphotericin B + fluconazole IV/PO 400 mg daily *or* fluconazole (400–800 mg daily) + flucytosine	Daily until CD4 >200 × 6 months
Disseminated histoplasmosis	Fever, fatigue, weight loss, hepatosplenomegaly, and lymphadenopathy. Cough, chest pain, and dyspnea occur in approximately 50% of patients.	*Histoplasma capsulatum*	≤150 for disseminated; < 300 for pulmonary alone	Histoplasma antigen in blood or urine is sensitive for disseminated disease (85%–95%) but insensitive for pulmonary infection Culture: blood, bone marrow, respiratory secretions, or other involved sites (+ in >85% of patients with AIDS) CXR: infiltrates, cavities, mediastinal/hilar lymphadenopathy	Lipid formulation of amphotericin B 3 mg/kg IV (6 mg/kg if CNS disease) for ≥2 weeks (or until clinical improvement), then oral itraconazole 200 mg tid for 3 days and then 200 mg bid for a total of >12 months	Itraconazole 200 mg daily can be considered for patients with CD4+ counts <150 cells/mcL and are at high risk due tooccupationalexposure or presence in an hyperendemic area for histoplasmosis (>10 cases./100 patient-years)

(continued)

TABLE 43.2 ■ Selected HIV-Related Diseases and Opportunistic Infections and Their Treatment or Prophylaxis   *(continued)*

Disease/Clinical Syndrome	Signs and Symptoms	Etiologic Agent	Typical CD4 Count (copies/mL)	Diagnosis, Lab Results, or Other Studies	Initial Treatments or Comments	Prophylaxis/Prevention
Coccidioidomycosis	Cough, fever, dyspnea, weight loss, night sweats CNS: headache, altered mental status	*Coccidioides immitis*	>200 focal pneumonia; disseminated: usually <50	CXR: focal or diffuse nodular infiltrate Sputum: stain or culture positive Blood: positive serology CSF: low glucose, elevated protein, mononuclear pleocytosis, eosinophils, positive antibody/culture	Focal pneumonia: fluconazole 400 mg PO daily (itraconazole and posaconazole have also been used) Diffuse pneumonia: amphotericin B 1 mg/kg/day IV daily until improvement, then fluconazole Meningitis: fluconazole 400–800 mg PO daily (alternative intrathecal amphotericin B)	Secondary: fluconazole 400 mg PO daily
Neoplastic						
Visceral KS	Pulmonary: subacute or chronic dyspnea, cough, hemoptysis GI: bleeding, dysphagia, pain Lymphadenopathy	HHV-8 or KSHV	Any	Pulmonary: perihilar nodular infiltrate on chest radiograph or CT, bronchoscopy with biopsy GI: endoscopy with biopsy	Systemic: liposomal doxorubicin or daunorubicin, paclitaxel	HAART

(continued)

TABLE 43.2 ■ Selected HIV-Related Diseases and Opportunistic Infections and Their Treatment or Prophylaxis *(continued)*

Disease/Clinical Syndrome	Signs and Symptoms	Etiologic Agent	Typical CD4 Count (copies/mL)	Diagnosis, Lab Results, or Other Studies	Initial Treatments or Comments	Prophylaxis/Prevention
Non-Hodgkin's lymphoma	Lymph node swelling, fevers/night sweats/weight loss (B symptoms), hepatosplenomegaly, anemia, bruising	EBV-diffuse large B cell, Burkitt, primary CNS HHV-8:body cavity lymphoma/ plasmacytic oral cavity lymphoma	<200	Blood: anemia, elevated LDH CT imaging: mediastinal and abdominal lymphadenopathy, hepatosplenomegaly Lymph node biopsy	Rituximab-based chemotherapy	

AFB, acid-fast bacillus; ARN, acute retinal necrosis; ART, antiretroviral therapy; BID, twice daily; CMV, cytomegalovirus; CN, cranial nerve; CNS, central nervous system; CSF, cerebrospinal fluid; CXR, chest x-ray; DOT, directly observed therapy; EBV, Epstein–Barr virus; GI, gastrointestinal; H&E, hematoxylin and eosin; HAART, highly active antiretroviral therapy; HHV, human herpesvirus; HHV-8, human herpesvirus 8; HPV, human papillomavirus; HSV, herpes simplex virus; IgG, immunoglobulin G; IGRA, interferon-gamma release assay; IV, intravenous; KS, Kaposi's sarcoma; KSHV, Kaposi sarcoma–associated herpesvirus; LDH, lactate dehydrogenase; LTBI, latent tuberculosis infection; MC, mucocutaneous; MSM, men who have sex with men; O&P, ova and parasites; OI, opportunistic infection; PCP, *Pneumocystis jirovecii* pneumonia; PCR, polymerase chain reaction; PI, protease inhibitor; PML, progressive multifocal leukoencephalopathy; PMN, polymorphonuclear leukocyte; PO, per os; PORN, progressive outer retinal necrosis; QD, daily; SMX, sulfamethoxazole; TB, tuberculosis; TID, three times per day; TMP, trimethoprim; VZV, varicella-zoster virus; WBC, white blood cell.

III. APPROACH TO THE PATIENT

A. **History.** Whether caring for a newly HIV-infected patient or an ART treatment–experienced infected patient, a thorough comprehensive history should be taken at the initial assessment. It should include *date of diagnosis, nadir* (the lowest) *CD4 count*, and *past HIV-related conditions*. The duration of HIV infection based on the dates of previous negative serologies, high-risk exposures (see the aforementioned risk factors), and acute illnesses suggestive of the acute retroviral syndrome can be valuable in understanding the state of the patient's disease. Knowledge of the source of the infection may be helpful in determining a possible infection with drug-resistant viruses.

Chronic medical conditions such as hepatitis, cardiovascular disease, renal disease, and gastroesophageal reflux disease likely to have an impact on the choice or efficacy of anti-HIV therapy should also be obtained. Social history and family history may also have an impact on when to start and the choice of ART.

B. **Physical Examination.** A comprehensive physical examination should be performed on initial evaluation including a careful eye, skin, and rectal examination. This can help to diagnose conditions that may indicate advanced HIV disease or AIDS. Areas to focus include:

1. **Head, eyes, ears, nose, and throat (HEENT) examination.** Funduscopic examination may suggest findings of CMV retinitis. Oral cavity lesions may suggest thrush, oral hairy leukoplakia, HSV (more commonly located on the vermilion border of the lip), or Kaposi's sarcoma.

2. **Dermatologic examination.** Many skin conditions can occur with advancing HIV disease; however, the most common ones to evaluate for are Kaposi's sarcoma lesions, cutaneous candidiasis, scabies, seborrheic dermatitis, molluscum contagiosum, and paronychia.

3. **Gastrointestinal examination.** Hepatomegaly, splenomegaly, and hepatosplenomegaly can give clues to systemic comorbid infections.

4. **Genitourinary examination.** A detailed anogenital inspection and examination can help uncover other sexually transmitted diseases such as human papillomavirus (HPV) and HSV infections (see Chapter 42, Sexually Transmitted Diseases).

5. **Lymph node examination.** Lymphadenopathy, localized or generalized, can help strengthen suspicions of OIs.

6. **Neurologic examination.** Level cognitive function and peripheral neurologic status should be determined.

C. **Laboratory Studies**

1. **Diagnosis.** The CDC recommends a policy of performing HIV testing routinely for everyone between ages 13 and 64 in healthcare settings.

   a. **Enzyme immunoassay (EIA)** is most commonly used and has a reported sensitivity and specificity of over 99%.

      i. **Positive or indeterminate EIA results** must be confirmed with a more specific assay such as the Western blot (WB).

      ii. **False-positive results** can occur with recent immunization (hepatitis B virus [HBV], influenza), autoimmune diseases (systemic lupus erythematosus [SLE]), pregnancy (due to antibodies to HLA antigens), multiple myeloma, and end-stage renal disease.

   iii. False-negative results can occur during acute HIV infection prior to antibody development (this can range from 12 to 22 days); this period is otherwise known as the *window phase*. False-negative results may also occur in cases of infection with certain genetic variants (HIV-2 or N and O group infections), and hypogammaglobulinemia.

   iv. The most recent EIA tests combine detection of antibodies with HIV p24 antigen to allow earlier diagnosis.

   v. Point of care rapid screening tests are available to screen in appropriate clinical situations *(e.g., patient in labor, source of needle-stick injury, acutely ill patient with possible* Pneumocystis pneumonia, *where the acuity of the condition warrants emergent diagnosis and treatment, or concern for lack of follow-up)* with results available in 30 to 60 minutes. ***A positive EIA test still needs confirmation with a WB.***

  b. WB: This is essentially an EIA test to detect specific HIV proteins after they are subject to electrophoresis with separation on a membrane. The false-positive rate without EIA is estimated at 2%.

   i. Positive WB is defined as reactive to gp 120/160 and either p24, gp 41, or both.

   ii. Indeterminate WB is common and can occur in as many as 15% to 20% of serum from patients without HIV infection. Indeterminate WB can also occur with very early or far-advanced HIV infection. An indeterminate WB is defined as the presence of one or more bands that do not meet the criteria for being positive. ***This is one of the major reasons why the WB alone is not suitable as a screening test.*** Indeterminate WB results should always be repeated.

  c. p24 antigen capture assay. Detects HIV-1 p24 protein in an EIA-based format. Only 30% to 90% sensitive.

  d. Direct detection of HIV. Three molecular techniques are available and include: reverse transcriptase polymerase chain reaction (PCR), branched DNA (bDNA), and nucleic acid sequence based amplification (NASBA).

   i. Can be used in making a diagnosis of primary HIV infection especially in the window period.

   ii. These tests are more useful in monitoring the effects of therapy (see the following).

2. Immunologic monitoring

  a. CD4 T lymphocyte counts are commonly determined by flow cytometry and are useful to stage disease, assess risk for OIs, diagnose AIDS, and monitor immunologic response to therapy. It's commonly measured at the time of diagnosis and every 3 to 6 months thereafter.

3. Virologic monitoring

  a. Standard assays use molecular methods and can detect as few as 20 to 40 copies of HIV RNA per milliliter of plasma.

    b. *Measure approximately 2 to 8 weeks after initiation of ART and then every 3 to 6 months to evaluate continued effectiveness. In most instances HIV RNA will drop to less than 50 copies per milliliter within 6 months after the initiation of antiretroviral treatment.*

4. Resistance testing

    a. Usually performed at baseline HIV evaluation (due to the frequency of transmission of resistant viruses) and in cases of virologic failure (persistent viral detection on a seemingly adequate regimen).

    b. *Generally must have a viral load greater than 1,000 copies/mL to obtain an accurate result.*

    c. Assay subtypes:

        i. *Genotypic assays*: reports the genomic sequence of the HIV obtained from patient's serum:

            (a) Must be interpreted by an experienced HIV provider.

            (b) Results come back faster, and the test is less expensive than the phenotypic assays.

        ii. *Phenotypic assays*: detects growth of viral isolates obtained from the patient and is then compared to reference strains of the virus in the presence or absence of different antiretroviral medications.

            (a) Reports fold change of the virus (similar to minimal inhibitory concentration for bacteria).

            (b) Easy to determine if drug is sensitive/resistant.

        iii. *Virtual phenotype*: Uses a database of matched genotypes and phenotypes to determine report from patient's genotype:

            (a) Easier to interpret.

            (b) The number of matches in the database determines the usefulness of a medication. It is of limited utility with new drugs or in patients with rare mutation patterns.

            (c) More expensive than genotype but cheaper than phenotype.

5. Laboratory tests prior to use of certain medications

    a. *Coreceptor tropism assays*: for the potential use of the CCR5 antagonist maraviroc.

        i. Assess which coreceptor the infecting virus uses to enter into CD4 positive cells. Maraviroc is only active when the virus is predominantly CCR5-tropic.

            (a) CCR5-tropic viruses predominate in early infection.

            (b) CXCR4-tropic viruses predominate later in disease.

    b. *HLA B5701 testing*: for the potential use of abacavir (ABC).

        i. With positive test, there is higher incidence of hypersensitivity reaction to ABC.

        ii. With negative test, risk of hypersensitivity is extremely low.

    c. *Glucose-6-phosphate dehydrogenase (G6PD):* for the potential use of dapsone. (Deficiency can be associated with increased risk of hemolytic anemia with dapsone.)

6. **Other baseline laboratory or screening tests**

   a. Complete blood count (CBC) with differential: baseline and every 3 to 4 months in those on ART.

   b. Complete metabolic and cholesterol panel (includes glucose, renal, liver, and lipid profiles): baseline and every 3 to 4 months in those on ART.

   c. Syphilis serology (i.e., rapid plasma reagin [RPR]): baseline and every 6 to 12 months.

   d. Gonorrhea and chlamydia screen: annually (see Chapter 42, Sexually Transmitted Diseases, for tests).

   e. Papanicolau smear should be performed for both men and women and includes the following:

      i. Vaginal/cervical: at baseline for all female patients. Repeat at 6 months, then annually if normal.

      ii. Anal: recommended by some experts in high-risk populations. Needs high-resolution anoscopy if abnormal.

   f. Purified protein derivative (PPD) or interferon-gamma release assay (IGRA): usually measured at baseline, then repeated following CD4 recovery for those whose tests were performed when the patient's initial CD4 count was below 200; repeat annually for high-risk populations (see Chapter 14, Tuberculosis).

   g. Hepatitis serology (A, B, and C): usually measured at baseline and annually in high-risk populations who have not been vaccinated (see Chapters 26–28, Hepatitis A, Hepatitis B, and Hepatitis C).

   h. Urinalysis (dipstick and microscopic).

D. **Radiography Studies.** Chest plain-film radiology is sometimes recommended *at baseline in patients* with certain risk factors for asymptomatic *Mycobacterium tuberculosis* (TB).

IV. MANAGEMENT OF HIV/AIDS

A. **Treatment of HIV Infection.** The treatment for HIV infection consists of using a combination of antiretroviral agents (usually a combination of three agents) with the goals of suppressing viral replication to undetectable levels, reducing HIV-associated morbidity, and prolonging the duration and the quality of the patient's life. The restoration and the preservation of the host immunologic functions as well as the prevention of HIV transmission by achieving a durable and optimal viral suppression are also goals of the treatment of HIV infection according to the most recent guidelines. Recommended antiretroviral treatment regimens have comparable efficacy; however, a regimen choice tailored to the patient and based on expected side effects, convenience, comorbidities, interactions with concomitant medications, and results of pretreatment genotypic drug-resistance testing among other factors offers the best chance of a durable regimen. ***Adherence counseling is a major prerequisite of starting HIV treatment.*** Usually, a physician trained in HIV care is consulted when ART is being started or changed.

B. **Indications for Starting ART**

   1. Prior to initiating any antiretroviral regimen, each patient's barriers to adherence including medical and social issues must be addressed.

2. The U.S. Department of Health and Human Services (DHHS) guidelines

   a. The DHHS recommends treatment in the following situations:

      i. Symptomatic disease

      ii. Pregnant women

      iii. HIV-associated nephropathy (HIVAN), hepatitis B coinfection, and patients at risk of transmitting HIV

      iv. Previously the recommendations were to start therapy for asymptomatic patients with a CD4 *less than* 500 cells/mL; however, the most recent recommendations state ***ART is recommended for all HIV-infected individuals, regardless of CD4 T lymphocyte cell count***, to reduce the morbidity and mortality associated with HIV infection.

      v. ***ART is also recommended for HIV-infected individuals to prevent HIV transmission***.

   b. Suggest that those with or having risk of cardiovascular disease be considered for treatment

3. Other guidelines similarly recommend treatment for symptomatic disease and comorbid conditions but vary on the CD4 count to start from *less than* 350 cells/mL in the British guidelines to *less than* 500 cells/mL in the International Antiviral Society—USA guidelines due to different interpretations of the incremental benefit of earlier treatment.

   a. Overall, the trend of most experts and guidelines is to treat patients earlier to minimize the risk of complications of HIV including cardiovascular disease and cancer and to reduce transmission.

C. **ART Regimens (In Treatment-Naïve Patients).** All the guidelines make recommendations based on available evidence, expert opinion, and toxicity. An antiretroviral regimen for a treatment-naïve patient generally consists of two nucleoside reverse transcriptase inhibitors (NRTIs) in combination with a third active antiretroviral drug from one of three drug classes: an integrase strand transfer inhibitor (INSTI), an NNRTI, or a protease inhibitor (PI) with a pharmacokinetic (PK) enhancer (booster) (cobicistat or ritonavir). This fact accounts for some of the variation seen. Alternative and acceptable agents may be used when the patient's individual situation warrants.

1. **DHHS-recommended regimens:**

   a. Dolutegravir/abacavir/lamivudine (DTG/ABC/3TC)—*if HLA-B 5701 negative*

   b. Dolutegravir plus either tenofovir disoproxil fumarate/emtricitabine (DTG/TDF/FTC) or tenofovir alafenamide/emtricitabine (DTG/TAF/FTC)

   c. Elvitegravir/cobicistat/tenofovir alafenamide/emtricitabine (EVG/c/TAF/FTC)

   d. Elvitegravir/cobicistat/tenofovir disoproxil fumarate/emtricitabine (EVG/c/TDF/FTC)—*in patients with CrCl >70 mL/min*

   e. Raltegravir plus either tenofovir disoproxil fumarate/emtricitabine (RAL/TDF/FTC) or tenofovir alafenamide/emtricitabine (RAL/TAF/FTC)

   f. Darunavir/ritonavir plus either tenofovir disoproxil fumarate/emtricitabine (DVR/r/TDF/FTC) or tenofovir alafenamide/emtricitabine (DVR/r/TAF/FTC)

2. **DHHS alternative agents:**

   a. Efavirenz/tenofovir disoproxil fumarate/emtricitabine (EFV/TDF/FTC)

   b. Efavirenz (EFV) plus tenofovir alafenamide/emtricitabine (TAF/FTC)

   c. Rilpivirine/tenofovir disoproxil fumarate/emtricitabine (RPV/TDF/FTC) or Rilpivirine/ tenofovir alafenamide/emtricitabine (RPV/TAF/FTC)

   d. Atazanavir/cobicistat (ATV/c) or atazanavir/ritonavir (ATV/r) plus either tenofovir disoproxil fumarate/emtricitabine (TDF/FTC) or tenofovir alafenamide/emtricitabine (TAF/FTC)

   e. Darunavir/cobicistat (DRV/c) or darunavir/ritonavir (DRV/r) plus abacavir/lamivudine (ABC/3TC)—*if HLA-B 5701 negative*

   f. Darunavir/cobicistat (DRV/c) plus either tenofovir disoproxil/ fumarate/ emtricitabine (TDF/FTC) or tenofovir alafenamide/emtricitabine (TAF/ FTC)

3. **DHHS acceptable agents:**

   a. Atazanavir/cobicistat (ATV/c) or atazanavir/ritonavir (ATV/r) plus abacavir/lamivudine (ABC/3TC)—*if HLA-B 5701 negative*

   b. Efavirenz (EFV) plus abacavir/lamivudine (ABC/3TC)—*if HLA-B 5701 negative*

   c. Raltegravir (RAL) plus abacavir/lamivudine (ABC/3TC)—*if HLA-B 5701 negative*

   d. Darunavir/ritonavir (DRV/r) plus raltegravir (RAL) twice daily

   e. Lopinavir/ritonavir (LPV/r) plus lamivudine (3TC) twice daily

D. **ART Regimens With Pregnancy (In Treatment-Naïve Patients).** All the guidelines make recommendations based on available evidence, expert opinion, and toxicity. In pregnant women, as in nonpregnant adults, ART with at least three agents is recommended. Recommendations for choice of antiretroviral drug regimen during pregnancy must be individualized according to a pregnant woman's specific antiretroviral history, the results of drug-resistance assays, and the presence of comorbidities. *In general, it is recommended that women who become pregnant while on a stable ART regimen with viral suppression remain on that same regimen, with the exception of regimens containing didanosine, stavudine, or treatment-dose ritonavir.* Transplacental passage of antiretroviral drugs is an important mechanism of infant pre-exposure prophylaxis. Thus, when selecting an antiretroviral regimen for a treatment-naïve pregnant woman, at least one nucleoside/nucleotide reverse transcriptase inhibitor agent with high placental transfer should be included as a component of the ART regimen. Alternative and acceptable agents may be used when the patient's individual situation warrants.

1. **DHHS-recommended regimens during pregnancy (*in treatment-naïve patients*).** An ART regimen including two NRTIs combined with a ritonavir-boosted PI or an integrase inhibitor is preferred:

   a. **Preferred NRTIs include:** Tenofovir disoproxil fumarate/emtricitabine (TDF/FTC) or tenofovir disoproxil fumarate/lamivudine (TDF/3TC) or abacavir/lamivudine (ABC/3TC)—*if HLA-B 5701 negative*

b. **Preferred PIs include:** Atazanavir/ritonavir (ATV/r) once daily or darunavir/ritonavir (DRV/r) twice daily

Use of an increased dose for ATV/r (400 mg ATV plus 100 mg RTV once daily with food) during the second and third trimesters results in plasma concentrations equivalent to those in nonpregnant adults on standard dosing. Although some experts recommend increased ATV dosing in all women during the second and third trimesters, the package insert recommends increased ATV dosing only for antiretroviral-experienced pregnant women in the second and third trimesters also receiving either TDF or an H2-receptor antagonist.

c. **Preferred integrase inhibitor(s) include:** Raltegravir (RAL) twice daily

2. **DHHS alternative agents during pregnancy (*in treatment-naïve patients*):**

a. **NRTI alternative(s) include:** Zidovudine/lamivudine (ZDV/3TC) plus either a preferred NNRTI agent, PI agent, or integrase inhibitor

b. **NNRTI alternative(s) include:** Efavirenz (EFV) plus a preferred NRTI combination

The Food and Drug Administration (FDA) advises women to avoid becoming pregnant while taking efavirenz and advises healthcare providers to avoid administration in the first trimester of pregnancy as fetal harm may occur. Although the limited data on first-trimester efavirenz exposure cannot rule out a two- or threefold increased incidence of a rare outcome, such as neural tube defects, the available data from a meta-analysis on more than 2,000 births suggest that there is not a large increase (e.g., a 10-fold increase to a rate of 1%) in the risk of neural tube defects with first-trimester exposure. As a result, the current Perinatal Guidelines do not include a restriction of use before 8 weeks' gestation.

c. **PI alternative(s) include:** Lopinavir/ritonavir (LPV/r) plus a preferred NRTI combination

LPV exposure is reduced in pregnant women receiving standard adult doses; increasing to *twice-daily dosing* results in exposure equivalent to that seen in nonpregnant adults receiving standard doses

3. **DHHS infant ART prophylaxis recommendations:** All HIV-exposed infants should receive postpartum antiretroviral drugs to reduce the risk of perinatal transmission of HIV (AI). Infant antiretroviral prophylaxis—at gestational age-appropriate doses—should be initiated as close to the time of birth as possible, preferably within 6 to 12 hours of delivery.

A 4-week neonatal zidovudine prophylaxis regimen can be used for full-term infants when the mother has received a standard ART regimen during pregnancy with sustained viral suppression and there are no concerns related to maternal adherence. Otherwise, a 6-week course as part of a combination infant prophylaxis regimen is recommended in consultation with a pediatric infectious diseases provider.

a. **Recommended infant zidovudine dosing (delivery at greater than 35 weeks' gestation):** Zidovudine (ZDV) 4 mg/kg orally twice daily within 6 to 12 weeks of delivery through 4 to 6 weeks of age (see the preceding).

b. **Recommended infant zidovudine dosing (delivery between 30 and 35 weeks' gestation):** Zidovudine (ZDV) 4 mg/kg orally twice daily within 6 to 12 weeks of delivery through 2 weeks of age, then 3 mg/kg orally twice daily through 4 to 6 weeks of age.

c. **Recommended infant zidovudine dosing (delivery at less than 30 weeks' gestation):** Zidovudine (ZDV) 2 mg/kg orally twice daily within 6 to 12 weeks of delivery through 4 weeks of age, then 3 mg/kg orally twice daily through 6 weeks of age.

E. HIV Treatment Failure

1. *Virologic failure:* failure of viral suppression with initial therapy or detectable viral load after achieving viral suppression.

   a. Confirm with second assay to ensure detectable viral load after viral suppression was achieved is not a blip or a laboratory error

   b. Assess adherence and address potential barriers to adherence

   c. Obtain a viral resistance assay if viral load >1,000 copies per milliliter

   d. Work with an HIV expert to develop a new regimen once barriers that led to failure have been addressed

2. *Immunologic failure:* persistent decline in CD4 count with concomitant decline in CD4 percentage and detectable viral load.

3. *Clinical failure:* development of OI/HIV disease progression. Regimen changes should be based on viral load information because an immune reconstitution inflammatory syndrome (IRIS) due to an undiagnosed OI or another condition can mimic virologic failure.

4. Discontinuing or briefly interrupting therapy should be *avoided* if possible in a patient with HIV viremia because it may lead to a rapid increase in HIV RNA, a decrease in CD4 cell count, and increases the risk of clinical progression.

F. Treatment of OIs (Table 43.2)

1. The risk of an OI is usually assessed by the patient's CD4 count with certain OIs occurring at very low counts (*Mycobacterium avium* complex, CMV, *Cryptococcus neoformans* spp, [progressive multifocal leukoencephalopathy]), while others may occur at any CD4 count (TB, bacterial pneumonia).

2. OIs may also occur during an acute HIV infection.

3. Prophylaxis for OIs is important for prevention (Table 43.2) especially for *Pneumocystis jirovecii* pneumonia (PCP), toxoplasmosis, *Mycobacterium avium complex*, and TB.

G. Immunizations

1. Live virus vaccines should *not* be given to HIV-infected patients with a CD4 count of less than 200 cells/mL.

2. Recommended vaccines for routine care includes:

   a. Hepatitis A vaccine: provided in high-risk groups (MSM, IDU, HBV, hepatitis C virus [HCV], liver disease)

   b. Hepatitis B vaccine: in those without past or present hepatitis B infection

   c. Influenza vaccine: provided annually

    d. Pneumococcal vaccine: vaccinate when CD4 is greater than 200 cells/mL; consider booster 5 years after initial immunization

    e. Tetanus toxoid: provided every 10 years

BIBLIOGRAPHY

Aberg JA, Kaplan JE, Libman H, et al. Primary care guidelines for the management of persons infected with human immunodeficiency virus: 2009 update by the HIV Medicine Association of the Infectious Diseases Society of America. *Clin Infect Dis.* 2009;49(5):651–681.

Bartlett JG, Gallant JE, Pham PA. Medical management of HIV infection 2012. Durham, NC: Knowledge Source Solutions; 2012.

Goldschmidt RH, Chu C, Dong BJ. Initial management of patients with HIV infection. *Am Fam Physician.* 2016;94(9):708–716.

Kaplan JE, Benson C, Holmes KH, et al. Guidelines for prevention and treatment of opportunistic infections in HIV-infected adults and adolescents: recommendations from CDC, the National Institutes of Health, and the HIV Medicine Association of the Infectious Diseases Society of America. *MMWR Recomm Rep.* 2009;58(RR-4):1–207.

Panel on Antiretroviral Guidelines for Adults and Adolescents. Guidelines for the use of antiretroviral agents in HIV-1-infected adults and adolescents. Department of Health and Human Services. 1–288. Retrieved from http://www.aidsinfo.nih.gov/ContentFiles/AdultandAdolescentGL.pdf

OBSTETRICS AND GYNECOLOGY-RELATED INFECTIONS

Jennifer Husson
Leonard A. Sowah

I. **INTRODUCTION.** The reproductive tract of the human female can be classified as lower and upper genital tracts by relation to the uterine cervix. In the healthy female, the upper genital tract is sterile and the lower genital tract is actively colonized by bacterial commensals. Infections of the lower genital tract are therefore due to either a disturbance in the normal bacterial flora or introduction of new pathogenic agents. Lower genital tract infections are sexually transmitted or associated with sexual activity and are described in Chapter 42, Sexually Transmitted Diseases. This chapter focuses on upper genital tract infections.

II. **UPPER GENITAL TRACT INFECTIONS.** Upper genital tract infections are closely related because of the close proximity and the interconnected nature of the female genital tract. **Pelvic inflammatory disease (PID)** is a collective terminology that typically incorporates the full spectrum of upper genital tract infections, which include: (a) endometritis (endomyometritis), (b) salpingitis, (c) tubo-ovarian abscess, (d) pelvic abscess or peritonitis, and (e) chronic pelvic pain syndrome.

A. **Risk Factors for PID.** The most common risk factors include:

1. Age of sexual debut (less than 18 years of age).

2. Multiple sexual partners (more than four partners in the past 6 months).

3. Lack of use of barrier contraception.

4. History of PID.

5. "Back-alley" abortions.

6. Prior history of infection with *Chlamydia trachomatis* or *Neisseria gonorrhoeae*.

7. Vaginal douching.

8. Intrauterine device (IUD) use.

9. History of bacterial vaginosis (BV).

10. History of HIV infection.

B. **Microbiology of PID.** PID is considered a polymicrobial infection involving aerobic and anaerobic organisms. In general, the majority of bacterial isolates are non–sexually transmitted disease (STD) related anaerobes and aerobes.

1. *C. trachomatis*

2. *Mycoplasma genitalium*

3. *Ureaplasma urealyticum*

4. N. *gonorrhoeae*

5. *Prevotella* spp

6. Peptostreptococcus spp

7. *Escherichia coli*

8. *Haemophilus influenzae*

9. *Mobiluncus* spp

10. *Bacteroides fragilis*

C. **Clinical Manifestations of PID.** While the presentation may be acute or sub-acute and vary among patients, a history of fever or chills was more commonly associated with PID. The *classic triad of fever, pelvic pain, and vaginal discharge* is infrequent (approximately 20% of cases). Common symptoms include:

1. Lower abdominal pain.

2. Fever (greater than 38.3°C) or chills.

3. Irregular or change in menses.

4. Dyspareunia.

5. Abnormal vaginal discharge.

6. Postcoital bleeding.

D. **History and Physical Examination.** A complete and accurate history should be obtained in all suspected cases of PID. The history should focus on the timing of events, risk factors, sexual contacts, birth control method, and menstrual cycle status. Additionally, a complete physical examination should always be performed; however, no single physical finding is characteristic of PID. Areas of the examination to focus on include:

1. Fever (greater than 38.3°C).

2. Abdominal tenderness.

3 Adnexal tenderness.

4. Cervical motion tenderness.

5. Mucopurulent cervical discharge.

E. **Diagnosis.** PID should be included in the differential diagnosis of any sexually active woman with fever, pelvic pain, and/or vaginal discharge. *The Centers for Disease Control and Prevention (CDC) minimum criteria for the diagnosis of PID* include:

1. Cervical motion tenderness.

2. Adnexal tenderness.

3. Uterine tenderness.

   The presence of these additional factors increases likelihood of PID:

4. Temperature greater than 101°F (greater than 38.3°C).

5. Vaginal or cervical mucopurulent discharge.

6. More than three white blood cells (WBCs) per high-power field on saline mount of vaginal fluid (smears without WBCs have a high negative predictive value for excluding PID).

7. Elevated inflammatory markers evidenced by high erythrocyte sedimentation rate (ESR; greater than 15 mm/hour) and C-reactive protein.

8. Evidence of cervical infection with *N. gonorrhoeae* or *C. trachomatis*.

Patients with adnexal mass on bimanual examination must be evaluated with imaging using either CT scans with oral and intravenous contrast or pelvic ultrasonography for tubo-ovarian abscess, pyosalpinx, or hydrosalpinx. Laparoscopy has been considered as a gold standard for diagnosis of PID; however, it is impractical for routine use and may not detect endometritis or fallopian tube abnormalities. Laparoscopy is very useful in the identification of tubo-ovarian abscess, hydrosalpinx, or pyosalpinx as well as provides therapeutic drainage. Thus, laparoscopy is usually reserved for ill patients with suspected abscess or patients with an unclear diagnosis for the following reasons:

   a. It is not easily available in most cases.

   b. It is an invasive and expensive test.

   c. In cases of isolated endometritis and mild salpingitis, laparoscopy may miss the diagnosis.

F. **Other Diagnostic Tools**

1. Transvaginal ultrasonography is useful to diagnose but not rule out PID.

2. Endometrial biopsy is both sensitive and specific; however, it is invasive and takes time for results.

G. **General Rules of Therapy.** While the majority of cases can usually be managed on an outpatient basis, the criteria for hospitalization include:

1. Severe illness with systemic symptoms (e.g., systemic inflammatory response syndrome [SIRS]/sepsis) or signs of peritonitis.

2. Pregnancy or seropositive for HIV.

3. Failure to respond to appropriate therapy within 48 to 72 hours or unable to tolerate oral therapy.

4. Inability to rule out surgical emergencies (e.g., acute appendicitis).

5. Adolescent patients (high likelihood of poor adherence to therapy).

6. Inability or low likelihood of follow-up.

7. Tubo-ovarian abscess.

H. **Antimicrobial Regimens.** Therapy should target the polymicrobial nature of the disease and also be directed to both *N. gonorrhoeae* and *C. trachomatis* infections. In general, the total duration of therapy is 14 days.

1. **Outpatient regimens** include:

   a. Ceftriaxone 250 mg IM once *plus* doxycycline 100 mg PO q12 with or without metronidazole 500 mg q12

   b. Cefoxitin 2 g IM once with probenecid 1 g once *plus* doxycycline with or without metronidazole 500 mg q12

2. **Hospital regimens** include:

a. Cefotetan 2 g IV q12 or cefoxitin 2 g IV q6 *plus* doxycycline 100 mg PO or IV q12

b. Clindamycin 900 mg IV q8 *plus* gentamicin 2 mg/kg load, then 1.5 mg/kg q8 (this is considered the preferred regimen for pregnant patients)

Parenteral treatment should be continued for at least 24 to 48 hours after clinical improvement and then changed to oral doxycycline to complete a total 14-day course of therapy. In cases of tubo-ovarian abscess, clindamycin or metronidazole should be included in the oral regimen to provide better anaerobic coverage.

I. **Partner Treatment.** In cases involving an STD, partner treatment at the time of diagnosis is essential and patients must be advised to abstain from sexual intercourse or use condoms to prevent reinfection until completing either the full therapy or 7 days after treatment with a single-dose regimen.

J. **Complications and Other Clinical Manifestations of PID**

1. **Tubo-ovarian abscess.** This is the most common early complication of PID and usually the result of delayed diagnosis and treatment. The diagnosis is usually established by ultrasound or CT scans. Current therapy is a combination of aggressive medical management with or without ultrasound-guided drainage (abscesses larger than 10 cm are more likely to require drainage).

2. **Pelvic abscess/peritonitis.** Most abscesses are due to the presence of tubo-ovarian abscesses, while most cases of peritonitis are due to ruptured tubo-ovarian abscesses.

3. **Fitz-Hugh and Curtis syndrome.** This syndrome is classically associated with right upper quadrant abdominal pain (e.g., pleurisy pain) in a female with a genital tract gonococcal or chlamydia infection. It is associated with fibrinous inflammation of the liver capsule and adjacent parietal peritoneum and often occurs in the setting of acute salpingitis; however, symptoms of salpingitis may be mild or absent. Current therapy is directed against gonorrhea and chlamydia.

4. **Secondary infertility.** Usually occurs secondary to scarring of the fallopian tubes and is more common in women with prior infection with *C. trachomatis.*

5. **Ectopic (tubal) pregnancy.** Usually presents with abdominal pain and vaginal bleeding in a patient with a delayed menses. Commonly due to fallopian tube scarring from a prior episode of PID.

6. **Chronic pelvic pain.** Approximately one third of women with PID will experience chronic pelvic pain; however, symptoms may vary widely. It is more likely to occur in those with multiple episodes of PID, lower socioeconomic status, and/or a history of psychiatric illness.

K. **IUD-Associated Infections**

1. **Acquisition of infections**

a. Upper genital tract infection associated with an IUD is temporally related to the initial insertion of the device; however, the risk of infection does not remain elevated for the duration of the IUD (the risk is most commonly confined to the first 20 days after insertion).

  b. The monofilament tail string *does not* pose an increased risk for infection.

  c. Insertion of an IUD during asymptomatic *N. gonorrhoeae* and *C. trachomatis* infection poses no increased risk of PID compared to asymptomatic patients without an IUD.

  d. Insertion of an IUD poses no increase in the rate of STD acquisition.

2. Treatment. In general, the IUD may be retained in the original position during and after treatment for upper genital tract infections. Antimicrobial therapy is directed at *N. gonorrhoeae* and *C. trachomatis*.

3. Complications. Tubal infertility is the most common complication and likely related to behavioral practices.

4. Prevention. Antimicrobial prophylaxis, such as a single dose of doxycycline, may be beneficial in decreasing infection rates (in areas of high prevalence of both PID and STD infections) following IUD insertion.

III. PUERPERAL INFECTIONS. This is a group of infections that occur in women within the first 6 weeks post partum. For the purpose of this chapter, we focus on infections related to the breast and the female genital tract.

  A. Puerperal Sepsis. The World Health Organization (WHO) defines puerperal sepsis as an infection of the genital tract occurring at any time between the onset of rupture of membranes or labor and the 42nd day postpartum in which *fever* and one or more of the following are present:

   1. Pelvic pain.

   2. Abnormal vaginal discharge.

   3. Abnormal odor of vaginal discharge.

   4. Delay in the rate of reduction of the size of the uterus.

  B. Endometritis. This is also known as *endomyometritis* or *endoparametritis* and is a common cause of sepsis in the puerperal period. Historically, Dr. Ignaz Semmelweis (1818–1865), a Hungarian physician, proved that proper hand-washing could reduce risk of puerperal infection by observing midwives and physicians.

   1. Risk factors. The most common risk factors are cesarean section delivery, prolonged labor, or prolonged rupture of membranes; however, additional risk factors include: BV, HIV infection, low socioeconomic status, anemia, and maternal colonization with group B *Streptococcus*.

   2. Clinical manifestations. Endometritis remains predominantly a clinical diagnosis; therefore, a complete and accurate history should always be obtained with a focus on the risk factors. ***Endometritis should be included in the differential diagnosis for any patient with a fever that commonly occurs 1 to 2 days post partum.*** Additional clinical manifestations include malaise, nonspecific abdominal pain, nausea, vomiting, and chills.

   3. Physical examination. A complete physical examination should always be performed; however, the examination should focus on a bimanual pelvic examination in order to determine the uterine size and tenderness as well as evaluate any discharge. Findings on examination include:

    a. Fever and tachycardia

    b. Uterine tenderness

    c. Purulent vaginal discharge or lochia; however, some infections, usually those involving beta-hemolytic streptococci, may be associated with an odorless lochia.

4. Microbiology. This is usually a polymicrobial infection; therefore, microorganisms commonly responsible for this condition include:

    a. Gram-positive bacteria. Beta-hemolytic streptococci (e.g., groups A, B, and D), *Staphylococcus epidermidis*, and *S. aureus*.

    b. Gram-negative bacteria. *Escherichia coli, Klebsiella pneumoniae, Citrobacter* spp, *Pseudomonas* spp, *Proteus mirabilis,* and *Haemophilus influenzae.*

    c. Anaerobic bacteria. *Prevotella* spp, *Peptostreptococcus* spp, *Bacteroides fragilis* group spp, *Clostridium* spp, and *Fusobacterium* spp.

    d. Miscellaneous bacteria. *Gardnerella vaginalis, C. trachomatis, Mycoplasma hominis,* and *Ureaplasma urealyticum.*

5. Laboratory tests. Endometritis remains predominantly a clinical diagnosis; therefore, laboratory testing is utilized to support the diagnosis. Commonly utilized laboratory investigations may include: *complete blood count (CBC) with differential, blood cultures* (20% of women may have positive blood cultures and, therefore, a culture should be obtained in all suspected cases), and *uterine cultures* (samples tend to also include colonizing vaginal bacteria). CT scanning or MRI of the abdomen and pelvis may be helpful to identify our etiologies for cases not responding to appropriate antimicrobial therapy.

6. Treatment

    a. Moderate-to-severe endometritis. This generally requires a combination of intravenous antimicrobial therapy, antipyretics, and supportive care.

        i. Gold standard: clindamycin 450 to 900 mg IV q8 *plus* gentamicin 3 to 5 mg/kg once daily

        ii. Alternative: cefoxitin 2 g IV q6–8 or cefotetan 2 g IV q12 or piperacillin–tazobactam 3.375 g IV q6

    b. Mild endometritis. This may be treated with oral antimicrobial therapy.

        i. Ciprofloxacin 500 mg PO q12 or clindamycin 300 mg PO q6 or doxycycline 100 mg PO q12

    c. Treatment considerations. If the patient fails to respond after 3 days of appropriate antimicrobial therapy, the patient must be evaluated with appropriate imaging for other etiologies requiring specific treatment such as ***septic pelvic vein thrombophlebitis*** (which is the most common cause of an unexplained fever despite appropriate antimicrobial therapy) or ***pelvic abscess***. Septic pelvic vein thrombophlebitis would require anticoagulation to a partial thromboplastin time (PTT) of 1.5 to 2.0 times the baseline.

7. Prevention. Common preventive measures include:

    a. A single intraoperative prophylactic dose of ampicillin 2 g following clamping of the umbilical cord

    b. Limiting the number of digital vaginal examinations after membrane rupture

    c. Standard prophylactic antimicrobial therapy for both preterm and premature rupture of membranes at term

    d. Early treatment of genital tract infections and asymptomatic bacteriuria in the prenatal period

C. Chorioamnionitis

  1. Definition. It is defined as inflammation of the umbilical cord, amniotic membranes, or placenta. Maternal fever greater than 100.4°F in association with one other clinical criterion including:

    a. Maternal tachycardia greater than 100 bpm or fetal tachycardia greater than 160 bpm

    b. Maternal leukocytosis greater than 15,000 cell/mm^3

    c. Uterine tenderness

    d. Foul amniotic fluid odor

  2. Pathogenesis. This is most commonly an ascending polymicrobial infection from the lower genital tract in the setting of either labor or prolonged rupture of membranes. Infection can also occur in the setting of intact membranes (organisms such as *Mycoplasma hominis* or *Ureaplasma urealyticum*), following obstetrical procedures (e.g., amniocentesis or chorionic villous sampling), and/or as the result of anterograde infection from the peritoneum through the fallopian tubes. Rarely, hematogenous spread may lead to infection (most commonly involving *Listeria monocytogenes*).

  3. Risk factors. While the most common risk factors are the duration of ruptured membranes (greater than 12 hours) and multiple vaginal examinations during labor (more than three increases the risk), other risk factors include:

    a. Prolonged labor (12 hours or more of active labor)

    b. Nulliparity

    c. Internal monitoring during labor

    d. Meconium-stained amniotic fluid

    e. Use of cigarettes, alcohol, and/or other drugs

    f. Group B *Streptococcus* colonization, BV, sexually transmitted infections, or *Ureaplasma* infection

    g. Immunocompromised status

    h. Use of epidural anesthesia

  4. Microbiology. Most infections are *polymicrobial* and include aerobes (e.g., *Escherichia coli*, group B *Streptococcus*, and *Viridans streptococcus* spp), genital *Mycoplasma* spp (e.g., *M. hominis, Ureaplasma urealyticum*), *Gardnerella vaginalis*, and anaerobes (e.g., *Bacteroides fragilis* spp, *Prevotella* spp, and *Peptostreptococcus* spp). *Listeria monocytogenes* can occasionally cause infection from a hematogenous source.

5. Clinical manifestations. Signs and symptoms may vary among patients; however, a maternal *fever* (greater than 100.4°F) in the third trimester is the most common manifestation. Other findings include:

   a. Maternal tachycardia (greater than 100 bpm) or fetal tachycardia (greater than 160 bpm)

   b. Maternal leukocytosis (greater than 15,000 cells/mm^3)

   c. Uterine tenderness on pelvic examination

   d. Foul amniotic fluid odor

   Women currently in labor may experience fever, tachycardia (including fetal tachycardia), fundal tenderness, and/or purulent amniotic fluid on rupture of membranes. Subclinical chorioamnionitis, usually occurring in the setting of intact membranes, may lack the typical clinical signs.

6. **Diagnosis**. Chorioamnionitis remains predominantly a clinical diagnosis; therefore, a complete and accurate history should always be obtained with a focus on the risk factors. ***Chorioamnionitis should be included in the differential diagnosis for any patient with a fever in the third trimester***. Additionally, a complete physical examination should always be performed, as the differential diagnosis to consider in a suspected case also includes: acute appendicitis, pyelonephritis, pneumonia, pelvic thrombophlebitis, round ligament pain, and epidural-associated fever.

7. **Laboratory tests**. Chorioamnionitis remains predominantly a clinical diagnosis; therefore, laboratory testing is utilized to support the diagnosis. Commonly utilized testing includes: *CBC with differential* (maternal leukocytosis occurs in 70% to 90% of cases) and *amniotic fluid testing* with Gram stain and culture. A pathologic diagnosis by histologic criteria may be useful for subclinical disease.

8. **Treatment.** Prompt antimicrobial therapy has been found to reduce the incidence of complications. Suggested antimicrobial regimens include:

   a. Ampicillin 2 g IV q4–6 *or* penicillin G 5 million units IV q6 *plus* gentamicin 3 to 5 mg/kg daily (once daily dosing is associated with lower risk of toxicity)

   b. Clindamycin 900 mg IV q8 is recommended for penicillin-allergic patients

   Only a single postpartum dose is required for the prevention of postpartum endometritis. A single dose of clindamycin is added for anaerobic coverage if delivery is via abdominal cesarean section.

   There is no evidence to support prolonged oral antibiotics postdelivery. Use of maternal steroid injection to promote fetal lung maturity in the setting of preterm premature rupture of membranes has not been shown to have any deleterious effects in the setting of chorioamnionitis.

9. **Complications of chorioamnionitis**. Complications are generally categorized as maternal or fetal. Maternal complications include increased risk of cesarean delivery, postpartum hemorrhage, and bacteremia, as well as increased risk of pelvic infections (e.g., endometritis, wound infection, pelvic abscess). Fetal complications include premature birth, low birth weight, neonatal respiratory distress, and neonatal sepsis.

10. **Prevention**. Common prevention measures include ampicillin prophylaxis (women colonized with group B *Streptococcus*), and induction of labor and delivery for prolonged rupture of membranes after 32 weeks reduces maternal infection rates and neonatal complications.

D. **Perineum and Surgical Wound Infections, Including Episiotomy Site.** This includes any infection at a surgical site within 30 days of surgery.

1. **Pathogenesis.** Most wound infections are due to endogenous flora or contamination introduced into a wound during the surgical procedure.

   a. Perineal infection. Generally associated with midline episiotomy or third- or fourth-degree laceration or may be caused by occult rectal injury.

2. **Microbiology.** In general, the microorganisms are the same pathogens that are associated with PID; however, additional microorganisms may include: *S. aureus*, group B *Streptococcus*, *Enterococcus* spp, and *Bacteroides fragilis* group spp.

   a. Endogenous flora: gram-negative rods, enterococci, group B *Streptococcus*, and anaerobes.

3. **Clinical manifestations.** Wound infections classically are associated with skin erythema, edema, warmth, and tenderness; however, additional manifestations include: fever, purulent drainage, and tissue separation (e.g., wound dehiscence).

4. **Diagnosis.** Perineal infections necessitate pelvic examination to identify a postoperative abscess (e.g., vaginal cuff abscess or pelvic/adnexal abscess) or rectovaginal fistulas. Vaginal cuff abscesses (an infected, foul-smelling hematoma) usually occur within 1 week of the postoperative period and are characterized by a vaginal fullness sensation. Pelvic or adnexal abscesses usually occur within 3 weeks of the postoperative period and are characterized by fever, abdominal pain, and tender pelvic mass.

5. **Treatment.** Uncomplicated localized perineal infections (without fascial disruption) may be managed with wound care (e.g., irrigation, wound debridement with wet-to-dry dressings 2–3 times per day) and sitz bath therapy alone. Antimicrobial therapy follows the same principles and practices as other skin and soft-tissue infections except therapy should be directed at the polymicrobial nature of the infection (both aerobes and anaerobes).

6. **Complications.** Surgical site infections can range from an uncomplicated cellulitis, abscess formation, to severe necrotizing fasciitis.

7. **Prevention. Perioperative handwashing with standard antimicrobial prophylaxis is the best preventive measure.** Other measures include preprocedural antiseptic and sterile technique (preoperative hair removal is often not necessary; however, depilatories or clippers are associated with lower rates of infection than standard shaving) and postprocedural wound care teaching.

E. **Mastitis.** Localized inflammatory reaction of the breast in a nursing mother that may be associated with systemic symptoms (e.g., fever and fatigue). Incidence is highest in lactating women with the peak incidence occurring in the second and third weeks post partum.

1. **Risk factors**. In general, risks are classified into two categories:

   a. Maternal factors include:

      i. Poor nutrition

      ii. Previous mastitis

      iii. Sore or cracked nipples

      iv. Tight-fitting undergarments, use of manual breast pump, and/or plastic breast pads

   b. Infant factors include:

      i. Poor latch and missed feedings

      ii. Cleft lip or palate and/or short frenulum

2. **Microbiology**. *S. aureus* (methicillin-susceptible *Staphylococcus aureus* [MSSA] and methicillin-resistant *Staphylococcus aureus* [MRSA]) is the most common isolate found in breast milk. Other pathogens include: coagulase-negative *Staphylococcus* spp, beta-hemolytic *Streptococcus* (e.g., group A *Streptococcus*), *Escherichia coli*, *Candida albicans*, and rarely, *Mycobacterium tuberculosis*.

3. **Clinical presentation.** Nursing women usually experience unilateral breast pain and erythema (V-shaped cellulitis) accompanied by fever, fatigue, body aches, and/or headaches. Inflammatory breast cancer should always be considered in the differential diagnosis, especially in a nonlactating female.

4. **Treatment.** In general, breastfeeding should continue from the affected breast as mother and infant are generally colonized with the same organisms. Additionally, draining breast milk thoroughly from the affected breast may prevent milk stasis (milk stasis is associated with abscess formation).

   Antimicrobial therapy typically includes an antistaphylococcal agent. *Breast milk should be obtained for Gram stain, culture, and antimicrobial susceptibilities.* The duration of therapy is generally **10 to 14 days** for uncomplicated mastitis.

   a. Dicloxacillin 250 to 500 mg PO q6

   b. Cephalexin 250 to 500 mg PO q6

   c. Amoxicillin–clavulanate 875 mg PO q12

   d. Clindamycin 300 mg PO q6–8

   e. Trimethoprim–sulfamethoxazole 160/800 mg PO q12

   Clindamycin or trimethoprim–sulfamethoxazole may also be used for cases involving MRSA; however, doxycycline should be avoided.

5. **Complications.** Abscess formation may rarely occur and is characterized by a firm area of induration with fluctuance. The diagnosis may be confirmed with the use of ultrasonography, while treatment involves a combination of antimicrobial therapy with surgical drainage. HIV transmission may occur in the presence of mastitis.

6. **Prevention.** While there remain no contraindications to breastfeeding during the treatment of mastitis, optimizing the breastfeeding technique continues to be an effective prevention measure.

BIBLIOGRAPHY

Biggs WS, Williams RM. Common gynecologic infections. *Prim Care.* 2009;36(1):33–51.

Fishman SG, Gelber SE. Evidence for the clinical management of chorioamnionitis. *Semin Fetal Neonatal Med.* 2012;17(1):46–50.

Gibbs RS. Severe infections in pregnancy. *Med Clin North Am.* 1989;73(3):713–721.

Grimes DA. Intrauterine device and upper-genital-tract infection. *Lancet.* 2000;356(9234):1013–1019.

Lareau SM, Beigi RH. Pelvic inflammatory disease and tubo-ovarian abscess. *Infect Dis Clin North Am.* 2008;22(4):693–708.

Tharpe N. Postpregnancy genital tract and wound infections. *J Midwifery Women's Health.* 2008;53(3):236–246.

Tita AT, Andrews WW. Diagnosis and management of clinical chorioamnionitis. *Clin Perinatol.* 2010;37(2):339–354.

Spencer JP. Management of mastitis in breastfeeding women. *Am Fam Physician.* 2008;78(6):727–731.

Sweet RL. Pelvic inflammatory disease: current concepts of diagnosis and management. *Curr Infect Dis Rep.* 2012;14:194–203.

INFECTIOUS KERATITIS

Jason Bailey
Anthony Amoroso
William F. Wright

I. INTRODUCTION

A. Definition. Inflammation of the cornea as a result of invasion by a microorganism. *Infectious keratitis is a vision-threatening condition that is considered a medical emergency.*

B. Pathogenesis. The cornea is an avascular transparent structure of the eye that is composed of five layers and normally functions to: (a) provide the eye with the capacity to focus light on the retina for vision, (b) filter ultraviolet sunlight, and (c) provide a barrier to protection. Additionally, tear film (contains antimicrobial enzymes) and mechanical blinking (reduces microbial adherence) provide corneal protection.

The five layers of the cornea include (from the external to internal eye):

1. **Epithelium.** Outermost layers that can regenerate *without* scarring within 24 hours if damaged or lost.

2. **Bowman layer.**

3. **Stroma.** Thickest inner layer that can regenerate *with* scarring if damaged or lost.

4. **Descemet's membrane.**

5. **Endothelium.** Innermost layer that *does not regenerate* if damaged or lost.

Any *defect in the corneal epithelium* may lead to invasion of a microorganism with a resultant inflammatory infiltration. Corneal inflammation can be either **ulcerative** (breach of the corneal epithelium) or **nonulcerative**.

C. Risk Factors. Usually associated with the disruption of the corneal epithelium and include:

1. **Ocular trauma** (e.g., burns, agricultural, or outdoor occupations).

2. **Conventional ocular contact lens use** (overnight or extended contact use is a common cause of corneal trauma as well as contamination of ocular solutions or contact lens storage device may be associated with infections).

3. **Ocular surface diseases** (e.g., keratoconjunctivitis, blepharitis).

4. **Ocular surgery** (e.g., laser-assisted in situ keratomileusis [LASIK] surgery).

5. **Systemic diseases** (e.g., diabetes mellitus, rheumatoid arthritis, Sjögren syndrome, Bell palsy, Graves disease, HIV, and Stevens–Johnson syndrome).

D. **Epidemiology.** The true incidence and prevalence of infectious keratitis are unknown; however, there is a slight male predominance (presumed due to ocular trauma from outdoor exposures).

II. **IMPORTANT CAUSES OF INFECTIOUS KERATITIS.** A list of the commonly important infectious pathogens implicated in infectious keratitis includes:

A. **Viral Pathogens.** Viral keratitis can result from primary infection or recurrent infections (e.g., herpes simplex virus 1 [HSV-1] or varicella-zoster virus [VZV]). Pathogens commonly implicated in keratitis include:

1. **HSV-1.** Recurrent infection is more common than primary infection. *This is the most common cause of corneal ulcers and blindness.*

2. **VZV.** Recurrent infection is more common.

3. **Adenovirus** (particularly adenovirus 8 and 19).

4. **Epstein–Barr virus (EBV) and cytomegalovirus (CMV).** Usually occur with immunocompromised host.

B. **Bacterial Pathogens.** Associated with 65% to 90% of infectious keratitis cases. Pathogens that can cause conjunctivitis can also cause infectious keratitis following invasion of the corneal epithelium. Some pathogens (e.g., *Neisseria gonorrhoeae, Listeria monocytogenes, Shigella* spp, and *Corynebacterium* spp) may penetrate the cornea by attaching and releasing proteolytic enzymes that destroy the corneal epithelial layer. Pathogens include:

1. **Gram-positive cocci**

   a. **Coagulase-negative staphylococcus** (CoNS; e.g., *Staphylococcus epidermidis*)

   b. **S. aureus** (both methicillin-susceptible *Staphylococcus aureus* [MSSA] and methicillin-resistant *Staphylococcus aureus* [MRSA])

   c. *Streptococcus pneumoniae*

2. **Gram-positive rods**

   a. **Nontuberculous mycobacteria (NTM).** (e.g., *Mycobacterium fortuitum, M. chelonae*). Commonly associated with laser-assisted subepithelial keratectomy (LASEK) surgery or trauma with soil contamination.

   b. *Mycobacterium tuberculosis*

   c. *Mycobacterium leprae*

   d. *Nocardia* spp

   e. *Propionibacterium acnes*

3. **Gram-negative cocci**

   a. *Neisseria gonorrhoeae*

4. **Gram-negative rods.** Typically related to contact lenses or comatose intubated critically ill patients.

   a. *Pseudomonas aeruginosa* (commonly associated with contact lenses)

   b. *Moraxella* spp (*M. liquefaciens*; commonly associated with malnourished patients in association with immunosuppression, diabetes, and/or alcoholism)

    c. *Haemophilus* **spp**

    d. **Enteric pathogens** (e.g., *Escherichia coli, Proteus* spp, *Klebsiella* spp)

    e. *Acinetobacter* **spp** (commonly associated with ocular burns)

C. Fungal Pathogens. These pathogens are considered rare causes of infectious keratitis with the majority of cases involving trauma (especially with vegetative matter), immunosuppression, and the use of ocular steroids for systemic conditions (e.g., uveitis). Pathogens may be inoculated into the cornea by trauma involving plant or vegetable matter, except for *Candida albicans*, which comes from the patient's own flora. Pathogens include:

    1. *Aspergillus* **spp**

    2. *Fusarium* **spp**

    3. *Curvularia* **spp**

    4. *Candida* **spp**

    5. *Cryptococcus neoformans*

D. Parasitic Pathogens. *Acanthamoeba*-related keratitis is the most common cause due to a parasite with the majority of cases involving wearers of soft contact lenses, contact lens solutions, or contact cases. Other less common parasites include:

    1. *Microsporidia* (can be associated with HIV or immunocompromised status)

    2. *Onchocerca* (Onchocerciasis, e.g., river blindness)

    3. *Leishmania* (Leishmaniasis)

Interstitial keratitis, otherwise known as *stromal* keratitis, is a nonulcerative corneal inflammation associated with HSV-1, *Mycobacterium tuberculosis*, *M. leprae*, and syphilis (e.g., *Treponema pallidum*). The majority of syphilis cases are congenitally acquired; however, noncongenital cases should be considered associated with HIV infection since a higher incidence of ocular syphilis occurs in HIV-seropositive patients.

III. CLINICAL MANIFESTATIONS OF INFECTIVE KERATITIS. Clinical manifestations are variable and can include acute and rapidly destructive infections or chronic and indolent infections. The major signs and symptoms include:

A. Classic Manifestations. Commonly associated with *miosis* (pupillary constriction), *photophobia, unilateral ocular erythema* (i.e., red eye), *ocular pain* (except HSV), *hyperlacrimation* (e.g., increased tearing), and *corneal defect* (most commonly a corneal ulcer).

B. Hypopyon. A visible layer of pus (seen as a gray fluid level) in the anterior chamber of the eye. As a general rule, bacterial ulcers usually have a sterile hypopyon unless rupture of Descemet's membrane occurs but fungal ulcers usually contain fungal elements with an associated hypopyon.

C. Loss of Corneal Transparency. A white corneal infiltrate associated with corneal inflammation or scarring.

D. Periorbital Rash or Vesicular Lesions. May be seen with HSV or VZV.

E. Mucous Membrane Lesion and/or Ulcers. May suggest a herpesvirus infection.

IV. APPROACH TO THE PATIENT

A. Patient History. The diagnosis of infectious keratitis can be difficult and should be included in the differential diagnosis of a patient evaluated for **a painful red eye (*pain out of proportion to examination findings is commonly associated with* Acanthamoeba), diminished vision, photophobia, ocular discharge, and/or foreign body sensation.** A complete history should be obtained, and it is important to obtain information about **risk factors** (see Section I.C) and the following:

1. **Timing of events.** Understanding the timing of symptoms in relation to ocular trauma, ocular surgery, or hospitalization may be helpful to identifying a possible pathogen.

2. **Contact lens use.** It is important to understand if the patient wears contact lenses, what type, and for what period of time each day.

3. **Recent travel and geographic location.** Can provide clues to risks of acquiring a particular pathogen endemic to a particular location (e.g., onchocerciasis and leishmaniasis).

4. **Comorbid illnesses.** May be helpful to identify conditions that predispose to corneal defects and immunosuppression (e.g., diabetes, rheumatoid arthritis).

5. **Occupational history.** An agricultural or outdoor occupation may be associated with infectious keratitis.

6. **Recent history of ocular surgery.** May be helpful to understanding a particular pathogen (e.g., LASIK surgery and NTM).

B. Physical Examination. While the general physical examination is unlikely to reveal the cause, both a complete examination and ocular examination should be performed. Areas of the examination for the physician to focus on include:

1. **Dermatologic examination** (to detect rashes or vesicular lesions).

   *A rash on the tip of the nose in association with herpes zoster ophthalmicus (e.g., **Hutchinson sign**) is associated with an increased risk of corneal involvement.*

2. **Ocular examination** (to detect focal changes or defects in the cornea).

   a. **Visual acuity examination.** *Single most important examination and most accurately tested using the Snellen chart.* The patient should stand 20 feet from the vision chart with testing of each eye (OD = right eye; OS = left eye; and OU = both eyes). The score is expressed as 20/X, where 20 equals 20 feet from the eye to the visual chart and X stands for the smallest print the patient can identify correctly. (X can range from 10 to 200, but normal is considered 20/20.)

   b. **Corneal examination.** General inspection of the cornea in keratitis is characterized by loss of corneal luster (seen as grayness of the cornea). Corneal ulceration can be visualized with the application of sodium *fluorescein* to the eye followed by illumination with a cobalt-blue filter light source (ulcerations or abrasions appear *green*).

   c. **Slit-lamp examination.** This examination is performed by an ophthalmologist with a powerful light source focused in a narrow slit upon the various layers of the cornea to obtain an accurate inspection of the areas of defect and inflammation.

The *general corneal ulcer morphologies seen on examination* that are associated with particular pathogens include:

i. Group A *Streptococcus*. Central ulcer with corneal infiltrate and edema associated with a large hypopyon.

ii. S. *pneumoniae*. A well-circumscribed ulcer that begins and spreads rapidly (24–48 hours) in many directions that is commonly associated with a hypopyon.

iii. *Staphylococcus* spp (CoNS, MSSA, MRSA). A centrally located ulcer that is both superficial and indolent in its course and may have a gray, well-defined stromal infiltrate with or without a hypopyon.

iv. Pseudomonas spp. A rapidly spreading ulcer from the site of injury that may involve a gray-yellow corneal infiltrate with a large hypopyon that may be blue-green.

v. *Moraxella* spp. An oval, inferior corneal ulcer that is indolent in its course and *not* usually associated with a hypopyon.

vi. NTM/*Nocardia*. An indolent ulcer with radiating edges that appears as a "cracked window" with or without a hypopyon.

vii. Fungal spp. An indolent ulcer with irregular edges and a gray stromal infiltrate with an associated hypopyon as well as satellite ulcers.

viii. HSV. A superficial ulcer arranged in a branching pattern with feathery edges and terminal bulbs (i.e., dendritic ulcer).

ix. VZV. A blotchy amorphous ulcer with occasional dendritic forms and stromal opacity.

x. Acanthamoeba. A stromal ring that is indolent in its course but extremely painful (pain out of proportion to examination findings).

C. Laboratory Studies

1. **Corneal scraping or biopsy.** Microbiology staining and culturing of a *corneal scraping* (using either a number 15 surgical blade or special ocular spatula to obtain a specimen from the ulcer base or edge) or *corneal biopsy* (surgically excising corneal tissue) on various culture media may yield a particular pathogen. *It is important to also culture the contact lens and lens case in suspected cases.*

2. **Blood cultures**. Routinely ordered but are of limited value.

3. **Complete blood count (CBC).** Routinely ordered but of limited value.

4. **Complete metabolic profile (CMP).** Usually nonspecific but may reveal comorbid illnesses (e.g., diabetes).

5. **HIV enzyme-linked immunosorbent assay (ELISA; serum).** Helpful in cases of noncongenital syphilis.

6. **Rapid plasma reagin (RPR; serum).** Helpful in cases suspected of syphilis.

7. **Thyroid-stimulating hormone (TSH), free T_3/T_4 (triiodothyronine/thyroxine).** May be helpful in cases associated with Graves disease.

8. **Erythrocyte sedimentation rate (ESR) and C-reactive protein (CRP).** May be helpful in cases associated with rheumatoid arthritis or other collagen vascular disorders.

D. Confocal Microscopy. A special in vivo microscopy examination method performed by an ophthalmologist that provides images of all corneal layers that can be used to both diagnose infections and monitor the response to treatment.

V. TREATMENT *(Antibiotic dosing listed assumes normal renal function.)*

A. *Infectious keratitis is a vision-threatening condition that is considered a medical emergency.* An ophthalmology consult should be obtained immediately.

B. Specific treatment should target the suspected or identified pathogen, and the duration of treatment should be determined in conjunction with an ophthalmologist.

C. Treatment recommendations for selected pathogens include:

1. **HSV/VZV.** Topical or systemic therapy may be used. Immunocompromised patients may benefit from a combination of both. Topical therapy may include 3% acyclovir ointment five times per day. Systemic therapy options include (in order of preference): (a) valacyclovir 1 g PO q12 for 7 to 10 days, (b) acyclovir 400 mg PO q8 for 10 days, *or* (c) famciclovir 250 mg PO q8 for 10 days.

2. **Bacterial pathogens.** Topical antibiotic eye preparations are capable of achieving high tissue levels and are the preferred treatment method. *Hospitalization* should be considered in selected patients (*e.g., vision-threatening condition, poor compliance, patients who live alone, or patients who do not readily have access to a clinic or hospital facility*) due to the risk of rapid necrosis or corneal thinning that can occur without adequate treatment. Treatment should be tailored to culture data (when available) and modified if the patient does not show clinical improvement within 48 hours.

   a. **Empirical treatment (covers most gram-positive and gram-negative pathogens).** Cefazolin (50 mg/mL) with tobramycin *or* gentamicin (9–14 mg/mL), *or* single-agent fluoroquinolones (e.g., ciprofloxacin 3 mg/mL *or* moxifloxacin 5 mg/mL) are the preferred topical treatments for empiric coverage when there is either no organism identified or multiple types of organisms.

   b. *Staphylococcus.* Topical cefazolin (50 mg/mL) for MSSA and topical vancomycin (50 mg/mL) for MRSA

   c. **NTM.** Topical amikacin and ciprofloxacin

   d. *Nocardia.* Topical ampicillin and sulfonamides

   e. *Pseudomonas.* Topical ticarcillin/piperacillin (50 mg/mL), gentamicin (15 mg/mL), ceftazidime (50 mg/mL), and ciprofloxacin (3 mg/mL) with systemic ciprofloxacin 500 mg PO q12

   f. **Gonococcus.** Ceftriaxone 1 to 2 g IV/IM q24 for 5 days

   g. *Streptococcus.* Topical cefazolin (50 mg/mL)

   h. *Moraxella.* Topical moxifloxacin (5 mg/mL) or ciprofloxacin (3 mg/mL)

3. **Parasite pathogens.** No consensus on treatment except for *Acanthamoeba* keratitis. Suggested treatment for *Acanthamoeba* includes a combination of biguanides and diamidines, although no agent is effective against the cyst stage:

    a. **Biguanides.** Polyhexamethylene biguanide (PHMB) 0.02% to 0.06% (200–600 mcg/mL) and chlorhexidine 0.02% to 0.2% (200–2,000 mcg/mL)

    b. **Diamidines.** Propamidine isethionate 0.1% (1,000 mcg/mL) and hexamidine 0.1% (1,000 mcg/mL)

4. **Fungal pathogens.** No consensus on treatment and may require a combination of topical and systemic agents.

    a. **Molds (e.g., *Aspergillus* spp).** While 5% natamycin is considered the first choice, 1% itraconazole *or* 0.15% amphotericin B can also be used and/or systemic voriconazole 200 mg PO q12.

    b. **Yeast (e.g., *Candida* spp).** Topical 0.15% amphotericin B *and/or* systemic fluconazole 50 to 100 mg PO daily.

BIBLIOGRAPHY

American Academy of Ophthalmology Retina Panel. Preferred Practice Pattern® Guidelines. Bacterial keratitis—limited revision. San Francisco, CA: American Academy of Ophthalmology; 2011. Retrieved from http://www.aao.org/ppp

Barnes, SD, Pavan-Langston D, Azar D. Keratitis. In GL Mandell, JE Bennett, R Dolin (Eds.), *Mandell, Douglas, and Bennett's Principles and Practice of Infectious Diseases*. 7th ed. Philadelphia, PA: Churchill Livingstone Elsevier; 2010: 1539–1551.

Garg P. Diagnosis of microbial keratitis. *Br J Ophthalmol*. 2010;94(8):961–962.

Sharma S. Keratitis. *Biosci Rep*. 2001;21(4):419–444.

Thomas PA, Geraldine P. Infectious keratitis. *Curr Opin Infect Dis*. 2007;20(2):129–141.

ENDOPHTHALMITIS

Adrian Majid
Anthony Amoroso
William F. Wright

I. INTRODUCTION

A. Definition. An inflammatory condition of the intraocular cavities (either the vitreous and/or aqueous humor; see Figure 46.1) as a result of the invasion by either a bacterial or fungal microorganism.

B. Pathogenesis. A breach, or disruption, in the integrity of the *ocular bulbus* provides the potential for the introduction of microorganisms that can then result in an intraocular infectious process. In general, endophthalmitis can arise from either an external introduction of microbes (**exogenous**) or hematogenous seeding of the eye (**endogenous**).

C. Risk Factors. Usually associated with the type of pathogenic mechanism (see the preceding) and include:

1. **Exogenous-source endophthalmitis.** Risk factors are mainly related to trauma and/or procedures that involve either the eye or external surrounding eye structures. The most common factors include:

   a. **Operative procedures** (e.g., glaucoma drainage surgery, intraocular lens implant, keratoplasty, trabeculectomy, strabismus surgery, and pterygium excision).

   b. **Intravitreal injections for systemic conditions** (e.g., uveitis).

   c. **Trauma and/or intraocular foreign body**.

   d. **Infectious keratitis.** Although rare, a chronic untreated corneal infection may result in corneal perforation with resultant intraocular spread.

2. **Endogenous-source endophthalmitis.** Risk factors are mainly related to the degree of immunosuppression and/or a predisposition that increases the risk of a blood-borne infection. The most common factors include:

   a. **Intravenous or indwelling catheter.**

   b. **Solid organ or stem cell transplantation.**

   c. **Malignancy, chemotherapy, and/or neutropenia.**

   d. **HIV infection.**

   e. **Intravenous drug use (IVDU).**

   f. **Diabetes mellitus.**

   g. **Chronic renal failure** (especially with hemodialysis).

FIGURE 46.1 Schematic diagram of the eye.

D. **Epidemiology.** In general, the incidence and prevalence of endophthalmitis are reported to be declining. Additionally, there is a *slight male predominance* (presumed due to ocular trauma from outdoor exposures). Most infections (90% of cases) are unilateral and due to an exogenous-source infection; however, endogenous-source infections (10% of cases) are also commonly unilateral, but as many as 25% of cases may be bilateral.

E. **Specific Categories of Endophthalmitis.** Categorizations are usually associated with the type of pathogenic mechanism (see the preceding) and include:

1. **Exogenous-source endophthalmitis.** These are mainly related to trauma and/or surgical procedures that involve either the eye or external surrounding eye structures and include:

   a. **Acute postoperative endophthalmitis.** This is the *most common form* of endophthalmitis. Approximately 90% of cases are due to cataract surgery (most common surgery) and usually *occur within 1 to 2 weeks of surgery*; however, patients can present up to 6 weeks after surgery. This form has an incidence of 0.08% to 0.7% with the estimated 2 million surgeries performed in the United States. The pathogenesis is related to contamination of the aqueous humor at the time of surgery with the patient's own periocular flora or with contaminated ocular irrigation fluids. While contamination can occur in an estimated 8% to 43% of all cases, very few progress to infection.

   b. **Chronic postoperative endophthalmitis.** While the true incidence is unknown, this form is less common than acute postoperative endophthalmitis and is characterized as an indolent infection occurring after intraocular surgery. Cases usually present greater than 6 weeks postsurgery. This form includes *chronic pseudophakic endophthalmitis*, a rare infection of the intraocular lens after cataract surgery.

c. **Bleb-related endophthalmitis**. This form is also called *filtering-bleb-associated endophthalmitis* or *post-trabeculectomy endophthalmitis* and *most commonly results from a glaucoma filtering surgery*. In other words, this is an infection of a surgically created defect in the sclera (bleb) used with glaucoma to allow aqueous humor to leak out of the anterior chamber and then be absorbed into the circulation (i.e., lowers intraocular pressure). The risk of infection is further increased with a bleb formation in an inferior rather than superior location. This form has an estimated incidence of 0.2% to 9.6% after glaucoma filtering surgeries and usually occurs days to years (mean time period of 19 months) after glaucoma filtering surgery.

d. **Posttraumatic endophthalmitis**. While this form can occur following either a *ruptured ocular globe or penetrating ocular injury*, it has an estimated incidence of 7% (higher incidence rates of 11%–30% are associated with intraocular foreign bodies). *Specific risk factors* associated with this infection include: (a) age greater than 50 years, (b) laceration with a metal object, (c) retained intraocular foreign body, (d) delay in presentation and/or primary closure of more than 24 hours, (e) contaminated wound, and (f) disruption of the lens.

2. **Endogenous-source endophthalmitis**. This form accounts for 2% to 8% of endophthalmitis cases. This form occurs when microorganisms in the bloodstream (most commonly bacteria and fungi) cross the blood–ocular barrier to infect intraocular tissue.

II. IMPORTANT MICROBIAL CAUSES OF ENDOPHTHALMITIS. A list of the important pathogens implicated in this infection are shown in the following table.

Type of Endophthalmitis	Common Pathogens
Acute postoperative endophthalmitis	**Coagulase-negative staphylococci (70%)**, *Staphylococcus aureus* (10%), streptococci (9%), various gram-negative bacilli (e.g., *Pseudomonas* spp, *Klebsiella* spp; 6%), other gram-positive cocci (e.g., *Enterococcus* spp; 5%)
Chronic postoperative endophthalmitis	*Propionibacterium* spp (63%), coagulase-negative staphylococci (16%), *Candida parapsilosis* (16%), *Corynebacterium* spp (5%). Rarer causes: *Actinomyces, Nocardia, Achromobacter, Cephalosporium, Acremonium, Paecilomyces, Aspergillus* spp
Bleb-related endophthalmitis	**Streptococci spp, coagulase-negative staphylococci,** *Staphylococcus aureus, Haemophilus influenzae, Moraxella catarrhalis*
Posttraumatic endophthalmitis	***Bacillus* spp, coagulase-negative staphylococci**, streptococci, gram-negative bacilli such as *Klebsiella* and *Pseudomonas*, molds (*Aspergillus* and *Fusarium* spp)
Endogenous endophthalmitis	North America and Europe: **streptococci (32%)**—*S. pneumoniae, S. anginosus*, group A and group B *Streptococcus* (30%–50% of cases), ***Staphylococcus aureus*** (25%), gram-negative bacilli (*Escherichia coli, Klebsiella* spp, *Serratia* spp), fungi (*Candida* spp most common), parasites (e.g., *Toxocara canis, Toxoplasma gondii*) Asia: gram-negative bacilli (*Klebsiella* spp, *E. coli*)

A. **Bacterial Pathogens.** In general, more virulent gram-negative bacteria and certain gram-positive bacteria (e.g., *Staphylococcus aureus, Streptococcus* spp) tend to produce infections with an earlier onset and worse outcome. Polymicrobial infections are more commonly found with posttraumatic endophthalmitis. Particular characteristics associated with certain pathogens include:

   1. ***Bacillus* spp (especially *B. cereus*).** This is a very virulent group of pathogens that are most commonly associated with IVDU (presumed contamination of injection drug paraphernalia and solutions) as well as following ocular trauma (especially with contaminated or soiled wounds).

   2. ***Propionibacterium acnes*.** A very low virulent organism that is most commonly associated with chronic postoperative infections.

B. **Fungal Pathogens.** In general, fungal pathogens most commonly cause endogenous endophthalmitis rather than exogenous endophthalmitis. Additionally, molds (e.g., *Aspergillus* and *Fusarium* spp) would be more likely to cause exogenous endophthalmitis rather than yeast (e.g., *Candida* spp). Particular characteristics associated with certain pathogens include:

   1. ***Candida* spp (particularly *C. albicans*).** This is the most common cause of endogenous endophthalmitis that is associated with IVDU, intravenous hyperalimentation, and/or indwelling catheters, immunosuppression medications.

   2. ***Aspergillus* spp**. Usually more virulent than *Candida*-related infections and tend to be associated with chronic pulmonary infections and IVDU.

   3. ***Fusarium* spp**. Usually associated with disseminated infection in immunocompromised patients.

C. **Parasitic Pathogens.** These pathogens are extremely rare as microbial causes of endophthalmitis.

III. **CLINICAL MANIFESTATIONS OF ENDOPHTHALMITIS.** Clinical manifestations are variable and can include acute and rapidly destructive infections or chronic and indolent infections. The major signs and symptoms include:

A. **Classic Manifestations.** Commonly associated with **vitritis** that is clinically characterized by a *visual deficit or loss, ocular pain*, and *hypopyon*.

B. **Hypopyon.** A visible layer of pus (seen as a gray fluid level) in the anterior chamber of the eye.

C. **Ocular Pain**

D. **Loss of Fundus Reflex.** A white infiltrate associated with retinal inflammation or scarring.

E. **Conjunctiva Erythema and/or Ocular Chemosis**

F. **Corneal Edema**

IV. **APPROACH TO THE PATIENT**

A. **Patient History.** The diagnosis of endophthalmitis can be difficult and should be included in the differential diagnosis of a patient evaluated for **a painful red eye, diminished vision, ocular discharge, and/or foreign-body sensation.** A complete history should be obtained, and it is important to obtain information about **risk factors** (see Section I.C) and the following:

1. **Timing of events.** Understanding the timing of symptoms in relation to ocular trauma, ocular surgery, or hospitalization may be helpful to identifying a possible pathogen.

2. **Contact lens use.** It is important to understand if the patient wears contact lenses, what type, and for what period of time each day.

3. **Recent travel and geographic location.** Can provide clues to risks of acquiring a particular pathogen endemic to a particular location (see the preceding table).

4. **Comorbid illnesses.** May be helpful to identify conditions that predispose to bloodstream infections and/or immunosuppression (e.g., diabetes, renal failure, malignancy).

5. **Occupational history.** An agricultural or outdoor occupation may be associated with traumatic ocular injuries with resultant infections.

6. **Recent history of ocular surgery.** May be helpful to understanding a particular pathogen (e.g., glaucoma surgery).

B. **Physical Examination.** While the general physical examination is unlikely to reveal the cause, both a complete physical examination and ocular examination should be performed. Areas of the examination for the physician to focus on include:

1. **Ocular examination** (to detect focal changes or defects in the eye). In bleb-related endophthalmitis, a purulent bleb may be present.

   a. **Visual acuity examination.** *Single most important examination.*

   Formally, visual acuity is most accurately tested using the ***Snellen chart*** (see Chapter 45, Infectious Keratitis); however, the most important determinant for identifying patients who would benefit from vitrectomy is to *determine light perception simply from hand-motion vision.* Hand motion is measured no closer than 2 feet with light originating from behind the patient.

   b. **Intraocular pressure examination.** Generally measured by an ophthalmologist using a tonometer with values reported as millimeters of mercury (mmHg). Normal intraocular pressures range from 10 to 20 mmHg.

   c. **Slit-lamp examination.** This examination is performed by an ophthalmologist with a powerful light source focused in a narrow slit upon the various layers of the cornea and retina to obtain an accurate inspection of the areas of defect and inflammation.

   The importance of an extended physical examination is to search for systemic infections that may suggest an endogenous-source infection. *The most common infections of origin include: liver abscesses, pneumonia, endocarditis, skin and soft-tissue infections, urinary tract infections, meningitis, and septic arthritis.*

2. **Dermatologic examination.** The findings of nail-bed splinter hemorrhages, Janeway lesions, and Osler nodes may suggest endocarditis.

3. **Abdominal examination.** Localized pain such as right upper quadrant (RUQ; biliary tract infection), right lower quadrant (RLQ; appendicitis), left lower quadrant (LLQ; diverticulitis), suprapubic discomfort (cystitis), and costovertebral angle (CVA) tenderness (pyelonephritis) may suggest a gastrointestinal or genitourinary cause for bacteremia.

4. **Cardiovascular examination.** A new diastolic murmur (indicating valvular regurgitation) or change with existing murmur may suggest endocarditis.

5. **Pulmonary examination.** To search for localized findings suggestive of pneumonia (see Chapter 11, Pneumonia).

6. **Neurologic examination.** Meningitis may be detected with findings of meningeal inflammation that is detected by testing for: (a) **Kernig** sign—positive test with flexion of hip and knee that produces neck pain, and (b) **Brudzinski** sign—positive test with flexion of neck.

7. **Musculoskeletal examination.** Septic arthritis may be indicated by *a single joint in association with rapid fluctuant swelling and joint pain and tenderness with diminished range of passive motion.*

C. **Laboratory Studies**

1. **Ocular cultures.** Samples should be obtained by an ophthalmologist with a 30-gauge needle on a tuberculin syringe after the eye is prepped with 5% povidone-iodine and then rinsed with sterile saline. Samples should be sent for Gram stain and fungal stains (e.g., periodic acid-Schiff stain [PAS], calcofluor white), bacterial and fungal culture, and antimicrobial susceptibility testing. Samples are optimally inoculated by the surgeon at the time they are obtained, and anaerobic cultures should be held for 14 days total (to detect *Propionibacterium acnes*). Vitreous samples provide a microbiological diagnosis more often than aqueous samples.

2. **Blood cultures.** Routinely ordered but are of limited value except in cases suspected of endogenous endophthalmitis.

3. **Complete blood count (CBC).** Routinely ordered but of limited value.

4. **Complete metabolic profile (CMP).** Usually nonspecific but may reveal comorbid illnesses (e.g., diabetes, renal failure, hepatic diseases).

5. **HIV enzyme-linked immunosorbent assay (ELISA; serum).** Helpful in cases of endogenous endophthalmitis.

6. **Beta-D-glucan and *Aspergillus* galactomannan (serum).** May be helpful in cases associated with fungal pathogens as well as to monitor the response to therapy.

D. **Radiology Studies.** Generally not useful in cases of endophthalmitis; however, a *B-scan type* (provides a two-dimensional image) *ocular ultrasound* may be helpful to show increased echogenicity of the vitreous due to intraocular inflammation, locate foreign bodies, or define the extent of infection (especially if the fundus is obscured).

V. TREATMENT

A. *Endophthalmitis is potentially a vision-threatening condition that is considered a medical emergency. An ophthalmology consult should be obtained immediately.*

B. Specific treatment should target the suspected or identified pathogen, and the duration of treatment should be determined in conjunction with an ophthalmologist. Retinal toxicity can occur with certain antimicrobials, especially aminoglycosides and amphotericin B.

C. **Medical Treatment Recommendations** for selected pathogens include:

1. **Bacterial pathogens.** In general, systemic antibiotics are *not* capable of achieving high tissue levels and therefore *intravitreal antibiotic injections* are the preferred treatment method. Systemic antimicrobial therapy with or without systemic or intravitreal steroids may be helpful but not routinely recommended. Treatment should be tailored to culture data (when available) and modified if the patient does not show clinical improvement within 36 to 48 hours, as it typically requires more than 24 hours to observe a response to the initial therapy.

   Current recommendations for empirical treatment (covers most gram-positive and gram-negative pathogens) include: **vancomycin 1.0 mg/0.1 mL intravitreal therapy *with* ceftazidime 2.25 mg/0.1 mL *or* amikacin 0.4 mg/0.1 mL intravitreal therapy.**

2. **Fungal pathogens.** No consensus on treatment and may require a combination of intravitreal and systemic therapy. *Current recommendations for empirical treatment include:* **amphotericin B (5–10 mg/0.1 mL) intravitreal therapy *with* fluconazole 12 mg/kg loading dose, then 4 mg/kg PO daily *or* voriconazole 6 mg/kg PO for 2 doses, then 4 mg/kg PO twice daily for a duration of 4 to 6 weeks.**

D. **Vitrectomy.** Certain types of endophthalmitis (e.g., chronic postsurgery, posttraumatic, foreign-body injury) or pathogens (e.g., *Bacillus cereus*) may respond better to this debridement procedure, which involves making an ocular surgical incision followed by aspiration of vitreous contents that are then replaced with a balanced salt solution.

BIBLIOGRAPHY

Durand ML. Endophthalmitis. In GL Mandell, JE Bennett, R Dolin (Eds.), *Mandell, Douglas, and Bennett's Principles and Practice of Infectious Diseases*, 7th ed. Philadelphia, PA: Churchill Livingstone Elsevier; 2010: 1553–1559.

Endophthalmitis Vitrectomy Study Group. Results of the Endophthalmitis Vitrectomy Study. A randomized trial of immediate vitrectomy and of intravitreous antibiotics for the treatment of postoperative bacterial endophthalmitis. *Arch Ophthalmol.* 1995;113(12):1479–1496.

Han DP, Wisniewski SR, Wilson LA, et al. Spectrum and susceptibilities of microbiologic isolates in the Endophthalmitis Vitrectomy Study. *Am J Ophthalmol.* 1996;122(6):1–17.

Lemley CA, Han DP. Endophthalmitis: a review of current evaluation and management. *Retina.* 2007;27(6):662–680.

Menikoff JA, Speaker MG, Marmor M, et al. A case-control study of risk factors for postoperative endophthalmitis. *Ophthalmology.* 1991;98(12):1761–1768.

SEPSIS AND SEPTIC SHOCK

John Vaz
Devang M. Patel
William F. Wright

I. INTRODUCTION

A. Definition. *Sepsis* is defined as a life-threatening organ dysfunction caused by a dysregulated host response to infection.

An appropriate physiologic reaction in association with a confirmed or strongly suspected infection or any other stimulus that activates inflammation is a systemic inflammatory response. This inflammatory response is commonly referred to as the *systemic inflammatory response syndrome* (SIRS) and is defined clinically by *two or more* of the following manifestations:

1. A core body temperature of greater than 38°C or less than 36°C

2. A heart rate above 90 beats per minute or greater than 2 standard deviations from the age-appropriate normal

3. A respiratory rate greater than 20 breaths per minute or hyperventilation (as evidenced by a $PaCO_2$ less than 32 mmHg)

4. A measured peripheral white blood cell (WBC) count of greater than 12,000 cells/mm^3 or less than 4,000 cells/mm^3

Sepsis, however, is no longer simply defined as infection or suspected infection plus *two or more* SIRS criteria alone.

The most recent established criteria for sepsis include the following:

1. **Quick Sepsis Organ-Failure Assessment (qSOFA).** This is defined by two of the following three variables: altered mentation, respiratory rate *greater* than 22 breaths per minute, and/or systolic blood pressure *less* than 100 mmHg. *This quick assessment tool is best applied to the identification of patients with sepsis outside the intensive care setting*.

2. **Sepsis Organ-Failure Assessment (SOFA).** This is defined by a score of *2 or greater* of the following variables from baseline (Table 47.1): alteration of PaO_2/FiO_2 ratio, worsening thrombocytopenia, escalating total bilirubin level, hypotension with or without the use of vasopressors, escalating serum creatinine and declining urinary output, and/or declining Glasgow coma scale score. *This assessment tool is best applied to the identification of patients with sepsis within the intensive care setting*.

B. Further Classifications. Terminology for the classification of sepsis syndrome must be applied carefully in order to further identify patients who may benefit from proven therapy options; therefore, further classifications include:

TABLE 47.1 ■ SOFA Scoring

System	Score = 0	Score =1	Score = 2	Score = 3	Score = 4
PaO_2/FiO_2, mmHg	>400	<400	<300	<200 with respiratory support	<100 with respiratory support
Platelets, x 10^3/ mcL	>150	<150	<100	<50	<20
Bilirubin, mg/ dL	<1.2	1.2–1.9	2.0–5.9	6.0–11.9	>12.0
Cardiovascular	MAP > 70 mmHg	MAP < 70 mmHg	Dopamine <5 or any dose dobutamine	Dopamine 5.1–15, epinephrine <0.1, or norepinephrine <0.1	Dopamine >15, epinephrine >0.1, or norepinephrine >0.1
Glasgow coma scale score	15	13–14	10–12	6–9	<6
Creatinine, mg/ dL and urine output, mL/ day	<1.2	1.2–1.9	2.0–3.4	3.5–4.9; urinary output less than 500	>5.0; urinary output less than 200

MAP, mean arterial pressure; SOFA, Sepsis Organ-Failure Assessment.

1. **Septic shock.** This is as defined as a *subset of sepsis* in which profound circulatory, cellular, and metabolic abnormalities are associated with a greater risk of mortality than with sepsis alone. *The most recent established criteria for this subset of sepsis are the need for vasopressors to maintain a mean arterial pressure (MAP) greater than 65 mmHg AND an elevated serum lactate greater than 2 mmol/L despite adequate fluid resuscitation.*

II. **PATHOGENESIS OF SEPSIS.** The pathogenesis of sepsis is complex and multifactorial; however, sepsis is generally considered a condition of hyperinflammation and hypercoagulation in the early stages with a shift toward a condition of hypoinflammation and immune suppression as sepsis persists. Some key components to the pathogenesis of sepsis include:

A. **Pattern Recognition Receptors (e.g., Toll-Like Receptors).** Innate immune cells (e.g., dendritic cells) recognize certain *pathogen-associated molecular patterns* that lead to the activation of a series of intracellular signaling pathways leading to an inflammatory state.

B. **Reactive Oxygen and/or Nitrogen Species.** These species are produced as part of the innate immune response to microorganisms but also have deleterious effects as they contribute to cardiovascular instability and organ dysfunction in sepsis.

C. **Hypercoagulation and Impaired Anticoagulation.** While this is most likely complex and multifactorial, *human activated protein C (APC)* is relatively deficient during sepsis and may contribute to both a hypercoagulation and hyperinflammatory state. (APC has anti-inflammatory properties.)

D. **Endothelial Dysfunction.** Alteration of the vascular endothelium occurs during sepsis (due to reduced nitric oxide) that results in an abnormal leukocyte response as well as both a hypercoagulation and a hyperinflammatory state.

E. **Mitochondrial Dysfunction.** Sepsis leads to abnormal oxygen utilization by mitochondria that may further contribute to cardiovascular instability and organ dysfunction.

F. **Apoptosis.** Sepsis leads to programmed cell death (e.g., apoptosis) of innate immune cells that eventually leads to an immunosuppressed state and reduced clearance of pathogenic microorganisms.

III. **MICROBIOLOGY OF SEPSIS.** While many microorganisms may be related to sepsis, the more commonly associated pathogens include:

A. **Gram-Positive Bacteria.** Predisposing factors for these pathogens usually include a normal or immunosuppressed host. Asplenia patients are particularly susceptible to encapsulated gram-positive bacteria such as *Streptococcus pneumoniae*. These pathogens are usually community-acquired (*Staphylococcus aureus* can also be hospital-acquired) and associated with skin and soft-tissue infections, pneumonia, or meningitis.

   1. *Staphylococcus aureus*
   2. *Streptococcus pyogenes* (group A)
   3. *Streptococcus agalactiae* (group B)
   4. *Streptococcus pneumoniae*
   5. *Listeria monocytogenes*

B. **Gram-Negative Bacteria.** Predisposing factors for these pathogens usually include immunosuppression (e.g., chronic corticosteroid use, chemotherapy, solid-organ or stem cell transplantation, neutropenia), chronic medical conditions (e.g., hemodialysis, diabetes, cirrhosis), or indwelling catheters. These pathogens are usually nosocomial in origin (e.g., hospital-acquired) and may be associated with multidrug resistance. Asplenia patients are particularly susceptible to encapsulated gram-negative bacteria such as *Neisseria* spp and *Haemophilus* spp.

   1. *Escherichia coli*
   2. *Klebsiella* spp (*K. pneumonia, K. oxytoca*)
   3. *Enterobacter* spp (*E. aerogenes, E. cloacae*)
   4. *Pseudomonas aeruginosa*
   5. *Acinetobacter* spp (*A. baumannii*)
   6. *Salmonella* spp (*S. enterica*)
   7. *Vibrio* spp (*V. vulnificus*)
   8. *Yersinia enterocolitica*
   9. Neisseria spp (*N. gonorrhoeae, N. meningitidis*)
   10. *Haemophilus* spp (*H. influenzae*)

C. **Anaerobic Bacteria.** Although uncommon, predisposing factors for these pathogens usually include traumatic injuries or invasive disease to cause necrotizing skin and soft-tissue infections.

1. *Clostridium* spp (*C. perfringens, C. septicum*). ***C. difficile is a pathogen strongly associated with recent antimicrobial use and recent history of diarrhea.***

2. *Fusobacterium* spp (*F. nucleatum, F. necrophorum*)

D. **Fungi.** Predisposing factors for these pathogens usually include immunosuppression (e.g., chronic corticosteroid use, chemotherapy, solid-organ or stem cell transplantation, neutropenia), chronic medical conditions (e.g., hemodialysis, diabetes), or indwelling catheters.

1. *Candida* spp (*C. albicans, C. glabrata, C. parapsilosis, C. tropicalis*)

2. *Aspergillus* spp (*A. fumigatus, A flavus, A. niger, A. terreus*)

3. *Pneumocystis jirovecii*

4. *Cryptococcus neoformans*

5. Zygomycetes (*Rhizopus* spp, *Mucor* spp)

6. *Fusarium* spp

E. **Viruses.** Predisposing factors for these pathogens usually include immunosuppression (see the preceding).

1. Cytomegalovirus

2. Herpes simplex virus

3. Varicella-zoster virus

4. Epstein–Barr virus

IV. **CAUSES OF SEPSIS.** As sepsis is defined as a dysregulated host response in association with a confirmed or strongly suspected infection, it is important to also systematically consider noninfectious causes that can mimic sepsis.

A. **Noninfectious Causes of Sepsis**

1. Trauma, surgery, or burns

2. Myocardial infarction or acute coronary syndrome

3. Severe pancreatitis

4. Thyroid storm or acute adrenal insufficiency

5. Acute leukemia or tumor lysis syndrome

6. Malignant hyperthermia (e.g., anesthetic-related halothane)

7. Malignant neuroleptic syndrome (e.g., haloperidol)

8. Pulmonary or deep venous thrombosis

9. Intracranial or subarachnoid hemorrhage (or any hematoma)

10. Solid-organ transplantation rejection

B. **Infectious Causes of Sepsis.** While a number of infections can result in sepsis, the major causes include:

1. Bacteremia (the major sources of bacteremia are intravascular devices, pulmonary infections, intra-abdominal infections, endovascular infections, or urinary tract infections)

2. Vascular access or intravascular device associated infection

3. Lower respiratory tract infection (e.g., pneumonia or empyema)

4. Intra-abdominal infection (e.g., peritonitis, cholecystitis, diverticulitis/abscess, pancreatic abscess, septic abortion or *Clostridium difficile* colitis)

5. Urinary tract infections (e.g., cystitis, pyelonephritis, renal abscess or Foley catheter–related infection)

6. Endovascular infections (e.g., endocarditis or vascular graft infections)

7. Skin and soft-tissue infections (e.g., necrotizing fasciitis, soft-tissue abscess, or surgical site infection)

V. **CLINICAL MANIFESTATIONS OF SEPSIS.** While the clinical manifestations associated with *sepsis* vary, manifestations typically reflect the underlying source of infection. **Common nonspecific clinical manifestations** include:

A. Fevers, chills, and/or rigors

B. Irritability, confusion, or lethargy

C. Tachypnea, hypoxia, acute respiratory distress, or respiratory failure

D. Hepatic and/or renal failure

VI. **APPROACH TO THE PATIENT WITH SEPSIS**

A. **History.** The most important initial approach to the patient with sepsis is a complete, accurate, and comprehensive history. **Physicians must be meticulous and systematic when obtaining information for the following key elements:**

1. **Age.** Certain illnesses may be more likely associated with particular age groups (e.g., urinary tract infections, pneumonia, and intra-abdominal abscess may be more likely in persons over the age of 50). Additionally, it is important to determine any attempted abortions in women of childbearing age.

2. **History of present illness.** It is important to establish in chronologic fashion the onset of symptoms and events that may be related to the sepsis syndrome.

3. **Past medical history.** This area should focus on any recent infection or chronic medical illness (e.g., inflammatory bowel disease, biliary tract disease, or underlying heart disease), any prior diagnosis of malignancy or chemotherapy, prior surgery (e.g., splenectomy or solid-organ transplantation) or complication related to surgery, any implanted prosthetic device (e.g., prosthetic valve, pacemaker or implantable defibrillator, cosmetic implanted surgical device, or implanted vascular graft) or indwelling venous catheter.

4. **Medications and allergies.** A complete list of prescription, over-the-counter, and herbal medications should be documented as well as medication- or antimicrobial therapy–related allergies.

a. **Beta-blockers** may falsely indicate relative bradycardia (see the following).

b. **Corticosteroids and nonsteroidal anti-inflammatory medications** may mask the signs and symptoms of infection.

5. **Social history.** This should include information about the patient's country of origin, immigration status, prior country or state of residence, travel history (with relevant exposure, vaccination, and prophylaxis history), vaccination status, occupation and occupational risks, smoking status, alcohol and drug exposure, hobbies or leisure activities, pet or animal exposure, and sexual activity that may place the patient at particular risk for infection.

B. **Physical Examination.** A complete physical examination should be performed with attention to all body systems. While physicians should be meticulous and conduct the examination in a systematic approach, repeat examinations are often helpful as diagnostic clues may be either atypical or obscure for the cause of sepsis. Some areas of the physical examination that require careful attention with common associations include:

1. **Vital signs.** While most vital signs are nonspecific to the cause of sepsis, *fever may be the first indication of sepsis* and the pulse should increase 15 to 20 beats/min for each 1 degree increase in core body temperature greater than 39°C. A lower than normal increase (or no increase) is termed *relative bradycardia.* Additionally, the *diastolic blood pressure* (DBP) usually decreases as a result of a sepsis-induced decrease in systemic vascular resistance. Impaired oxygenation and tachypnea may also be present but is generally nonspecific.

2. **Dermatologic examination.** Surgical sites, traumatic wounds, pressure ulcers, and vascular access sites should be examined for signs of infection (e.g., erythema, edema, warmth, tenderness, and purulent drainage). **Greater than 4 mm of erythema surrounding a vascular access site has been associated with infection.**

Petechiae and bleeding from vascular access sites may suggest disseminated intravascular coagulation (DIC).

Janeway lesions, Osler nodes, and proximal nail-bed splinter hemorrhages may suggest endocarditis.

Purpuric macules, papules, or bullae may suggest disseminated infection with *S. aureus, N. gonorrhoeae,* or *N. meningitidis. Pseudomonas aeruginosa* can be associated with *ecthyma gangrenosum* (oval–circular skin lesion with surrounding erythema and a central ulcer with or without eschar). Candidiasis may be associated with diffuse erythematous nodules.

Furuncles or intravenous (IV) drug injection sites should also be sought and may indicate deep skin and soft-tissue infections or endocarditis.

3. **Head, eyes, ears, nose, and throat (HEENT) examination.** A funduscopic examination may reveal *Roth spots* suggestive of systemic candidiasis. While *jaundice* is nonspecific in sepsis, its presence may suggest a biliary tract infection (e.g., ascending cholangitis) or a *Clostridium* spp deep-wound infection (usually in association with red blood cell [RBC] hemolysis). Additionally, conjunctiva petechial lesions may suggest endocarditis.

Findings of *gingival inflammation and poor dentition* may suggest a head and neck infection (e.g., odontogenic infection) or a necrotizing pneumonia (especially with a history of aspiration and respiratory symptoms).

4. **Cardiovascular examination.** A new diastolic murmur or change with existing murmur may suggest endocarditis.

5. **Pulmonary examination.** Impaired oxygenation, tachypnea, and signs of pulmonary consolidation may suggest pneumonia, complicated parapneumonic effusion, or empyema.

6. **Abdominal, pelvic, and rectal examination.** The abdominal examination should begin with a general inspection for *prior surgical scars* (e.g., splenectomy, cholecystectomy, hysterectomy, or appendectomy) in order to assist with the differential diagnosis of an intra-abdominal infection. *Abdominal tenderness, guarding, rebound, and absent bowel sounds* may suggest peritonitis (from a ruptured viscus or abscess).

   While both an internal and external rectal examination may reveal a perirectal abscess, findings of a *swollen and tender prostate* on internal examination may suggest prostatitis.

   A bimanual pelvic examination should be performed in women to exclude the possibility of pelvic inflammatory disease (PID).

7. **Neurologic examination.** An altered mental status is commonly observed in elderly patients with infection but is nonspecific; however, findings of a stiff neck (e.g., Kernig sign and Brudzinski sign) may suggest meningitis.

8. **Musculoskeletal examination.** While *bone tenderness* on palpation may suggest osteomyelitis, a *warm, tender joint with an effusion and decreased range of motion* may suggest septic arthritis. A *prior joint-space surgical scar* should also be sought that may indicate a prosthetic joint infection.

C. **Laboratory Studies.** There is no diagnostic gold standard workup for the etiology of sepsis. While the following represents a minimum diagnostic evaluation, laboratory testing or imaging should be guided by findings from a complete history and physical examination.

   1. **Complete blood count (CBC) with differential cell count.** Leukocytosis may suggest infection; however, an elevated neutrophil count (e.g., left shift) lacks sufficient sensitivity to differentiate infectious from noninfectious etiologies for sepsis. Thrombocytosis (greater than 600,000 mm^3) may be associated with infections due to yeast or molds.

   2. **Basic metabolic panel.** Routinely ordered but nonspecific; however, results of the serum creatinine level may affect antimicrobial dosing.

   3. **Liver enzymes and coagulation tests (prothrombin time/partial thromboplastin time/international normalized ratio [PT/PTT/INR]).** Biliary tract infections may be associated with elevated alkaline phosphatase and total bilirubin levels. Coagulation studies can be abnormal with sepsis but nonspecific with elevated values suggesting DIC (especially with a decreased fibrinogen level).

   4. **Serum lactate.** Levels greater than 2 mmol/L may suggest tissue hypoperfusion and the need for fluid resuscitation; however, sepsis is associated with increased glycolysis and increased serum lactate production.

5. **Urine microscopy and urine culture.** Fever and/or urinary tract infection symptoms (e.g., urinary frequency, dysuria, urgency, or costovertebral angle tenderness) in association with *hematuria*, significant *pyuria* (at least 10 WBCs per cubic millimeter), and *bacteriuria* (traditionally defined as 10^5 colony-forming units per milliliter) may suggest cystitis, pyelonephritis, or renal abscess.

6. **Blood cultures.** Routinely ordered as two sets of blood cultures (10 mL of blood per blood culture bottle) prior to the initiation of antimicrobial therapy. One set should be obtained through a percutaneous site (using standard skin preparation methods) and one set should be obtained through each vascular access site that has been in place for greater than 48 hours.

7. **Sputum Gram stain and culture.** A valid sputum sample should be evaluated by Gram stain and routine culture in patients with sepsis and purulent respiratory secretions.

8. **Wound or abscess cultures.** *Superficial swab cultures are not recommended*. Needle-aspirated contents from intact bullae or vesicles as well as deep cultures from abscesses, surgical wounds, or pressure ulcers are most helpful to identify a causative pathogen.

9. **Stool studies.** A stool sample should be evaluated for *Clostridium difficile* colitis.

10. **Erythrocyte sedimentation rate (ESR), C-reactive protein (CRP), and procalcitonin (PCT).** Nonspecific tests that are elevated with infections or inflammation; however, systemic PCT production has been observed to be relatively specific to bacterial infections and sepsis. PCT levels between 0.5 and 2.0 ng/mL make sepsis possible as these levels are also associated with noninfectious conditions (e.g., *trauma, postsurgical, burns, heat stroke, mesenteric infarction, and pancreatitis*) while levels between 2.0 and 10.0 ng/mL are suggestive of sepsis. Alternatively, a serum PCT value less than 0.5 ng/mL may serve best to identify those patients without sepsis rather than identify those for whom infection has actually been detected.

11. **Chromogranin A (CgA).** An acidic glycoprotein that belongs to the granin family and is present in the secretory dense-core granules that function in the storage of peptide hormones and catecholamines in all endocrine and neuroendocrine cells. During the past decade, a growing body of evidence has demonstrated that CgA is released in abnormal amounts by many neoplastic neuroendocrine cells as well as during sepsis-related shock that is associated with cardiovascular dysfunction. Elevated serum circulating CgA levels (a level >6.6 nmol/) have been suggested to be a helpful biochemical marker for the prognosis of patients in septic shock but its practicability for the clinical management of septic shock is still debatable.

D. **Radiography Studies.** The need for transportation to the radiology suite for certain diagnostic imaging methods should be balanced by the clinical status and safety of the patient.

1. **Plain-film abdominal and chest imaging.** These imaging modalities rarely yield a diagnosis; however, a single-view chest image may be helpful to identify pneumonia. Additionally, plain films of the abdomen may indicate free air

(suggesting bowel perforation with peritonitis) or the presence of gas within an abscess cavity.

2. **CT scan.** Imaging of the abdomen and chest with contrast is more sensitive than plain films or ultrasonography and of importance early in the evaluation as two of the most common causes of sepsis include pneumonia and intra-abdominal abscesses.

3. **Echocardiography.** Transthoracic or transesophageal imaging in association with the review of Duke criteria is important for the evaluation of endocarditis (see Chapter 7, Infective Endocarditis).

4. **Ultrasonography.** A noninvasive imaging study that may be helpful to evaluate biliary tract or pelvic etiologies for sepsis.

VII. **TREATMENT.** The treatment for sepsis consists of immediate efforts to stabilize the patient followed by identifying the underlying cause and formulating a treatment plan for that particular condition. Guidelines have been developed for the treatment of sepsis that involves three main components:

A. **Early Goal-Directed Therapy and Initial Resuscitation.** Guidelines suggest that reduced mortality in sepsis can occur with a combination of sequential supportive therapy (along with appropriate antimicrobial therapy) that is directed at the following measures:

1. **Initial fluid resuscitation** should be initiated with persistent hypotension (*defined as absolute systolic blood pressure less than 90 mmHg or a relative systolic blood pressure less than 40 mmHg of the baseline*) and/or serum lactate level greater than 2 mmol/L in order to improve cardiovascular support and perfusion. **Goals to therapy should include the following:**

   a. **Maintain a central venous pressure (CVP) of 8 to 12 mmHg.** For patients with cardiovascular history (e.g., diastolic heart failure) or mechanical ventilation, the CVP should be maintained at 12 to 15 mmHg.

   b. **Maintain an MAP of greater than 65 mmHg.** For patients with sepsis-induced hypoperfusion, infuse 30 mL/kg of IV crystalloid within 3 hours with additional fluid replacement based on frequent reassessments.

   c. **Maintain central venous oxygenation at greater than 70% (mixed venous oxygenation greater than 65%).**

2. **Vasopressor and inotropic support** to further improve cardiovascular status and perfusion. Norepinephrine followed by dopamine are the preferred agents with the goals for therapy as in the preceding.

3. **Corticosteroid therapy.** Some data suggest that patients with persistent hypotension despite initial fluid resuscitation and vasopressor and inotropic support may benefit from corticosteroid therapy for functional adrenal insufficiency. Suggested agents include: **hydrocortisone 50 mg IV q6 *or* fludrocortisone 50 mcg PO daily** (if hydrocortisone is not available). Corticosteroid therapy should be weaned off following the discontinuation of vasopressor and inotropic support.

4. **Blood product administration.** Transfuse packed RBCs if the hemoglobin is less than 7.0 g/dL. Platelets should be transfused for any significant bleeding episode or if the platelet count is less than 5,000 cells/mm^3.

5. **Glucose control.** Insulin therapy should be initiated to maintain glucose levels between 140 and 180 mg/dL (this improves neutrophil function).

6. Other supportive measures include ***renal replacement therapy*** (continuous veno-venous hemofiltration [CVVH] or intermittent hemodialysis can both be considered), ***mechanical ventilation support*** (tidal volume target should be *6 mL/kg* of predicted body weight with a goal plateau pressure *LESS* than *30 cm of water*), ***deep venous thrombosis prophylaxis,*** and ***stress ulcer prophylaxis*** (either an H_2-blocker or proton-pump inhibitor can be used).

7. Mechanically ventilated patients should be maintained with the **head of the bed between 30 degrees and 45 degrees** in order to help prevent ventilation-associated pneumonia (VAP).

B. **Antimicrobial Therapy.** *(Antibiotic dosing listed assumes normal renal function.)* Prompt initiation of broad-spectrum antimicrobial therapy (e.g., a combination regimen that covers both gram-positive and gram-negative pathogens) *within the first hour* of sepsis recognition is paramount to patient survival.

Obtain anatomical infection source control as rapidly as clinically practical. Assess patients daily for de-escalation of antimicrobial therapy and/or narrow therapy based on culture data and/or clinical improvement.

While no standard empirical regimen exists, suggested combination regimens may include:

1. **Ceftazidime 2 g IV q8** *or* **cefepime 2 g IV q8** *or* **doripenem 500 mg IV q8** *or* **meropenem 500 mg IV q8** *or* **piperacillin–tazobactam 3.375 to 4.5 g IV q6**. *Metronidazole 15 mg/kg IV loading dose followed by 7.5 mg/kg IV q6-8 maintenance dosing* should be used with regimens containing ceftazidime or cefepime; however, the addition of metronidazole is *NOT* required for doripenem, meropenem, or piperacillin–tazobactam; *plus*

2. **Daptomycin 6 mg/kg IV q24** (*daptomycin should **NOT** be used if the infection is suspected from a central nervous system [CNS] or pulmonary source due to inadequate penetration*) **or linezolid 600 mg IV q12** *or* **vancomycin 15 mg/kg IV q12–24** (*dosing for vancomycin should be adjusted to a goal serum level between 15 and 20 mcg/mL*).

3. While guidelines suggest an estimated *duration of antimicrobial therapy for sepsis be 7 to 10 days,* therapy should be monitored daily and adjusted for renal function and comorbid conditions, drug intolerances or interactions, susceptibility pattern of isolated pathogens, and the underlying infectious disease process.

C. **Source Identification and Control.** *Within the first 6 hours* of sepsis the source should be identified if possible in order to identify patients who may benefit from a timely and effective intervention (e.g., percutaneous or surgical drainage). Conditions that may benefit from early intervention include:

1. *Prompt removal of an infected vascular access device* (e.g., central venous catheter, urinary Foley catheter).

2. *Percutaneous or surgical drainage of deep space infection* (e.g., intra-abdominal, intrathoracic, or intracranial abscess, joint-space infection, or necrotizing skin and soft-tissue infection).

BIBLIOGRAPHY

Bone RC, Balk RA, Cerra FB, et al. American College of Chest Physicians/Society of Critical Care Medicine Consensus Conference: definitions for sepsis and organ failure and guidelines for the use of innovative therapies in sepsis. *Crit Care Med.* 1992;20(6):864–874.

Cinel I, Dellinger RP. Advances in pathogenesis and management of sepsis. *Curr Opin Infect Dis.* 2007;20(4):345–352.

Cohen J, Brun-Buisson C, Torres A, et al. Diagnosis of infection in sepsis: an evidence-based review. *Crit Care Med.* 2004;32(11 suppl):S466–494.

Levy MM, Fink MP, Marshall JC, et al. 2001 SCCM/ESICM/ACCP/ATS/SIS International Sepsis Definitions Conference. *Crit Care Med.* 2003;31(4):1250–1256.

Peake SL, Delaney A, Bailey M, et al. Goal-directed resuscitation for patients with early septic shock. *N Engl J Med.* 2015;371(16):1496–1506.

Rhodes A, Evans L, Alhazzani W, et al. Surviving Sepsis Campaign: international guidelines for the management of sepsis and septic shock: 2016. *Crit Care Med.* 2017;45(3):486-552. doi:10.1097/CCM.0000000000002255

Rosjo H, Nygard S, Kaukonen KM, et al. Prognostic value of chromogranin A in severe sepsis: data from the FINNSEPSIS study. *Intensive Care Med.* 2012;38(5):820–829.

Singer M, Deutschman CS, Seymour CW, et al. The Third International Consensus Definitions for Sepsis and Septic Shock (Sepsis-3). *JAMA.* 2016;315(8):801–810.

48

HEMATOPOIETIC STEM CELL TRANSPLANT INFECTIONS

Michael Tablang
David J. Riedel

I. INTRODUCTION

A. Definition. Infectious complications after hematopoietic stem cell transplants (HSCTs) are common and depend on the degree of immunosuppression, presence of tissue and organ damage, and environmental exposures.

B. Classification. Different types of infections occur in a fairly predictable sequence based on time elapsed since myelosuppressive regimen used in HSCT.

1. **Pre-engraftment phase (less than 30 days).** The two major risk factors for infection in this period are neutropenia and altered defense barriers resulting from mucositis and cutaneous damage as a consequence of the myelosuppressive conditioning regimen.

2. **Early postengraftment phase (31–100 days).** This period is characterized by resolution of profound neutropenia and early recovery of cell-mediated immunity. Infections are determined by impaired cellular and humoral immunity, immunomodulating viruses, and diminished phagocyte function. Allogeneic HSCT recipients have an added risk for infection due to the possibility of graft-versus-host disease (GVHD) or its treatment.

3. **Late postengraftment phase (greater than 100 days).** During this period, cellular and humoral immunity has recovered. Infections are unusual in the absence of chronic GVHD. Among allogeneic HSCT recipients with chronic GVHD, infections arise from mucocutaneous damage and immunodeficiency from GVHD and its required therapy.

II. MICROBIAL CAUSES OF HSCT INFECTIONS. HSCT recipients can be infected by various organisms based on different phases of immunosuppression after transplantation (see Table 48.1.).

A. Pre-Engraftment Phase. Bacterial infections predominate during this period, usually as a result of indwelling central venous catheters and mucositis. Gram-positive bacteria include coagulase-negative staphylococci, *Staphylococcus aureus*, and viridans streptococci. Common gram-negative bacteria include *Pseudomonas aeruginosa*, Enterobacteriaceae, and *Stenotrophomonas maltophilia*. *Candida* spp are the most common fungal infection agent, but as neutropenia is prolonged, the risk of *Aspergillus* and other filamentous fungal infections increases. In the absence of prophylaxis, herpes simplex virus (HSV) reactivation occurs in the majority of HSCT seropositive recipients.

TABLE 48.1 ■ Infections After Hematopoietic Stem Cell Transplantation

Pre-Engraftment Period (Less Than 30 Days)
Gram-positive bacteremia (related to venous catheters)
Gram-negative bacteremia (related to mucosal injury and neutropenia)
Clostridium difficile
Candida (related to mucosal injury and neutropenia)
HSV (if seropositive)
Early Postengraftment (31–100 Days)
Gram-positive bacteremia (related to venous catheters)
Gram-negative bacteremia (related to mucosal injury and venous catheters)
CMV (if seropositive)
VZV (if seropositive)
Aspergillus
Pneumocystis jirovecii
BK virus
Late Postengraftment (Greater Than 100 Days)
Encapsulated bacteria
Nocardia
CMV (if seropositive)
VZV (if seropositive)
Aspergillus
Pneumocystis jirovecii
Time Independent (May Occur in Any Risk Period)
HHV-6
Epstein–Barr virus
Legionella spp
Mycobacterium spp
Encapsulated bacteria
Respiratory viruses

CMV, cytomegalovirus; HHV-6, human herpesvirus 6; HSV, herpes simplex virus; VZV, varicella-zoster virus.

B. Early Postengraftment Phase. The most important pathogens during this period are the herpesviruses, especially cytomegalovirus (CMV). CMV may reactivate in seropositive patients or may be acquired by seronegative recipients from seropositive donors. CMV infections can manifest as pneumonitis, hepatitis, and colitis. Other infections during this period are *Pneumocystis jirovecii* and opportunistic mycoses including *Aspergillus* spp, *Fusarium* spp, and Zygomycetes.

C. Late Postengraftment Phase. Chronic GVHD with its concomitant immunosuppression predisposes to viral infections, particularly CMV and varicella-zoster virus (VZV). Functional asplenia from chronic GVHD increases risk of infection from encapsulated bacteria such as *Neisseria* and *Streptococcus pneumoniae*. Invasive aspergillosis may also occur.

III. CLINICAL MANIFESTATIONS OF HSCT INFECTIONS

A. **Febrile Neutropenia (FN).** Fever in neutropenic patients is considered a medical emergency and should always prompt an evaluation for infection. Fever is defined as a single temperature greater than 38.3°C or a temperature greater than 38°C sustained over a 1-hour period. Neutropenia is classified based on absolute neutrophil count (ANC) as mild (ANC less than 1,500), moderate (ANC less than 1,000), or severe (ANC less than 500).

B. **Pneumonia Syndromes.** Pneumonia is the most common infection after transplantation. Classic symptoms of fever, cough, and dyspnea may be absent. Hypoxemia may be the only presenting feature. Noninfectious pulmonary complications, such as pulmonary edema, diffuse alveolar hemorrhage, or drug reactions, may have similar manifestations.

C. **Hepatitis.** Clinical hepatitis in HSCT recipients can present with fever, abdominal pain, and jaundice.

D. **Gastroenteritis.** Diarrhea after transplantation is primarily noninfectious, although *Clostridium difficile* is becoming increasingly common. Patients may present with fever, abdominal pain, nausea, or vomiting.

E. **Typhlitis.** Fever with abdominal pain and right lower quadrant pain during periods of neutropenia may reflect typhlitis, or neutropenic enterocolitis.

F. **Rash.** Dermatologic diseases may be local or disseminated manifestations of infections. The morphology of infectious skin lesions is usually atypical in immunocompromised patients and of limited diagnostic value.

G. **Central Nervous System Infections.** Clinical manifestations of central nervous system infections include altered mental status, fever, headache, seizures, or focal neurologic signs.

IV. APPROACH TO THE PATIENT

A. **History.** A thorough history in HSCT recipients should be performed with an emphasis on the following information:

1. **Timeline posttransplantation.** Different infections in HSCT occur based on the degree of immunosuppression after transplantation and can guide differential diagnosis.

2. **Type of stem cell transplantation.** Allogeneic HSCT has greater risk of infections compared to autologous HSCT because of extended period of immune system recovery and added risk of GVHD. Other transplant characteristics influencing the risk of infection include source of stem cells, myeloablative regimen, the degree of HLA matching, and GVHD treatment regimen.

3. **Prophylactic antimicrobials.** Infections among HSCT recipients receiving prophylactic antimicrobials should raise concern for resistant pathogens and alter empiric treatment.

4. **Prior infections.** HSCT candidates are routinely screened for prior infections that may reactivate after transplantation such as HSV, VZV, hepatitis B and C. History and serologic examinations are key.

5. **Noninfectious syndromes.** Many noninfectious complications of HSCT may mimic infections such as drug reactions, transfusion reactions, pulmonary infiltrates, veno-occlusive disease, GVHD, and thromboembolic disease.

B. **Physical Examination.** A comprehensive and careful physical examination may reveal focal and localizing signs of infections in HSCT recipients particularly in the absence of demonstrable fever. Special considerations include:

1. **Neurologic examination.** Complete neurologic and ophthalmologic examinations should be performed to elicit signs of meningitis, encephalitis, or focal brain lesions.

2. **Skin and mucosal examination.** Cutaneous and subcutaneous lesions are a valuable source of information though they are rarely pathognomonic. Viral and fungal infections are the leading causes of skin lesions in solid-organ transplant recipients.

3. **Endovascular infections.** Careful evaluation for cardiac murmurs and peripheral stigmata of endovascular and embolic infections (e.g., splinter hemorrhages, petechiae) should be performed.

4. **Hardware and devices.** Signs of inflammation around vascular catheters, prosthetic hardware, and cardiac devices are suggestive of infection, although their absence does not exclude infection.

C. **Laboratory Studies.** Specific blood, urine, and imaging studies can enhance diagnostic evaluation for infection.

1. **Complete blood count (CBC).** Neutropenia, particularly the ANC, will reflect degree of infectious risk. Leukocytosis is observed in infected HSCT patients.

2. **Complete metabolic profile (CMP) and liver function tests (LFTs).** Renal function, electrolyte abnormalities, and elevated liver enzymes can be essential in identifying a source of infection and assessing severity of organ dysfunction.

3. **Blood cultures.** Blood cultures should always be obtained prior to instituting empiric antimicrobials. At least two sets of blood cultures from separate venipuncture sites should be sent. If a central venous catheter is present, a separate set should be collected from each lumen.

4. **Bronchoscopy.** Lower respiratory tract specimens from bronchoalveolar lavage (BAL) are essential in patients with pulmonary infiltrates of uncertain etiology. Gram stain, cultures, and polymerase chain reaction (PCR) assays of different organisms can be tested.

5. **Viral screening.** HSCT recipients should be evaluated for viral infections based on their symptoms. PCR of respiratory viruses (e.g., influenza, parainfluenza) from nasal wash or BAL is recommended in patients with respiratory complaints. Serum CMV PCR can be obtained to detect CMV viremia that, if present, is predictive of tissue-invasive disease.

6. **Stool studies.** *C. difficile*–associated diarrhea is common among HSCT recipients. Enzyme immunoassay (EIA) for detecting toxins A and B has moderate sensitivity and excellent specificity. PCR detection of gene toxin has both excellent sensitivity and specificity. A negative EIA result requires repeat testing, while a single negative or positive PCR test is sufficient to rule out disease.

7. **Histology.** Biopsy and histopathologic examination of lesions (skin, lymph nodes, lungs, gastrointestinal) may be necessary for definitive diagnosis.

D. Radiographic Studies. Evaluation for an infectious process can be augmented with radiographic imaging as clinically indicated.

1. **Chest radiograph.** This should be obtained even in patients without respiratory symptoms to evaluate for infection in the lungs.

2. **CT scan.** CT scan of the chest and abdomen may be necessary for optimal definition of any abnormalities such as pneumonia, colitis, abscesses, and pyelonephritis.

3. **Ultrasonography.** Examination of local fluid collections and the hepatobiliary system can be further delineated.

4. **MRI.** MRI is the best modality when examining bone and spinal infections.

V. MANAGEMENT OF HSCT INFECTIONS

A. Medical Management

1. FN is a medical emergency, and patients require immediate empiric intravenous antipseudomonal beta-lactam antibiotics (e.g., cefepime, carbapenem, or piperacillin–tazobactam).

2. Vancomycin can be added in patients with hemodynamic instability, known methicillin-resistant *Staphylococcus aureus* (MRSA) colonization, suspected catheter-related or skin and soft-tissue infection.

3. Initial antimicrobial regimen should be modified based on available clinical and microbiological data. If a specific organism has been isolated, antibiotics should be adjusted based on susceptibility patterns.

4. Persistent or recurrent fever greater than 3 days despite empiric antimicrobials should prompt a thorough reevaluation for an infection, including repeat blood cultures and imaging of new or worsening focus of infection. Empiric antiyeast or antimold therapies can be considered particularly if prolonged neutropenia is anticipated.

5. Fluoroquinolone prophylaxis should be considered for patients with prolonged (greater than 7 days) and severe neutropenia (ANC less than 100). Levofloxacin and ciprofloxacin have been studied extensively and are considered equivalent.

B. Surgical Management

1. Surgical indications in HSCT recipients are similar to nontransplant population. Platelet transfusions may be required prior to surgery in patients with severe thrombocytopenia.

2. Early involvement of surgeons and proper timing of surgical management can prevent detrimental outcomes.

BIBLIOGRAPHY

Dummer JS, Thomas LD. Risk factors and approaches to infections in transplant recipients. In GL Mandell, JE Bennett, R Dolin (Eds.), *Mandell, Douglas, and Bennett's Principles and Practice of Infectious Diseases*, 7th ed. Philadelphia, PA: Churchill Livingstone Elsevier; 2010: 3809–3819.

Freifeld AG, Rolston KV, Bow EJ, et al. Clinical practice guideline for the use of antimicrobial agents in neutropenic patients with cancer: 2010 update by the Infectious Diseases Society of America. *Clin Infect Dis.* 2011;52(4):e56–e93.

Leather HL, Wingard JR. Infections following hematopoietic stem cell transplantation. *Infect Dis Clin North Am*. 2001;15(2):483–520.

Tomblyn M, Chiller T, Hermann E, et al. Guidelines for preventing infectious complications among hematopoietic cell transplant recipients: a global perspective. *Bone Marrow Transplant*, 2009;44(8):453–558.

Wingard JR, Hsu J, Hiemenz JW. Hematopoietic stem cell transplantation: an overview of infection risks and epidemiology. *Infect Dis Clin North Am*. 2010;24(2):257–272.

Young JH. Weisdorf DJ. Infections in recipients of hematopoietic cell transplantation. In GL Mandell, JE Bennett, R Dolin (Eds.), *Mandell, Douglas, and Bennett's Principles and Practice of Infectious Diseases*, 7th ed. Philadelphia, PA: Churchill Livingstone Elsevier; 2010: 3821–3837.

SOLID-ORGAN TRANSPLANT INFECTIONS

Michael Tablang
Charles E. Davis

I. INTRODUCTION

A. Definition. Infections in solid-organ transplant (SOT) recipients are determined by the net state of immunosuppression—a concept to describe the dynamic interaction of all the factors that contribute to the patient's risk of infection.

B. Classification. SOT infections can be divided into four overlapping categories: donor-derived infections, recipient-derived infections, community-acquired infections, and healthcare-associated infections.

1. **Donor-derived infections.** Transplanted organs can transmit latent or active infections from organ donors. Most of these infections have been prevented by molecular assay, serologic and culture-based organ donor screening, and routine surgical antimicrobial prophylaxis. However, screening is limited by the technology and short time period available during organ procurement (Table 49.1).

   a. **Latent infection.** Clusters of infections not routinely screened for have been reported, such as lymphocytic choriomeningitis virus, West Nile virus (WNV), rabies virus, HIV, human herpesvirus 8, human T-cell lymphotropic disease, and Chagas disease.

   b. **Active infection.** Bacteremia or viremia undiscovered during organ procurement and nosocomial organisms resistant to routine surgical prophylaxis (e.g., vancomycin-resistant enterococci or azole-resistant *Candida* spp) can be transmitted to the recipient.

2. **Recipient-derived infections.** Transplant candidates are screened for prior infections, unique exposures, residence in regions with endemic fungi or parasites, and travel history (Table 49.1).

   a. **Latent infection.** Common infections that need treatment to prevent reactivation include *Mycobacterium tuberculosis*, endemic fungi (e.g., *Histoplasma capsulatum*, *Coccidioides immitis*), and certain parasites (e.g., *Strongyloides stercoralis* and *Trypanosoma cruzi*).

   b. **Active infection.** SOT recipients may have active infections related to complications of organ failure. Renal transplant candidates may have infected hemodialysis catheters and liver transplant candidates may have spontaneous bacterial peritonitis.

3. **Community-acquired infections.** Compared to a normal host, community-associated infections in SOT recipients may lead to infections that have an atypical presentation and increased severity.

TABLE 49.1 ■ Common Donor-Derived Infections and Standard Pretransplant Evaluation of Both Donor and Recipient

Common Donor-Derived Infections	
Viruses	Herpesviruses (CMV, EBV, HHV-6, HSV, VZV), HTLV-I and -II, HIV, West Nile virus, rabies, LCMV
Bacteria	Mycobacterium tuberculosis Nontuberculous mycobacteria Meningococcus Syphilis Bacteremia at the time of donation (many organisms)
Fungi	*Candida* spp *Aspergillus* spp Endemic mycoses (*Histoplasma capsulatum, Coccidioides* spp) *Cryptococcus gattii* *Cryptococcus neoformans*
Parasites	*Toxoplasma gondii* *Trypanosoma cruzi* Malaria (e.g., *Plasmodium falciparum*) *Babesia* *Strongyloides stercoralis*

Standard Pretransplant Evaluation

CMV antibody

EBV antibody panel: EBV viral capsid antigen, early antigen, nuclear antigen levels

HSV antibody

HIV antibody and viral load

HBV serologies: HBsAg, HBsAb, HBcAb

HCV antibody

HTLV-I/II antibody

Latent TB: tuberculin skin test or interferon-gamma release assay

Syphilis (TPHA or TPPA or FTA-Abs or RPR)

Toxoplasma gondii antibody (in heart transplant donors)

VZV antibody

Other Screening Tests

Coccidioides immitis (for recipient in endemic areas)

Histoplasma capsulatum (for recipient in endemic areas)

Sputum cultures for bacteria, mycobacteria, and fungi (in lung transplant candidates)

Strongyloides stercoralis serology (for recipient in endemic areas)

Trypanosoma cruzi (for recipient in endemic areas)

Urinalysis and urine culture (for kidney transplants)

Urine ova and parasites (1 cystoscopy) for *Schistosoma* spp (for kidney transplants)

CMV, cytomegalovirus; EBV, Epstein–Barr virus; FTA-Abs, fluorescent treponemal antibody absorption; HBV, hepatitis B virus; HCV, hepatitis C virus; HHV-6, human herpesvirus 6; HSV, herpes simplex virus; HTLV, human T-cell lymphotropic virus; LCMV, lymphocytic choriomeningitis virus; RPR, rapid plasma reagin; TB, tuberculosis; TPHA, *Treponema pallidum* hemagglutination; TPPA, *Treponema pallidum* particle agglutination; VZV, varicella-zoster virus.

4. **Healthcare-associated infections.** Transplant candidates are at risk for colonization with antimicrobial-resistant nosocomial organisms, including methicillin-resistant *Staphylococcus aureus*, vancomycin-resistant enterococcus, azole-resistance *Candida* spp, *Clostridium difficile*, or multidrug-resistant, gram-negative bacilli.

II. MICROBIAL CAUSES TO SOLID-ORGAN TRANSPLANT INFECTIONS. The timeline of posttransplant infections occurs in a generally predictable pattern and can be used to establish the infectious syndrome at different stages after transplantation. The timeline is delayed by antimicrobial prophylaxis and reset with treatment of graft rejection or intensification of immunosuppressive therapy.

A. **Early Posttransplant Period (1–4 Weeks).** Donor- or recipient-derived infections predominate in this period. Patients are also at greatest risk for nosocomial infections, which are often procedure- or device-related (e.g., catheter-associated infections) or surgical complications (e.g., wound infections, anastomotic leaks, and ischemia). Opportunistic infections are uncommon with effective suppressive antimicrobials.

B. **Middle Posttransplant Period (1–6 Months).** Viral pathogens and graft rejection constitute the majority of febrile episodes in this period. Infectious pathogens are selected for by presence or absence of prophylactic antimicrobials against *Pneumocystis jirovecii*, cytomegalovirus (CMV), or hepatitis B. The preventive antimicrobials should also prevent some urinary tract infections and other opportunistic infections such as *Listeria, Toxoplasma,* and *Nocardia* spp.

C. **Late Posttransplant Period (Greater Than 6 Months).** Risk of infection is determined by intensity of immunosuppression, allograft function, and residual infections. In this period, SOT recipients fall in one of three unique groups:

1. **Adequate allograft function and no allograft rejection**. Infectious risk is diminished as immunosuppression is tapered. Community-acquired bacterial and viral infections are most common. There is low risk for opportunistic infections.

2. **Chronic viral infections**. Concurrent viral infections including BK polyomavirus, adenovirus, recurrent hepatitis C, human papillomavirus (HPV), and HIV can cause allograft dysfunction.

3. **Allograft rejection or recurrent infections**. Intensified immunosuppressive therapy due to allograft rejection increases risk for opportunistic infections with *P. jirovecii, Nocardia, Rhodococcus, Cryptococcus neoformans,* and invasive fungal pathogens (e.g., *Aspergillus* spp and *Mucor* spp).

III. CLINICAL MANIFESTATIONS OF SOLID-ORGAN TRANSPLANT INFECTIONS

A. **Bacterial Infections.** Bacterial pathogens are the most common infection in SOT recipients similar to the general population. Clinical manifestations are diverse and depend on site of infection and have included the following:

1. **Gram-negative and gram-positive bacteria** can present as pneumonia, urinary tract, intra-abdominal, bloodstream, and wound infections.

2. *Mycobacterium tuberculosis* can manifest as a pulmonary or disseminated disease. It is also a well-known cause of fever of unknown origin (FUO).

3. *Nocardia* typically causes pneumonia but can involve the joints, skin, and brain.

B. **Viral Infections.** Viral pathogens are associated with specific syndromes and may serve as copathogens to many opportunistic infections.

1. **CMV** infection is the most important infection that causes significant mortality and morbidity in SOT recipients. *CMV-seronegative recipients of allograft from CMV-seropositive donors have the highest risk of CMV infection.* CMV-seropositive recipients are also at risk for disease reactivation. Besides non-specific febrile illness and myelosuppression (CMV syndrome), CMV can cause the following:

   a. **Direct effects**. Tissue invasive disease can present as pneumonitis, gastrointestinal disease (e.g., gastritis, esophagitis, colitis), hepatitis, and pancreatitis.

   b. **Indirect effects**. Immunomodulatory effects of CMV can result in graft rejection, predisposition to opportunistic infection (e.g., pneumocystis), and oncogenesis.

2. **Herpes simplex virus (HSV) and varicella-zoster virus (VZV)** infections represent reactivation of latent virus. HSV most commonly presents as an orolabial or genital ulcer while VZV as a painful dermatomal vesicular rash. Disseminated disease may manifest as pneumonitis, hepatitis, or encephalitis.

3. **Epstein–Barr virus (EBV)** infections consist of all EBV-driven lymphoproliferative syndromes such as infectious mononucleosis and *posttransplant lymphoproliferative disease (PTLD)*.

C. **Fungal Infections.** Fungal pathogens may present as a colonization or true infection. Recognition of a true infection is based on compatible clinical signs and symptoms.

1. *Candida* **spp and** *Aspergillus* **spp** are the most common fungal pathogens in SOT recipients. *Candida* may present as superficial infections (e.g., thrush, mucositis, and wound infections) or invasive disease (e.g., bloodstream infections, endocarditis, or hepatosplenic candidiasis). *Aspergillus*-related infections usually present as lung nodules but may also cause disseminated disease (e.g., brain abscess, bone marrow).

2. *Pneumocystis jirovecii* remains an important life-threatening pathogen that causes pneumonitis in SOT recipients. Subtle presentations include low-grade fever, nonproductive cough, dyspnea, and hypoxemia.

D. **Parasitic Infections.** Parasitic infections, although uncommon, should be considered in SOT recipients who are immigrants or had extensive travel history.

1. **Toxoplasmosis** may present as primary or reactivation disease. Fever and lymphadenopathy are common manifestations, but could progress to pneumonia or neurologic disease.

2. *Strongyloides stercoralis* may cause larval accumulation in the lungs resulting in eosinophilic pneumonia (Loeffler syndrome) or gram-negative bacteremia after larval gut penetration to cause a hyperinfection syndrome.

IV. APPROACH TO THE PATIENT

A. **History.** A detailed medical history in SOT recipients should be solicited with the following important considerations:

1. **Timeline of posttransplantation.** Review of the time frame and specific infections occurring in a particular period can establish a differential diagnosis for a causative infectious process.

2. **Epidemiologic exposures.** Important historical clues may be obtained from remote or recent travel, employment or lifestyle, and residence in areas with endemic fungi or parasites. Recent hospitalization or surgeries may point to healthcare-associated infections.

3. **Transplant-specific infections.** Specific types of infection are more common in specific types of transplantation, such as candidiasis in liver transplants and aspergillosis in lung transplants.

4. **Organ-specific symptoms.** Organ-based symptoms (dyspnea, altered mental status, abdominal pain) should prompt a focused evaluation with consideration to most significant bacterial or viral pathogen that could cause such presentations.

5. **Noninfectious syndromes.** Drug fever, allograft rejection, PTLD, and graft-versus-host disease should be considered.

B. **Physical Examination.** A methodical physical assessment is critical to recognize even the subtle manifestations of infections in SOT recipients. Special considerations should be given to the following:

1. **Neurologic examination.** Complete neurologic and ophthalmologic examinations should be performed to elicit signs of meningitis, encephalitis, or focal brain lesions.

2. **Skin and mucosal examination.** Cutaneous and subcutaneous lesions are valuable sources of information. Viral and fungal infections are the leading causes of skin lesions in SOT recipients.

3. **Endovascular infections.** Careful evaluation for cardiac murmurs and peripheral stigmata of endovascular and embolic infections (e.g., splinter hemorrhages, petechiae) should be performed.

4. **Hardware and devices.** Signs of inflammation around vascular catheters, prosthetic hardware, and cardiac devices are suggestive of infection, although their absence does not exclude infection.

5. **Surgical sites.** Surgical wounds, especially those complicated by hematoma or dehiscence, are a common source of infection.

C. **Laboratory and Radiologic Studies.** Laboratory examination should be tailored based on a possible causative infectious pathogen.

1. **Fever without localizing findings.** At minimum, urinalysis, urine culture, blood cultures, chest x-ray (CXR), and CMV-quantitative polymerase chain reaction (PCR) should be obtained.

2. **Patients with pulmonary findings.** Evaluation of interstitial or alveolar CXR infiltrates includes sputum Gram stain and culture, sputum acid-fast bacillus

(AFB) smear and mycobacterial culture (DNA probes if available), blood cultures, and urine *Legionella* and pneumococcal antigens. Urine *Histoplasma* antigen and *Coccidioides* serology may be obtained in endemic areas or suggestive travel. Serum cryptococcal and *Aspergillus* antigens may be useful, if suggested clinically or radiographically. Bronchoscopy with transbronchial biopsy may be considered when fever persists or during atypical presentation. Bronchoalveolar lavage (BAL) should be sent for bacterial, viral, fungal, AFB stains and cultures, *Legionella and Nocardia cultures, Pneumocystis jirovecii* pneumonia (PCP) smear, CMV PCR, and cytology.

3. **Patients with altered mental status.** Evaluation for causes of altered mentation includes brain MRI and lumbar puncture. Cerebrospinal fluid (CSF) analysis includes cell count with differential, glucose, protein, cytology, and cultures for bacterial, viral, fungal, and AFB organisms. Cryptococcal antigen and PCR for other pathogens (CMV, EBV, HSV, VZV, and WNV) may be considered.

4. **Patients with abdominal findings.** Hepatobiliary evaluation includes liver function tests and right upper quadrant (RUQ) ultrasound. Evaluation of diarrhea includes stool leukocytes and cultures, stool ova and parasites, *Clostridium difficile* antigen or preferably PCR, if available; endoscopic evaluation with biopsy and CMV staining and abdominal CT scan if warranted.

5. **Patients with lymphadenopathy.** Biopsy of involved lymph nodes to exclude PTLD and occult infections (e.g., mycobacterial infections). Tissue should be sent for histologic examination and cultures. CT scan of body areas may be useful to determine extent of nodal involvement.

V. **DIAGNOSTIC CRITERIA.** Special consideration will be given to diagnosis of CMV—the most important pathogen to cause mortality and morbidity in SOT recipients.

A. **CMV Status.** Serologic status of both transplant donor and recipient determines risk of CMV disease.

1. **CMV-positive donor, CMV-negative recipient (D1/R2).** Risk of CMV disease is highest in this group, developing in 70% to 90% of SOT recipients without prophylaxis.

2. **CMV-negative donor, CMV-positive recipient (D2/R1).** Reactivation of latent CMV develops in 20% of SOT recipients without prophylaxis.

3. **CMV-positive donor, CMV-positive recipient (D1/R1).** Reactivation of latent CMV or superinfection with a new viral strain can occur.

4. **CMV-negative donor, CMV-negative recipient (D2/R2).** CMV disease is lowest in this group, and no antiviral prophylaxis is recommended.

B. **Diagnosis of CMV Infection.** CMV is prevalent in the general population. Lifelong latency is established after primary infection.

1. **CMV infection.** Evidence of CMV replication regardless of symptoms.

2. **CMV disease.** Evidence of CMV infection with compatible symptoms. It can manifest as CMV syndrome (fever with myelosuppression) or CMV invasive disease (pneumonitis, hepatitis, gastritis, or colitis).

VI. **MANAGEMENT**

A. **Medical Management.** Empiric antimicrobials are given based on most likely pathogens and adjusted if the patient is colonized with nosocomial multidrug-resistant organisms. *(Antimicrobial agents listed presume normal renal function.)*

B. **Surgical Management.** Surgical indications are the same as in the general population. Emphasis is given to source control of infections in SOT recipients due to their decreased immune function.

C. **Prevention/Prophylaxis.** Antimicrobial prophylaxis has altered the incidence and severity of SOT infections. Preventive strategies include vaccinations, universal prophylaxis, and preemptive therapy.

1. **Vaccination.** Antibody response to immunization decreases with greater degree of immunosuppression. Inactivated vaccines are generally safe following SOT. Live vaccines should be given at least 4 weeks before SOT and generally avoided following transplantation. The American Society of Transplantation has published guidelines (December 2009) for vaccination of SOT candidates and recipients.

2. **Universal Prophylaxis.** Antimicrobial therapies are administered for prolonged periods to all SOT recipients, irrespective of their risk of infection. Major limitations of this approach include cost, drug toxicity, and emergence of resistance (see Table 49.2).

TABLE 49.2 ■ Antimicrobial Therapy for Treatment and Prophylaxis of Common Pathogens in Solid-Organ Transplant Recipients

MRSA	Vancomycin—dosing based on weight and renal function
VRE	Linezolid 600 mg PO or IV twice daily Daptomycin 6 mg/kg IV q24–48 based on renal function Quinupristin/dalfopristin 7.5 mg/kg IV q8
ESBL-producing Enterobacteriaceae	Carbapenem: imipenem/cilastatin 500 mg IV q6, meropenem 1–2 g IV q8, ertapenem 1 g IV once daily, doripenem 500–1,000 mg IV q8
MDR *Pseudomonas aeruginosa*	Combination therapy: antipseudomonal beta-lactam or aminoglycoside ± fluoroquinolone
MDR *Acinetobacter baumannii*	Imipenem/cilastatin 500 mg IV q6 h, meropenem 1–2 g IV q8; doripenem 500–1,000 mg IV q8, ampicillin/sulbactam 3 g IV q6 (Consider combination therapy with an aminoglycoside or colistin if beta-lactam resistance is suspected.)
Stenotrophomonas maltophilia	TMP/SMX 10–15 mg/kg (TMP) PO or IV in divided doses given every 6–8
Cytomegalovirus	Ganciclovir 5 mg/kg IV twice daily—preferred in patients with impaired intestinal absorption or in severe/life-threatening disease Valganciclovir 900 mg PO twice daily
Influenza virus	Oseltamivir 75 mg PO twice daily (active against influenza A and B)
Pneumocystis jirovecii	TMP/SMX 10–15 mg/kg (TMP) PO or IV in divided doses given every 6–8 h

(continued)

TABLE 49.2 ■ Antimicrobial Therapy for Treatment and Prophylaxis of Common Pathogens in Solid-Organ Transplant Recipients (*continued*)

Candida spp –For less severe illness, no recent azole exposure –For bloodstream and other severe infections, recent azole exposure	Fluconazole 800 mg loading dose, then 400 mg IV or PO Echinocandin: caspofungin 70 mg 3 1, then 50 mg IV daily, micafungin 100 mg IV daily, anidulafungin 200 mg × 1, then 100 mg IV daily
Aspergillus spp	Voriconazole 6 mg/kg q12 PO or IV loading dose for two (2) doses, then 4 mg/kg PO or IV twice daily
Prophylaxis for Common Pathogens	
Cytomegalovirus	Valganciclovir 900 mg PO once daily Ganciclovir 5 mg/kg IV once daily (CMV-IVIG may be added to antivirals in heart and lung transplants.)
Pneumocystis jirovecii	TMP/SMX SS or DS daily or three times weekly
Candida spp	Fluconazole 400 mg PO or IV daily
Aspergillus spp	Voriconazole 200 mg PO or IV twice daily

ESBL, extended-spectrum beta-lactamase; IV, intravenous; IVIG, intravenous immunoglobulin; MDR, multidrug-resistant; MRSA, methicillin-resistant *Staphylococcus aureus*; SMX, sulfamethoxazole; TMP, trimethoprim; VRE, vancomycin-resistant *Enterococcus*.

3. **Preemptive Therapy.** Antimicrobial therapies are directed only toward high-risk SOT recipients. Sensitive and quantitative assays (e.g., PCR or molecular antigen detection) are monitored at specific intervals to detect early infection. Positive assays prompt initiation of antimicrobial therapy to prevent progression to symptomatic and invasive disease (Table 49.2).

BIBLIOGRAPHY

Bouza E, Loeches B, Munoz P. Fever of unknown origin in solid organ transplant recipients. *Infect Dis Clin North Am.* 2007;21:1033–1054.

Danzinger-Isakov L, Kumar D, AST Infectious Diseases Community of Practice. Guidelines for vaccination of solid organ transplant candidates and recipients. *Am J Transplant.* 2009;9(suppl 4):S258–S262.

Fishman JA. Infection in solid-organ transplant recipients. *N Engl J Med.* 2007;357:2601–2614.

Fishman JA, AST Infectious Diseases Community of Practice. Introduction: infection in solid organ transplant recipients. *Am J Transplant.* 2009;9(suppl 4):S3–S6.

Fishman JA, Issa NC. Infection in organ transplantation: risk factors and evolving patterns of infection. *Infect Dis Clin North Am.* 2010;24:273–283.

Grim SA, Clark NM. Management of infectious complications in solid-organ transplant recipients. *Clin Pharmacol Ther.* 2011;90(2):333–342.

Grossi PA, Fishman JA, AST Infectious Disease Community of Practice. Donor-derived infections in solid organ transplant recipients. *Am J Transplant.* 2009;9(suppl 4):S19–S26.

Humara A, Snydman D, AST Infectious Diseases Community of Practice. Cytomegalovirus in solid organ transplant recipients. *Am J Transplant.* 2009;9(suppl 4):S78–S86.

Kotton CN, Kumar D, Caliendo AM, et al. International consensus guidelines on the management of cytomegalovirus in solid organ transplantation. *Transplantation.* 2010;89:779–795.

LYME DISEASE

William F. Wright

I. INTRODUCTION

A. Definition. A tick-borne illness caused by the bacterium *Borrelia burgdorferi* and transmitted primarily by the deer tick (*Ixodes scapularis*; *Ixodes pacificus* on the West Coast).

B. Epidemiology and Life Cycle. The disease is more common in the following states: Connecticut, Delaware, Maine, Maryland, Massachusetts, Minnesota, New Hampshire, New Jersey, New York, Pennsylvania, Rhode Island, and Wisconsin. Lyme disease can occur in both sexes and at any age; however, it occurs primarily in males, and the peak ages of incidence are 5 to 9 years and 55 to 59 years.

Lyme disease is acquired by the transmission of *B. burgdorferi* to humans through the bite of an infected tick of the *Ixodes* species. The tick has a 2-year, three-stage life cycle and feeds once during each stage. The cycle begins when larvae hatch in the summer. Larvae stage (first stage) ticks are usually uninfected with *B. burgdorferi* because transovarial transmission of the spirochete is rare. Larvae emerge then the following spring after molting into the nymphal stage (second stage). Subsequently then the tick may become infected at any stage of its life cycle by feeding on a host, usually a small mammal (in particular the white-footed mouse, *Peromyscus leucopus*). The nymphal-stage tick is most likely to transmit the infection to humans, presumably because it is so small it is difficult to identify the bite and to remove the tick in a timely manner. In addition, because it is small it becomes engorged more quickly than do adult ticks (engorgement is necessary before the organism can be transmitted). Moreover, nymphs are prevalent during spring and summer, when humans frequently enter habitats in which ticks thrive. The nymphs then molt to adults in the fall. The females lay their eggs the following spring before they die and the 2-year life cycle begins again.

C. Classification. There are three well-recognized clinical stages of Lyme disease.

1. **Early localized disease.** Most commonly characterized by the erythema migrans (EM) skin lesion (see Section V.B) and typically begins 1 to 2 weeks after a tick bite.

2. **Early disseminated disease.** Characterized by multiple EM lesions or involvement of the cardiac, musculoskeletal, or neurologic systems.

3. **Late disease.** Characterized predominantly by involvement of the musculoskeletal or neurologic systems and typically begins 6 to 12 months after a tick bite.

II. PATHOGENESIS OF LYME DISEASE

A. **Bacterium-Vector Survival Mechanism, Bacterial Transmission, and Host Immune Response Theory.** The most widely held theory concerning the cause of Lyme disease is that the host immune response is important for the pathogenesis of disease. Expression of outer surface proteins (Osps) by the bacterium is important for both survival in the tick and for infection in humans (see Section III). OspA is required for bacterial adherence to the tick midgut. Its expression decreases during tick blood meal engorgement as the spirochete leaves the midgut for the tick salivary glands and subsequent injection into the mammalian host. During this period, the expression of OspC increases and it therefore has been postulated that OspC plays a role in migration of and infection by the bacterium. The ability to spread through skin and other tissues may also be facilitated by the binding of OspC to human plasminogen.

In general, it takes hours for the mouthparts of ticks to implant fully in the host and much longer (days) for the tick to become fully engorged with a blood meal. The bites of these ticks are painless, in part because they secrete enzymes (such as bradykininases) that break down mediators of inflammation. Experiments have shown that both nymphal and adult ticks must feed for approximately 36 to 48 hours or longer before the risk of transmission of *B. burgdorferi* becomes substantial. *How long the tick is attached and whether it is engorged are two of the most important factors to consider when assessing the risk of bacterium transmission.*

During early localized Lyme disease, characterized by the EM lesion, there involves an infiltrate of both macrophages and T cells to produce both inflammatory and anti-inflammatory cytokines. Dissemination within humans involves the bacterium attaching to certain host integrins eliciting a proinflammatory response, which includes production of both matrix glycosaminoglycans and extracellular-matrix proteins, which may explain the organism's tropisms for particular tissues (e.g., collagen fibrils in the extracellular matrix in the heart, nervous system, and joints). Adaptive T-cell and B-cell responses in lymph nodes during disseminated infection results in the production of antibodies against many components of the spirochete.

Dissemination from the site of the tick bite, via the bloodstream, produces the systemic symptoms that may be associated with early localized Lyme disease as well as the clinical manifestations of early disseminated and, ultimately, of late Lyme disease.

III. MICROBIOLOGY OF LYME DISEASE

A. **Basic Microbiology Characteristics.** The microbiology is best illustrated as a gram-negative organism that is 10 to 30 mm long and 0.2 to 0.25 mm wide. It grows best at 30 to 34°C in a microaerophilic atmosphere, dividing every 8 to 12 hours during log-phase growth. It is routinely grown in liquid cultures in Barbour–Stoenner–Kelly II (BSK II) medium.

B. **Ultrastructural Microbiology Characteristics.** *B. burgdorferi* resembles other spirochetes in the genus *Borrelia*, with 7 to 11 periplasmic flagella that are attached subterminally to the protoplasmic cylinder and overlap in the center of the cell. The main structural component of the flagella is flagellin, a 41-kDa protein. The outer membrane contains an abundance of Osps anchored to the outer membrane via lipid moieties at their amino termini (some may also extend to the cytoplasmic membrane). These include OspA, OspB, and OspC (lipoproteins of approximately 32, 34, and 24 kDa, respectively). Another antigen of *B. burgdorferi* is the 60-kDa antigen, which has been termed "common antigen" and belongs to the heat-shock protein family. Unlike other spirochetes, *B. burgdorferi* has linear chromosomes and 4–9 linear and circular plasmids. The genes that encode the major Osps of *B. burgdorferi* are located on plasmids.

IV. **CLINICAL MANIFESTATIONS OF LYME DISEASE.** The clinical manifestations of Lyme disease are classified into stages of illness: early localized disease, early disseminated disease, and late disease.

A. **Early Localized Disease.** Characterized by the EM rash that is classically reported as a single lesion. It most commonly appears as a uniform erythematous oval to circular rash with a median diameter of 16 cm (range of 5–70 cm). Approximately 19% of EM rashes are associated with a "bull's-eye" appearance. EM is usually asymptomatic but may be pruritic or painful. EM may also be accompanied by systemic findings such as fever, malaise, headache, regional lymphadenopathy, stiff neck, myalgia, or arthralgia.

B. **Early Disseminated Disease.** The most common manifestation of early disseminated Lyme disease in the United States is multiple EM lesions. The secondary skin lesions, which usually appear from 3 to 5 weeks after the tick bite, consist of multiple annular erythematous lesions similar to, but usually smaller than, the primary EM lesion. Other common manifestations of early disseminated Lyme disease include:

1. **Musculoskeletal symptoms** are the most common extracutaneous manifestations of disseminated disease and may include transient oligoarticular symptoms of arthralgia or myalgia that may include joint swelling.

2. **Neurologic symptoms**, affecting up to 15% of untreated patients, can include lymphocytic meningitis, a seventh cranial nerve (Bell) palsy (primarily unilateral, but rarely bilateral, facial nerve palsy), motor or sensory radiculoneuropathy, mononeuritis multiplex, cerebellar ataxia, and myelitis.

3. **Cardiac symptoms** usually occur within 1 to 2 months after infection (range of less than 1 week to 7 months). Lyme carditis is a less common complication of systemic disease, occurring in approximately 4% to 10% of patients. It may present as chest pain, dyspnea on exertion, fatigue, palpitations, or syncope, and often includes some form of atrioventricular block.

C **Late Disease.** Arthritis is usually a manifestation of late disease, and occurs in up to 60% of untreated patients. Patients typically present approximately 6 months after infection with joint pain and swelling, and synovial fluid findings that suggest an inflammatory process.

V. **APPROACH TO THE PATIENT**

A. **History.** A complete and chronologically accurate history should be obtained in all suspected cases of Lyme disease. The history should focus on the timing of events, risk factors, comorbid conditions, medication allergies, recent infections, and recent antimicrobial therapy. *Lyme disease should be included in the differential diagnosis of any patient who presents with a known* Ixodes *species tick exposure, a seventh cranial nerve (Bell) palsy in endemic areas, and/or EM rash.*

B. **Physical Examination.** A complete physical examination should be performed, but areas of focus include:

1. **Vital signs.** Findings are usually normal or nonspecific; however, a fever response is variable and the pulse and blood pressure measurements may or may not demonstrate abnormalities unless the patient has cardiac involvement.

2. **Cutaneous examination.** Examination should focus on searching for EM lesions. Also, certain skin and soft-tissue manifestations of Lyme disease, such as *acrodermatitis chronica atrophicans* and *lymphocytomas*, usually caused by *B. afzelii* or *B. garinii*, are seen in Europe but are extremely rare in the United States

3. **Cardiac examination.** Lyme carditis may be associated with third-degree atrioventricular block, some form of second- or first-degree atrioventricular block, or no conduction abnormalities.

4. **Musculoskeletal examination.** Evaluation should search for a painful joint on range-of-motion testing and/or significant joint effusion.

5. **Neurologic examination.** Lyme disease may manifest with meningitis, cranial neuropathies, motor or sensory radiculoneuropathy (*e.g., seventh cranial nerve [Bell] palsy*), mononeuritis multiplex, cerebellar ataxia, and/or myelitis.

C. **Laboratory Studies.** EM rash is the only clinical manifestation sufficient to make the diagnosis of Lyme disease in the absence of laboratory confirmation. Currently, the standard laboratory recommendation for the diagnosis of Lyme disease without the identification of an EM lesion is a two-tier protocol using an enzyme-linked immunosorbent assay (ELISA) initially, followed by the more specific Western immunoblot to confirm the diagnosis when the assay samples are positive or equivocal.

If the ELISA result is negative, an immunoblot is not indicated. Immunoblots should not be ordered without a simultaneously ordered ELISA. The ELISA provides a quantitative estimate of the concentration of antibodies against *B. burgdorferi*. The immunoblot provides information about the specificity of the antibodies; positive "bands" mean that antibodies against specific protein antigens of *B. burgdorferi* are present. Most authorities require the presence of antibodies against at least either 2 of 3 bands for immunoglobulin M (IgM) or 5 of 10 bands for immunoglobulin G (IgG) specific proteins of *B. burgdorferi* for the immunoblot to be considered positive.

With Lyme-related symptoms lasting 4 weeks or less for which first-step ELISA is positive, separate IgM and IgG Western blot testing should be utilized. However, for symptoms of greater than 4 weeks' duration for which first-step ELISA is positive the IgG Western blot test should be utilized.

Other ELISA-based antigens of *B. burgdorferi* that may assist with the standard two-tier testing include the C6 peptide and PepC10.

The utility of other laboratory investigations include:

1. **Complete blood count (CBC).** Routinely ordered but nonspecific for Lyme disease.

2. **Basic metabolic panel (BMP).** Routinely ordered but nonspecific for Lyme disease.

3. **Blood cultures**. Commonly two sets are ordered but are of low yield.

4. **Molecular studies (e.g., polymerase chain reaction [PCR])**. Should be obtained in patients with disease manifestations such as arthritis or meningitis.

5. **Gram stain and routine cultures** are very unlikely to yield results beneficial to guide further antimicrobial therapy in complicated disease (e.g., arthritis, carditis, or meningitis).

6. **12-lead ECG**. Commonly ordered to identify any cardiac conduction abnormalities.

D. **Radiologic Studies**. Radiologic studies are not, in general, required when evaluating patients suspected of Lyme disease.

VI. MANAGEMENT OF LYME DISEASE

A. **Medical Management**. Appropriate antimicrobial therapy is the mainstay of treatment for Lyme disease. *Doxycycline is the preferred agent of therapy because of its activity against other tick-borne illnesses (e.g., Borrelia miyamotoi, B. mayonii, human granulocytic anaplasmosis, human monocytic ehrlichiosis, Ehrlichia muris, or Rickettsia-related infections), which can occur in up to 10% of patients with Lyme disease. Doxycycline is contraindicated in pregnant and breastfeeding women and in children younger than 8 years.*

Coinfection with **Babesia microti** (e.g., babesiosis) should be considered in patients with Lyme disease who have fever for more than 48 hours while receiving appropriate antimicrobial therapy or with unexplained leukopenia, thrombocytopenia, and/or anemia. The diagnosis of babesiosis is best obtained by using a specific PCR assay or thin blood smear examination of blood for parasites. While mild infection is treated using azithromycin (500 mg once followed by 250 mg daily for 7–10 days) plus atovaquone (750 mg twice daily for 7–10 days), severe infection requires clindamycin 300 to 600 mg intravenously every 6 hours plus quinine 650 mg every 6 to 8 hours for 7 to 10 days.

General Lyme antimicrobial therapy recommendations include (dosing assumes normal renal function):

1. **Early localized disease**

   a. **Erythema migrans**

      i. **Adults**. Doxycycline, 100 mg orally twice per day or amoxicillin, 500 mg orally three times per day or cefuroxime axetil (Ceftin), 500 mg orally twice per day or azithromycin (Zithromax), 500 mg orally once per day.

      ii. **Children**. Doxycycline, 4 mg per kg orally per day in two divided doses (maximum of 100 mg twice per day) in children 8 years or older or amoxicillin, 50 mg per kg orally per day in three divided doses (maximum of 500 mg per dose) or cefuroxime axetil, 30 mg per kg orally per day in two divided doses (maximum of 500 mg per dose) or azithromycin, 10 mg per kg orally per day (maximum of 500 mg per day).

      iii. **Duration of therapy** (both adults and children) is range of 7 to 10 days for azithromycin, 10 to 21 days for doxycycline, and 14 to 21 days for amoxicillin or cefuroxime axetil.

2. **Early disseminated disease**

   a. **Cardiac or neurologic involvement.** Hospitalization and parenteral antibiotic therapy are recommended for patients with first-degree atrioventricular block and PR interval greater than 30 milliseconds, as well as for patients with second- or third-degree atrioventricular block.

      Patients with an isolated facial nerve palsy and normal cerebrospinal fluid examination can be treated with a 14-day course of the same antibiotics used to treat EM (see the preceding).

      i. **Adults.** Ceftriaxone (Rocephin), 2 g intravenously per day or cefotaxime (Claforan), 2 g intravenously every 8 hours or doxycycline, 200 to 400 mg orally in two divided doses per day.

      ii. **Children.** Ceftriaxone, 50 to 75 mg per kg intravenously per day (maximum of 2 g per dose) or cefotaxime, 150 to 200 mg per kg intravenously per day in three or four divided doses (maximum of 6 g per day) or doxycycline, 4 to 8 mg per kg intravenously in two divided doses per day in children 8 years or older (maximum of 100 to 200 mg per dose).

      iii. **Duration of therapy** (both adults and children) is 14 to 21 days for ceftriaxone or cefotaxime and 10 to 28 days for oral doxycycline.

3. **Late disease.** Same oral antibiotics as used for EM. Same intravenous antibiotics as used for neurologic symptoms of early disseminated disease. Duration of therapy (both adults and children) is 14 to 28 days. Patients with persistent or recurrent joint swelling following initial therapy may be retreated with another 4-week course of oral antibiotics (or 2–4-week course of intravenous ceftriaxone).

B. **Surgical Management.** The primary treatment of Lyme disease is appropriate antimicrobial therapy (see the preceding).

VII. PREVENTION

A. Removal of ticks within 24 hours of attachment can usually prevent acquisition of Lyme disease. Fine-tipped forceps are generally recommended for tick removal, with care taken to grasp the tick as close to the skin as possible without compressing the body.

B. Avoiding areas with high tick burdens (e.g., wooded or grassy areas with a large deer population) is the best preventive measure. For persons living in endemic areas, additional recommended measures include wearing light-colored protective clothing, performing frequent body checks for ticks and bathing following outdoor activities, and instituting environmental landscape modifications (e.g., grass mowing, deer exclusion fencing, removing leaf litters and woodpiles) to reduce the tick burden.

C. Tick and insect repellants (e.g., diethyltoluamide [DEET]) applied to the skin provide additional protection, but require reapplication every 1 to 2 hours for maximum effectiveness. Use of products with concentrations of DEET greater than 30% is not necessary and increases the risk of adverse effects. DEET should be applied sparingly only to exposed skin, but not to the face, hands, or skin that is either irritated or abraded. After one returns indoors, skin that was treated should be washed with soap and water. Permethrin (a synthetic pyrethroid) is available in a spray for application to clothing only and is particularly effective because it kills ticks on contact.

BIBLIOGRAPHY

Sanchez E, Vannier E, Wormser GP, Hu LT. Diagnosis, treatment, and prevention of Lyme disease, human granulocytic Anaplasmosis, and Babesiosis: a review. *JAMA*. 2016;315(16):1767–1777.

Wormser GP, Dattwyler RJ, Shapiro ED, et al. The clinical assessment, treatment, and prevention of Lyme disease, human granulocytic anaplasmosis, and babesiosis: clinical practice guidelines by the Infectious Diseases Society of America. *Clin Infect Dis*. 2006;43(9):1089–1134.

Wormser GP. Clinical practice. Early Lyme disease. *N Engl J Med*. 2006;354(26):2794–2801.

Wright WF, Riedel DJ, Talwani R, Gilliam BL. Diagnosis and management of Lyme disease. *Am Fam Physician*. 2012;85(11):1086–1093.

51

TRAVEL MEDICINE

Susan L. DeBiase
William F. Wright

I. INTRODUCTION

A. Definition. Travel medicine is also known as *emporiatrics* and is a specialty branch of medicine that deals primarily with the prevention and treatment of diseases acquired through international travel.

B. Epidemiology. International travel is markedly increased for reasons that are mainly for tourism, business, and education; however, in some regions of the world, migrant workers and refugees contribute substantially to international migration. More than half of international travelers to developing countries become ill during their trip, and less than 20% are estimated to seek medical care in a designated certified travel clinic for a travel-associated illness either before, during, or after travel. The most common destinations from which ill travelers returned were sub-Saharan Africa, Southeast Asia, south-central Asia, and South America. The most frequently identified illness categories are gastrointestinal, febrile, and dermatologic conditions.

C. Categories of Travelers. These are general categories of travelers based on risk of infection.

1. **Immigrants visiting friends and relatives (immigrant VFRs).** These are persons who originally had been immigrants but who are returning to their country of origin to visit friends and relatives. Immigrant VFRs tend to seek less pretravel medical advice, acquire more travel-related infections, and more often require hospitalization for these illnesses.

2. **Travelers visiting friends and relatives (traveler VFRs).** These are persons who originally had *not* been immigrants but who are returning to their country of ancestry to visit friends and relatives.

3. **Tourism, education, and/or employment travelers.** These are persons traveling from a developed country or region of the world to an underdeveloped country or region of the world for the purpose of tourism, education, and/or employment. These travelers usually seek more pretravel medical advice, acquire fewer travel-related infections, and rarely require hospitalization after travel.

II. PRETRAVEL CONSULTATION.
In general, the approach to travel medicine involves a *triad* of the traveler, the trip, and the proposed health interventions. The pretravel clinical evaluation involves risk identification, stratification, and counseling to improve patient awareness of travel risks. This evaluation takes into consideration the travel destination itinerary, travel history, preexisting medical conditions, immunization history, behavioral risk factors, and biological health threats that

should preferably be performed 4 to 6 weeks prior to travel. Pretravel topics for review with each traveler should include:

A. **Travel Destination Itinerary, Mode of Transportation, and Duration.** Effective counseling begins with assessment of intended travel destinations, mode of travel (e.g., air, boat, train, or car), and duration, which improves an understanding of patient's risk to travel-related infections or conditions. Strategies for minimizing the risk of transportation-related illness include keeping mobile and wearing compression stockings to prevent deep vein thrombosis (DVT) during air travel (especially air travel greater than 8 hours' duration), avoiding caffeine during air travel to decrease jet lag, and staying hydrated. Risk factors for travel-associated DVT include: smoking, obesity, oncology and inflammatory diseases (rheumatoid arthritis, Crohn's disease, and systemic lupus), hereditary clotting disorders (e.g., Factor V Leiden), pregnancy, use of supplemental estrogens (e.g., oral contraceptives), advanced age, and disorders of blood vessels (e.g., venous stasis).

B. **Preexisting Patient Medical Conditions and Medication History.** Factors such as age, chronic medical conditions, medications, immune status, and pregnancy potentially influence the epidemiologic risk associated with specific destination-related infections.

C. **Immunization History.** This is the most common reason for patients seeking pretravel medical evaluation. Immunizations for the traveler are categorized as routine, recommended, and required for travel. A review of all routine childhood immunization schedules should be performed. Depending on the destination, immunizations may be required (e.g., yellow fever) or recommended based on individual risk.

D. **Animal and Insect Avoidance.** Effective prevention of animal or vector-borne diseases involves avoiding stray animals, use of proper clothing, minimizing skin exposure, use of insecticide-impregnated bednets, and use of insect repellents with at least 30% of N,N-diethyl-m-toluamide (DEET).

E. **Food and Water Precautions.** Gastrointestinal diarrheal disease can be prevented by avoiding foods that cannot be cooked thoroughly, boiled, or peeled. Additional prevention measures include avoiding ice in beverages, brushing teeth with tap water, and drinking only treated water (e.g., bottled, boiled, iodinated, microfiltered, and carbonated).

F. **Environmental Precautions.** Remind travelers to follow preventive measures regarding temperature and altitude extremes, sun exposure, swimming-related risks, and accidents. Solar burns are best avoided with use of proper protective clothing and use of sunscreen with a sun protection factor of at least 30. Travelers to altitudes above 8,000 feet are recommended to ascend slowly (1,000 feet per day). Additional protective measures include use of seat belts, helmets, traveling in pairs or small groups, and staying hydrated.

III. **ROUTINE STANDARD IMMUNIZATIONS.** These are standard immunizations that should be considered for all travelers regardless of the travel destination.

A. **Hepatitis A (Hepatitis A Virus [HAV]).** A very common preventable disease among travelers.

1. **Geographic infection risk.** Worldwide distribution with highest risk of non-immune travelers to developing countries.

2. **Transmission and incubation period.** Fecal–oral transmission route with a 28-day incubation period.

3. **Clinical manifestations.** Characterized by abrupt onset of fever, malaise, nausea, and abdominal pain followed by the onset of jaundice.

4. **Vaccine and schedule.** Available vaccines are inactivated virus components for intramuscular (IM) administration in a two-dose series (baseline primary dose and 6-month to 5-year duration for the second booster dose; average is 6 to 12 months for the booster). The dose is 0.5 to 1.0 mL IM injection. Seroconversion at 4 weeks after administration of the primary dose is 95% to 100%.

   A combined HAV and hepatitis B virus (HBV) vaccine is available for IM administration in a three-dose series (baseline primary dose, 1- and 6-month duration for the booster dose). An accelerated administration schedule is available with impending travel that is expected to occur in less than 28 days (baseline primary dose, 7- and 28-day duration for the booster doses). The dose is 1.0 mL IM injection. Seroconversion at 4 weeks after administration of the primary dose is 95% to 100%.

5. **Prevention.** Avoid, boil, or fully cook potentially contaminated food or water.

B. **Hepatitis B (HBV).** Routine hepatitis B vaccination efforts were incorporated into the childhood immunization schedule in 1990; therefore, anyone born before this time may require the full vaccination series.

1. **Geographic infection risk.** Worldwide distribution with high prevalence rates among sex workers and injection drug users with highest risk of nonimmune travelers to the Caribbean as well as Africa and eastern Asian countries.

2. **Transmission and incubation period.** Transmission routes occur through injection or transfusion of contaminated blood products, injection drug use, sexual intercourse, and perinatally from infected mother to fetus with a 45-day to 6-month incubation period (average of 4 months).

3. **Clinical manifestations.** Characterized by abrupt onset of fever, malaise, nausea, and abdominal pain followed by the onset of jaundice.

4. **Vaccine and vaccine schedule.** Available vaccines are single-antigen formulation to contain 10 to 40 mcg of hepatitis-B surface antigen (HBsAg)/mL for IM administration in a three-dose series (baseline primary dose, 1-month dose, and 6-month dose). The dose is 1.0 mL IM injection. A protective antibody response occurs in approximately 30% to 55% of healthy adults after the first dose, 75% after the second dose, and over 90% after the third dose. After age 40 years, the proportion of persons who have a protective antibody response after a three-dose vaccination regimen declines below 90%, and by age 60 years, protective levels of antibody develop in only 75% of vaccinated persons. Alternative vaccination schedules (e.g., 0, 1, and 4 months or 0, 2, and 4 months) have been demonstrated to elicit dose-specific and rates of seroprotection similar to those obtained on the standard 0-, 1-, 6-month schedule.

   Adults over the age of 20 years with immunocompromising medical conditions (e.g., HIV) and/or the requirement for renal replacement therapy (e.g., hemodialysis) should receive a 2.0 mL IM injection dose (e.g., 40 mcg).

   A combined HAV and HBV vaccine is available for IM administration in a three-dose series (baseline primary dose, 1- and 6-month duration for the booster dose). An accelerated administration schedule is available with impending travel that is expected to occur in less than 28 days (baseline primary dose, 7- and 28-day duration for the booster doses). The dose is 1.0 mL IM injection.

5. **Prevention.** Measures include vaccination, safe-sex practices, and avoiding contaminated needles and blood products.

C. **Influenza.** During the influenza season travelers should be offered vaccination against influenza according to standard recommendations.

1. **Geographic infection risk.** Worldwide distribution with higher risk of non-immune travelers to the northern hemispheres from November to April and in the southern hemispheres from April to September.

2. **Transmission and incubation period.** Airborne droplet transmission route with a 1- to 4-day incubation period (average of 2 days).

3. **Clinical manifestations.** Characterized by abrupt onset of fever, fatigue, nausea and abdominal pain, joint and muscle aches, nonproductive cough, shortness of breath, sore throat, and/or headache.

4. **Vaccine and vaccine schedule.** There are four types of influenza virus known as A, B, C, and D. The majority of infections are caused by types A and B. Two glycoproteins of the influenza virus membrane, hemagglutinin (HA) and neuraminidase (NA), both recognize sialic acid on respiratory epithelial cells. Initiation of virus infection involves multiple HAs binding to sialic acids on carbohydrate side chains of cell-surface glycoproteins and glycolipid.

   Available vaccines against influenza are single-antigen formulation to contain 15 mcg of inactivated or recombinant viral HA of the most common circulating strains of virus for IM administration in a one-dose annual series (e.g., deltoid muscle). Available vaccines are either trivalent (two influenza A and one influenza B) or quadrivalent (two influenza A and two influenza B). The dose is 0.5 to 1.0 mL IM injection. A protective antibody response (defined as a hemagglutination inhibition test titer greater than or equal to 40) occurs in approximately 30% to 60% of healthy adults. The estimated duration of immunity is for 6 to 8 months.

5. **Prevention.** Frequent handwashing and avoiding crowded environments are recommended.

D. **Measles–Mumps–Rubella (MMR).** Travelers should be offered vaccination according to standard recommendations.

1. **Geographic infection risk.** Worldwide distribution with higher risk of non-immune travelers to countries with insufficient vaccination coverage.

2. **Transmission and incubation period.** Airborne droplet transmission route with a 7- to 21-day incubation period (average of 14 days) for measles, a 12- to 25-day incubation period (average of 16–18 days) for mumps, and a 12- to 23-day incubation period (average of 14 days) for rubella.

3. **Clinical manifestations.** Measles manifest as fever, nonproductive cough, nasal congestion, and rash. Mumps is characterized by salivary gland swelling (particularly the parotid gland), testicular pain or swelling, and headache. Rubella is characterized by fever, generalized lymphadenopathy, and rash in children but primarily generalized arthralgias in adults.

4. **Vaccine and vaccine schedule.** Available vaccines are a reconstituted sterile liquid suspension of live attenuated viruses that have been propagated in

chick embryo cell cultures for subcutaneous (SQ) administration in a one-dose series. Each dose contains 1,000 $TCID_{50}$ (tissue culture infectious doses) of measles virus, 12,500 $TCID_{50}$ of mumps virus, and 1,000 $TCID_{50}$ of rubella virus. Each dose of the vaccine also contains sorbitol (14.5 mg), sodium phosphate, sucrose (1.9 mg), sodium chloride, hydrolyzed gelatin (14.5 mg), recombinant human albumin (less than 0.3 mg), fetal bovine serum (less than 1 part per million), and approximately 25 mcg of neomycin. The dose is 0.5 mL SQ injection.

Adults born after 1957 without evidence of serum immunity to MMR should receive 1 dose of MMR vaccine unless they have a medical contraindication to the attenuated live-virus vaccine (e.g., pregnancy or immunodeficiency). The vaccine is also contraindicated in individuals with an allergy history to neomycin.

5. **Prevention.** Frequent handwashing and avoiding crowded environments are recommended.

E. **Diphtheria/Tetanus/Pertussis (*Corynebacterium* diphtheriae, *Clostridium tetani*, and *Bordetella pertussis*).** Travelers should be offered vaccination according to standard recommendations.

1. **Geographic infection risk.** Worldwide distribution with higher risk of non-immune travelers.

2. **Transmission and incubation period.** *Bordetella pertussis* is transmitted from infected respiratory mucosa through droplets with an incubation period of 7 to 10 days. *Clostridium tetani* spores are transmitted from the soil to open wounds with an incubation period of 7 to 10 days. *Corynebacterium diphtheriae* is transmitted from infected respiratory mucosa through droplets with an incubation period of 2 to 5 days.

3. **Clinical manifestations.** Diphtheria can manifest in two forms, respiratory or cutaneous, and is characterized by sore throat, fever, hoarseness, fatigue, and/or a nonspecific pustular skin rash. The respiratory form is characterized classically by a gray pharyngeal membranous growth (i.e., pseudomembrane) consisting of necrotic tissue and fibrin.

Pertussis is characterized into three stages that can last as long as 12 weeks: (a) catarrhal stage (weeks 1–2)—highly contagious initial stage characterized by runny nose, fever, and cough; (b) paroxysmal stage (weeks 3–8)—characterized by rapid nonproductive coughs followed by a "whoop" sound and associated vomiting; and (c) convalescent stage (weeks 9–12)—characterized by lessening nonproductive coughs.

Tetanus is characterized by stiffness and muscle spasms, particularly of the jaw muscles (i.e., lockjaw).

4. **Vaccine and vaccine schedule.** Available vaccines are a sterile liquid suspension of inactivated toxins and acellular bacterial components absorbed onto aluminum phosphate as the adjuvant for IM administration in a one-dose series. Each dose contains 5 Lf tetanus toxoid, 2 Lf diphtheria toxoid, and acellular pertussis antigens (2.5 mcg detoxified PT, 5 mcg FHA, 3 mcg pertactin, 5 mcg FIM). Lf is known as limes flocculation (i.e., the smallest amount of toxin that, when mixed with one unit of antitoxin, yields the most rapid flocculation in the Ramon test). Flocculation, also known as precipitation from

solution, indicates a neutralized mixture of toxin and antitoxin. The dose is 0.5 mL IM injection. Adults who have not received tetanus and diphtheria toxoids and acellular pertussis vaccine (Tdap) or for whom pertussis vaccination status is unknown should receive 1 dose of Tdap followed by a tetanus and diphtheria toxoids (Td) booster every 10 years.

5. **Prevention.** Frequent handwashing, avoiding crowded environments, and proper wound care are recommended.

F. **Pneumococcus (*Streptococcus* pneumoniae).** Travelers should be offered vaccination according to standard recommendations.

1. **Geographic infection risk.** Worldwide distribution.

2. **Transmission and incubation period.** Airborne droplet transmission route with a 1- to 3-day incubation period.

3. **Clinical manifestations.** Characterized by abrupt onset of fever, chills or shakes (e.g., rigors) and chest discomfort, mucopurulent productive cough, and shortness of breath. Occasionally associated with nausea, vomiting, and/ or headache.

4. **Vaccine and vaccine schedule.** Available vaccines against pneumococcus are multiple-antigen formulations to contain either 2.2 to 4.4 mcg each of 13 polysaccharides (1, 3, 4, 5, 6A, 6B, 7F, 9V, 14, 18C, 19A, 19F, and 23F) conjugate with a diphtheria protein or 25 mcg of purified capsular polysaccharides (1, 2, 3, 4, 5, 6B, 7F, 8, 9N, 9V, 10A, 11A, 12F, 14, 15B, 17F, 18C, 19F, 19A, 20, 22F, 23F, and 33F) for IM administration in a two-dose series (e.g., deltoid muscle). Available vaccines are either 13-valent (conjugate protein; PCV13) or 23-valent (polysaccharide; PPSV23). For immunocompetent adults who previously received PPSV23 when aged less than 65 years and for whom an additional dose of PPSV23 is indicated when aged greater than 65 years, this subsequent PPSV23 dose should be given 1 year after PCV13 and 5 years after the most recent dose of PPSV23. For adults aged greater than 65 years with immunocompromising conditions, functional or anatomic asplenia, cerebrospinal fluid leaks, or cochlear implants, the recommended interval between PCV13 followed by PPSV23 is 8 weeks. The dose is 0.5 mL IM injection.

5. **Prevention.** Frequent handwashing and avoiding crowded environments are recommended.

IV. **VACCINE-PREVENTABLE DISEASES.** Immunizations for the traveler are categorized as routine (see the preceding), recommended, and required for travel.

A. **Required Immunizations.** Some destinations demand proof of vaccination to certain infectious disease prior to entry. Some destinations also require proof of vaccination upon reentry from an endemic region.

1. **Yellow fever virus (YFV).** A viral disease that has caused life-threatening epidemics throughout the last 500 years of human civilization. The liver is often affected, which eventually leads to jaundice, the symptom that gave the disease its name. Previously also known as "yellow jack" because of the yellow quarantine flag on 19th century merchant ships; the disease terrorized populations and severely disrupted trade. Max Theiler, PhD (1899–1972) received the Nobel Prize in Physiology or Medicine in 1951 for his discovery of an effective vaccine against yellow fever.

a. **Geographic infection risk.** Vaccination may be required for travelers to certain urban and rural areas of Africa and Central and South America.

b. **Transmission and incubation period.** Mosquito-to-human transmission route with a 3- to 6-day incubation period. Primary vectors are virus-infected *Aedes* and *Haemagogus* mosquitoes. The mosquitoes primarily reside indoors and are most active approximately 2 hours after sunrise and several hours before sunset.

c. **Clinical manifestations. The disease is caused by a single-stranded RNA virus of the genus** *Flavivirus*. Early manifestations are characterized by sudden onset of fever, chills, myalgias, fatigue, headache, nausea, vomiting, and bradycardia. Late manifestations occur in approximately 15% of infected individuals and are associated with a resurgence of fever, onset of jaundice (elevated total bilirubin), abdominal pain, nausea, vomiting, and hemorrhagic complications due to thrombocytopenia and shock (usually 1–2 days after onset of infection). Treatment is supportive care as there are no licensed antiviral treatment regimens.

d. **Vaccine and vaccine schedule.** Available vaccines are live attenuated virus formulations for SQ injection in individuals over 9 months of age and travelers at least 10 days prior to travel. Each 0.5 mL dose is formulated to contain not less than 4.74 to 5.04 log_{10} plaque-forming units (PFU) of either the 17D-204 or 17DD strain of YFV propagated in living avian leukosis virus–free (ALV-free) chicken embryos. Sustained lifelong protective immunity is over 90% after a single SQ dose. However, some countries may require for entry evidence of a valid yellow fever vaccination within the previous 10 years for certain individuals, depending on current and prior travel itinerary. *Vaccination in patients greater than 60 years of age and/or immunosuppression is associated with a higher risk of post-vaccination encephalitis and nonspecific multiorgan system failure that can be similar to fulminant yellow fever disease caused by wild-type YFV, with liver failure and internal bleeding, leading to death.*

e. **Prevention.** Personal protective measures against mosquito bites.

2. **Meningococcus.** A contagious infection caused by the bacteria *Neisseria meningitidis*, particularly serogroups A, B, C, W, X, and Y.

a. **Geographic infection risk.** Worldwide distribution; however, vaccination may be required for travelers to the sub-Saharan meningitis belt during the dry season as well as pilgrims visiting Mecca for the Hajj or Umrah.

b. **Transmission and incubation period.** Person-to-person transmission through respiratory droplets with a 3- to 4-day incubation period (average 2–10 days).

c. **Clinical manifestations.** Characterized by abrupt onset of fever, intense headache, photophobia, neck stiffness, nausea, and vomiting. Occasionally associated with systemic infection that is characterized by sepsis and hemorrhagic skin lesions (e.g., bullae).

d. **Vaccine and vaccine schedule.** Available vaccines against meningococcus are usually a 0.5 mL sterile solution of multiple-antigen formulations to contain at least 4.0 mcg each of four polysaccharides (A, C, Y, and W-135) conjugated with at least 48.0 mcg of a diphtheria toxoid carrier protein for primarily IM administration. A recombinant (or chimeric) meningococcal group B vaccine is available for a 0.5 mL IM dose as a sterile solution formulated to contain 50 mcg each of recombinant proteins *Neisseria* adhesin A (NadA), Neisserial Heparin Binding Antigen (NHBA), and factor H binding protein (fHbp) as well as 25 mcg of outer membrane vesicles (OMVs), 1.5 mg aluminum hydroxide, 3.125 mg sodium chloride, 0.776 mg histidine, and 10 mg sucrose at pH 6.4 to 6.7. Primary vaccination is usually initiated in children as early as 2 to 7 months in a multidose series (e.g., deltoid muscle). Young adults aged 16 to 23 years of age may be vaccinated with a two-dose series (e.g., day 0 and 6 months). *Travelers to certain countries may be required to have a one-time booster that should be administered after 5 years of age and every 5 years thereafter if they travel to a hyperendemic area and at least 10 days prior to travel.*

  e. **Prevention.** Frequent handwashing as well as avoiding overcrowding in confined spaces.

3. **Poliomyelitis (polio).** The term derives from Ancient Greek referring to gray (polio) matter or spinal cord inflammation (myelitis) causing paralysis. It is also sometimes referred to as *infantile paralysis.*

  a. **Geographic infection risk.** Vaccination may be required for travelers to Afghanistan, Burma (Myanmar), Guinea, Laos, Madagascar, Nigeria, Pakistan, and the Ukraine.

  b. **Transmission and incubation period.** Fecal–oral transmission route with a 7- to 21-day incubation period.

  c. **Clinical manifestations.** The disease is caused by any three of the single-stranded RNA virus genotypes from the genus *Enterovirus*, family Picornaviridae. While the majority of individuals are asymptomatic, clinical manifestations are best characterized by acute flaccid paralysis involving a single limb, quadriplegia, and/or respiratory failure. Treatment is supportive care as there are no licensed antiviral treatment regimens. Infection can result in long-term serious neurologic sequelae.

  d. **Vaccine and vaccine schedule.** Available vaccines against polio are either live attenuated virus or multiantigen inactivated virus formulations. The live attenuated virus vaccine is a four-dose oral administration series at these ages: birth, 6 weeks, 10 weeks, and a booster dose at 14 weeks. The inactivated virus vaccine requires IM administration in a four-dose series (e.g., deltoid muscle) at these ages: 2 months, 4 months, 6 to 18 months, and a booster dose at 4 to 6 years. *Travelers to certain polio-endemic countries may be required to have a one-time booster administered 10 years after the aforementioned primary series and at least 4 weeks prior to travel.*

  For the live attenuated virus vaccine each oral dose is a sterile solution formulated to contain not less than $10^{6.0}$ $TCID_{50}$ for type 1, $10^{5.0}$ $TCID_{50}$ for type 2, and $10^{5.8}$ $TCID_{50}$ for type 3 live attenuated Sabin strains of polioviruses produced in MRC5 human diploid cells. One dose of vaccine (0.1 mL) is delivered in two drops. Immunity by oral vaccination elicits predominantly an immunoglobulin A (IgA) response (gut lymphoid tissue) as well as an immunoglobulin G (IgG) response. Long-term protective immunity (defined as greater than 5–10 years) is over 90% after ingestion of all doses. $TCID_{50}$ is the tissue culture infectious dose that will infect 50% of the cell monolayers challenged with the defined inoculum. In vaccine manufacturing, $TCID_{50}$ is the standard titration method accepted by regulatory authorities for setting batch release, virus stability, and dose determination for clinical use. ***The oral vaccine has a risk of causing vaccine-associated paralytic polio (VAPP) and should not be used during acute illness and/or in pregnant or immunocompromised patients.***

For the inactive virus vaccine each IM dose is a sterile formulation to contain 40 D antigen units of type 1 (Mahoney strain), 8 D antigen units of type 2 (Middle Eastern Forces 1 strain), and 32 D antigen units of type 3 poliovirus (Saukett strain) propagated in Vero cells. Each dose (0.5 mL) of trivalent vaccine also contains 0.5% of 2-phenoxyethanol and 0.02% of formaldehyde as preservatives as well as 5 ng neomycin, 200 ng streptomycin, 25 ng polymyxin B, and less than 50 ng of calf bovine serum albumin. Long-term protective immunity (defined as greater than 5–10 years) is over 90% after IM injection of all doses. Vero cells are derived from the kidney of an African green monkey (*Cercopithecus aethiops*) and are a common mammalian continuous cell line used in medical research as well as for the licensed production of viral vaccines. The D antigen unit is a poliovirus type–specific unit in determining the potency of vaccine. The D antigen of poliovirus is the component of the virus involved in eliciting neutralizing antibodies, and therefore a D antigen assay has become a simple in vitro method for assessing the antigenic potency of polio vaccines.

   e. **Prevention.** Frequent handwashing as well as avoiding, boiling, or fully cooking potentially contaminated food or water.

B. **Recommended Immunizations.** These immunizations are recommended to provide protection against certain infectious diseases endemic to the traveler's intended destination.

1. **Typhoid.** *Salmonella enterica* serotypes Typhi and Paratyphi A, Paratyphi B (tartrate negative), and Paratyphi C cause a protracted bacteremic illness referred to respectively as typhoid and paratyphoid fever, and collectively as enteric fever.

   a. **Geographic infection risk.** Vaccination should be recommended for travelers to many Asian, African, and Latin American countries.

   b. **Transmission and incubation period.** Fecal–oral transmission route by contaminated food or water with a 6-day to 1-month incubation period (average 8–14 days).

   c. **Clinical manifestations.** Characterized by insidious onset of fever, fatigue, headache, decreased appetite, and transient macular rash. Occasionally associated with intestinal hemorrhage and/or intestinal perforation (usually 2–3 weeks after infection).

   d. **Vaccine and vaccine schedule.** Available vaccines against typhoid are either live attenuated mutant bacteria or single-antigen formulations (capsular polysaccharide) for a four-dose oral administration series or IM administration in a single-dose series (e.g., deltoid muscle).

The oral vaccine is an enteric-coated capsule that contains 2.0–10.0 × 10^9 viable *Salmonella enterica* serotype Typhi Ty21a and 5–50 × 10^9 nonviable *Salmonella enterica* serotype Typhi Ty21a. The enteric-coated capsule must be refrigerated and is taken 1 hour before meals over a 1-week duration (day 0, 2, 4, and 6) with a boosting interval of every 5 years. Immunity by oral vaccination elicits predominantly an IgA response (gut lymphoid tissue) as well as an IgG response. Protective immunity is over 65% for a duration of approximately 7 years after ingestion of all doses.

Each IM vaccine dose is a sterile solution formulated to contain 0.025 mg of purified Vi capsular polysaccharide, preserved with phenol (Vi simply stands for virulence). The dose is a single 0.5 mL IM injection 2 weeks prior to travel. The boosting interval is every 2 years. Seroconversion at 4 weeks after administration of the primary dose is greater than 90% for a duration of 2 years.

   e. **Prevention.** Frequent handwashing and avoiding, boiling, or fully cooking potentially contaminated food or water.

2. **Japanese encephalitis virus (JEV).** In 1871 the first clinical case of encephalitis was described in Japan. The virus was first isolated in 1935 and is a member of the genus *Flavivirus*, family Flaviviridae, and is transmitted between vertebrate hosts by mosquitoes, principally by *Culex tritaeniorhynchus*.

   a. **Geographic infection risk.** Vaccination should be recommended for travelers to Southeast Asia, India, China, Korea, Japan, Taiwan, Indonesia, Singapore, Papua New Guinea, and the Philippines. The risk of infection peaks during the summer and fall seasons.

   b. **Transmission and incubation period.** Mosquito-to-human transmission route with a 5- to 15-day incubation period. Primary vectors are virus-infected *Culex* mosquitoes. The mosquitoes primarily reside outdoors in agricultural rural settings (e.g., rice cultivation and flood irrigation) and are most active approximately 2 hours after sunrise and several hours before sunset (e.g., daytime biting). However, short-term travelers (less than 1-month duration) restricted to major urban areas have minimal risk of transmission.

   c. **Clinical manifestations.** The disease is caused by any four of the single-stranded RNA virus genotypes. Early manifestations are characterized by sudden onset of fever, fatigue, headache, nausea, and vomiting. Late manifestations are associated with a parkinsonian syndrome (e.g., mask-like facies, tremor, cogwheel rigidity, and choreoathetoid movements), mental status changes, motor weakness, and/or seizures (usually 3–5 days after onset of infection). Treatment is supportive care as there are no licensed antiviral treatment regimens. Infection can result in long-term serious neurologic, cognitive, and/or psychiatric sequelae.

   d. **Vaccine and vaccine schedule.** Available vaccines against JEV are either inactivated Vero cell–derived, live attenuated and/or live recombinant formulations for IM or SQ administration in a single-dose or two-dose series (e.g., deltoid muscle). Inactivated mouse brain–derived vaccines are no longer recommended. The boosting interval is every 1 to 2 years.

For the Vero cell–derived vaccine each IM dose is a sterile solution formulated to contain 6 mcg of inactivated JEV strain SA14-14-2, produced in Vero cells and adsorbed on 0.25 mg of hydrated aluminum hydroxide as a two-dose series 28 days apart (e.g., day 0 and day 28). Vero cells are derived from the kidney of an African green monkey (*Cercopithecus aethiops*) and are a common mammalian continuous cell line used in medical research as well as for the licensed production of viral vaccines. Each injection is either a single 0.25 mL dose for children 2 months to 3 years of age or a single 0.5 mL dose for individuals greater than 3 years of age as an IM injection 2 weeks prior to travel. Seroconversion at 1 week after administration of the second dose is greater than 95% for a duration of 2 years.

For the live attenuated vaccine, each SQ dose is a sterile solution formulated to contain not less than 5.7 log PFU per mL of attenuated JEV strain SA14-14-2, produced in primary hamster kidney cells as a single-dose series. Each injection is a single 0.5 mL dose for individuals greater than 8 months of age as an SQ injection. Seroconversion at 1 week after administration of the primary dose is greater than 95% for a duration of 5 years.

For the live attenuated recombinant (or chimeric) vaccine, each SQ dose is a sterile solution formulated to contain not less than 4.0 to 5.8 log PFU per ml of attenuated chimeric JEV strain SA14-14-2, produced using recombinant DNA technology by replacing the premembrane (prM) and envelope (E) coding sequences of the yellow fever live attenuated 17D vaccine virus with the SA 14-14-2 live attenuated JE vaccine virus. Each injection is a single 0.5 mL dose for individuals greater than 9 months of age as an SQ injection. Seroconversion at 4 weeks after administration of the primary dose is greater than 95% for a duration of 3 years.

Live attenuated virus vaccines should not be used during acute illness and/or in pregnant or immunocompromised patients.

e. **Prevention.** Personal protective measures against mosquito bites.

3. **Rabies.** The first written reference to this disease is when Hector was compared to an enraged dog in Homer's epic poem *The Iliad*. It is a zoonotic illness of "bullet-shaped" RNA viruses with 1 to 7 serotypes belonging to the genera *Lyssavirus*, family *Rhabdoviridae*, and order *Mononegavirales*. The term derives from Ancient Latin referring to infection of the central nervous system (CNS) causing madness, rage, and fury. In 1885, the first successful vaccine was developed by two French scientists, Louis Pasteur and Emile Roux, and used for a young boy named Joseph Meister.

a. **Geographic infection risk.** Worldwide distribution, except Antarctica. Vaccination may be considered for travelers who may come in contact with wild or domestic animals such as dogs, foxes, raccoons, mongooses, and bats. High-risk travelers may include campers, cavers, veterinarians, and wildlife professionals.

b. **Transmission and incubation period.** Animal-to-human transmission route with a 20- to 60-day incubation period. Transmission can occur from licks, bites, or scratches.

c. **Clinical manifestations.** Early manifestations are characterized by fever, fatigue, headache, and sensory changes at the site of entry. Additional manifestations include hallucinations, abnormal fear of drafts of air (aerophobia), and fear of water (hydrophobia) due to spasms of the swallowing muscles. Late manifestations are associated with delirium, mental status changes, convulsions, and/or seizures followed by death. Treatment is supportive care as there are no licensed antiviral treatment regimens. Postexposure prophylaxis is best managed by appropriate wound cleansing (e.g., soap and water). Two doses of modern cell culture vaccine should be given on days 0 and 3 after the exposure in travelers who received pretravel vaccination. For travelers without pretravel vaccination the administration of human rabies immunoglobulin (RIG) is at a dose of 20 IU/kg and four doses of IM vaccination, one each on days 0, 3, 7, and 14 (day 28 if immunocompromised).

d. **Vaccine and vaccine schedule.** Available vaccines against rabies are either human diploid cell or purified chick embryo cell formulations for IM administration in a multiple dose series (e.g., deltoid muscle).

For the purified chick embryo vaccine, each IM dose is a sterile freeze-dried formula to contain at least 2.5 IU rabies antigen of the fixed-virus strain Flury LEP, produced in primary chicken fibroblasts as a pretravel multiple-dose series, one each on days 0, 7, and 21 or 28. The final vaccine also contains neomycin at less than 10 mcg, chlortetracycline at less than 200 ng, and amphotericin B at less than 20 ng per dose. Each injection is a single 1.0 mL dose for individuals greater than 2 years of age as an IM injection. Seroconversion at 4 weeks after administration of the primary dose series is greater than 95% for a duration of 2 years.

For the cell-derived vaccine each IM dose is a sterile solution formulated to contain at least 2.5 IU rabies antigen of the strain PM-1503-3M virus, produced in MRC5 human diploid cells as a pretravel multiple-dose series, one each on days 0, 7, and 21 or 28. The final vaccine also contains neomycin at less than 150 mcg, human albumin at less than 100 mg and betapropiolactone at less than 50 parts per million per dose. Each injection is a single 1.0 mL dose for individuals greater than 2 years of age as an IM injection. Seroconversion at 4 weeks after administration of the primary dose series is greater than 95% for a duration of 2 years.

A booster dose for each vaccine should be administered if the neutralizing antibody titer falls below the minimum antibody titer accepted as seroconversion (defined as complete inhibition in the rapid fluorescent focus inhibition test [RFFIT] at 1:5 dilution as specified by the Centers for Disease Control and Prevention [CDC] or ≥0.5 IU per milliliter (mL) as specified by the World Health Organization [WHO]). *Vaccination should be avoided in pregnant women or individuals with immunosuppressive conditions.*

e. **Prevention.** Frequent handwashing and avoiding wild or unknown domestic animals.

4. **Cholera.** A contagious infection caused by *Vibrio cholerae* bacteria serogroups O1 and O139. The term is first mentioned in the writings of Hippocrates and is used to describe a disease characterized by diarrhea.

a. **Geographic infection risk.** Vaccination should be recommended for travelers to many countries of Asian and African as well as the Dominican Republic and Haiti.

b. **Transmission and incubation period.** Fecal–oral transmission route by contaminated food or water with a 1- to 5-day incubation period (average 2–3 days).

c. **Clinical manifestations.** Characterized best by the onset of watery diarrhea in mild cases. Occasionally associated with severe diarrhea characterized as "rice-water stools" associated with nausea, vomiting, and dehydration. Rarely the condition could lead to severe dehydration, hypovolemic shock, and/or death. The cornerstone of treatment involves adequate and timely rehydration measures in combination with doxycycline antimicrobial therapy.

d. **Vaccine and vaccine schedule.** Available vaccines are live attenuated bacterial formulations containing 4×10^8 to 2×10^9 colony-forming units (CFUs) of the *V. cholerae* strain CVD 103-HgR in a sterile suspension for oral administration in a single-dose series for travelers 18 to 64 years of age. This attenuated strain was produced from the serogroup O1 classical Inaba strain 569B by deleting both genetic copies of the catalytic domain sequence preventing the synthesis of active cholera toxin. Each single reconstituted 100 mL vaccine dose must be taken 1 hour before or after meals within 10 days of travel. Immunity by oral vaccination elicits predominantly an IgA response (gut lymphoid tissue) as well as an IgG response. Protective immunity is over 90% for serogroup O1 (*not effective for serogroup O139*) approximately 10 days after ingestion of a single dose. The vaccine should not be administered to pregnant women, patients with immunosuppressive conditions, and to patients who have received oral or parenteral antibiotics within 14 days prior to vaccination.

e. **Prevention.** Frequent handwashing and avoiding, boiling, or fully cooking potentially contaminated food or water.

V. NON-VACCINE-PREVENTABLE DISEASES

A. **Malaria.** The term originates from Medieval Rome and the notion that this disease resulted from the "bad air" of swamp marshes. In 1880, French army surgeon Charles Louis Alphonse Laveran first discovered these parasites in the blood of patients suffering from this disease. British officer Ronald Ross, in 1897, demonstrated that mosquitoes transmitted the malaria parasites. Malaria in humans is caused by several species of the *Plasmodium* protozoan parasite (*P. falciparum, P. vivax, P. ovale, P. malariae* and *P. knowlesi*).

1. **Geographic infection risk.** Travelers to many countries of Asian, African, and South America as well as the Dominican Republic, Haiti, Southeast Asia, India, China, Korea, Japan, Taiwan, Indonesia, Singapore, Papua New Guinea, and the Philippines. The risk of infection peaks during the rainy seasons.

2. **Transmission and incubation period.** Mosquito-to-human transmission route with a 9- to 14-day incubation period for *P. falciparum*, 12- to 18-day incubation period for *P. vivax* and *P. ovale*, and 18- to 40-day incubation period for *P. malariae*. Primary vectors are virus-infected female *Anopheles* mosquitoes. The mosquitoes primarily reside outdoors in agricultural rural settings and are most active approximately 2 hours before sunrise and several hours after sunset (e.g., nighttime biting).

3. **Clinical manifestations.** Characterized by abrupt onset of fever and chills that occur in cyclic intervals. Fever cycles occur every second day with the "tertian" parasites (*P. falciparum, P. vivax,* and *P. ovale*) and every third day with the "quartan" parasite (*P. malariae*). Additional symptoms include intense headache, sweats, myalgias, and malaise. Severe disease may include altered mentation, seizures, coma, acute respiratory distress syndrome, jaundice, renal failure, and/or death.

4. **Treatment.** Infection caused by *P. falciparum* is considered a medical emergency that can result in a serious, life-threatening illness and treatment should begin immediately. Treatment options also depend on the species of malaria, the likelihood of drug resistance (based on where the infection was acquired), the age of the patient, pregnancy status, and the severity of infection.

   Treatment recommendations include (the following regimens are based on adult dosing for individuals over 35 kg weight):

   a. **Complicated or severe malaria.** Severe malaria is most often caused by *P. falciparum*. Manifestations of more severe disease are travelers with one or more of the following clinical criteria: impaired consciousness/coma, severe normocytic anemia, renal failure, pulmonary edema, acute respiratory distress syndrome, circulatory shock, disseminated intravascular coagulation, spontaneous bleeding, acidosis, hemoglobinuria, jaundice, repeated generalized convulsions, and/or parasitemia of greater than 5%.

      i. **First-line therapy.** Artesunate 2.4 mg/kg intravenous administration at 0, 12, 24, and 48 hours *plus* either atovaquone–proguanil 200 mg/100 mg, four tablets orally daily for 3 days, doxycycline 100 mg orally twice daily for 7 days, clindamycin 6–7 mg/kg orally three times daily for 7 days *or* mefloquine 750 mg salt oral loading dose followed by 500 mg salt orally 6 to 12 hours after the loading dose. (Mefloquine may be associated with QT interval prolongation.)

      ii. **Second-line therapy.** Quinidine gluconate 10 mg/kg salt intravenous loading dose administered over 1 to 2 hours followed by 0.02 mg/kg/min salt continuous intravenous infusion for 24 hours. (Quinidine infusion may be associated with infusion-related hypotension, QT interval and/or QRS complex prolongation, torsades de pointes arrhythmia, and/or hypoglycemia.) Once the patient has clinical improvement or percentage parasitemia of less than 1% then switch to quinine 625 mg salt orally three times a day for 7 days if infected in Southeast Asia (3 days if not infected in Southeast Asia) *plus* either doxycycline 100 mg orally twice daily *or* clindamycin 20 mg base/kg orally three times daily for 7 days.

   b. **Uncomplicated *P. falciparum***

      i. **Chloroquine-sensitive (travelers to the Dominican Republic and/or Haiti).** Chloroquine phosphate 1,000 mg salt oral loading followed by 500 mg salt orally at 6, 24, and 48 hours *or* hydroxychloroquine 800 mg salt oral loading followed by 400 mg salt orally at 6, 24, and 48 hours (retinal toxicity is unlikely with short-term administration).

      ii. **Chloroquine-resistant.** Atovaquone–proguanil 200 mg/100 mg, four tablets orally daily for 3 days *or* artemether–lumefantrine 20 mg/120 mg, four tablets loading dose followed by four tablets at 8 hours, then four tablets twice daily for 2 days *or* mefloquine 750 mg salt oral loading dose followed by 500 mg salt orally 6 to 12 hours after the loading dose (mefloquine may be associated with QT prolongation). Another option may be quinine sulfate 650 mg salt orally three times a day for 7 days if infected in Southeast Asia (3 days if not infected in Southeast Asia) *plus* either doxycycline 100 mg orally twice daily *or* clindamycin 20 mg base/kg orally three times daily for 7 days.

c. **Uncomplicated *P. ovale* and/or *P. vivax***

   i. Chloroquine-sensitive. Chloroquine phosphate 1,000 mg salt oral loading followed by 500 mg salt orally at 6, 24, and 48 hours *or* hydroxychloroquine 800 mg salt oral loading followed by 400 mg salt orally at 6, 24, and 48 hours (retinal toxicity is unlikely with short-term administration). Primaquine phosphate 30 mg base orally once daily for 14 days should be administered after either treatment option in the preceding. (Primaquine may be associated with hemolytic anemia if there is a history of G6PD deficiency.)

   ii. Chloroquine-resistant **(travelers to Papua New Guinea and/or Indonesia).** Quinine sulfate 650 mg salt orally three times a day for 7 days if infected in Southeast Asia (3 days if not infected in Southeast Asia) *plus* either doxycycline 100 mg orally twice daily *or* clindamycin 20 mg base/kg orally three times daily for 7 days. Other options may be either atovaquone–proguanil 200 mg/100 mg, four tablets orally daily for 3 days *or* mefloquine 750 mg salt oral loading dose followed by 500 mg salt orally 6 to 12 hours after the loading dose. (Mefloquine may be associated with QT prolongation.) Primaquine phosphate 30 mg base orally once daily for 14 days should be administered after either treatment option in the preceding. (Primaquine may be associated with hemolytic anemia if there is a history of G6PD deficiency.)

d. **Uncomplicated *P. knowlesi* and/or *P. malariae*.** Chloroquine 1,000 mg salt oral loading followed by 500 mg salt orally at 6, 24, and 48 hours *or* hydroxychloroquine 800 mg salt oral loading followed by 400 mg salt orally at 6, 24, and 48 hours (retinal toxicity is unlikely with short-term administration).

Atovaquone–proguanil, artemether–lumefantrine, and doxycycline should not be used for pregnant women infected with malaria.

Treatment options for pregnant women include:

   i. *Complicated or severe malaria. Quinidine gluconate plus clindamycin followed by quinine sulfate plus clindamycin or mefloquine (see dosing in the preceding).*

   ii. *Uncomplicated malaria.*

      (1) *Chloroquine-sensitive. Chloroquine or hydroxychloroquine (see dosing in the preceding).*

      (2) *Chloroquine-resistant. Quinine sulfate plus clindamycin or mefloquine (see dosing in the preceding).*

   5. Prevention. Chemoprophylaxis (Table 51.1) and personal protective measures against mosquito bites.

B. Dengue. The term "dengue" is Spanish for fastidious (or slow and careful), which was used to describe the walking gait of a person suffering from bone pain.

   1. Geographic infection risk. Dengue is endemic throughout the tropics and subtropics, predominantly Africa, Southeast Asia, Latin America, and the Caribbean.

   2. Transmission and incubation period. Mosquito-to-human transmission route with a 4- to 10-day incubation period. Primary vectors are virus-infected *Aedes aegypti* and *Aedes albopictus* mosquitoes. The mosquitoes primarily reside indoors and are most active approximately 2 hours after sunrise and several hours before sunset.

   3. Clinical manifestations. The disease is caused by one of four *Flavivirus* serotypes. The disease is caused by any four of the single-stranded RNA virus genotypes. While the majority of individuals are asymptomatic, early clinical manifestations are characterized by sudden onset of fever, fatigue, headache, retro-orbital pain, nausea, vomiting, myalgias and arthralgias, and petechial rash. Late manifestations are associated with severe infection that is characterized by shock, respiratory distress, severe bleeding, and/or severe organ impairment.

TABLE 51.1 ■ Chemoprophylactic Agents for Malaria

Agent	Destination	Dose	Adverse Effects
Atovaquone–proguanil	Short-term travelers worldwide	250 mg atovaquone + 100 mg proguanil PO daily, starting 2 days pre-exposure and continuing for 7 days postexposure	Mild gastrointestinal disturbances
Chloroquine	Travelers to the Caribbean and Haiti	500 mg salt (300 mg base) PO weekly, starting 2 weeks pre-exposure and continuing for 4 weeks postexposure	Retinal toxicity with long-term use
Doxycycline	Long-term and short-term travelers worldwide	100 mg PO daily starting 2 days pre-exposure and continuing 4 weeks postexposure	Esophageal irritation/ ulceration. Nausea and abdominal discomfort. Skin photosensitivity.
Mefloquine	Long-term and short-term travelers worldwide	250 mg salt (228 mg base) PO weekly, starting 2–3 weeks pre-exposure, and continuing 4 weeks postexposure	Neuropsychiatric effects

Atovaquone–proguanil is contraindicated in pregnant women.
Chloroquine is contraindicated in patients with a history of psoriasis or epilepsy.
Doxycycline is contraindicated in pregnant women but it is effective for travelers at risk for leptospirosis and rickettsial infections.
Mefloquine should be avoided for patients with a history of psychiatric disorder.

4. Treatment. Supportive care as there are no licensed antiviral treatment regimens.

5. Prevention. Personal protective measures against mosquito bites (appropriate clothing, indoor insecticides, and repellents).

C. Chikungunya. The term "chikungunya" is a Makonde (language of northern Mozambique and southeast Tanzania) phrase meaning "that which bends up" which was used to describe the severe arthritis pain of a person suffering from the disease.

1. Geographic infection risk. Chikungunya is endemic mostly during the rainy seasons throughout the tropics and subtropics, predominantly Africa, Southeast Asia, islands in the Indian and Pacific Oceans, Latin America, and the Caribbean.

2. Transmission and incubation period. Mosquito-to-human transmission route with a 1- to 12-day incubation period (average 3–7 days). Primary vectors are virus-infected *Aedes aegypti* and *Aedes albopictus* mosquitoes. The mosquitoes primarily reside indoors and are most active approximately 2 hours after sunrise and several hours before sunset.

3. Clinical manifestations. The disease is caused by a single-stranded RNA virus within the family Togaviridae. The majority of infected individuals are symptomatic and best described as a sudden onset, acute, febrile illness (temperature is typically greater than 102°F [39°C]) with severe bilateral symmetric joint pains (most commonly of the hands and feet). Additional symptoms may include a maculopapular rash, headache, conjunctivitis, nausea, and/or vomiting.

4. Treatment. Supportive care as there are no licensed antiviral treatment regimens.

5. Prevention. Personal protective measures against mosquito bites (appropriate clothing, indoor insecticides, and repellents).

D. Zika. The term is Luganda for overgrown and describes the Zika forest of Uganda to which the virus was first isolated in 1947.

1. Geographic infection risk. Zika is associated with sporadic epidemics throughout the tropics and subtropics, predominantly Africa, Southeast Asia, Pacific Islands, Latin America, and the Caribbean.

2. Transmission and incubation period. Mosquito-to-human transmission route with a 3- to 12-day incubation period. Primary vectors are virus-infected *Aedes aegypti* and *Aedes albopictus* mosquitoes. The mosquitoes primarily reside indoors and are most active approximately 2 hours after sunrise and several hours before sunset.

3. Clinical manifestations. The disease is caused by a single-stranded RNA virus within the family Flaviviridae. While the majority of infected individuals are asymptomatic, symptoms are best described as a mild, febrile illness with a maculopapular rash, arthralgias, and conjunctivitis. Additional symptoms may include myalgias and headaches. The infection is also associated with fetal microcephaly and spontaneous abortions in pregnant women.

4. Treatment. Supportive care as there are no licensed antiviral treatment regimens.

5. Prevention. Personal protective measures against mosquito bites (appropriate clothing, indoor insecticides, and repellents).

E. Leptospirosis. A zoonotic disease caused by obligate aerobic, gram-negative spirochetes of the genus *Leptospira*.

1. **Geographic infection risk.** Worldwide distribution; however, travelers to the tropics and subtropics during the rainy season are at higher risk. Travelers to Southeast Asia, Oceania, sub-Saharan Africa, Latin America, the Caribbean, Hawaii, and Puerto Rico participating in recreational freshwater activities, such as swimming or boating, are at higher risk.

2. **Transmission and incubation period.** Transmission to humans through environmental surface waters contaminated by the urine of chronically infected mammals, particularly dogs. The incubation period is 2 to 30 days (average 3–14 days).

3. **Clinical manifestations.** Originally described in the 19th century as Weil's disease that was historically characterized by a triad of fever, jaundice, and splenomegaly. Currently the term "Weil's disease" refers to fever, jaundice, and renal failure and is often considered synonymous with severe leptospirosis.

   While the majority of infected individuals are asymptomatic, early manifestations are abrupt onset of fever and chills, headache, myalgia, anorexia, nausea, and vomiting. Additional symptoms may include a maculopapular rash, conjunctival suffusion (red eyes without exudate), nonproductive cough, and/or diarrhea. Severe manifestations of leptospirosis include any combination of jaundice, renal failure, hemorrhage (most commonly pulmonary), myocarditis, and hypotension refractory to fluid resuscitation.

4. **Treatment.** Treatment involves supportive measures in combination with appropriate antimicrobial therapy. Options include:

   a. **Severe infection.** Penicillin G 1.5 MU intravenously every 6 hours for 7 days.

   b. **Mild infection, nonpregnant.** Doxycycline 100 mg orally every 12 hours for 7 days.

   c. **Mild infection, pregnant, and/or child under the age of 12 years.** Amoxicillin 500 mg orally every 8 hours for 7 days.

5. **Prevention.** Frequent handwashing as well as avoiding potentially contaminated food or water and potentially infected animals or their body fluids (particularly urine).

VI. SELF-TREATABLE TRAVEL-RELATED CONDITIONS

A. Traveler's Diarrhea. Characteristics are classically defined as passage of more than three unformed stools in a 24-hour period with one or more accompanying symptoms of enteric disease, such as nausea, vomiting, abdominal cramps, fever, tenesmus, or bloody stool. It also includes episodes of diarrhea that occur during the first 7 to 10 days after the traveler returns home.

1. **Geographic infection risk.** Travelers to Central and South America, Africa, Asia, the Middle East, and Mexico have the highest risk of infection. Travelers to the Caribbean, Eastern Europe, and South Africa have an intermediate risk of infection.

2. **Microbiology.** While enterotoxigenic *Escherichia coli* is the most common bacterial cause, *Campylobacter jejuni, Shigella* and *Salmonella* species, *Aeromonas* and *Plesiomonas* species as well as enterotoxigenic *Bacteroides fragilis* group species bacteria may also cause disease. Viral pathogens most commonly involve astrovirus, norovirus, and rotavirus. The main parasite pathogen is *Giardia lamblia.*

3. **Transmission and incubation period.** Fecal–oral transmission route with a 6- to 72-hour incubation period for bacteria and viral pathogens. The incubation period may be 1 to 2 weeks for parasite pathogens.

4. **Clinical manifestations.** Characterized by abrupt onset of mild cramps and diarrhea in mild cases. More severe disease may include the abrupt onset of fever, nausea, vomiting, and abdominal pain followed by the onset of bloody diarrhea as well as dehydration. Illness due to parasitic infection generally involves an insidious onset of abdominal cramps and diarrhea (ranging from 2 to 5 diarrhea stools per day).

   Untreated bacterial or viral illness resolves within 2 to 7 days. Untreated parasite illness may persist for more than 2 weeks.

5. **Treatment.** The cornerstone of treatment involves adequate and timely rehydration measures in combination with antimicrobial therapy.

   Antibiotic regimen(s) include: azithromycin 1,000 mg as a single dose, azithromycin 500 mg once daily for 3 days, ciprofloxacin 500 mg twice daily for 3 days, or rifaximin 200 mg daily for 3 days.

   Antiparasite regimen(s) include: metronidazole 250 mg three times daily for 5 days.

   Loperamide has antimotility and antisecretory effects and considered safe when combined with antimicrobial therapy. It is administered as two 2 mg tablets after the first loose stool, followed by one tablet after each subsequent loose stool (maximum of 8 mg in 24 hours for 2 days).

6. **Prevention.** Frequent handwashing and avoiding, boiling, or fully cooking potentially contaminated food or water. Prophylactic antimicrobial therapy such as ciprofloxacin 250 mg once daily for no more than 21 days total may be considered for short-term travelers who are high-risk hosts (e.g., pregnant women and immunosuppressed patients). Bismuth subsalicylate administered as two tablets four times daily for no more than 21 days total also may be considered. However, it is not recommended for individuals taking certain anticoagulants or other salicylates and should not be taken by travelers using doxycycline for malaria prophylaxis due to interference with absorption. Adverse reactions associated with bismuth subsalicylate are transient blackening of tongue and stools, constipation, tinnitus, and nausea.

VII. BLOOD-BORNE AND SEXUALLY TRANSMITTED INFECTIONS

Prevention of sexually transmitted diseases (STDs) as well as blood-borne pathogens (e.g., HIV and hepatitis B) should be a priority among travel clinic services. Several factors are associated with a higher frequency of casual sexual intercourse during travel, particularly: male sex, single status, age of less than 20 years, traveling without a partner, having had more than two sexual partners in the previous 2 years, being a casual user of illicit drugs, or being an abuser of alcohol. Additionally, travelers who make trips with the intention to visit an area in which sex is for sale (e.g., "sexual tourist") are at increased risk. Primary prevention is based on recommendations regarding safer sex practices such as limiting the number of new sexual partners, consistent and proper use of condoms during sexual activity, and limiting the use of alcohol and/or illicit drugs. Travelers with high-risk sexual exposures or the development of genital symptoms should seek professional medical care (see Chapter 42, Sexually Transmitted Diseases).

VIII. POST-TRAVEL CARE

The most common clinical presentations after travel include systemic febrile illness, diarrheal illness, and dermatologic conditions. A complete and chronologically accurate history should be obtained in all suspected cases of illness among travelers returning home. The history should focus on the destination(s) and timing of recent travel, onset of illness in relation to recent travel, comorbid medical conditions, medication(s) and allergies, pretravel immunizations, travel-related chemoprophylaxis and adherence (e.g., malaria), recent infections, and antimicrobial therapy. The history should also include a review of the relevant individual risk factors. A complete physical examination should also be performed, but both clinical and epidemiologic considerations in relation to recent travel must guide appropriate testing and treatment.

BIBLIOGRAPHY

Freedman DO, Chen LH, Korarsky PE. Medical considerations before international travel. *N Engl J Med*. 2016;375(3):247–260.

Hill DR, Ericsson CD, Pearson RD, et al. The practice of travel medicine: guidelines by the Infectious Diseases Society of America. *Clin Infect Dis*. 2006;43(12):1499–1539.

Lo Re V 3rd, Gluckman SJ. Fever in the returned traveler. *Am Fam Physician*. 2003;68(7):1343–1350.

Ryan ET, Wilson ME, Kain KC. Illness after international travel. *N Engl J Med*. 2002;347(7):505–516.

Sanford CA, Fung C. Illness in the returned international traveler. *Med Clin North Am*. 2016;100(2):393–409.

Sanford C, McConnell A, Osborn J. The pretravel consultation. *Am Fam Physician*. 2016;94(8): 620–627.

Sanford CA, Jong EC. Immunizations. *Med Clin North Am*. 2016;100(2):247–259.

BASIC APPROACH TO INFECTION CONTROL AND EPIDEMIOLOGY

Clare Rock
Surbhi Leekha

I. INTRODUCTION AND DEFINITIONS

A. Healthcare-Associated Infection. *A healthcare-associated infection (HAI) is an infection developing in an individual receiving care at a healthcare facility (such as a hospital, nursing home, or receiving outpatient care in a dialysis or infusion center), and no evidence suggests that the infection was present or incubating at the time of presentation to the healthcare facility.* Commonly recognized HAIs are central line–associated bloodstream infections, surgical-site infections, pneumonia (including ventilator-associated pneumonia), catheter-associated urinary tract infection, and *Clostridium difficile* infection.

B. Multidrug-Resistant Organisms. *Multidrug-resistant organisms (MDROs) are defined as organisms, usually bacteria, that are resistant to more than one class of antimicrobials generally used to treat that organism,* although in practice most MDROs are resistant to many classes of antimicrobials. Commonly encountered MDROs include methicillin-resistant *Staphylococcus aureus* (MRSA), vancomycin-resistant *Enterococcus* (VRE), and multidrug-resistant gram-negative bacteria (such as *Pseudomonas aeruginosa, Acinetobacter baumannii,* and *Klebsiella pneumoniae*). Recent increases in MDR gram-negative bacteria have been particularly concerning: they were responsible for one third of all HAIs in 2006 and 2007; they exhibit multiple resistance mechanisms that can be upregulated under antimicrobial selection pressure; newer strains with carbapenemases and other beta-lactamases that make them resistant to a broad range of beta-lactams are spreading worldwide; they survive well in the hospital environment and are easily transmissible. Finally, there are no new gram-negative antibiotics on the horizon, making treatment very difficult.

Factors common to development of HAIs and colonization with MDROs include:

1. Presence of invasive devices

2. Loss of normal host defenses and barriers against infection

3. Biofilm formation enabling bacterial colonization of devices and body sites

4. Broad-spectrum antimicrobial use and selection for antimicrobial-resistant pathogens

In 2002, the estimated number of HAIs in U.S. hospitals was approximately 1.7 million and was associated with nearly 100,000 deaths. In 2006 and 2007,

16% of all HAIs in acute care hospitals reporting surveillance data to the Centers for Disease Control and Prevention (CDC) National Healthcare Safety Network (NHSN) were associated with MDROs. A 2009 CDC report estimated that the overall annual direct medical costs of HAI to U.S. hospitals ranges from $35 billion to $45 billion. Therefore, there is a clear need for an infection prevention and control program in each healthcare facility.

II. **THE INFECTION PREVENTION AND CONTROL/HOSPITAL EPIDEMIOLOGY PROGRAM.** *The aim of such a program is to decrease the risk of HAI for patients, healthcare personnel (HCP), and visitors.* The science of healthcare epidemiology deals with identifying risk factors for HAIs so that they can be prevented. A hospital epidemiology program generally consists of one or more hospital epidemiologists, infection preventionists, and a multidisciplinary infection control committee. The infection control committee has representatives from hospital administration, nursing, physicians including critical care and infectious-disease specialists, pharmacy, microbiology, surgical services, employee health, housekeeping, and facilities maintenance.

Functions of the hospital epidemiology program include:

1. Surveillance

2. Development of routine infection prevention policies and procedures

3. Implementation of specific evidence-based interventions aimed at HAI prevention

4. Outbreak investigation

5. Monitoring antimicrobial use and resistance rates

6. Education of HCP on infection control principles

7. Research in healthcare epidemiology

8. New product evaluation

A. **Surveillance.** Surveillance in hospital epidemiology is used primarily to establish the rate of HAIs in a facility or a unit and forms the backbone of the program. To be most effective, surveillance should be continuous, generate data that are meaningful to participating units and facilities, provide the basis for intervention, and lead to measurable reduction in HAI events (see Figure 52.1).

1. **Uses of surveillance**

   a. Estimate the burden and distribution of HAIs and MDROs

   b. Evaluate risk factors for HAIs and MDROs

   c. Allocate resources for infection prevention interventions

   d. Evaluate the impact of those interventions

   e. Identify possible outbreaks

2. **Types of surveillance**

   a. *Passive versus active surveillance.* Passive surveillance relies on bedside clinicians to report, leading to the possibility of underreporting and bias. Under active surveillance, defined data elements are collected periodically, thereby providing more complete and unbiased data.

FIGURE 52.1 ■ Elements of effective surveillance in hospital epidemiology.
HAI, healthcare–associated infection.

    b. *Prospective/concurrent versus retrospective surveillance.* Prospective
surveillance provides real-time data and is better suited for detecting
outbreaks and finding opportunities for behavior change but is more
resource intensive. Retrospective surveillance is relatively inexpensive but
relies on the completeness and accuracy of existing data, and it may be
too late to intervene by the time the data are analyzed and a problem is
recognized. Most facilities utilize a combination of prospective and retrospective surveillance.

    c. *Hospitalwide versus targeted surveillance.* When resources are limited,
surveillance may be focused on units with patients at high risk for HAIs
and MDRO colonization, such as intensive care units and hematology–
oncology units. However, surveillance is becoming increasingly hospital-
wide. Electronic records have made surveillance much easier to conduct
and require less time than previously when chart records would have
been reviewed to get the required information.

3. Role of active surveillance for MDROs. Active surveillance for MDRO colonization may be of benefit in selected situations (e.g., during an outbreak,

or screening for MRSA prior to major surgery) but routine screening of all patients via active surveillance cultures and subsequent contact precautions (see the following) remains controversial. Moreover, there could be potential negative consequences and increase in noninfectious adverse events associated with contact precautions. Although the effectiveness of this strategy continues to be debated, active surveillance, particularly for MRSA, is required by legislative mandates in several states in the United States. The CDC's NHSN allows hospitals to compare their institutional rates with that of a large group of hospitals nationwide. Surveillance also meets requirements of regulatory agencies such as the Joint Commission, and contributes to measures of quality of care being increasingly reported to the public to allow comparisons between hospitals.

B. **Outbreak Investigation.** *An outbreak of an HAI or epidemiologically significant organism is defined as an occurrence of cases that are or appear to be in excess of the normal expectancy.* While the terms "cluster" and "epidemic" are sometimes used interchangeably with "outbreak," the number of cases constituting an outbreak may vary depending on the organism or disease. In some instances, a single case can constitute an outbreak (e.g., smallpox, healthcare–associated Legionnaires disease). An outbreak investigation is broadly divided into preliminary and definitive investigations.

1. **Preliminary/initial investigation (descriptive study)**

    a. Verify diagnosis of patients/healthcare workers (HCWs) suspected to have the condition

    b. Perform quick review of medical records, available literature, and create a case definition

    c. Notify the microbiology laboratory and save all isolates that might be part of the outbreak

    d. Develop methodology to maximize detection rate of additional cases

    e. Create a line list and, when possible, graph an epidemic curve

    f. When available, compare with historical data to verify the existence of an outbreak

    g. Alert appropriate clinical staff and other stakeholders (e.g., hospital administration, health department)

    h. Institute emergency interim prevention and control measures based on initial impression

2. **Definitive/follow-up investigation (comparative study)**

    a. Perform a detailed review of medical records of case patients

    b. Perform a review of published literature for any existing association of practices and procedures with the type of outbreak under investigation

    c. Refine the case definition and determine the at-risk population

    d. Develop hypotheses to explain the likely cause(s) or source(s)

    e. Determine the need for outside consultation (e.g., state health department, CDC)

   f. Perform one or more of the following depending on the type of outbreak and available resources:

     i. *Observational studies, including HCW interviews and surveys (e.g., operating room practices)*

     ii. *Microbiologic or laboratory studies (e.g., surveillance cultures on clinically uninfected patients): If transmission of a single organism (e.g., MRSA) is suspected, molecular typing (e.g., using pulse-field gel electrophoresis) may be utilized to determine strain relatedness*

     iii. *Case–control or cohort study if source remains unclear and outbreak is ongoing*

   g. Arrive at conclusions about the cause(s) or source(s) of the outbreak

   h. Develop and execute an action plan. This includes:

     i. *Communicate results and plan to all stakeholders*

     ii. *Use a timeline and give priority to the simplest possible corrective measure*

     iii. *Perform periodic audits to ensure compliance with recommended measures*

     iv. *Continue enhanced surveillance*

     v. *Provide education to HCP as necessary*

III. INFECTION CONTROL MEASURE FOR MDROs. Two broad categories of strategies are recognized to help contain the MDRO burden in hospitals:

A. Measures to Prevent Transmission of Infectious Agents Including MDROs

   1. Hand hygiene. It is well known that the hands of HCP play a significant role in patient-to-patient transmission of MDROs. *Hand hygiene (handwashing with soap and water or use of alcohol-based hand rub) is considered the cornerstone of prevention of transmission of infectious agents including MDROs in the healthcare environment.* Alcohol-based hand rubs should be used preferentially as they require less time, increase compliance with hand hygiene, and are more effective than handwashing for nonsoiled hands. For *C. difficile* infection, handwashing with soap and water may be preferred (particularly during outbreaks) to mechanically remove the bacteria, as alcohol does not adequately kill *Clostridium* spores. In nonoutbreak situations, the use of alcohol-based hand rubs has not been associated with increases in the rates of *C. difficile*.

   2. Isolation. Patients infected or colonized with MDROs can be isolated to prevent transmission via HCW hands, apparel, equipment, and environment. The CDC's Healthcare Infection Control Practices Advisory Committee (HICPAC) has developed a system for isolation that has two basic precaution types: standard precautions and transmission-based precautions.

     a. *Standard precautions.* *Standard precautions apply when caring for all patients and aim primarily to reduce risk to HCP from pathogens transmitted via body fluids.* This approach acknowledges that there are many patients who have undiagnosed blood-borne pathogens and therefore all patients are considered potentially infectious. **Standard precautions include gloves for contact with blood (whether or not they are visibly bloody), all body fluids, and secretions except sweat, nonintact skin, and mucous membranes. It includes hand hygiene before and after patient contact and immediately after glove removal.** Masks, eye protection, and gowns should be worn during activities likely to generate splashes or sprays of blood, body fluids, secretions, and/or excretions.

b. ***Transmission-based precautions***. Transmission-based precautions are specific to the patient and a known or suspected microorganism that is being contained. *There are three major categories of transmission-based precautions: contact, airborne, and droplet* (see Table 52.1). For diseases with multiple routes of transmission, more than one category may be used, and these are always used in addition to standard precautions.

3. ***Environmental cleaning***. It is known that MDRO transmission is related to contamination of equipment such as blood pressure cuffs and near-patient surfaces such as bedside tables. Use of dedicated patient care equipment and thorough cleaning of the environment and reusable equipment are additional measures in the prevention of MDRO transmission. Monitoring systems

TABLE 52.1 ■ Requirements and Indications for Transmission-Based Precautions

	Contact	Airborne	Droplet
Context of use	Prevent transmission of organisms, including MDROs, which are spread by direct or indirect contact with the patient or patient's environment	Prevent transmission to organisms that remain infectious over long distances when suspended in the air	Prevent transmission of organisms spread through close respiratory or mucous membrane contact; pathogens do not remain infectious over long distances
Examples of infections requiring precautions	Colonization or infection with MDRO, *Clostridium difficile*, infectious diarrhea, RSV, adenovirus, SARS	*Mycobacterium tuberculosis*, measles, smallpox, varicella (chickenpox), disseminated zoster, SARS	Influenza, *Neisseria meningitides*, *Bordetella pertussis*, group A streptococcus, adenovirus, SARS
Single-patient room	Preferred; can cohort patients with same organism if single room not available	Necessary, with negative pressure with HEPA filtration or exhaust directly to outside	Preferred; spatial separation of 3 feet when single room not available
Mask	Not routine	N95 or PAPR on entry	Surgical mask and eye shield on entry
Gown	Required on entry	Not routine*	Not routine*
Gloves	Required on entry	Not routine*	Not routine*

*Should be used when standard precautions are indicated.

HEPA, high-efficiency particulate air; MDRO, multidrug-resistant organism; PAPR, powered air-purifying respirator; RSV, respiratory syncytial virus; SARS, severe acute respiratory syndrome.

such as fluorescent markers and adenosine triphosphate (ATP) assays are being increasingly used to evaluate the quality of cleaning and cleanliness in healthcare facilities, and novel disinfection mechanisms such as hydrogen peroxide vapor and ultraviolet light are being investigated for routine hospital use.

B. **Antimicrobial Stewardship to Limit Emergence of MDROs.** *Antimicrobial stewardship involves selecting an appropriate drug, at the correct dose, and for the correct duration to cure an infection while minimizing toxicity and preventing emergence of resistant bacterial strains.* There are many different antimicrobial stewardship strategies. One of the most widely used strategies is the restriction and preauthorization strategy. An example of a strategy with little restriction is the "unrestricted but closed formulary" strategy: The prescriber can chose any antimicrobial from the formulary, but the formulary only contains antimicrobial approved by the hospital drugs and therapeutics committee. Another is the "infectious-diseases consultation required" strategy: If the prescriber wishes to use a restricted antimicrobial, an infectious-diseases consult is automatically generated. A multidisciplinary antimicrobial management team, usually led by infectious-diseases physicians and/or infectious-diseases pharmacists, is responsible for the implementation of antimicrobial stewardship strategies.

IV. **THE FUTURE OF INFECTION CONTROL.** Infection prevention in hospitals has been under great scrutiny in the past few years, and this is expected to increase with wider availability of HAI data to the public. As delivery of healthcare continues to shift heavily into the outpatient arena, there will be increasing focus on the appropriate practice of infection prevention measures in ambulatory settings. While the emergence of technologies to enhance and monitor the quality of healthcare practices (e.g., environmental cleaning) holds promise, the promotion of hand hygiene and other routine practices in all healthcare settings through behavioral engineering and education will remain the cornerstone of a successful infection control and hospital epidemiology program.

BIBLIOGRAPHY

Duncan R, Lawrence K. Improving use of antimicrobial agents. In Lautenbach E, Woeltje K, Malani P, eds. *Practical Healthcare Epidemiology*, 3rd ed. The Society for Healthcare Epidemiology of America; 2010: 228–246.

Edmond MB, Wenzel RP. Organization for infection control. In Mandell GL, Bennett JE, Dolin R, eds. *Principles and Practice of Infectious Diseases*, 7th ed. Philadelphia, PA: Churchill Livingstone; 2005: 3669–3672.

Hebert C, Weber SG. Common approaches to the control of multidrug-resistant organisms other than methicillin-resistant *Staphylococcus aureus* (MRSA). *Infect Dis Clin North Am.* 2011;25(1):181–200.

Siegel JD, Rhinehart E, Jackson M, et al. Healthcare Infection Control Practices Advisory Committee 2007 Guideline for Isolation Precautions: preventing transmission of infectious agents in healthcare settings. 2007. http://www.cdc.gov/ncidod/dhqp/gl_isolation.html

Srinivasan A, Jarvis WR. Outbreak investigation. In Lautenbach E, Woeltje K, Malani P, eds. *Practical Healthcare Epidemiology*, 3rd ed. The Society for Healthcare Epidemiology of America; 2010: 143–155.

INDEX